Anesthesia and Perioperative Care of the High-Risk Patient

Third Edition

Edited by

Ian McConachie MB ChB FRCA FRCPC

Associate Professor

Department of Anesthesia & Perioperative Medicine

Western University,

London, Ontario, Canada

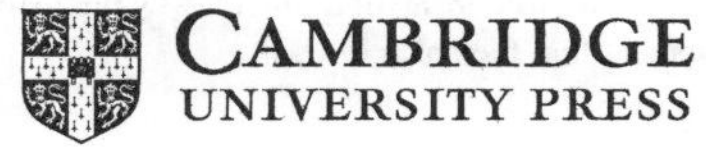

CAMBRIDGE
UNIVERSITY PRESS

University Printing House, Cambridge CB2 8BS, United Kingdom

Cambridge University Press is part of the University of Cambridge.

It furthers the University's mission by disseminating knowledge in the pursuit of education, learning and research at the highest international levels of excellence.

www.cambridge.org
Information on this title: www.cambridge.org/9781107690578

First edition published 2002
Second edition published 2009
Third edition published 2014

Printed in the United Kingdom by Clays, St Ives plc

A catalogue record for this publication is available from the British Library

Library of Congress Cataloging-in-Publication Data
Anesthesia for the high risk patient
Anesthesia and perioperative care of the high-risk patient / edited by I. McConachie. – Third edition.
p. ; cm.
Preceded by: Anesthesia for the high risk patient / edited by Ian McConachie. 2nd ed. 2009.
Includes bibliographical references and index.
ISBN 978-1-107-69057-8 (Pbk.)
I. McConachie, Ian, editor of compilation. II. Title.
[DNLM: 1. Anesthesia–adverse effects–Handbooks. 2. Anesthesia–methods–Handbooks. 3. Perioperative Care–methods–Handbooks. 4. Risk Factors–Handbooks. WO 231]
RD82.2
617.9′6–dc23 2014004589

ISBN 978-1-107-69057-8 Paperback

Table of contents

Contributors

A. Adams, MB ChB BSc FRCS FRCA
Consultant, Department of Anaesthesia, Lancashire Teaching Hospitals NHS Foundation Trust, Preston, UK

P.J.D. Andrews, MD MB ChB FRCA
Professor, Centre for Clinical Brain Sciences, University of Edinburgh, Edinburgh, UK

A. Antoniou, MD FRCPC
Assistant Professor, Department of Anesthesia & Perioperative Medicine, Western University, London, Ontario, Canada

D. Bainbridge, MD FRCPC
Associate Professor and Director, Cardiac Anesthesia Program, Department of Anesthesia & Perioperative Medicine, Western University, London, Ontario, Canada

M. Banasch, MD
Department of Anesthesia & Perioperative Medicine, Western University, London, Ontario, Canada

R. Blank, MD
Assistant Professor of Anesthesiology, University of Michigan Medical Center, Ann Arbor, MI, USA

J.M. Blum, MD
Assistant Professor of Anesthesiology, University of Michigan Medical Center, Ann Arbor, MI, USA

J. Brookes, MB ChB FRCA
Assistant Professor, Department of Anesthesia & Perioperative Medicine, Western University, London, Ontario, Canada

C.H. Brown IV, MD
Assistant Professor, Department of Anesthesiology and Critical Care Medicine, Johns Hopkins University, Baltimore, MD, USA

I. Bruni, MD FRCPC
Assistant Professor, Department of Anesthesia & Perioperative Medicine, Western University, London, Ontario, Canada

A. Cave, MD FRCPC
Assistant Professor, Department of Anesthesia & Perioperative Medicine, Western University, London, Ontario, Canada

E.H.L. Chau, MD
Department of Anaesthesiology, Toronto Western Hospital, University Health Network University of Toronto, Toronto, Ontario, Canada

D. Cheng, MD MSc FRCPC FCAHS CCPE
Distinguished University Professor and Chair, Department of Anesthesia & Perioperative Medicine, Western University, London, Ontario, Canada

M. Chin, MD
Department of Anesthesia & Perioperative Medicine, Western University, London, Ontario, Canada

F. Chung, MB BS FRCPC
Professor, Department of Anaesthesiology, Toronto Western Hospital University Health Network, University of Toronto, Toronto, Ontario, Canada

C. Clarke, MD FRCPC
Assistant Professor, Department of Anesthesia & Perioperative Medicine, Western University, London, Ontario, Canada

J. Cooke, MD
Division of Pulmonary & Critical Care Medicine, Rush University Medical Center, Chicago, IL, USA

P. Cowie, MBChB FRCA
Department of Anaesthetics, Royal Infirmary of Edinburgh, Edinburgh, UK

A. Dhir, MB BS MD FRCA FRCPC
Associate Professor, Department of Anesthesia & Perioperative Medicine, Western University, London, Ontario, Canada

S. Dhir, MD FRCPC
Associate Professor, Department of Anesthesia & Perioperative Medicine, Western University, London, Ontario, Canada

G. Evans, MD FRCPC
Assistant Professor, University of Ottawa, Ottawa, Ontario, Canada

L. Fleisher, MD
Robert Dunning Dripps Professor of Anesthesiology and Critical Care, University of Pennsylvania, Philadelphia, PA, USA

G.M. Flood, MB BS FRCA
Consultant Anaesthetist, Mater Misericordiae University Hospital, Dublin, Ireland

M.P.W. Grocott, BSc MBBS MD FRCA FRCP FFICM
Professor of Anaesthesia and Critical Care, University of Southampton NIHR Respiratory Biomedical Research Unit, University Hospital Southampton NHS Foundation Trust, Integrative Physiology and Critical Illness Group, Clinical and Experimental Sciences, Faculty of Medicine, University of Southampton, Southampton, UK

C. Harle, MB ChB FRCA FRCPC
Associate Professor, Department of Anesthesia & Perioperative Medicine, Western University, London, Ontario, Canada

A. Howie, BM BCh FRCA
Consultant, Department of Anaesthesia, Lancashire Teaching Hospitals NHS Foundation Trust, Preston, UK

S. Jack, MSc PhD
Consultant Clinician Scientist, Integrative Physiology and Critical Illness Group, Clinical and Experimental Sciences, Faculty of Medicine, University of Southampton, University Hospital Southampton NHS Foundation Trust, Southampton, UK

G. Jarvis, RN
Department of Palliative Care, The Ottawa Hospital Regional Cancer Centre, The Ottawa Hospital, Ottawa, Ontario, Canada

R. Kishen, MB FRCA
Department of Anaesthesia and Intensive Care, Salford Royal NHS Foundation Trust, Salford, UK (Retired)

M. Koutra, MB BS FRCA
Department of Anaesthesia, The Royal Marsden NHS Foundation Trust, London, UK

L. Loughney, BSc MSc
Clinical Exercise Physiologist, Integrative Physiology and Critical Illness Group, Clinical and Experimental Sciences, Faculty of Medicine, University of Southampton, University Hospital Southampton NHS Foundation Trust, Southampton, UK

N. Ludwig, MD
Department of Anesthesia & Perioperative Medicine, Western University London, Ontario, Canada

I. McConachie, MB ChB FRCA FRCPC
Associate Professor, Department of Anesthesia & Perioperative Medicine, Western University, London, Ontario, Canada

A. McLeod, MB BS FRCA
Consultant Anaesthetist, The Royal Marsden NHS Foundation Trust, London, UK

M. McFarling, MD
Department of Anesthesia & Perioperative Medicine, Western University London, Ontario, Canada

S. Morrison, MD FRCPC
Assistant Professor, Department of Anesthesia & Perioperative Medicine, Western University, London, Ontario, Canada

M. Pariser, MD
Department of Anesthesia & Perioperative Medicine, Western University London, Ontario, Canada

S. Patel, MD FRCA
Consultant Anaesthetist, Pennine Acute Hospitals NHS Trust, Oldham, UK

C. Railton, BSc PhD MD FRCPC
Associate Professor, Department of Anesthesia & Perioperative Medicine, Western University, London, Ontario, Canada

L.R. Rochlen, MD
Assistant Professor of Anesthesiology, University of Michigan Medical Center, Ann Arbor, MI, USA

A. Schlachter, MD
Division of Pulmonary & Critical Care Medicine, Rush University Medical Center, Chicago, IL, USA

V. Schulz, MD FRCPC
Palliative Medicine Consultant, Associate Professor, Department of Anesthesia & Perioperative Medicine, Western University, London, Ontario, Canada

F. Sieber, MD
Professor of Anesthesiology and Critical Care Medicine, Department of Anesthesiology and Critical Care Medicine, Johns Hopkins University Baltimore, MD, USA

P.M. Singh, MD
Department of Anaesthesia, All India Institute of Medical Sciences, Delhi, India

A.C. Sinha, MD PhD
Professor and Vice Chair (Research), Anesthesiology and Perioperative Medicine, Drexel University College of Medicine, Philadelphia, PA, USA

C. Smyth, MD PhD FRCPC
Complex Cancer Pain Consultant, Department of Anesthesia, The Ottawa Hospital, Ottawa, Ontario, Canada

A. Suphathamwit, MD FRCA (Thailand)
Attending Anesthesiologist, Siriraj Hospital, Bangkok, Thailand, Clinical Transplant, Anesthesia Fellow, Department of Anesthesia & Perioperative Medicine, Western University, London, Ontario, Canada

J. Vergel de Dios, MD
Department of Anesthesia & Perioperative Medicine, Western University London, Ontario, Canada

M. West, MD MRCS
Preoperative Cardiopulmonary Exercise Testing Clinical Lead, Aintree University Teaching Hospitals NHS Foundation Trust, University of Liverpool, Institute of Ageing and Chronic Disease, Department of Musculoskeletal Biology, Liverpool, UK

J. Wong, MD FRCPC
Assistant Professor, Department of Anaesthesiology, Toronto Western Hospital, University Health Network, University of Toronto, Toronto, Ontario, Canada

M. Yoder, MD
Assistant Professor, Division of Pulmonary & Critical Care Medicine, Rush University, Medical Center, Chicago, IL, USA

Z. Zafirova, MD
Assistant Professor, Department of Anesthesiology, Mount Sinai Hospital New York, NY, USA

Foreword

The current practice of anesthesia, pain, perioperative, and critical care medicine is increasingly characterized by high-risk patients with advanced age and comorbidity for an ever-growing spectrum of surgical interventions in and out of the operating rooms. Anesthesia management has advanced with preoperative admission screening and tests, cardiac medications guidelines, and predictive risk assessment and optimization; intraoperative monitoring, safer anesthetic agents, regional anesthesia techniques, and blood management; postoperative pain, and fast-track recovery management. These perioperative developments and team-based care have contributed to the remarkable safety and very low mortality and morbidity rate in modern anesthesia, despite a higher prevalence of high-risk patients.

This comprehensive, concise, and practical book edited by Dr. Ian McConachie is updated from the Second Edition and provides a useful guide to the anesthesia management and postoperative care of high-risk adult patients undergoing elective and emergency surgery. This book provides a succinct, problem-oriented source of practical information, based on current best evidence and the content–expert experience of leading clinicians. The outstanding and unique contributors selected by Dr. McConachie from both sides of the Atlantic have presented a full spectrum of preoperative, intraoperative, and postoperative management of high-risk surgical patients undergoing anesthesia care; in particular, patients with specific diseases have been highlighted in individual chapters.

All practitioners will benefit from refreshing and acquiring new knowledge of the principles and advanced perioperative anesthesia management presented in these chapters with the goal of improving the care of high-risk surgical patients.

Davy Cheng, MD, MSc, FRCPC, FCAHS, CCPE
Distinguished University Professor & Chair/Chief
Department of Anesthesia & Perioperative Medicine
London Health Sciences Centre and St. Joseph's Health Care London
University of Western Ontario
London, Ontario
Canada

Preface to the third edition

This text:

- is aimed primarily at trainees in anesthesia although more experienced practitioners may find it useful as a refresher in recent concepts and advances. A basic knowledge of physiology, pharmacology, and anesthesia is assumed.
- may be a useful *aide memoire* for postgraduate examinations in anesthesia.
- exclusively discusses adult anesthesia. Pediatric and neonatal anesthesia is outside the scope of this text.
- aims to provide practical information on the management of high-risk patients presenting for surgery as well as sufficient background information to enable understanding of the principles and rationale behind their anesthetic and perioperative management. We hope it will prove useful but we would emphasize that this, or any other book, is no substitute for experienced supervision, support, and training.
- is not a substitute for the major anesthetic texts but concentrates on principles of management of the most challenging anesthetic cases.
- has a slightly changed title in this third edition, to emphasize the importance of a coordinated approach to the high-risk surgical patient in the perioperative period and to highlight the role of the anesthetist as perioperative physician. We aim to "bridge the gap" between the operating room and the intensive care unit and to provide guidance to manage patients in the perioperative period in line with modern concepts of critical care.
- emphasizes cardiovascular risk and cardiac disease and its management as these undoubtedly are the most important aspects of perioperative anesthetic risk.
- incorporates a selective choice of topics but should appeal and be useful to the majority of practitioners. Important information not readily available in similar texts is also included.
- is designed so that the format provides easy access to information presented in a concise manner. We have tried to eliminate all superfluous material. Selected important or controversial references are presented. The styles of the chapters vary. This is deliberate. Some relate more to basic principles, physiology, pharmacology, etc. – bookwork. Others are more practical in nature, discussing the principles of anesthetic techniques for certain high-risk situations.
- was written by authors who are all experienced practitioners working with high-risk patients presenting for both elective and emergency surgery. The authors are committed to providing a high level of perioperative care of patients undergoing anesthesia. We make no apologies for repetition of important principles and facts – a second perspective on a subject is often useful.
- incorporates contributions from a multinational team, enlisted by the editor from institutions on both sides of the Atlantic. The contributors are active in both practice and training. The aim therefore has been to produce a text of international relevance.
- builds, in this third edition, on the success of the second and contains several new chapters as well as revisions of older chapters.

- by way of disclosure, includes many drugs discussed and many trials reported and discussed that involve use of drugs in "off label" situations. Use of drugs in such situations is at the discretion of individual physicians after full evaluation of the circumstances at that time. Similarly, dosages presented in this text represent those commonly found in the literature but physicians should always seek guidance from appropriate pharmaceutical literature.

Ian McConachie

Abbreviations

AAA abdominal aortic aneurysm
AAGBI Association of Anaesthetists of Great Britain and Ireland
ABG arterial blood gases
ABW actual body weight
ACC American College of Cardiology
ACCF American College of Cardiology Foundation
ACCP American College of Chest Physicians
ACE angiotensin-converting enzyme
ACRM Anesthesia Crisis Resource Management
aCS acute coronary syndrome
ACS American College of Surgeons
ACS NSQIP American College of Surgeons National Surgical Quality Improvement Program
ACTH adrenocorticotropic hormone
ADH antidiuretic hormone
ADHD attention deficit hyperactivity disorder
ADL activities of daily living
ADP adenosine diphosphate
ADQI acute dialysis quality initiative
AF atrial fibrillation
AHA American Heart Association
AHI Apnea–Hypopnea Index
AHRQ Agency for Healthcare Research and Quality
AI aortic incompetence
AICD automated implantable cardiac defibrillator
AIMS Anaesthetic Incident Monitoring Study
AKI acute kidney injury
AKIN acute kidney injury network
AL anastomotic leak
ALI acute lung injury
ANH acute normovolemic hemodilution
APACHE acute physiology and chronic health evaluation
APS Acute Pain Service
APT antiplatelet therapy
aPTT activated partial thromboplastin time
AR aortic regurgitation
ARA angiotensin receptor antagonist
ARB angiotensin receptor blocking
ARDS acute respiratory distress syndrome
AS aortic stenosis
ASA American Society of Anesthesiologists
ASRA American Society of Regional Anesthesia
ATN acute tubular necrosis
ATP adenosine triphosphate
AUC area under the curve
AV arteriovenous
A-V atrioventricular
AVF arteriovenous fistula
AVG arteriovenous graft
AVPU alert, voice, pain, unresponsive
AVR aortic valve replacement
AWS alcohol withdrawal syndrome
BARI Bypass Angioplasty Revascularization Investigation
BART Blood Conservation Using Antifibrinolytics in a Randomized Trial
BIPAP bilevel positive airway pressure
BIS bispectral index score
BMI Body Mass Index
BMS bare-metal stent
BNP brain natriuretic peptide
BPI bactericidal permeability increasing (protein)
BPInv Brief Pain Inventory
BRAN (Benefits, Risks, Alternatives, Nothing)
BUN blood urea nitrogen
CABG coronary artery bypass grafting
CCB calcium channel blockers
CaO_2 arterial oxygen content
CAD coronary artery disease
CAM Confusion Assessment Method
CARP Coronary Artery Revascularization Prophylaxis trial
CAS carotid artery stenting

CASE Comprehensive Anaesthesia Simulation Environment system
CASS Coronary Artery Surgery Study
CBF cerebral blood flow
CC creatinine clearance
CCF congestive cardiac failure
CCOT critical care outreach team
CCRT continuous renal replacement therapy
CCTA coronary computed tomography angiography
CEA carotid endarterectomy
CEPOD Confidential Enquiry into Peri-Operative Deaths
CG control group
CHD congenital heart disease
CHF congestive heart failure
CI cardiac index
CI_{95} 95% confidence interval
CIN contrast-induced nephropathy
CKD chronic kidney disease
CMR cardiac magnetic resonance
CMV cytomegalovirus
CNA central neuraxial analgesia
CNI calcinurin inhibitor
CNS central nervous system
CNST Clinical Negligence Scheme for Trusts
CO cardiac ouput
COETT cuffed oral endotracheal tube
COPD chronic obstructive pulmonary disease
COX cyclooxygenase
CP cricoid pressure
CPAP continuous positive airway pressure
CPB cardiopulmonary bypass
CPET cardiopulmonary exercise testing
CPK creatine phosphokinase
CPP cerebral perfusion pressure
CPR cardiopulmonary resuscitation
CPX cardiopulmonary exercise
Cr creatinine
CRI Cardiac Risk Index
CRRT continuous renal replacement therapy
CRT cardiac resynchronization therapy
CSF cerebrospinal fluid
CT computed tomography
CTA computed tomographical angiography
CV closing volume
CVA cardiovascular accident
CVD cardiovascular disease
CvO_2 venous oxygen content
CVP central venous pressure
CXRs chest X-rays
DAI diffuse axonal injury
DAPT dual antiplatelet therapy
DASI Duke Activity Status Index
DCCT Diabetes Control and Complications Trial
DCLB diasprin cross-linked hemoglobin
DES drug-eluting stent
DLCO diffusion capacity of the lung for carbon monoxide
DM diabetes mellitus
DNAR do not attempt resuscitation
DNR do not resuscitate
DO_2 oxygen delivery
DPG diphosphoglycerate
DSE dobutamine stress echocardiography
DT delirium tremens
DTI direct thrombin inhibitors
DVD degenerative valve disease
DVT deep vein thrombosis
EA epidural analgesia
EBV Epstein–Barr virus
ECG electrocardiograph
ECOG Eastern Cooperative Oncology Group
EDH extradural hematoma
EEG electroecephalography
EF ejection fraction
EG exercise group
eGFR estimated glomerular filtration rate
EMG electromyograph
EN enteral nutrition
EPO erythropoietin
ER emergency room
ERAS enhanced recovery after surgery
ERP enhanced recovery protocols
ERV expiratory reserve volume
ESA European Society of Anaesthesiology
E-SA erythropoiesis-stimulating agents

ESAS Edmonton Symptom Assessment Scale
ESC European Society of Cardiology
ESLD end-stage liver disease
ESRD end-stage renal disease
EuSOS European Surgical Outcomes Study
EWS Early Warning Score
FDA Food and Drug Administration
FDP fibrin degradation products
FEV forced expiratory volume
FFP fresh, frozen plasma
FiO_2 inspired oxygen concentration
FOI fiberoptic intubation
FRC functional residual capacity
FVC forced vital capacity
GA general anesthesia/anesthetic
GABA γ-aminobutyric acid
GCS Glasgow Coma Scale
G-CSF granulocyte colony-stimulating factor
GD goal-directed
GDT goal-directed therapy
GFR glomerular filtration rate
GI gastrointestinal
HABR hepatic arterial buffer response
Hb hemoglobin
HBOCs hemoglobin-based oxygen carriers
HCC hepatocellular carcinoma
Hct hematocrit
HDU high-dependency unit
HE hepatic encephalopathy
HF heart failure
HIV human immunodeficiency virus
HMG 3-hydroxy-3-methyl-glutaryl
HOCM hyperthrophic obstructive cardiomyopathy
HPS hepatopulmonary syndrome
HRO high-reliability organization
HRR heart rate reserve
HRS hepatorenal syndrome
HTN hypertension
IABP intra-aortic balloon pump
IADL instrumental activities of daily living
IAP intra-abdominal pressure
IBF intestinal blood flow
IBW ideal body weight
ICD implantable cardioverter-defibrillators
ICP intracranial pressure
ICU intensive care unit
IDDS intrathecal drug delivery system
IE infective endocarditis
IHD ischemic heart disease
IL interleukin
IMT inspiratory muscle training
INR international normalized ratio
IPPV intermittent positive pressure ventilation
ISB interscalene block
ITP intrathoracic pressure
ITS iontophoretic transdermal system
IV intravenous
IVRA intravenous regional analgesia
IYDT if you do not treat
KIM1 kidney injury molecule 1
LAt left atrium
LA local anesthetic
LMA laryngeal mask airway
LoS length of stay
LV left ventricular/ventricle
LVEDP left ventricular end-diastolic pressure
LVEDV left ventricular end-diastolic volume
LVH left ventricular hypertrophy
LVOT left ventricle outflow tract
M3G morphine-3-glucuronide
M6G morphine-6-glucuronide
MAC minimum alveolar concentration
MACE major adverse cardiac events
MAMC mid-arm muscle circumference
MAP mean arterial pressure
MBT massive blood transfusion
MDEA 3,4-methylenedioxyethamphetamine
MDMA methylenedioxymethamphetamine
MDPV methylenedioxypyrovalerone
MELD model for end-stage liver disease
MEP motor evoked potentials
mEq milliequivalents
MEq metabolic equivalent
MERIT Medical Early Response Intervention and Therapy
MET medical emergency team
MEWS Modified Early Warning System

MI myocardial infarction
MMA multimodal analgesia
MMF mycophenolate mofetil
MODS multi-organ dysfunction syndrome
MR mitral regurgitation
MRA magnetic resonance angiogram
MRI magnetic resonance imaging
MS mitral stenosis
mTAL medullary thick ascending part of the loop of Henlé
mTOR mammalian target-of-rapamycin
MUST malnutrition screening tool
MVR mitral valve replacement
NAC neoadjuvant chemotherapy
NARC neoadjuvant chemoradiotherapy
NASH non-alcoholic steatohepatitis
NCCG Non-Consultant Career Grade
NCEPOD National Confidential Enquiry into Perioperative Deaths
NDMR non-depolarizing muscle relaxants
NEWS National Early Warning System
NG nasogastric
NHS National Health Service
NICE National Institute for Health and Clinical Excellence
NIRS near infrared spectroscopy
NK natural killer (cells)
NMDA N-methyl-D-aspartate
NNH number needed to harm
NNM number needed to monitor
NNT number needed to treat
NO nitric oxide
N_2O nitrous oxide
NRI nutritional risk index
NRS numerical rating scale
NRT nicotine replacement therapy
NSAIDs non-steroidal anti-inflammatory drugs
NSCLC non-small cell lung cancer
NT pro-BNP N-terminal pro-brain natriuretic peptide
NYHA New York Heart Association
OCP oral contraceptive pill
ODC oxyhemoglobin dissociation curve
OHS obesity hypoventilation syndrome
OR odds ratio
ORm operating room
OSA obstructive sleep apnea
OSAS obstructive sleep apnea syndrome
PA pulmonary arteries
PAC pulmonary artery catheter
PACU post-anesthesia care unit
PAFC pulmonary artery flotation catheter
PAI plasminogen activator inhibitor
PAOP pulmonary artery occlusion pressure
PAP positive airway pressure
PART patient-at-risk team
PASP pulmonary artery systolic pressure
PBW predicted body weight
PC palliative care
PCA patient-controlled analgesia
PCC prothrombin complex concentrate
PCEA patient-controlled epidural analgesia
PCI percutaneous coronary intervention
pCO_2 arterial carbon dioxide tension/partial pressure of carbon dioxide
PCT proximal convoluted tubule
PCWP pulmonary capillary wedge pressure
PE pulmonary embolism
PEEP positive end expiratory pressure
PEM protein energy malnutrition
PFC perfluorocarbon
PFT pulmonary function test
PHTN pulmonary hypertension
PIP peak inspiratory pressure
PMI perioperative myocardial infarction
PNS peripheral nerve stimulator
pO_2 partial pressure of oxygen/arterial oxygen tension
POC point-of-care
POCD postoperative cognitive dysfunction
POISE Perioperative Ischemic Events Trial
PONV postoperative nausea and vomiting
PORIF perioperative renal insufficiency and failure
POSSUM Physiological and Operative Severity Score for the Enumeration of Mortality and Morbidity
PPC perioperative pulmonary complications
PPO predicted postoperative
PPV pulse pressure variation
PR pulmonary rehabilitation
PSS physiological scoring system

PT prothrombin time
PTLD post-transplant lymphoproliferative disorder
PTT partial thromboplastin time
PVB paravertebral block
PVR pulmonary vascular resistance
QoL quality of life
RA regional anesthesia
RAt right atrium
RAS renin–angiotensin system
RBCs red blood cells
RBF renal blood flow
RCRI Revised Cardiac Risk Index
RCT randomized controlled trial
RER respiratory exchange ratio
rFVIIa recombinant activated factor
RHD rheumatic heart disease
RIFLE risk, injury, failure, loss, and end-stage kidney disease
RM recruitment maneuver
ROC receiver operating characteristic
ROS reactive oxygen species
RPP renal perfusion pressure
RR relative ratio
RRS rapid response system
RRTs rapid response teams
RRTh renal replacement therapy
RSII rapid sequence induction and intubation
RV right ventricular/ventricle
RVol residual volume
RVR renal vascular resistance
SABA short-acting β-agonist
SAH subarachnoid hemorrhage
SAM systolic anterior motion
SAPS simplified acute physiology score
SaO_2 arterial oxygen saturation
SCAI Society for Cardiovascular Angiography Interventions
SCC squamous cell carcinoma
SCI spinal cord injury
SCLC small cell lung cancer
SCPP spinal cord perfusion pressure
SCr serum creatinine
$ScvO_2$ central venous blood oxygen saturation
SDH subdural hematoma
SDM substitute decision makers
SEP somatosensory evoked potentials
SGA subjective global assessment
SGD upraglottic airway device
SIADH syndrome of inappropriate antidiuretic hormone
SIRS systemic inflammatory response syndrome
SLIP surgical lung injury prediction
S-MPM Surgical Mortality Probability Model
SpA spinal anesthesia
SP stump pressure
SpO_2 oxygen saturation via pulse oximetry
SSI surgical site infection
SSRI selective serotonin reuptake inhibitor
ST stent thrombosis
SV stroke volume
SVC superior vena cava
SVI stroke volume index
SVO_2 mixed venous oxyhemoglobin saturation
SVR systemic vascular resistance
TAA thoracic aorta aneurysm
TACE transarterial chemoembolization
TAPB transversus abdominis plane block
TBI traumatic brain injury
TCA tricarboxylic acid
TCD transcranial Doppler
TEA thoracic epidural analgesia
TEE transesophageal echocardiography
TEG thromboelastography
TEVAR thoracic endovascular aortic repair
TF tissue factor
TGF tubuloglomerular feedback
THC tetrahydrocannabinol
ThRCRI Thoracic Revised Cardiac Risk Index
TIMI thrombosis in myocardial infarction
TIPS transjugular intrahepatic portosystemic shunt
TIVA total intravenous anesthesia
TLC total lung capacity
TNF tumor necrosis factor
tPA tissue plasminogen activator

TPN total parenteral nutrition
TRALI transfusion-related acute lung injury
TRBF total renal blood flow
TRICC Transfusion Requirements in Critical Care
TRIM transfusion-related immune modulation
TSF triple skin fold thickness
TXA tranexamic acid
UO urine output
US ultrasound
VAD ventricular assist device
VAE venous air embolism
VC vital capacity
vCJD human variant Creutzfeldt–Jacob disease
VEGF vascular endothelial growth factor
VHD valvular heart disease
VILI ventilator-induced lung injury
VIP ventilation, infusion, and perfusion
VO_2 oxygen consumption
VRE vancomycin-resistant enterococcus
VSAQ Veterans Specific Activity Questionnaire
VTE venous thromboembolism/ thromboembolic disease
WFNS World Federation of Neurosurgical Societies
WHO World Health Organization

Risk and risk assessment

A. Howie and A. Adams

What is risk?

- Risk is a concept that denotes a potential negative impact to an asset or some characteristic of value that may arise from some present process or future event.
- Implicitly negative, risk is suggestive of potential danger or hazard and therefore is associated with discomfort and loss and not gain or well-being.
- *Risk* is often used synonymously with the *probability* of a known loss.
- Paradoxically, a probable or possible loss may be uncertain and relative in an individual event, but may be much more certain over an aggregate of multiple events.
- Risk is the probability of an event occurring that will have an impact on the achievement of objectives. Risk is measured in terms of impact and likelihood.
- In 1983, the Royal Society in the U.K. defined *risk* as "the probability that a particular event occurs during a stated period of time or results from a particular challenge." They defined a *hazard* as a situation that could lead to harm. The chance or likelihood of this occurring is its associated *risk* [1].
- Risk is part of life whether we like it or not [2]. All medical interventions carry risks but anesthesia is often perceived to be especially risky, although in general, the risks of anesthesia are small. Risk communication, understanding, and perception are fundamental to all decision making, including consent for surgical operation.
- Risk evaluation by individuals is not a purely statistical phenomenon. It is widely accepted that individuals tend to evaluate risk not solely on statistical data but on many other subjective qualitative aspects of risk. This means that the assessment and perception of risk may incorporate subconscious, subjective, personality-dependent factors and may not follow any rational or methodical pattern [3].

Identifying risk

There are numerous potential hazards and we have many ways of predicting and quantifying the risks associated with these hazards. Experience of each procedure undertaken gives us an idea of the hazards associated with it. Pooled experience within a department gives us the experience of our colleagues as well, but this requires openness and a platform from which this information can be shared. Peer-reviewed journals and specialist literature, freely available now on the internet, allows us to evaluate not only our own practice, but that of others throughout the world.

Anesthesia and Perioperative Care of the High-Risk Patient, Third edition, ed. Ian McConachie.
Published by Cambridge University Press.

Frequently occurring adverse events are fairly straightforward to identify simply because they are common. The rarer an event, the less likely it is that an individual practitioner will encounter such an event during his/her practice. Without accurate reporting, these events may go undocumented and lead to inaccuracies in the pooled data. For a very rare event, this will cause large discrepancies in the estimated risk level for that event.

For very rare adverse events or for procedures that are not performed regularly, it may be difficult to recruit enough patients for a study to be adequately powered to show anything meaningful. For this reason one must be cautious in interpreting the results of many smaller studies. Multi-center co-operation is increasingly being organized to produce data from large numbers of patients that could not possibly be recruited from a single center.

An alternative method of producing some relevant conclusion from a number of smaller studies, which themselves do not show anything statistically significant, is to conduct a meta-analysis. This pools the patient numbers from smaller studies so as to give a number large enough to reach significance. One must be wary in interpreting these results as often it is difficult to find studies that are similar enough to be comparable.

The timing of an adverse outcome will affect both our ability to identify and report it, and the way in which patients will perceive it. Immediate events are identifiable by staff caring for patients in the postoperative period, either in the operating room (ORm), the post-anesthesia care unit (PACU), or on the wards. Immediate adverse outcomes will also be reported by the patients themselves. Later complications may be reported less frequently by the patient especially if deemed not to be too serious. If there is a long lead-time between treatment and complication, the association may go unnoticed.

Perceiving risk [4]

The timing of the event can have an effect on the way risk is perceived. Early complications, for example, often have a greater impact than those that are delayed. These tend to have a diminished perceived risk value.

The duration of an adverse event can also affect risk perception. Similarly, the ease with which something can be treated will reduce the severity of risk perceived. The possibility of postoperative pain or nausea is usually transient and easily treated, and therefore is perceived as having lower risk severity than a possible longer term or irreversible disability.

Many studies have been done to evaluate the particular aspects thought relevant to the way risk is perceived and many mental biases exist to prejudice our view [5]. These characteristics include both conscious and subconscious elements:

- magnitude
- severity
- vulnerability
- controllability
- familiarity
- acceptability
- framing effect

Risk probability or magnitude

This is usually expressed as a mathematical probability. As already mentioned, these numbers come from our personal experiences and from published data from previous studies.

The populations investigated by previous studies may not be comparable to your population. There may be medical, age, gender, or ethnic differences that need to be considered before the data presented is accepted as applicable to your population.

The magnitude of the risk can be biased. There are two types of error known as availability and compression bias.

- Availability bias is also known as exposure bias or publication bias. This results in an overestimation of risk due to over exposure and increased publicity associated with a rare but catastrophic event. When rare events are sensationalized in the media, the perception of risk associated with them increases. The perceived frequency is also increased.
- The general public are increasingly worried about terrorism, but the chance of being involved in a terrorist attack is very low. As these events command high profile media coverage, the perceived risk is greatly exaggerated. Similarly, airline accidents command dramatic and sensational media coverage, which increases public anxiety. However, car travel is vastly more dangerous in terms of fatalities per kilometer traveled.
- Common events are, by definition, less dramatic, and therefore are perceived to occur less frequently.
- Compression bias occurs because in many cases we do not know exactly how frequently something occurs. Usually there will be a range of probabilities and this range may be vast for rarer events. Patients tend to overestimate small risks and underestimate large ones. To use the earlier example here, compression bias causes the risk of dying in a car crash to be underestimated, but the risk of dying in a plane crash to be overestimated.

Risk severity

This may be thought of as a combination of the actual probability and the weight or perceived impact that the event may have on the patient. Therefore, this entity is subjective. The worst outcomes, death or permanent disability, will have great impact on the way the risk is perceived, even if the probability is low.

A mathematical concept used in the past in an attempt to analyze the process of risk perception was to compare different risks using an expectation value [6]. This is only of use, though, if a numerical value can be assigned to severity:

expectation value = probability × severity

This is an over-simplification of the processes involved in risk perception and evaluation. For example, risks with a very low probability but high severity, such as death or disability, are perceived worse than risks with a higher probability and less severe outcome even though they have the same expectation value.

- An example of events with the same expectation value: if people are offered the choice of being given £5000 or of winning £10 000 on the toss of a coin, the majority will choose the £5000 certainty rather than the uncertain alternative. This has been interpreted as evidence that, if possible, people will try to avoid risk and uncertainty.

Vulnerability

Vulnerability is the extent to which people believe an event could happen to them, or alternatively it is the degree of immunity one possesses to a risk. Generally, we tend to exhibit unrealistic optimism and a feeling of immunity or invincibility; thus, people tend to not behave cautiously. Feeling invulnerable, we underestimate or downgrade our own risk but overestimate the risk to others.

- For example, one might fear more the catastrophic but rare risk of nuclear accident than the common but minor risk of passive smoking.

Controllability

As we like to be in control of things that affect us, the possibility of something happening that cannot be controlled tends to magnify the perceived severity of the risk. The perception of being in control or having choice downgrades the perceived severity of the risk [4].

- Risky pastimes, e.g., skiing, diving, parachuting, etc. all have major risks associated with the undertaking of that activity, including death. The individuals involved are aware of the risk, but because they are in some control of their outcome, they perceive the risk to be lower. The likelihood of accepting higher risk is greater when people have the choice whether to participate.
- Involuntary or imposed risks are significantly less acceptable and incite resentment.

Familiarity

Repeated exposure to a risk induces overconfidence and familiarity. This in turn desensitizes us to the risks present. On the contrary, unfamiliar risks incite a much greater degree of fear and dread. This is known as miscalibration bias.

Acceptability

This is another very subjective issue. Individual attitudes resulting from upbringing, class, ethnic, religious, and cultural background can significantly affect the concept of acceptability or non-acceptability of the risk.

Characteristics of the hazard affect the acceptability including how severe, transient, controllable, familiar, and vulnerable or immune the patient perceives themselves to be.

Risk comparison may help the patient reach a conclusion as to the acceptability of a risk. This is achieved by comparing the risk in question with an alternative event more familiar to the patient that has a similar numerical level of risk. This shows them that they have accepted similar risks in the past.

There are many other variables including the trust the patient has in the team responsible for his/her care and any support network, including family, that are close to the patient.

Framing effect or framing bias

This is how the presentation of the risk information can affect the perception.

- It is well recognized that differences in the presentation of risk information can strongly affect the perception of risk in both lay people and doctors, and thereby influence decision making [7].
- The order in which clinicians discuss advantages and disadvantages of treatment may have an impact on a patient's perception and final decision.
- Emphasizing positive aspects before discussing risks may be more likely to persuade an individual to accept a particular treatment.

- A therapy reported to be 60% effective would be evaluated more favorable than one with a 40% likelihood of failure, although the two statements mean the same thing.
- Similarly, a treatment with a 10% mortality will be more positively perceived if phrased as having a 90% chance of survival.

This is called positive framing.

- One study[8] compared the way in which a treatment option for cholesterol lowering and hypertension was presented to patients. Relative risk reduction, absolute risk reduction, number needed to treat (NNT), average gain in disease-free years, and stratified gain in disease-free years were the methods compared. Relative risk reduction was the most likely to persuade patients to agree to treatment whereas the NNT was the least persuasive.

Communicating risk levels

As the assessment of risk and therefore the prediction of risk is not an exact science, it is almost impossible to convey an accurate picture of what an individual's clinical risk actually is. There is no way of translating population risk data into specific data for an individual [9].

The range of probabilities when expressing risk can be large, due to the lack of accurate data and to patient individuality and variability. This leaves us with the difficult issue of trying to be as accurate as we can but also communicating this to the patient in a way that is best understood. When several orders of magnitude are covered by the range, integer logarithmic scales are often used as a way of presenting information in a manageable format for the patient.

- Examples of logarithmic scales in everyday use are the Richter scale for earthquake magnitude, the pH scale for hydrogen ion concentration, and the decibel scale for sound intensity.
- Logarithmic scales may be helpful to some people, but they simply replace very large numbers with smaller ones, sometimes with the effect of overestimating very small risk.
- By substituting a word or a descriptive phrase instead of a number, Calman's verbal scale [3] and the community cluster classification [4] goes some way to being more meaningful to the layperson (Table 1.1). It is quite easy to visualize one person in a street where you live, or one person in a small town compared with one person in a large city.

Table 1.1. Risk scales

Risk level 1 in:	Calman's verbal scale	Calman's descriptive cluster	Community scale
1–9	Very high		
10–99	High	Frequent, significant	Family
100–999	Moderate		Street
1000–9999	Low	Tolerable, reasonable	Village
10 000–99 999	Very low		Small town
100 000–999 999	Minimal	Acceptable	Large town
1 000 000–9 999 999	Negligible	Insignificant, safe	City

Other analogies more meaningful to the layperson have been sought. The U.K. Lotto, formerly U.K. National Lottery, and the probability of winning has been used [10]:

3 balls	1 in 57
4 balls	1 in 1032
5 balls	1 in 55 491
5 balls + bonus	1 in 2 330 636
6 balls	1 in 13 983 816

Number needed to treat

This is a concept introduced by Laupacis et al. in 1988 [11]. It is a method used to compare the efficacy of treatments and is calculated from the reciprocal of the absolute risk reduction. In other words, it is the number of patients needed to be treated for one patient to benefit.

- It has been used to compare analgesics and a league table has been drawn up. This has been helpful to clinicians as NNT is said to convey both statistical and clinical significance [12]. Paracetamol (acetaminophen) and ibuprofen have NNTs of 3.6 and 2, respectively, and are therefore effective, whereas codeine has a rather poor NNT of 18 in comparison.

This concept has evolved when looking at risk to number needed to harm (NNH) and if you do not treat (IYDT). The same principle calculates the number of patients needed to treat before one patient suffered the adverse effect in question.

- The higher the NNH, the safer the treatment.
- IYDT gives a number of patients from whom treatment is withheld before an adverse incident occurs.

An extension into anesthetic practice would be the number needed to monitor (NNM) to prevent one anesthetic-related death.

- This number may be very high, but is worthwhile to preserve the safety of anesthesia [13].

While trying to communicate risk to a patient, it must be remembered that what is actually perceived may not be the same as was intended. Differing knowledge base and past personal experience may result in the two people essentially "coming from opposite directions" and misunderstandings should be expected and predicted. As there are clearly many methods of trying to convey actual levels of risk to our patients, it is likely that their ability to understand is very variable and more than one approach may well be required for many patients.

If booklets are used as a way of conveying information, it must be remembered that factual information is not the only thing that is communicated. The patient will respond on an emotional level as well and this is all too often neglected by doctors. It could be that this is because we fail to appreciate the importance or are not comfortable with the way the patient might be feeling.

What is high-risk ?

When evaluating risk, we have already said it is difficult to convey a probability in terms that mean something to the layperson. Using an actual number may be misleading as well.

- When asked, 85% of the population thought they had a better than average sense of humor.
- Many patients, however, are disturbed to learn that 49% of doctors show below average performance.

We need to find a way to give a meaning to a number. When a likely risk, or a numerical probability, is displayed directly alongside a series of day-to-day events corresponding to the same probability of occurring, then the impact is greater and has some relevant meaning [14]. Figure 1.1 shows this as a risk ladder.

- A risk level of 1 in 100 000 has been deemed *acceptable* [4] and a risk level of 1 in 1 000 000 is deemed *safe*.
- The risk of death by road traffic accident in the U.K. in one year is 8000 – a risk that a large proportion of us take every day on our way to and from work. This corresponds to a risk level less than 1 in 1000, which is deemed *tolerable* or *reasonable* [3].
- There are those who do not believe that any degree of risk is universally acceptable [2].
- When evaluating risk perception, we have already seen that there are numerous subjective criteria to be considered alongside the numerical magnitude of risk.

When considering overall risk, one must consider the baseline risk and then add on, or superimpose, the relevant additional risk to reach the real risk.

- For example, we all have a risk of dying every day. This baseline risk increases as we get older. Any other risk of premature death such as smoking or murder need to be added to the baseline to see the actual risk of death for that day.
- In anesthesia, the number given as baseline for death under anesthesia is 1 in 185 000. We all know that this is an artificial figure as people are generally not given anesthetics without some operation or procedure also happening to them.
- The risk of death after surgery is much greater than this figure because the surgery, the patient, the surgeon, and the anesthetist all have a little extra risk to add on.
- The extra risk may not always be quantifiable, but will be additive.
- The more closely we can form a personalized estimate of risk for an individual, the more the gap between population-based data and the subjective experience of the patient will narrow and the more informed that patient's decision will be [15].

Relative and absolute risk

These two terms can be used solely or together to convey risk. When used solely, the relative risk of an event can be very misleading.

- If the absolute risk of an event occurring is very small, say 1 in 1 000 000, this is often perceived quite correctly as a very unlikely occurrence. If the absolute risk were 2 in 1 000 000, most observers would still perceive the risk as very unlikely.
- When described in terms of relative risk, we can say that the risk has doubled or is twice as likely, or has increased by 100%. All of these terms tend to be more alarming and likely to result in the perception of a greatly increased risk.

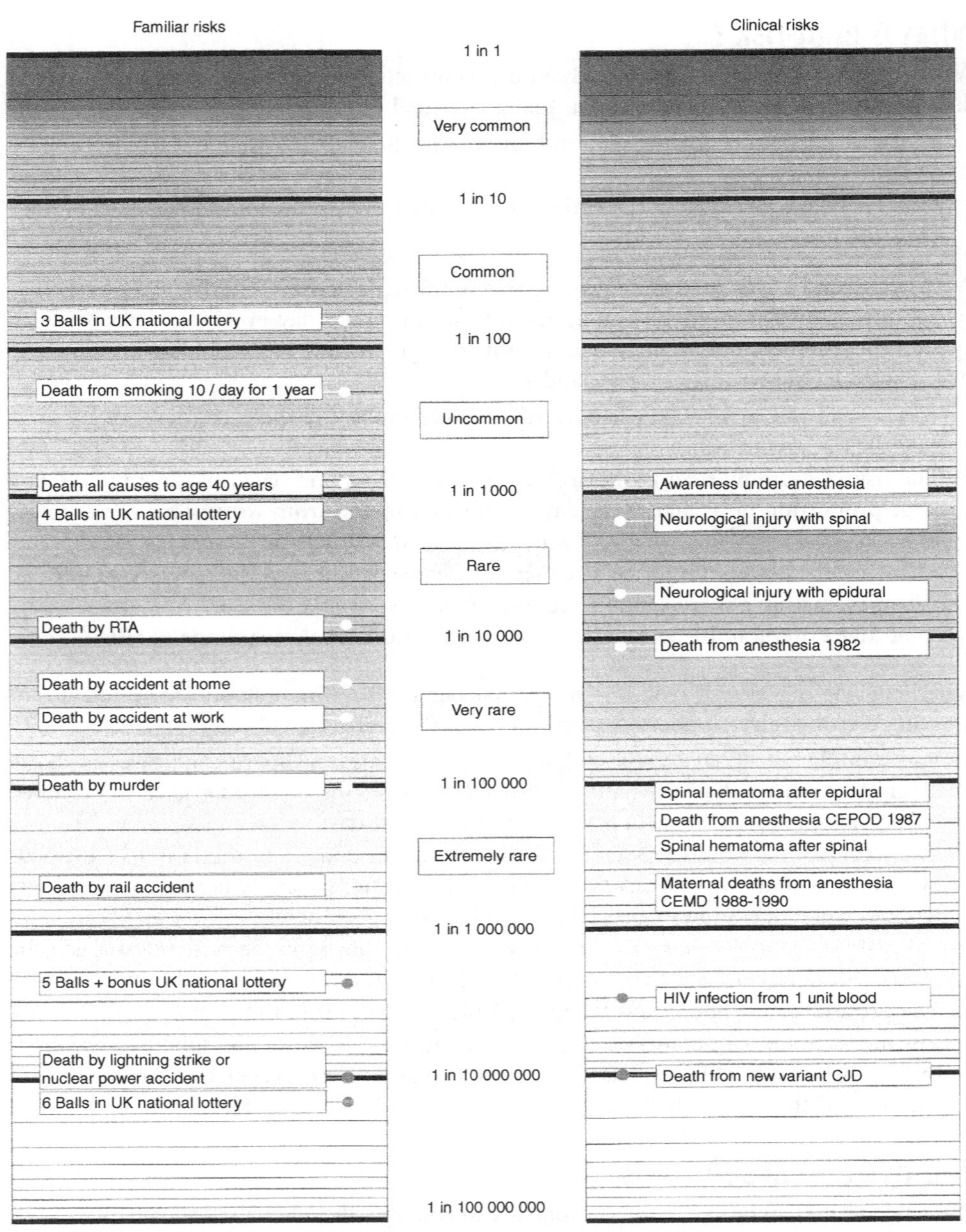

Figure 1.1. Risk ladder.

This is a method the media use frequently to over-dramatize a story.

- A very good example of this is the risk of venous thromboembolism (VTE) while taking a "low-dose" third-generation oral contraceptive pill (OCP) [15]. The press revealed accurate but misleading relative risk figures without adequately stressing the absolute risk.

- This was further compounded by the general public, and many medical professionals, not having extra information to put these figures into context.
- The actual risk of VTE when pregnant is higher again and the risk to someone not on either pill does not equal zero.

	Incidence of VTE per million women per year	Mortality; deaths per million women per year
No oral contraceptive	50	0.5
2nd-generation OCP	150	1.5
3rd-generation OCP	300	3.0
Pregnancy	600	6.0

Risk–benefit analysis

In the U.K., the General Medical Council has issued guidance on consent, which entitles patients and doctors to make decisions together [16]. It makes the points that:

- All efforts should be made to involve the patient in the decision making process and that assumptions should not be made about what they would and would not want.
- Patients should be given sufficient information before deciding to give their consent and must be warned of serious risks before proceeding even if they do not want to know detailed information regarding the treatment.
- It states that information should be personalized to each patient as much as possible and presented in a way that s/he can understand and be given time to reflect on the information presented before coming to a decision.
- If a patient states that s/he does not want information, this must be documented clearly in the medical notes and it be made clear that s/he can change her/his mind and have more information at any time.

We have moved from a concept of "the reasonable doctor," where the doctor knew what was best for the patient and decided what the patient needed to be told, to the concept of "the reasonable patient."

- Doctors now are expected to give much more information as a matter of course so the patient is empowered fully to decide what happens to her/him. But is this always in the patients' best interests?
- Although patients have the power to make decisions about their healthcare, it brings with it a significant amount of responsibility that many patients simply do not want or cannot deal with.
- Furthermore, the giving of information, some of which will have negative implications, may well frighten a patient just at the time when s/he is looking for reassurance and comfort.
- Is it justifiable that we scare our patients so that we can satisfy ourselves that we have disclosed all the risks?

The subject of consent throws into conflict two important ethical principles:

- autonomy (the individual having the right to determine what happens to her/him)
- beneficence (the obligation for doctors to do only good for the patient)

Doctors may exercise "therapeutic privilege," which allows us to withhold certain information if it is deemed that it would be contrary to the patient's best interests, cause harm to the patient, or deter the patient from proceeding with a therapeutic procedure considered essential. All risks discussed and those not discussed, with the reasons for not doing so, should be documented in the patient's notes [17].

The "reasonable" patient who is fully informed may sometimes turn out to be an "unreasonable" patient.

- Patients sometimes choose the option that the doctor would not choose for the patient [18]. If a patient states a preference for a procedure that increases the risks for the patient (e.g., a patient requesting general anesthesia [GA] for an elective cesarean section instead of a spinal technique), does this mean the patient has made a wrong choice?
- Should the anesthetist accept the decision and proceed while managing the extra risk, or should the anesthetist have the right to refuse to treat the patient on the grounds that she is putting herself at unnecessary extra risk?

When making an assessment of risk acceptability, there needs to be a complete assessment of all the risks and benefits.

- Perception of the advantages of an event versus the disadvantages of the hazards associated with the event are personal to each individual.
- This is an unpredictable process and it is often surprising what patients are prepared to accept in terms of high-risk for what might appear to be little gain.
- Conversely, some individuals will refuse treatment that is likely to have a positive outcome because of fears about something we perceive to be quite trivial.
- Our duty is to be as honest and as accurate as we can with the information we have and allow the patient time to perform her/his own individual risk–benefit analysis.
- Depending on the urgency, this process can take months and sometimes even years.

The mnemonic BRAN (Benefits, Risks, Alternatives, Nothing) offers a useful way of approaching this analysis. This covers the benefits and risks associated with a course of action. It also prompts us to think of alternative treatments and what would happen if nothing were done.

What are the benefits?

- Identify the benefits.
- Assess the likelihood of benefit.
- Assess the perceived value of the benefit.
- How soon could benefit occur?
- Is the benefit permanent or temporary?

What are the risks?

- Identify the risks.
- Assess the likelihood or probability of risk.
- Assess the perceived magnitude of the risk.
- How soon could the risk occur?
- Is the risk permanent or temporary?

What are the alternatives?

- Are there alternative courses of action?
- Is there a new treatment on the horizon?
- Is there a less efficacious, but more acceptable alternative?

What if you do nothing?

- Remember *primum non nocere* – firstly do no harm.
- In the modern era with medical and surgical advances pushing the boundaries of what is achievable, it must not be forgotten that although we may be able to undertake a course of action, it does not always mean that we should.

The BRAN mnemonic may be useful in anesthetic practice to help direct discussion and thought; however, one must know what the risks are before it can be applied to individual patients.

What are the risks?

When patients present for surgery, there are a number of potential hazards with associated risks. These risks can be divided into categories:

- risks associated with a hospital admission
- risks associated purely with the anesthetic
- risks associated with the proposed surgery

The degree of risk associated with all of these categories will vary from patient to patient, depending on a number of factors. These include whether the surgery is elective or emergency and whether the patient has any premorbid conditions (chronic disease, obesity, etc.) or any lifestyle habits (smoking cigarettes or drinking alcohol) that may increase the risk involved. These are known as patient factors.

There are some risks present during an anesthetic irrespective of what the proposed surgery is. Not all of these risks are down to anesthesia. A significant risk is delivered by the surgery and by the patient her/himself, which the anesthetist partly has a role in managing. The magnitude of risk can be difficult to quantify and has been one of the aims of the U.K. National Audit Projects in Anesthetics.

Risks associated with a hospital admission

Appropriately trained staff

- The aviation industry is one that the medical profession looks to frequently and is compared to when it comes to errors, accidents, and near misses. The training systems in place within the aviation industry do not focus solely on the captain, but include the crew and the whole corporation. All are encouraged to spot potential problems before they occur and an open reporting system, which does not apportion blame on an individual but looks at the system itself and how it can be improved, has certainly increased airline safety [19].
- A rigorous critical incident reporting system is needed to record and subsequently investigate any incident that causes patient harm as well as the near misses that may have caused harm. This type of reporting system is effective only if all incidents and near

misses are reported. This will occur only if the reporter does not fear blame as a repercussion for bringing the incident to light. This "no blame" culture is gradually becoming accepted as part of the culture in many countries.

- Studies have shown that training, experience, and competence of the team have an effect on outcome. The team includes all the staff from the surgeon, anesthetist, and ORm team through to the nurses, physical therapists and rehabilitation team involved in postoperative care and follow-up clinics. Individual surgeon workload has been shown to influence outcome in colorectal and pancreatic surgery [20].
- Although the volume for surgeons may be important, it has been shown that a high-volume hospital may compensate partially for low-volume surgeons [21].
- Surgeons have been studied extensively, but not so the anesthetist. There have been few studies that have effectively shown the role of the anesthetist to have any effect on risk and outcome. One study looking at coronary artery bypass surgery showed that the only non-patient related factors influencing outcome were cardiac bypass time and the anesthetist [22].
- A more recent study looking at daycase surgery demonstrated that consultant anesthetists had lower unplanned admission rates and reduced adverse outcome reporting than staff specialists or trainees [23].
- The hierarchical structure of operating theater teams has been proposed to be a potential barrier to patient safety, with one study showing that residents were unlikely to correct and indeed would support a senior colleague who they knew to be making a mistake [24].

Timing of surgery

The National Confidential Enquiry into Perioperative Death (NCEPOD) in the U.K. has shown that surgery performed at night, when staff are more likely to be fatigued, is more hazardous and contributes to increased mortality [25]. As a result, emergency surgery is increasingly being performed during the day, with a reduction in adverse incidents.

Risks associated with the anesthetic

- The process of anesthesia has been compared with the aviation industry in that it demonstrates high dynamism, time pressure, uncertainty, complex human–machine interactions, and risk.
- Because the rare events are catastrophic (a plane crash or an anesthetic-related death), both of these professions have developed mechanisms for safety promotion. Anticipating complications and dealing with them prior to any potential untoward incident has become second nature.
- Death is the complication both anesthetists and patients fear most, whether it results from surgical complications or directly as a result of the anesthetic. However, more than 90% of deaths that occur perioperatively are not caused directly by the anesthetic [26].
- It is generally accepted that anesthesia is safer now than it was 30 years ago, and the report by the U.S. Institute of Medicine supports this [27].
- Comparing mortality figures is not an exact science as the nature of surgical patients and the operations performed upon them have also changed. More complex procedures are now performed more frequently on sicker, more elderly patients.

- Giving patients information leaflets specific to their surgery and their anesthetic, and by seeing them preoperatively in specifically designed clinics helps to allay some common misconceptions and also gives the medical team an opportunity to impress upon the patient some of the rarer, but more serious risks.

Risks associated with the surgery

- The number of surgery-related deaths identified each year by NCEPOD in the U.K. has changed very little between 1989 and 2011 [28,29].
- Approximately 3 000 000 surgical procedures are performed every year in the U.K. and over 20 000 patients will die as a result of undergoing this surgery.
- The mortality rates in the U.K. are slightly higher than for similar patients in the U.S. [30].
- In the U.K. there are 0.6 critical care beds per 10 000 patients compared to 4.4 per 10 000 patients in the U.S.
- The NCEPOD report in 2011 [29] reviewed the perioperative care of surgical patients. This report highlighted the increasing complexity of cases and increasing comorbidities of patients undergoing elective and emergency surgery. Identification of high-risk patients is clearly key; however, 20% of patients classed by the anesthetist as high-risk had not been seen preoperatively. The postoperative mortality was significantly different in the groups that had been seen (0.7%) and those that had not (4.8%), and highlights the importance of surgical preassessment.
- In those patients where discharge location was seen as not ideal by the anesthetist, the mortality rate was 5.0% compared to 1.4% where there were no concerns over discharge location; 6.7% of patients were discharged to critical care (22.1% of high-risk cases). Therefore, over 75% of high-risk patients were discharged back to the ward. Patients who were discharged to the ward and who subsequently required critical care had a poor outcome.
- Just over 20% of patients in this study were judged to be high-risk. There was a suggestion that invasive monitoring and specifically cardiac output monitoring was underutilized in the high-risk group.
- This high-risk population accounts for 77% of deaths in the NCEPOD study.
- Careful preoperative risk assessment is vital to guide appropriate utilization of postoperative critical care beds, and several scoring systems have been used for this purpose [31].
- It is recommended that an estimate of mortality should be undertaken preoperatively, communicated with the patient, and an appropriate package of care initiated (NCEPOD). The Department of Health and Royal College of Surgeons in their report in 2011 highlight the need for consultant presence in any case where predicted mortality is >10% and patients with a predicted mortality of >5% should be classed as high-risk [32].
- The evidence for surgical procedures is that risk is reduced through robust systems for preoperative assessment, risk stratification, and optimal peri- and postoperative management.
- A huge change resulted from the widespread international adoption of surgical safety checklists after the publication of a paper by Gawande and colleagues in 2009 [33].

In study hospitals worldwide the use of this checklist resulted in large reductions in perioperative mortality and surgical site infections. However, the majority of survival and other benefits were seen in the centers studied that were located outside the developed world. Nevertheless, the benefits of improved communication in the surgical environment are generally accepted by all.

Patient factors

- Many patient factors are beyond the control of the anesthetist. Some are beyond the control of the patient as well!
- We may be able to modify some of these factors, with the help of the patient. This requires early access to the patient and a means by which the patient may be fully informed. This may take the form of preoperative clinics where advice and support may be given or specific leaflets prepared for the proposed procedure.

Gender

- Females tend to recover from anesthesia quicker than males. When the differences in baseline characteristics, duration, and extent of surgery and anesthetic drug administration were adjusted for, it was found that females had a higher bispectral (BIS) score intraoperatively, woke up quicker, and were discharged from the PACU sooner than males. This study speculates than females therefore are less sensitive to the hypnotic effects of anesthetic drugs than males [34].
- Females, however, have been found to be more sensitive to muscle relaxant effects of rocuronium and vecuronium, although not to cisatracurium [35], and to opioid receptor agonists [36].
- Females have significantly better outcomes including mortality and recurrence rates from melanomas [37].
- The incidence of septic shock requiring intensive care is significantly less in females – but females have a worse outcome! [38].
- Females have a worse outcome following vascular surgery [39].

Ethnic group

This is an area that is poorly understood and is a difficult area to investigate. It is a highly sensitive issue and any actual or perceived differences may be seen to reflect prejudice or the ability to access medical care.

There are, however, observed differences in ethnic incidences for some disease processes.

- Differences in drug responses have long since been recognized in the treatment of hypertension.
- One retrospective study has found black race to be an independent risk factor for complications and death following hip and knee arthroplasty [40].
- A study in the pediatric population has found increased sensitivity and complications from opioid analgesia in white children and increased analgesic requirement in African American children following tonsillectomy [41].

Genetic predisposition

The understanding of genetic factors affecting risk of sepsis or cardiac prognosis is poor. It is almost certain that the inflammatory process and the response to infection is, at least in part, genetically predetermined.

References

1. Royal Society. *Risk Assessment: Report of a Royal Society Working Party, 1983.* London: Royal Society, 1983.
2. Keeney RL. Understanding life-threatening risks. *Risk Anal* 1995; **15**: 627–37.
3. Calman KC. Cancer: science and society and the communication of risk. *BMJ* 1996; **313**: 799–802.
4. Calman KC, Royston HD. Risk language and dialects. *BMJ* 1997; **315**: 939–42.
5. Bogardus ST, Holmboe E, Jekel JF. Perils, pitfalls and possibilities in talking about medical risk. *JAMA* 1999; **281**: 1037–41.
6. Broadbent DE. Psychology of risk. In: Cooper MG, ed. *Risk: Man-made Hazards to Man.* Oxford: Clarendon Press, 1985.
7. Malenka DJ, Baron JA, Johansen S, et al. The framing effect of relative and absolute risk. *J Gen Intern Med* 1993; **8**: 543–8.
8. Hux JE, Naylor CD. Communicating the benefits of chronic preventative therapy: does the format of efficacy data determine patients' acceptance of treatment? *Med Decis Making* 1995; **15**: 152–7.
9. Edwards A, Prior L. Communication about risk - dilemmas for general practitioners. *Br J Gen Prac* 1997; **47**: 739–42.
10. Barclay P, Costigan S, Davies M. Lottery can be used to show risk (letter). *BMJ* 1998; **316**: 124.
11. Laupacis A, Sackett DL, Roberts RS. An assessment of clinically useful measures of the consequences of treatment. *N Engl J Med* 1988; **318**: 1728–33.
12. Cook RJ, Sackett DL. The number needed to treat: a clinically useful measure of treatment effect. *BMJ* 1995; **310**: 452–4.
13. Adams AM, Smith AF. Risk perception and communication: recent developments and implications for anaesthesia. *Anaesthesia* 2001; **56**: 745–55.
14. Smith A, Adams A. Risk communication and anaesthesia. In: Lack AJ, Rollin A-M, Toms G, et al., eds. *Raising the standard: Information for patients.* London: Royal College of Anaesthetists, 2003; 77–86.
15. McPherson K. Third generation oral contraception and venous thromboembolism. *BMJ* 1996; **312**: 68–9.
16. General Medical Council. *Consent: Patients and Doctors Making Decisions Together.* London: General Medical Council, 2008.
17. Smith R. The discomfort of patient power (editorial). *BMJ* 2002; **324**: 497–8.
18. General Medical Council. *Seeking Patients' Consent: The Ethical Considerations.* London: General Medical Council, 1998; 7.
19. Helmreich RL. On error management: lessons from aviation. *BMJ* 2000; **320**: 781–5.
20. Archampong D, Borowski D, Wille-Jørgensen P, et al. Workload and surgeon's specialty for outcome after colorectal cancer surgery. *Cochrane Database SystRev* 2012; **3**: CD005391.
21. Harmon JW, Tang DG, Gordon TA, et al. Hospital volume can serve as surrogate for surgical volume for achieving excellent outcomes in colorectal resection. *Ann Surg* 1999; **230**: 404–11.
22. Merry AF, Ramage MC, Whitlock RM, et al. First-time coronary artery bypass grafting: the anaesthetist as a risk factor. *Br J Anaesth* 1992; **68**: 6–12.
23. Hanousek J, Stocker ME, Montgomery JE. The effect of grade of anaesthetist on outcome after day surgery. *Anaesthesia* 2009; **64**: 152–5.
24. Sydor DT, Bould MD, Naik VN, et al. Challenging authority during a life-threatening crisis: the effect of operating

theatre hierarchy. *Br J Anaesth* 2013; **110**: 463–71.

25. Cullinane M, Gray AJG, Hargreaves CMK, et al. *Who Operates When II*. London: NCEPOD, 2003.
26. Department of Health. *NHS Performance Indicators*. London: Department of Health, 2002.
27. Committee on Quality of Health Care in America IOM. *To Err is Human: Building a Safer Health Care System*. Kohn L, Corrigan J, Donaldson M, eds. Washington, DC: National Academy Press, 1999; 241.
28. Campling EA, Devlin HB, Lunn JN. *Report of the National Confidential Enquiry into Perioperative Deaths, 1989*. London: NCEPOD, 1990.
29. Findlay GP, Goodwin APL, Protopapa A, et al. *Knowing the Risk. A review of the Perioperative Care of Surgical Patients*. London: NCEPOD, 2011.
30. Bennett-Guerrero E, Hyam JA, Shaefi S, et al. Comparison of P-POSSUM risk-adjusted mortality rates after surgery between patients in the USA and the UK. *Br J Surg* 2003; **90**: 1593–8.
31. Neary WD, Prytherch D, Foy C, et al. Comparison of different methods of risk stratification in urgent and emergency surgery. *Br J Surg* 2007; **94**: 1300–5.
32. Royal College of Surgeons and Department of Health. *The Higher Risk Surgical Patient. Towards Improved Care for a Forgotten Group*. London: Royal College of Surgeons and Department of Health, 2011.
33. Haynes AB, Weiser TG, Berry WR, et al. A surgical safety checklist to reduce morbidity and mortality in a global population. *N Engl J Med* 2009; **360**: 491–9.
34. Buchanan F, Myles P, Leslie K, et al. Gender and recovery after general anaesthesia combined with neuromuscular blocking drugs. *Anesth Analg* 2006; **102**: 291–7.
35. Adamus M, Gabrhelik T, Marek O. Influence of gender on the course of neuromuscular block following a single bolus dose of cisatracurium or rocuronium. *Eur J Anesthesiol* 2008; **25**: 589–95.
36. Ueno K. Gender differences in pharmacokinetics of anesthetics. *Masui* 2009; **58**: 51–8.
37. Stidham KR, Johnson JL, Seigler HF. Survival superiority of females with melanoma. A multivariate analysis of 6383 patients exploring the significance of gender in prognostic outcome. *Arch Surg* 1994; **129**: 316–24.
38. Sakr Y, Elia C, Mascia L, et al. The influence of gender on the epidemiology of and outcome from severe sepsis. *Crit Care* 2013; **17**: R50.
39. Norman PE, Semmens JB, Lawrence-Brown M, et al. The influence of gender on outcome following peripheral vascular surgery: a review. *Cardiovasc Surg* 2000; **8**: 111–15.
40. Adelani MA, Archer KR, Song Y, et al. Immediate complications following hip and knee arthroplasty: does race matter? *J Arthroplasty* 2013 **28**: 732–5.
41. Sadhasivam S, Chidambaran V, Ngamprasertwong P, et al. Race and unequal burden of perioperative pain and opioid related adverse effects in children. *Pediatrics* 2012; **129**: 832–8.

Perioperative mortality and cardiac arrest

D. Bainbridge and D. Cheng

One of the first reported anesthetic deaths occurred shortly after the discovery and use of chloroform as a general anesthetic (GA). On January 22, 1848, Hannah Green died under anesthesia while having an ingrown toenail removed. Then, as today, the case caused great consternation. Since then, much effort has been directed at reducing perioperative death from anesthesia. The purpose of this chapter is to review the trends in mortality, risks for perioperative cardiac arrest, and mechanisms to reduce adverse outcomes.

Historical perspective

From one of the first investigations in 1848 on the death of Hannah Green to a seminal article by Beecher [1] in 1954 on perioperative mortality, the confidential inquiry into perioperative mortality in 1986 in the U.K. [2], and the crucial paper on pulse oximetry monitoring in 1993 [3,4], there has been a continuous focus on safety in anesthesia with the aim of reducing adverse events.

Has the mortality risk from anesthesia declined over the years?

- Mortality risks have declined over the past 60 years [5].
- Event rates for mortality solely attributable to anesthesia have decreased from roughly 300 per million before 1970 to 30 per million anesthetics today (Figure 2.1a).
- Event rates for early postoperative mortality have also declined from roughly 10 000 events per million in the pre-1970s to roughly 1000 per million anesthetics today (Figure 2.1b).

Causes of perioperative death

Historically, causes of perioperative death under anesthesia have been divided into patient, surgical, and anesthetic factors. This reflected the high rates of death caused by errors of surgical or anesthetic delivery. While the risk of surgical or anesthetic errors have declined, it is important to remember that anesthetic and surgical miscalculations are usually entirely preventable and represent avoidable mortality. Often patient-related factors in perioperative death are caused by underlying disease and therefore may represent either an acceleration of or a natural history for the underlying disease process. However, this trend toward greater patient-related factors has led to a growing focus on risk stratification of patient illness.

Anesthesia and Perioperative Care of the High-Risk Patient, Third edition, ed. Ian McConachie. Published by Cambridge University Press.

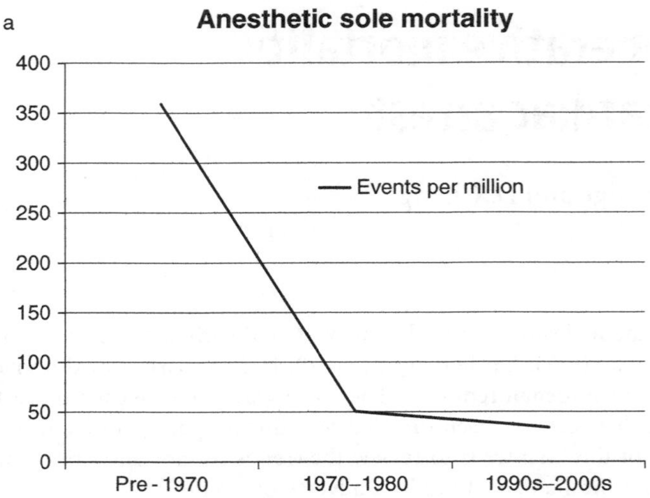

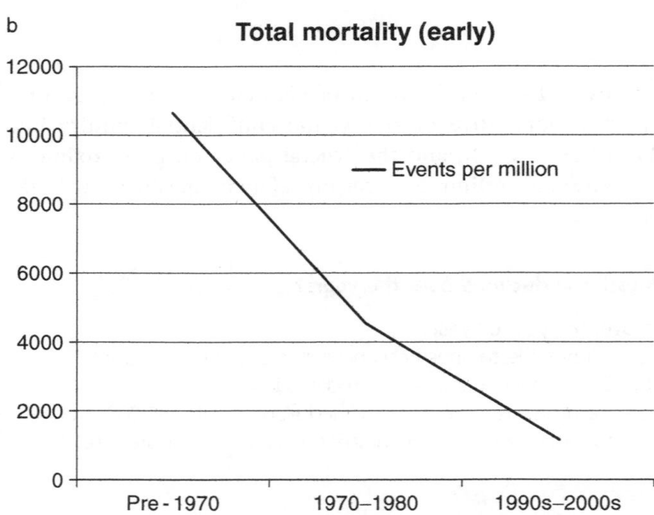

Figure 2.1a and 2.1b. Anesthetic and total early mortality. Adapted from Bainbridge et al. [5].

Anesthesia factors

- Traditionally, focus was on safety of anesthetic agents.
- Historically, errors frequently were related to inadequate monitoring, airway management issues, inadequate training.
- Steady improvement and standardization of equipment and approaches to patients (American Society of Anesthesiologists' [ASA] airway algorithm, surgical checklist) are important.
- Thus, anesthetic-related mortality and mortality in general (especially early mortality of <48 h) have decreased steadily.
- Recently, more focus has been on system errors including team work, communication, etc.

Patient factors

Causes of death

- Cardiovascular mortality accounts for approximately 60% of perioperative deaths [6,7].
- Thus, non-cardiovascular causes account for 40% of deaths, which is often under-appreciated.

Prediction–risk scoring

Reflected in many perioperative scoring systems:

- One of the earliest scoring systems was the Goldman Cardiac Risk Index (CRI), later followed by Detsky [8,9].
- It became the Revised Cardiac Risk Index (RCRI) [10]
- However, these are cardiac risk scores and not mortality risk scores and hence perform poorly for predicting mortality [11]. This is likely related to the high-risk of non-cardiovascular causes of death [6].

Mortality-specific scores

- Historically, there were few mortality scoring systems.
- Tiret identified the ASA score, age, type of surgery, and emergency surgery as mortality risks [12]. A high ASA score, the type of surgery (major versus minor), and planned versus urgent or emergency cases are all considerations in risk prediction.
- The Surgical Risk Scale was developed in 2002 with essentially the same factors [13].
- Many scoring systems, including the American College of Surgeons National Surgical Quality Improvement Program (ACS NSQIP) [14–16], the Agency for Healthcare Research and Quality (AHRQ) [17], and in the U.K., the Physiological and Operative Severity Score for the Enumeration of Mortality and Morbidity (UK POSSUM) [18] are used more as administrative or research tools and are not practical bedside scoring tests.
- The Surgical Mortality Probability Model (S-MPM) is a large practical scoring system again based on ASA status, procedure risk (surgical type), and procedure urgency [19].

Risk factor	Points assigned
ASA physical status	
I	0
II	2
III	4
IV	5
V	6
Procedure risk	
Low-risk	0
Intermediate-risk	1
High-risk	2
Emergency	
Non-emergent	0
Emergency surgery	1

- Mortality risk based on classification from S-MPM

Class	Point	Total mortality
I	0–4	<0.50%
II	5–6	1.5%–4.0%
III	7–9	>10%

Effect of patient age on mortality

Few studies have identified age as an independent factor contributing to death [12]. Hamel [20], in a comparison of over 80- versus under-80-year-olds, found:

- more associated comorbidities in the elderly
- independent functional status in only 67% of >80-year-olds (versus 86% in <80-year-olds)
- an independent increase in mortality of 5% for each year over 80 years (i.e., and 85-year-olds risk is 25% higher than 80-year-olds)
- mortality up substantially in the presence of postoperative complications

Surgical factors

As previously discussed, most risk prediction models have identified as surgical risk factors:

- the type of surgery (usually classified as minor, intermediate, or major)
- the urgency of surgery (elective, urgent, emergency)

The degree to which surgery contributes to mortality risk may be underestimated as we tend to subcategorize surgical procedures – the most obvious being non-cardiac from cardiac surgery.

Time frame – when do perioperative deaths occur?

Historically, the time frame for death from surgery (anesthesia-, surgery-, or patient-related) has been considered over short time periods of one to seven days. This again tended to reflect the early demise of patients caused by surgical or anesthetic complications or errors, and to some extent, on the limitations of our ability to track long-term events. Frequently, the risk related to surgery may extend beyond this early time point. However, other unrelated factors may contribute to mortality at later time points.

Early mortality (<48 h)

- Early mortality was the focus in the 1950s to 1980s.
- Early mortality may be more specific for errors or adverse events from surgery, anesthesia, or patient factors.
- As perioperative care has improved, many patients survive for longer periods, shifting perioperative mortality into the weeks following surgery; therefore, it is likely that we underestimate the impact of surgery on patient survival.

Late mortality

- Using 30-day or hospital discharge mortality may reflect the risk associated with surgery better.
- Risk of death, uniform over the first 20 days, starts to decline to stable levels up to 30 days [6,7].
- In one large non-cardiac surgical observational trial, roughly one quarter of deaths occurred at a median of 11 days after hospital discharge [7].

Natural history of patients

When following mortality over longer time frames, the natural history of sick patients becomes a cofounding factor:

- In nonsurgical elderly patients admitted to hospital, the in-hospital mortality and one-month mortality was 7.6% and 11%, respectively [21]. There was a similar rate of out-of-hospital deaths with one quarter of the mortality occurring after hospital discharge.
- Annual mortality in U.S. actuarial tables for anyone aged 75 years is 4.0% for males and 2.8% for females.
- At age 80 years, the risk increases to 6.4% for males and 4.6% for females.
- At age 85 years, the risk is 10.1% for males and 7.8% for females – add roughly 1% mortality per month for males.
- By age 95 years, mean life expectancy (all comers) is 2.75 years for males and 3.26 years for females (Available from: http://www.ssa.gov/oact/STATS/table4c6.html [Accessed May 3, 2013]).

Perioperative cardiac arrest

If mortality represents the end result to those who suffered either critical errors or poor care during the perioperative period, would there be a better marker of near misses than death? Would acute events like cardiac arrests represent a better surrogate of this than absolute mortality? Most deaths are preceded by cardiac arrest but not all these patients go on to die. Causes of cardiac arrest may also give clues as to causes of death and may aid in preventive measures.

Have the rates of perioperative cardiac arrest been declining?

- Not surprisingly, the rates of perioperative cardiac arrest appear to have declined in a manner similar to mortality from approximately 1800 events per million anesthetics in the 1970s and 1980s to approximately 700 events per million anesthetics in the 1990s and 2000s [5,22].

What are the predictors of perioperative cardiac arrest ?

- Similar to mortality, the ASA score seems to play a strong role in predicting who is at risk for cardiac arrest. In addition, the urgency of surgery was found to be a factor [2,23–26.]

What are the causes of perioperative cardiac arrest?

The use of perioperative ultrasound (US) in the operating room for pre-arrest and arrest situations has led to some interesting insights into the causes of intraoperative cardiac arrest [27–30].

- Severe left ventricular (LV) dysfunction is the most frequently found cause in pre-arrest and arrest situations, followed by right ventricular (RV) dysfunction.
- Thromboembolism appears quite commonly.
- Hypovolemia and tamponade as diagnoses during arrest and pre-arrest appear less commonly.

The role of US monitoring to diagnose and to treat intraoperative pre-arrests and arrests is evolving and is likely to play an increasing role in the management of these patients. Few studies are published currently to report on the benefit of echocardiography in this setting.

What is the mortality following perioperative cardiac arrest?

- Survival rates (hospital discharge) of 30%–40% are typically reported following intraoperative cardiac arrest [22,31].
- A multivariate model looking at predictors of survival found bleeding/hypovolemia (versus cardiac or other causes) was associated with decreased survival. Cardiac arrest during working hours (07h00 to 20h00) had improved survival versus arrests after hours. Protracted hypotension and diabetes mellitus were also associated with worse outcomes [22].
- Overall, perioperative cardiac arrest mirrors mortality in patients who are at risk and the overall mortality over time. Survival rates following arrests in the perioperative period seem to be equal to or better than those occurring in hospitalized patients.

Systems to reduce errors

There are many different approaches to changing the system of delivering care to improve outcomes by focusing on the reduction of medical errors. Some examples include:

- Focus on communication and team work [32] can be defined broadly by behaviors including briefing, information sharing, inquiry, assertion, vigilance, and awareness, and contingency management.
- A surgical safety checklist [33–35] provides a more structured approach to team work by ensuring that communication occurs prior to and throughout the procedure.
- A standardized order entry/computer entry [36–38] as the physician ordering is responsible for 50% of all medication errors.
- The Institute of Medicine identifies medication errors as a threat to patient safety.
- 80% of studies show reductions in prescribing errors with computer order entry. In these studies, reductions of errors by 60% were noted after inititation of computer order entry [36].
- Drug labels [39–42] – error rates of drug administration during anesthesia are roughly 1 in 1300 medication administrations. Harm rates from drug errors, while low (1 in 3000 to 1 in 6000), are typically preventable.
- Currently, the international standard (ISO 26825:2008) for labeling medications aims to reduce drug errors.

Improving care – intensive monitoring

If identification through risk modeling is possible, is intensive monitoring in a critical/high intensity care area beneficial?

Currently, evidence supporting intensive monitoring of high-risk patients to improve mortality is limited. There is indirect evidence supporting intensive monitoring:

- A study comparing the use of the POSSOM risk model for predicting death showed higher rates of mortality in the U.K. cohort vs the U.S. cohort (U.K.: predicted 10.2, observed 9.9; U.S. predicted 7.8, observed 2.1). Most of the deaths in the U.K. cohort occurred during the first two days. Reduced utilization of beds in the intensive care unit (ICU) was postulated as one possible difference (lower in the U.K.) [43].
- A randomized study of high-risk general surgical patients showed improved outcomes (fewer complications, shorter hospital stay) in patients who received goal-directed therapy (fluids and inotropes to increase oxygen delivery) versus ICU admission alone. However, no difference in mortality was observed [44].

Evidence against intensive monitoring:

- In a trial of over 3000 high-risk surgical patients randomized to pulmonary artery catheter (PAC) and goal-directed therapy versus standard of care, no improvement in mortality was seen [45].

No clear evidence exists that intensive postoperative care has an impact on mortality. Given the time frame of death postoperatively, it may be difficult to have a substantial impact with limited intensive care admissions alone. Use of an integrated system of intensive care for high-risk patients on the floor followed by intensive monitoring in a high-dependency unit and the use of clinical outreach teams [46] may contribute to the system of improved care. This is considered further elsewhere in this text.

Improving care – type of anesthetic

Are there substantial differences in the mortality rates based on the type of anesthetic given?

- Numerous trials have looked at rates of death or cardiac arrest based on the anesthetic provided. Figure 2.2 provides a summary of these studies.
- Most of these studies are observational and did not account for differences in patient populations within each anesthetic type.
- Some studies group regional and neuraxial anesthesia together.

From the figure, neuraxial anesthesia appears to be the safest while monitored anesthesia care/local anesthesia (LA) appears to be the highest risk. However, patient selection has a strong impact on mortality and patients undergoing monitored anesthesia care/LA are likely felt to be too sick to survive GA. This suggests that patient factors have a greater impact on adverse outcome than the choice of anesthesia per se.

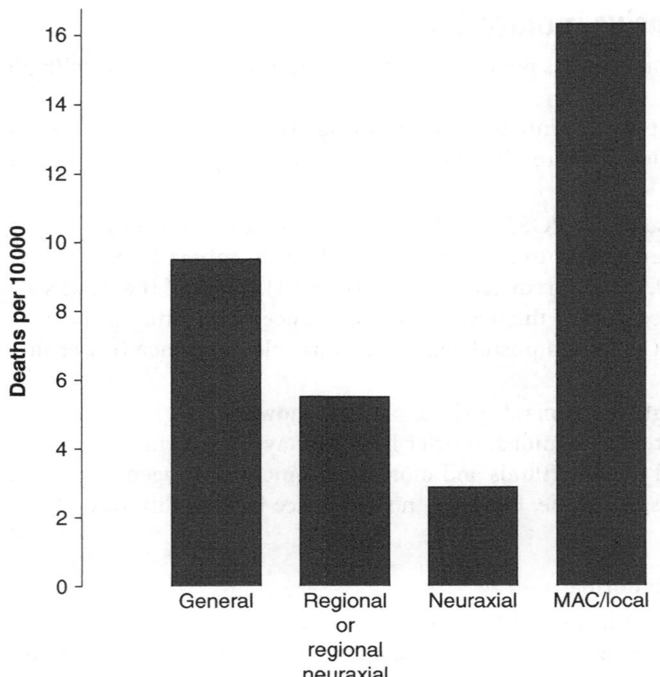

Figure 2.2. Average rates of death or cardiac arrest from observational studies [22][25][47–52].

The big picture – informed consent

The American Medical Association describes informed consent as:

> "In the communications process, you, as the physician providing or performing the treatment and/or procedure (not a delegated representative), should disclose and discuss with your patient:
>
> - The patient's diagnosis
> - The nature and purpose of a proposed procedure
> - The risks and benefits of the procedure
> - Alternatives
> - The risks and benefits of the alternatives
> - The risks and benefits of not receiving the procedure." [53].

Therefore, having an appreciation of the risk of (a) the procedure, (b) patient risk, and (c) anesthetic risk is essential to allow informed decision making.

Over and above risk estimates, the physician needs to be aware of risk perception when discussing anesthetic risk, particularly observed biases in risk, which may impact the perioperative period, including:

- Immediacy: the perception of reduced risk to events are delayed (myocardial infarction [MI] postoperatively) as opposed to immediately "dying on the table."
- Familiarity: familiar risks (car accident) are more acceptable then unfamiliar risks (dying in hospital).

- Rare yet catastrophic: people are more concerned about rare yet catastrophic complications than the more frequent yet more mundane (death vs dental injury).
- Trust: the more individuals or the team is trusted, the lower the perceived risk.

The concepts of risk are further explored in a separate chapter.

The big picture – is anesthesia safe enough?

The question of how safe is safe enough is difficult to answer. We often benchmark surgical safety against transportation safety including air travel and car travel. Air travel has shown consistent improvements over time as has motor vehicle safety.

- Airline accidents: civil aviation accidents have fallen from rates of approximately six per million flights in 2000 to three per million flights in 2009 [54].
- Car safety: Figure 2.3 shows fatalities per million miles traveled. From 1.6 deaths per million miles traveled in 1991 to 1.2 million deaths in 2011 [55].

The risks of transportation fatalities are controllable (we do not deal with sick aircraft), and usually elective (we do not have to fly to live), which is unlike the situation faced by healthcare providers and patients. However, while flying and car travel are felt to be very safe both now and 10 years ago, clearly incremental improvements have led to further safety gains, and this should be the aim of anesthesia as a speciality.

A global perspective

It is important to identify that the majority of publications on perioperative mortality focus on developed countries. Few discuss the issue of perioperative mortality in the developing world. Preventable mortality may be comparable between countries but there are issues related to patient health (likely younger patients with less chronic diseases) and types of illness (trauma, or infectious diseases in developing countries), making direct comparisons difficult. In addition, available infrastructure – not only hospital infrastructure but roads, access to cars/ambulances, presence or absence of lines of communication

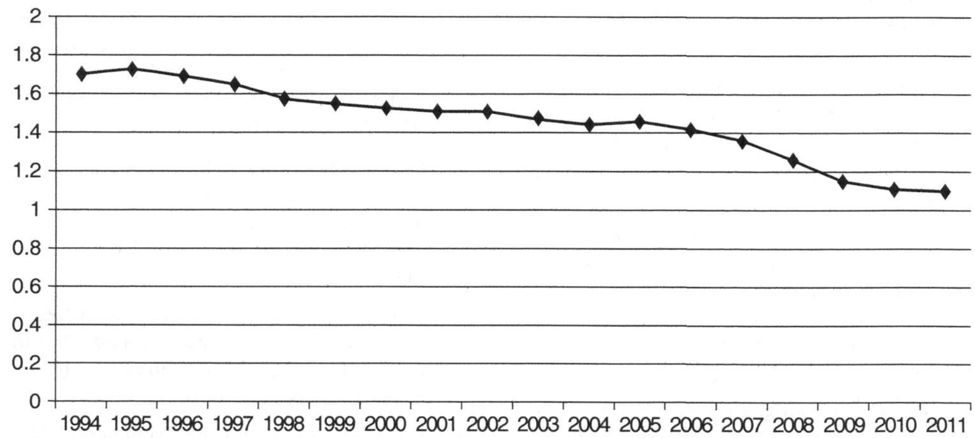

Figure 2.3. Car fatalities per million miles traveled. From NHTSA, 2013.

(one number for emergencies, etc. – may limit the presentation of patients in a timely fashion. However, improvements in developing countries still lag behind those in developed countries over the last 30 to 40 years [5]. Thus, generalization of findings from developed countries should be applied to the developing world with caution.

Conclusion

Despite increasing patient baseline risk, perioperative mortality has declined significantly over the past 50 years, with the greatest reduction in developed countries. Mortality solely attributable to anesthesia declined over time, from 357 per million before the 1970s to 52 per million in the 1970s–1980s, and 34 per million in the 1999s–2000s. The total perioperative mortality also decreased over time, from 10 603 per million before the 1970s, to 4533 per million in the 1970s–1980s, and 1176 per million in the 1990s–2000s.

Mortality in the perioperative period has seen a gradual shift away from the immediate perioperative period and toward the extended recovery phase of days to weeks. This likely reflects both an improvement in the care provided and an increase in the number of patients presenting with severe underlying medical conditions. Future work will need to be done to improve our identification of these patients and of potential interventions that will result in prolonged survival. As the population ages, the number of patients presenting with pre-existing conditions will increase, placing further pressure on scarce healthcare resources. The best evidence-based approaches provide the only rational approach to the management and care of these individuals.

References

1. Beecher HK, Todd DP. A study of the deaths associated with anesthesia and surgery: based on a study of 599,548 anesthesias in ten institutions 1948–1952, inclusive. *Ann Surg* 1954; **140**: 2–35.

2. Lunn JN, Devlin HB. Lessons from the Confidential Enquiry into Perioperative Deaths in three NHS regions. *Lancet* 1987; **2**: 1384–6.

3. Moller JT, Pedersen T, Rasmussen LS, et al. Randomized evaluation of pulse oximetry in 20,802 patients: I. Design, demography, pulse oximetry failure rate, and overall complication rate. *Anesthesiology* 1993; **78**: 436–44.

4. Moller JT, Johannessen NW, Espersen K, et al. Randomized evaluation of pulse oximetry in 20,802 patients: II. Perioperative events and postoperative complications. *Anesthesiology* 1993; **78**: 445–53.

5. Bainbridge D, Martin J, Arango M, et al. Evidence-based peri-operative clinical outcomes research: G. Perioperative and anaesthetic-related mortality in developed and developing countries: a systematic review and meta-analysis. *Lancet* 2012; **380**: 1075–81.

6. Group PS, Devereaux PJ, Yang H, et al. Effects of extended-release metoprolol succinate in patients undergoing non-cardiac surgery (POISE trial): a randomised controlled trial. *Lancet* 2008; **371**: 1839–47.

7. Devereaux PJ, Chan MT, et al. Association between postoperative troponin levels and 30-day mortality among patients undergoing noncardiac surgery. *JAMA* 2012; **307**: 2295–304.

8. Detsky AS, Abrams HB, McLaughlin JR, et al. Predicting cardiac complications in patients undergoing non-cardiac surgery. *J Gen Int Med* 1986; **1**: 211–19.

9. Goldman L, Caldera DL, Nussbaum SR, et al. Multifactorial index of cardiac risk in noncardiac surgical procedures. *N Engl J Med* 1977; **297**: 845–50.

10. Lee TH, Marcantonio ER, Mangione CM, et al. Derivation and prospective validation

of a simple index for prediction of cardiac risk of major noncardiac surgery. *Circulation* 1999; **100**: 1043–9.

11. Ford MK, Beattie WS, Wijeysundera DN. Systematic review: prediction of perioperative cardiac complications and mortality by the revised cardiac risk index. *Ann Int Med* 2010; **152**: 26–35.
12. Tiret L, Hatton F, Desmonts JM, et al. Prediction of outcome of anaesthesia in patients over 40 years: a multifactorial risk index. *Stat Med* 1988; **7**: 947–54.
13. Sutton R, Bann S, Brooks M, et al. The Surgical Risk Scale as an improved tool for risk-adjusted analysis in comparative surgical audit. *Br J Surg* 2002; **89**: 763–8.
14. Khuri SF, Daley J, Henderson W, et al. The Department of Veterans Affairs' NSQIP: the first national, validated, outcome-based, risk-adjusted, and peer-controlled program for the measurement and enhancement of the quality of surgical care. National VA Surgical Quality Improvement Program. *Ann Surg* 1998; **228**: 491–507.
15. Cohen ME, Bilimoria KY, Ko CY, et al. Effect of subjective preoperative variables on risk-adjusted assessment of hospital morbidity and mortality. *Ann Surg* 2009; **249**: 682–9.
16. Birkmeyer JD, Shahian DM, Dimick JB, et al. Blueprint for a new American College of Surgeons: National Surgical Quality Improvement Program. *J Am Coll Surg* 2008; **207**: 777–82.
17. Glance LG, Osler TM, Mukamel DB, et al. Impact of the present-on-admission indicator on hospital quality measurement: experience with the Agency for Healthcare Research and Quality (AHRQ) Inpatient Quality Indicators. *Med Care* 2008; **46**: 112–19.
18. Copeland GP. The POSSUM system of surgical audit. *Arch Surg* 2002; **137**: 15–19.
19. Glance LG, Lustik SJ, Hannan EL, et al. The Surgical Mortality Probability Model: derivation and validation of a simple risk prediction rule for noncardiac surgery. *Ann Surg* 2012; **255**: 696–702.
20. Hamel MB, Henderson WG, Khuri SF, et al. Surgical outcomes for patients aged 80 and older: morbidity and mortality from major noncardiac surgery. *J Am Geriatr Soc* 2005; **53**: 424–9.
21. Espallargues M, Philp I, Seymour DG, et al. Measuring case-mix and outcome for older people in acute hospital care across Europe: the development and potential of the ACMEplus instrument. *QJM* 2008; **101**: 99–109.
22. Sprung J, Warner ME, Contreras MG, et al. Predictors of survival following cardiac arrest in patients undergoing noncardiac surgery: a study of 518,294 patients at a tertiary referral center. *Anesthesiology* 2003; **99**: 259–69.
23. Marx GF, Mateo CV, Orkin LR. Computer analysis of postanesthetic deaths. *Anesthesiology* 1973; **39**: 54–8.
24. Newland MC, Ellis SJ, Lydiatt CA, et al. Anesthetic-related cardiac arrest and its mortality: a report covering 72,959 anesthetics over 10 years from a US teaching hospital. *Anesthesiology* 2002; **97**: 108–15.
25. Biboulet P, Aubas P, Dubourdieu J, et al. Fatal and non fatal cardiac arrests related to anesthesia. *Can J Anaesth* 2001; **48**: 326–32.
26. Vacanti CJ, VanHouten RJ, Hill RC. A statistical analysis of the relationship of physical status to postoperative mortality in 68,388 cases. *Anesth Analg* 1970; **49**: 564–6.
27. Denault AY, Couture P, McKenty S, et al. Perioperative use of transesophageal echocardiography by anesthesiologists: impact in noncardiac surgery and in the intensive care unit. *Can J Anaesth* 2002; **49**: 287–93.
28. Memtsoudis SG, Rosenberger P, Loffler M, et al. The usefulness of transesophageal echocardiography during intraoperative cardiac arrest in noncardiac surgery. *Anesth Analg* 2006; **102**: 1653–7.
29. Suriani RJ, Neustein S, Shore-Lesserson L, et al. Intraoperative transesophageal echocardiography during noncardiac surgery. *J Cardiothorac Vasc Anesth* 1998; **12**: 274–80.

30. Shillcutt SK, Markin NW, Montzingo CR, et al. Use of rapid "rescue" perioperative echocardiography to improve outcomes after hemodynamic instability in noncardiac surgical patients. *J Cardiothorac Vasc Anesth* 2012; **26**: 362–70.

31. Girardi LN, Barie PS. Improved survival after intraoperative cardiac arrest in noncardiac surgical patients. *Arch Surg* 1995; **130**: 15–18.

32. Mazzocco K, Petitti DB, Fong KT, et al. Surgical team behaviors and patient outcomes. *Am J Surg* 2009; **197**: 678–85.

33. Lingard L, Regehr G, Orser B, et al. Evaluation of a preoperative checklist and team briefing among surgeons, nurses, and anesthesiologists to reduce failures in communication. *Arch Surg* 2008; **143**: 12–17.

34. Haynes AB, Weiser TG, Berry WR, et al. A surgical safety checklist to reduce morbidity and mortality in a global population. *N Engl J Med* 2009; **360**: 491–9.

35. de Vries EN, Prins HA, Crolla RM, et al. Effect of a comprehensive surgical safety system on patient outcomes. *N Engl J Med* 2010; **363**: 1928–37.

36. Shamliyan TA, Duval S, Du J, et al. Just what the doctor ordered. Review of the evidence of the impact of computerized physician order entry system on medication errors. *Health Serv Res* 2008; **43**: 32–53.

37. Khajouei R, Jaspers MW. The impact of CPOE medication systems' design aspects on usability, workflow and medication orders: a systematic review. *Methods Inf Med* 2010; **49**: 3–19.

38. Manias E, Williams A, Liew D. Interventions to reduce medication errors in adult intensive care: a systematic review. *Br J Clin Pharmacol* 2012; **74**: 411–23.

39. Merry AF, Shipp DH, Lowinger JS. The contribution of labelling to safe medication administration in anaesthetic practice. *Best Pract Res Clin Anaesthesiol* 2011; **25**: 145–59.

40. Webster CS, Merry AF, Larsson L, et al. The frequency and nature of drug administration error during anaesthesia. *Anaesth Intensive Care* 2001; **29**: 494–500.

41. Glavin RJ. Drug errors: consequences, mechanisms, and avoidance. *Br J Anaesth* 2010; **105**: 76–82.

42. Llewellyn RL, Gordon PC, Wheatcroft D, et al. Drug administration errors: a prospective survey from three South African teaching hospitals. *Anaesth Intensive Care* 2009; **37**: 93–8.

43. Bennett-Guerrero E, Hyam JA, Shaefi S, et al. Comparison of P-POSSUM risk-adjusted mortality rates after surgery between patients in the USA and the UK. *Br J Surg* 2003; **90**: 1593–8.

44. Pearse R, Dawson D, Fawcett J, et al. Early goal-directed therapy after major surgery reduces complications and duration of hospital stay. A randomised, controlled trial. *Crit Care* 2005; **9**: R687–93.

45. Sandham JD, Hull RD, Brant RF, et al. A randomized, controlled trial of the use of pulmonary artery catheters in high-risk surgical patients. *N Engl J Med* 2003; **348**: 5–14.

46. Hillman K, Chen J, Cretikos M, et al. Introduction of the medical emergency team (MET) system: a cluster-randomised controlled trial. *Lancet* 2005; **365**: 2091–7.

47. Braz LG, Modolo NS, do Nascimento P Jr, et al. Perioperative cardiac arrest: a study of 53,718 anaesthetics over 9 yr from a Brazilian teaching hospital. *Br J Anaesth* 2006; **96**: 569–75.

48. Aubas S, Biboulet P, Daures JP, et al. [Incidence and etiology of cardiac arrest occurring during the peroperative period and in the recovery room, apropos of 102,468 anesthesia cases]. *Ann Fr Anesth Reanim* 1991; **10**: 436–42.

49. Kawashima Y, Seo N, Morita K, et al. [Annual study of perioperative mortality and morbidity for the year of 1999 in Japan: the outlines – report of the Japan Society of Anesthesiologists Committee on Operating Room Safety]. *Masui* 2001; **50**: 1260–74.

50. Kubota Y, Toyoda Y, Kubota H, et al. Frequency of anesthetic cardiac arrest and death in the operating room at a single general hospital over a 30-year period. *J Clin Anesth* 1994; **6**: 227–38.

51. Morita K, Kawashima Y, Irita K, et al. [Perioperative mortality and morbidity in the year 2000 in 520 certified training hospitals of Japanese Society of Anesthesiologists: with a special reference to age – report of Japanese Society of Anesthesiologists Committee on Operating Room Safety]. *Masui* 2002; **51**: 1285–96.

52. Turnbull KW, Fancourt-Smith PF, Banting GC. Death within 48 hours of anaesthesia at the Vancouver General Hospital. *Can Anaesth Soc J* 1980; **27**: 159–63.

53. http://www.ama-assn.org/ama/pub/physician-resources/legal-topics/patient-physician-relationship-topics/informed-consent.page (Accessed May 27, 2013.)

54. National Transportation Safety Board. Review of U.S. Civil Aviation Accidents ARNA-W, DC. *Review of U.S. Civil Aviation Accidents, 2007–2009.* Washington, DC: National Transportation Safety Board, 2011.

55. NHTSA, 2013. http://www-fars.nhtsa.dot.gov/Main/index.aspx (Accessed May 28, 2013.)

Assessment of cardiovascular disease

G.M. Flood and L. Fleisher

The American College of Cardiology Foundation (ACCF)/American Heart Association (AHA) and the European Society of Cardiology (ESC) (endorsed by the European Society of Anaesthesiology [ESA]) have published guidelines on perioperative cardiovascular evaluation before non-cardiac surgery [1,2]. The ACCF/AHA 2009 guidelines were updated from the 2007 guidelines with regard to perioperative β-blockade and the ESC guideline dates from 2009. These two guidelines differ in their advice on β-blockade perioperatively, and this area of perioperative risk prevention has recently been thrown into contention yet again with concerns over the validity of some published and widely cited European work.

Cardiovascular disease and perioperative major adverse cardiac events (MACE) carry a considerable burden of morbidity and mortality during non-cardiac surgery.

- In the European Surgical Outcomes Study (EuSOS), in-hospital mortality after inpatient non-cardiac surgery varied across Europe and on average was higher than previously documented at 4.0% [3].
- The VISION trial included 15 133 patients undergoing non-cardiac surgery with 1.9% thirty-day overall mortality [4].
- The Perioperative Ischemia Events (POISE) Trial showed that patients with or at risk of atherosclerotic disease undergoing inpatient non-cardiac surgery had an overall mortality of 2.3%–3.1%, with cardiovascular death accounting for approximately 60% of these mortalities [5].

However, mortalities are merely the tip of a morbidity "ice-berg" and in socioeconomic terms carry a much higher burden of cost. Consequently, the perioperative assessment and care of the patient with cardiovascular disease remains an important and relevant topic for anesthesiologists. It is understood now that alterations in perioperative care can potentially influence longer-term patient outcome. Engagement with medical services during the perioperative period offers a unique opportunity to alter a patient's risk profile, thereby impacting not only perioperative but also long-term outcome with potential future cost savings.

Perioperative risk

Attempts to identify patients at high surgical risk and quantify individual risk have been published for more than fifty years. In 1962, the American Society of Anesthesiologists

Anesthesia and Perioperative Care of the High-Risk Patient, Third edition, ed. Ian McConachie. Published by Cambridge University Press.

(ASA) adopted a five-point classification system based on the patient's physical status to characterize perioperative mortality risk.

- The ASA Risk Index, while being simple and widely used in everyday practice, is far from perfect and is not designed to identify cardiovascular risk, although cardiovascular morbidity is the leading cause of perioperative mortality.
- It does highlight that the more incapacity a patient has, caused by comorbid disease, the higher the perioperative risk.
- It also appears to be a relatively simple risk adjustment for overall mortality, which, given the partial subjective nature of the index, may reflex the anesthesiologists ability to risk stratify.

The first Cardiac Risk Index (CRI) for non-cardiac surgery was designed in 1977 by Goldman et al. [6]. It identified nine risk factors for cardiac mortality, and of these factors, evidence of decompensated congestive cardiac failure (CCF) was the single factor weighted most heavily. The original CRI was later modified and subsequently revised (RCRI) and simplified by Lee et al. [7] to include six equally weighted factors:

- high-risk surgery
- history of ischemic heart disease (IHD)
- history of cerebrovascular disease
- history of CCF
- diabetes mellitus treated with insulin
- preoperative serum creatinine >2 mg/dL.

The more the accumulated risk factors, the higher the risk of perioperative MACE. The RCRI remains poor at identifying exactly which patients of those with multiple risk factors will actually suffer MACE. Three or more factors give a MACE incidence of >11% and the index offers no treatment intervention to reduce risk.

Despite this, the RCRI is widely quoted and risk indices remain useful, encouraging focus on relevant patient comorbidities associated with an increased risk of MACE. As identified in the original CRI, CCF remains an important risk factor.

- In the EuSOS study, a diagnosis of CCF had the second highest in-hospital perioperative mortality at 7.71% behind only a diagnosis of cirrhosis [3].

The American College of Surgeons (ACS) National Surgical Quality Improvement Programme (NSQIP) prospective database collects data on outcome of care surgical measures from more than 250 U.S. hospitals that have signed up to this quality improvement program voluntarily.

The 2007 database was interrogated to identify five predictors of perioperative myocardial infarction (MI) or cardiac arrest. A risk model was developed and validated using the 2008 database. The resulting index and risk calculator were shown to outperform the RCRI when used on the 2008 validation cohort. The five predictors included:

- ASA class
- dependent functional status
- age
- abnormal creatinine (>1.5 mg/dL)
- type of surgery, with aortic, intracranial neurosurgery, and foregut/hepatopancreatobiliary surgeries carrying the highest odds ratio (OR) for perioperative MI or cardiac arrest [8].

It is important to note that patient-specific risk in terms of comorbidities form only half of the clinical risk picture; surgery type, both in terms of specialty and grade, along with urgency are very important factors in determining the incidence of perioperative cardiovascular mortality and morbidity:

- The highest overall EuSOS in-hospital mortality was associated with upper gastrointestinal (GI) surgery (6.96%), with vascular surgical mortality the next highest (5.89%).
- Surgery graded as major (high-risk) carried a 5.63% risk of in-hospital death compared to 3.33% and 3.58% for moderate (intermediate-risk) and minor (low-risk) surgeries, respectively.
- Increasing urgency of surgery is also associated with increasing mortality [3].
- The same surgery types were associated with increased mortality in the ACS NSQIP dataset, with the addition of intra-cranial neurosurgery [8].

The problem for risk prediction models is that every patient is subtly different in terms of the number, severity, and treatment of comorbidities, along with urgency, grade, and specialty of surgery.

We know that the location of surgery in terms of center volume of specific surgeries performed, along with individual surgical and anesthetic experience also affect perioperative risk.

- Considerable variation in mortality risk for Medicare patients undergoing fourteen different surgery types has been shown, with surgical mortality decreasing as center volume increases [9].
- The magnitude of risk reduction varied between procedures but was more pronounced for upper GI surgeries. This fact is sometimes the "elephant in the room."
- If we are serious about optimizing patient outcomes, altering the surgeon, anesthetist, or planned surgery/surgical technique to ensure the "team," as well as the patient, are maximally optimized must be explored.

Patient assessment

The goals of the ideal preoperative risk assessment involve obtaining the answers to four clinical questions:

- Is the patient fit enough to survive and benefit from the intended surgical procedure?
- What is the risk to the patient if the surgery goes ahead as planned?
- Is the patient in the best possible condition for surgery, or can s/he be optimized further, and consequently, the perioperative risk reduced?
- What level of postoperative care should the patient receive; level 1 (care that can be delivered on a standard ward); level 2 (high dependency; single-organ support); level 3 (intensive care; advanced respiratory support or $\geq$2-organ support)?

A thorough patient history remains the cornerstone of individual cardiovascular risk assessment. Symptoms of undiagnosed or unoptimized CCF, IHD, valvular heart disease (VHD), cardiac arrhythmias, pulmonary hypertension, and/or right heart failure must be sought.

Surgical urgency carries paramount importance in this setting. Emergency surgery allows little time for investigation or preoperative optimization, but identifying evidence

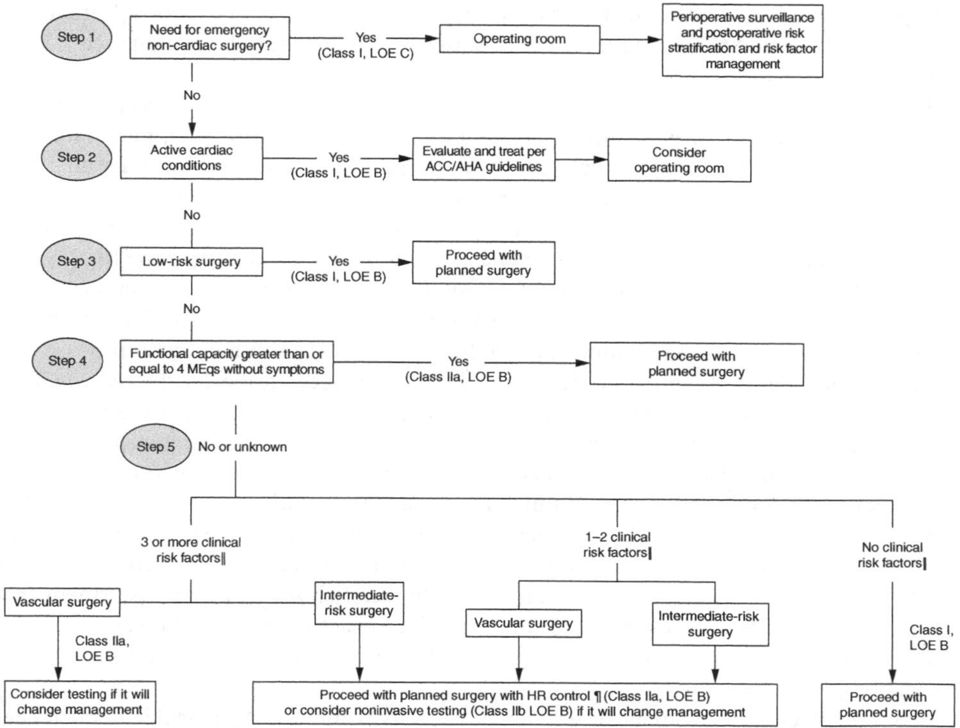

Figure 3.1. Approach to cardiovascular assessment. Reproduced from Fleisher et al. [1], with permission.

of cardiovascular disease from the patient history remains crucial. All factors that can be should be optimized within the preoperative and intraoperative time frame as dictated by the surgical condition.

The ACCF/AHA guidelines recommend a step-wise approach to patient assessment and contain a flow chart (Figure 3.1) [1].

- Step 1 requires determination of the urgency of surgery. Those patients at high cardiovascular risk, as dictated by their history, who have not been assessed previously but require emergency or very urgent surgery, may not be able to undergo full cardiovascular investigation and optimizsation preoperatively but warrant appropriate postoperative investigation. The location of postoperative care needs to be carefully considered in these patients to ensure optimal delivery of care in the event of MACE. In this particular patient group, appropriate interventions that should be instigated to optimize the patient and minimize perioperative risk include maintenance of chronic medications where possible, correction of anemia, acid–base and electrolyte abnormalities, optimization of fluid status, control of arrhythmias and tachycardia, maintenance of good perfusion pressure and normal oxygenation, along with the provision of optimal anesthesia and excellent analgesia. Correct interpretation of appropriate intraoperative monitoring is vital, as is the choice of postoperative care location, given the associated limitations on monitoring and interventions.

- Step 2 necessitates an assessment of the presence of active cardiac conditions. If there are active cardiac conditions, and time permits, optimization should be sought (see following discussion).
- If no active cardiac conditions are found, assessment of the grade of surgery forms Step 3. The grade of surgical insult and therefore risk–minor (low-risk), moderate (intermediate-risk), or major (high-risk) is important in determining whether an assessment of functional capacity is necessary. The estimated risk of MI and cardiac death within 30 days of surgery was categorized as low-risk (<1%), intermediate-risk (1%–5%), and high-risk (>5%) by Boersma et al. during the validation of the RCRI [10]. Low-risk surgeries include endoscopic or superficial procedures, cataract surgery, and breast surgery. Day-case or ambulatory surgeries generally are considered to be low-risk; however, as more complex procedures are deemed "ambulatory," the physiological derangement associated with the surgery needs to be considered when assessing the risk of the surgery. Whether it is appropriate to perform surgery in the "ambulatory" setting in a particular individual must be considered. High-risk surgeries include aortic and other major vascular and peripheral vascular surgery; however, there is evidence that upper GI surgery should be viewed as potentially high-risk surgery [3,8]. All other non-cardiac surgeries are deemed to be intermediate-risk. The patient with no active cardiac conditions undergoing low-risk (minor) surgery can proceed to surgery without delay. However, for intermediate- and higher-risk surgeries, an assessment of functional capacity is recommended. Importantly, the actual risk may be very institution-specific and therefore knowing local complication rates may aid in the decision process.
- Step 4 involves an assessment of functional capacity, which is of particular importance when considering intermediate- or high-risk surgical procedures. Some centers use cardiopulmonary exercise testing (CPET) to better quantify a patient's functional capacity, and may even use the results to determine suitability for surgical treatment versus modified surgery or a non-operative option and to assist planning the postoperative care location. This is discussed fully elsewhere in this text. If CPET is unavailable or not feasible within the time constraints of surgery, self-reported exercise tolerance in terms of the ability to perform everyday activities, such as climbing flights of stairs, has been shown to be predictive of perioperative myocardial ischemia, and serious cardiovascular and neurological events [11]. The metabolic equivalents (MEq) scale can be used to assess the oxygen consumption of day-to-day activities. Basal or resting oxygen consumption is 3.5 mL/kg/min, equivalent to 1 MEq; poor exercise tolerance would be rated at <4 MEq and would equate to an inability to bicycle at 10 mph, walk at 3.5 mph, or climb a flight of stairs. The Duke Activity Status Index (DASI) is a twelve-point questionnaire of everyday activities that has been shown to correlate with peak oxygen uptake [12]. Activities listed in the DASI have been graded according to their MEq value, and this can provide a useful assessment of exercise tolerance from the patient's history. Actual observation of the patient walking or climbing stairs can be very informative and more objective than self-reported patient activity. A problem arises in assessing cardiopulmonary functional capacity for those patients limited in their exercise tolerance by musculoskeletal disease. A higher index of suspicion for poor exercise tolerance has to be applied in these cases.
- Step 5 involves the further assessment of clinical risk factors for those patients with poor or unknown functional capacity scheduled to undergo intermediate- or high-risk

surgery. Clinical risk factors should be assessed using the RCRI. If a patient has no clinical risk factors, surgery can proceed as planned, as long as other comorbid non-cardiovascular conditions are fully optimized. If the patient has one or more clinical risk factors, consideration should be given to noninvasive cardiac testing, as long as the result may potentially change management. The over-riding ethos of whether a preoperative test should be performed is whether the result will alter perioperative management.

Active cardiac conditions

Active cardiac conditions include acquired cardiovascular disease, CCF, IHD, VHD, cardiac arrhythmias, pulmonary hypertension, and also congenital heart disease.

- Systemic arterial hypertension in the absence of other cardiovascular morbidities is not a risk factor for MACE [13].
- However, for those patients with stage 3 hypertension where systolic blood pressure is ≥180 mmHg and diastolic blood pressure ≥110 mmHg, optimization of blood pressure prior to surgery has to be carefully weighed against the risk of delaying non-cardiac surgery.
- If there are serious concerns that secondary hypertension may be present, it may be prudent to delay surgery to investigate further.

For those patients with active cardiac conditions where a lack of optimization is identified, this should be corrected prior to surgery, where possible. This correction may necessitate delaying surgery and could involve further investigation to guide the maximization of ventricular function, optimization of fluid status, stabilization of ischemia, the maintenance of normal sinus rhythm, heart rate control, and reduction in pulmonary vascular resistance, all without compromising renal function.

- Investigations must be used wisely to focus on not only potential new diagnoses but also the etiology of such; for example, the etiology of heart failure, thereby directing optimization therapies.
- Likewise, if there has been any new deterioration in the symptoms of a known diagnosis, then investigations may be indicated to identify potential areas for optimization.
- Investigations should only be performed preoperatively where the results will potentially change perioperative management and improve patient optimization, as tests may carry potential morbidity and the risk of a false positive result.
- Investigations and optimization must be carried out within the time frame necessitated by the surgical condition.

If the patient has suffered MI recently, the ACC/AHA taskforce recommended in 2006 that elective non-cardiac surgery should be delayed for four to six weeks, but did recognize that this recommendation lacked validation by randomized controlled trials (RCTs).

- Livhits at al. analyzed the records of over half a million patients undergoing five different types of non-cardiac surgery over a six-year period and identified a subgroup of patients undergoing surgery after acute MI. Thirty-day mortality was higher the closer surgery was performed to the MI; 0–30 days, 14.2%; 31–60 days, 1.5%; 61–90 days, 10.5%; 91–180 days, 9.9%. The postoperative MI rate was 32.8% for those operated

on within 30 days of the original MI, gradually reducing to 5.9% if surgery was performed 91–180 days after the initial MI [14].
- It appears that elective non-cardiac surgery should be delayed preferably a minimum of eight weeks after acute MI and this delay should allow time for optimal medical management to be achieved.

There may be situations where different diagnoses compete for priority, comorbid versus surgical condition. In these difficult cases, multidisciplinary input is vital to ensure the severity and risks of a comorbid condition are appropriately balanced against the risks of the surgical condition, and that the consequences of alternatives to surgery, surgical modification of technique, or surgical delay are fully understood. Multidisciplinary consultation and consensus on perioperative management is to be advocated in all challenging cases. It is important that the patient is fully informed of risks versus benefits in these discussions.

Noninvasive testing

- The resting preoperative electrocardiograph (ECG) is only a potentially useful investigation for patients with cardiovascular disease or risk factors for cardiovascular disease. It is not recommended for patients who lack risk factors [1,2]. An abnormal ECG is a risk factor for cardiac death postoperatively; however, it lacks specificity and sensitivity [15].
- Routine tests of resting left ventricular (LV) function are not indicated or helpful for the assessment of ischemia in the absence of signs of CCF. Patients >40 years of age who underwent resting echocardiography prior to intermediate- or high-risk non-cardiac surgery showed no benefit in terms of reduced mortality or shorter hospital length of stay [16], and the routine assessment of LV function has limited predictive value for perioperative outcome. Consequently, resting echocardiography is recommended only for the identification of abnormal valvular function or LV dysfunction in the presence of symptoms that have not been assessed previously. Symptomatic severe valvular heart disease may warrant treatment prior to elective non-cardiac surgery, therefore assessment is recommended, but there is no role for testing to identify mild valvular heart disease in the absence of symptoms.
- Detection of myocardial ischemia requires a technique that images during cardiovascular stress. This stress may be pharmacologically or exercise induced.

Detection of myocardial ischemia

Physiological exercise probably provides a better assessment of true ischemic potential. However, if a patient is unable to reach their ischemic threshold due to limited exercise capacity, pharmacological stress (dipyridamole, adenosine, or dobutamine) testing with either nuclear perfusion imaging or echocardiography may be more suitable.

- A population-based cohort study of patients who underwent noninvasive stress testing in the six months prior to non-cardiac surgery showed benefits in terms of one-year survival and hospital length of stay for those with at least one RCRI factor. The more RCRI factors, the greater the benefit, with maximum benefit seen in those with more than three RCRI factors [17].

- Dipyridamole thallium-201 scanning and dobutamine stress echocardiography (DSE) appear comparable in their prognostic value, but DSE has advantages in the ability to assess resting LV ejection fraction and potential valvular abnormalities [11].
- Cardiac magnetic resonance (CMR) imaging is rapidly becoming the myocardial imaging technique of choice if available. It consists of several different techniques that can be used to assess cardiac morphology, myocardial perfusion reserve, and scar detection. The ability of dobutamine CMR to detect ischemic but viable myocardium is superior to DSE, given the issues with poor echocardiographic acoustic windows in some patients. Contrast-enhancement CMR has the potential to be even more sensitive in the detection of viable myocardium, especially in areas of severe ventricular dysfunction [18]. Dobutamine CMR was used in patients undergoing major non-cardiac surgery in one study [19]. However, no study has yet randomized patients to risk stratification and resultant change in management using CMR prior to non-cardiac surgery.
- Coronary computed tomography angiography (CCTA) can be used to detect coronary calcium load, which reflects coronary atherosclerosis, and is therefore useful to exclude a diagnosis of coronary artery disease (CAD) with a high negative predictive value. However, the positive predictive value of CCTA and its role in providing useful information about the degree of stenosis and ischemia is less clear [20].

Biomarkers

Biomarkers of cardiovascular risk could potentially add value to the ACCF/AHA clinical evaluation algorithm by improving risk stratification. Within the population–risk epidemiological research setting, many different biomarkers have been investigated for long-term prognostic utility, but few biomarkers have been scrutinized within the perioperative setting.

- C-reactive protein, an acute phase reactant, has been shown to have utility within the community setting but lacks the necessary sensitivity for cardiovascular disease within the perioperative setting [21,22].
- Troponins have far greater tissue specificity, and even small rises in postoperative serum concentrations of fouth generation troponin-T have been shown to be prognostic for 30-day mortality following non-cardiac surgery [23]. Focused postoperative troponin monitoring in those patients at moderate- or high-risk of cardiovascular complications may be useful to predict postoperative MI [24], although efficacy and cost effectiveness have yet to be proven.
- Preoperative troponin concentrations have been shown to be effective in predicting postoperative cardiac events, with 20% of patients undergoing vascular surgery who sustained MACE perioperatively having a preoperative troponin level greater than the upper reference limit, compared to only 1% who did not sustain MACE. However, despite this, the authors did not recommend the routine use of preoperative troponin concentrations as a screening test in those at high clinical risk, as a subgroup of patients who sustained MACE were incorrectly reclassified from high- to low-risk on the basis of their preoperative troponin concentration.
- Brain-type natriuretic peptide (BNP) and its precursor N-terminal pro-BNP (NT pro-BNP) are produced by cardiac myocytes in response to increasing myocardial wall

stress. Preoperative BNP concentrations are an independent predictor of MACE and significantly improve risk stratification of patients with and without MACE [22]. Within the nonsurgical setting, they have been shown to be good prognostic indicators in patients with not only CCF but also acute coronary syndromes and stable CAD [24]. Preoperative plasma BNP and NT pro-BNP concentrations have prognostic value for early postoperative cardiac events, as well as intermediate- and longer-term mortality after major elective and emergency non-cardiac surgery [25,26]. Currently, American guidelines do not mention the use of plasma BNP or NT pro-BNP to aid risk stratification. ESC guidelines do not recommend routine preoperative biomarker sampling for all patients to prevent cardiac events, but do state that BNP or NT pro-BNP measurements should be considered to obtain independent prognostic information for perioperative and late cardiac events in high-risk patients [2]. It is likely that the utility of BNP will be addressed in the new guidelines under revision. The true utility of preoperative plasma BNP or NT pro-BNP concentrations for risk stratification will only be realized when a well-designed trial, randomizing patients to a change in perioperative management according to a preoperative BNP/NT pro-BNP concentration versus standard care, shows evidence of benefit.

Assessment of optimization

Coronary artery revascularization

Multiple studies have shown no long-term survival benefit for coronary artery revascularization by either coronary artery bypass grafting (CABG) or percutaneous coronary intervention (PCI) over optimal medical therapy [27]. Whether coronary revascularization is protective prior to non-cardiac surgery has always been a contentious issue, with many studies published prior to the era of optimal medical therapy.

- Subgroup analysis of the Coronary Artery Surgery Study (CASS) registry showed that those who had undergone non-cardiac surgery following surgical coronary revascularization had a reduced mortality of 1.7% versus 3.3%, and postoperative MI incidence of 0.8% versus 2.7%, when compared to those who were known to have CAD but did not undergo surgical revascularization, respectively [28].
- However, the CASS registry was non-randomized and patients were enrolled between 1974 and 1979. There were concerns raised that to gain any mortality benefit from surgical revascularization, the mortality of the initial cardiac surgery, which was not insignificant, needed to be added to the mortality of the subsequent non-cardiac surgery.
- Mortality after CABG is now significantly reduced with U.K. 2004–2005 data reporting first-time CABG mortality at 1.8% [29].
- In the Coronary Artery Revascularization Prophylaxis (CARP) trial, patients scheduled for elective vascular surgery with evidence of one or more coronary artery stenosis >70% on coronary angiography were eligible for randomization to revascularization or medical therapy prior to their vascular surgery [30]. Patients with left main stem stenosis >50%, severe aortic stenosis, LV ejection fraction <20%, severe co-existing disease, and evidence of recurrence of ischemia following prior revascularization were excluded. Essentially, patients with stable CAD were randomized to revascularization or medical therapy. Revascularization consisted of CABG in 49% and PCI in 61%;

however, insertion of a coronary artery stent and stent type (bare metal versus drug eluting) was not reported. Mortality at 2.7 years was not significantly different between those randomized to revascularization versus those who received medical therapy. Postoperative MI was also not significantly different between the two groups.

- In a subsequent analysis of patients who underwent coronary angiography in both the randomized and non-randomized portion of the CARP trial, the subset of patients with unprotected left main disease showed a benefit with preoperative coronary revascularization [31].
- The ACCF/AHA guidelines [1] state that coronary revascularization prior to non-cardiac surgery is useful in patients with high-risk unstable angina, MI, or stable angina and significant left main stenosis, three-vessel disease or two-vessel disease, including significant proximal left anterior descending artery stenosis and an ejection fraction of <50% or demonstrable ischemia on noninvasive testing.
- Therefore, there is no evidence that revascularizing patients with stable angina in the absence of left main stem or severe multi-vessel stenosis, or LV dysfunction, is beneficial, whether the patient requires non-cardiac surgery. It is important to ensure that these patients have stable symptoms and are fully medically optimized preoperatively.
- Given the concerns with delay to non-cardiac surgery following coronary artery revascularization, it is interesting to note that the median time to non-cardiac surgery following revascularization was 54 days (mean delay of 50 days for CABG and 42 days for PCI) in the CARP trial. Ward et al. performed subgroup analysis of the revascularized patients in the CARP trial and demonstrated that the postoperative MI rate in those who received PCI was 16.8% versus 6.6% in those who underwent CABG. In the discussion, inappropriate timing of non-cardiac surgery following PCI was not felt to be a related issue [32].
- When considering the optimal timing of non-cardiac surgery following revascularization, there appears to be a window of reduced risk. This window is far enough from the revascularization for MACE risk to have dropped but not long enough to allow the recurrence of ischemic symptoms. The optimum time for non-cardiac surgery following coronary revascularization is dependent partly on the method of revascularization.
- Surgical revascularization usually does not necessitate dual antiplatelet therapy (DAPT) for a prescribed duration, and currently it is recommended that non-cardiac surgery is delayed for six weeks following CABG [33].
- The clinical picture is less clear for the optimal time delay from coronary artery stent implantation to non-cardiac surgery. The prospective RECO study showed an incidence of 10.9% MACE and 9.5% for patients undergoing non-cardiac surgery following coronary artery stent implantation, and found the rate of stent thrombosis (ST) was higher when surgery was performed within twelve months of stent placement [34].
- Retrospective work has shown a gradual reduction in the incidence of ST and all MACE with increasing time from coronary artery stent implantation to non-cardiac surgery [35]. However, the first 42 days post-stent implantation has been identified as a period of particularly high-risk; with a study of more than 2300 patients undergoing surgery following coronary artery stent placement showing a 30-day MACE rate of 9% if surgery were performed within 42 days of stent implantation versus 2% if performed after 42 days [36]. Interestingly, stent type–bare metal stent (BMS) versus drug-eluting stent (DES) appears to have little impact on ST and MACE incidence.

- Percutaneous revascularization involving coronary artery stent implantation requires a mandatory period of DAPT. This is potentially a disadvantage when compared to CABG, especially when the recent ASCERT trial showed no difference in mortality at one year post-CABG or PCI, and 20% survival benefit was seen for CABG after four years [37]. The Bypass Angioplasty Revascularization Investigation (BARI) showed a more complete revascularization associated with a reduced incidence of angina at one year post-CABG compared to PCI [38].

In 2007, a significant incidence of late ST with DES was identified and the ACC/AHA/SCAI (Society for Cardiovascular Angiography Interventions) 2005 guidelines were updated, increasing the advised duration of DAPT from six months to twelve months following DES implantation [39].

- This guideline had significant implications for non-cardiac surgery performed within the first twelve months after DES implantation, as the challenges inherent in the perioperative management of DAPT were realized.
- The 2007 guideline recommended a minimum of one month DAPT duration following BMS implantation [39].
- Therefore, it is recommended if non-cardiac surgery, associated with significant potential blood loss precluding its performance on DAPT, is known to be required within one year of coronary stent implantation, and consideration should be given to BMS if non-cardiac surgery can wait one month, or balloon angioplasty if surgery is more urgent, instead of DES implantation [1,2].
- This guideline remains in place, but recently the literature has indicated that the risk of ST with third generation coronary artery stents may be less, due to biodegradable polymer platforms and new anti-proliferative agents with reduced endothelial toxicity [40].
- Some work has shown that three to six months of DAPT potentially may be sufficient with these newer stents [41,42]. However, the incidence of ST in the original DES trials was lower than that seen in "real world" applications; thus, these studies must be interpreted with caution.

When assessing patients with recently (within one year) implanted stents, current guidelines highlight the need to assess both the patient and the procedure-specific thrombotic and bleeding risk [43]. Comprehensive assessment of thrombotic risk necessitates an understanding of the patient's stent anatomy; the type, number, length, and position of stents, including their proximity to arterial bifurcations, the thrombosis in MI (TIMI) flow achieved, and any potential stent under-sizing [44].

- The age and associated comorbidities of the patient are also important. Increasing age has been identified as a risk factor for ST [45], but more recent work identified that younger age was a risk factor [44].
- Other patient factors implicated in ST include diabetes mellitus, renal impairment, active malignancy, and a low cardiac output state, as well as thrombophilias [44,45].
- Perioperative bleeding risk is greater in those with increased age, thrombocytopenia, coagulopathy, CCF, renal impairment, and advanced liver failure [46].
- The urgency of surgery, the bleeding potential of the surgery, and any modifications to surgical technique to reduce bleeding potential all need to be considered when forming a perioperative DAPT management plan.

If surgery can be delayed until the indication for DAPT has passed, this is the preferential management. Problems arise when the surgery cannot wait.

- An assessment of the bleeding risk of surgery should be made in this case.
- If possible, the surgery should be performed on DAPT; however, if the bleeding risk is too high, the surgery should proceed, where possible, on single agent aspirin with the second antiplatelet agent being stopped for the minimum time possible, as dictated by the bleeding risk of surgery.
- For those patients at extremely high-risk of ST with risk factors for ST, complex stent anatomy, and/or stents less than 42 days implanted, consideration should be given to bridging the patient to surgery with a shorter-acting intravenous antiplatelet agent.

Drug therapies

β-blockade

Perioperative β-blocker therapy was potentially considered a standard of care for all patients with or at risk of cardiovascular disease. After much controversy and multiple publications, it is clear that β-blockers, when appropriately prescribed, titrated, and monitored, do reduce the risk of perioperative MI in patients defined at risk by two or more RCRI factors [47]. However, if used inappropriately in patients at low-risk of perioperative MI and not individually titrated and carefully monitored, they risk causing harm by producing significant hypotension, bradycardia, and cerebrovascular events [5]. Guidelines recommend that β-blockade should be considered in the setting of all acute coronary syndromes; unstable angina, non-ST elevation MI, and ST-elevation MI. They also have utility in patients with a prior history of MI, stable angina pectoris, LV dysfunction, uncontrolled atrial fibrillation, and as second- or third-line therapy for uncontrolled hypertension (especially if in association with heart failure or IHD).

The literature is clear that there are risks inherent in stopping chronic β-blockade. Outside of the perioperative period, the risks associated with acute β-blocker withdrawal have been long recognized, with rebound deterioration in anginal symptoms, increased risk of MI, and a reduction in LV ejection fraction [48,49]. The perioperative period has the potential for significant cardiovascular stress, and intuitively it does not seem to be a good time to provoke a rebound deterioration in symptoms. Continuation of chronic β-blocker therapy during the perioperative period is recommended in both the ACCF/AHA and ESC guidelines [1,2].

Perioperative β-blockade is discussed in more detail in the chapter on cardiac drugs.

α_2 agonists

Meta-analysis has shown potential benefits in vascular surgery for perioperative α_2-adrenergic agonist therapy, with reductions in both mortality and MI [50]. However, the total number of patients included in this meta-analysis was relatively small – 1648 patients from seven studies, and the results were dominated by one study [51]. The beneficial effects were not translated to non-cardiac, nonvascular surgery, where a slight increase in MI incidence in the treated group was observed. The POISE-2 trial is a large RCT aiming to examine the effect of the α_2-adrenergic agonist clonidine, administered orally preoperatively and by transdermal patch for 72 hours postoperatively, on all-cause mortality and non-fatal MI at 30 days and one year postoperatively in 10 000 patients with or at risk of cardiovascular disease [52]. Until the results of this trial are known, there is currently not enough evidence of benefit to justify routine administration of α_2-adrenergic blockers to patients perioperatively for risk prevention.

Statin therapy

Outside of the perioperative period, statin therapy has been clearly shown to provide cardiovascular and cerebrovascular protection with reductions in MACE, requirement for coronary revascularization, and stroke [53,54]. Statin therapy also provides symptom relief from anginal symptoms and is therefore recommended for risk reduction in all patients with coronary and other atherosclerotic vascular disease [55]. More recently, concerns have been raised about the risks of statin therapy outside of the perioperative setting. These concerns relate to potentially accelerated cognitive decline, cancer risk, and an increased incidence of type 2 diabetes mellitus. Only a slightly increased risk of type 2 diabetes mellitus with long-term statin usage appears proven [56], and this increased risk is felt to be offset by the cardio- and cerebroprotective effects of statin therapy. Concerns about the risk of statins in those with early-stage chronic kidney disease and the risk of rhabdomyolysis perioperatively appear unfounded [57]. Given this evidence, it is sensible that patients with indications of atherosclerotic disease processes are prescribed statin therapy irrespective of their impending non-cardiac surgery. Acute discontinuation of chronic statin therapy may be detrimental to vascular function, and therefore should be avoided perioperatively [58].

Antiplatelet agents

DAPT is recommended following acute coronary syndrome and coronary artery stent implantation. The management of patients taking antiplatelet therapy necessitates knowledge of the indication and recommended duration of DAPT as well as the pharmacology of the antiplatelet agents taken. The combination of aspirin and a platelet ADP-receptor antagonist remains the bedrock of DAPT.

- The second-generation thienopyridine, clopidogrel, is still a popular choice of second antiplatelet therapy. However, clopdiogrel is a pro-drug with a resultant delay to peak effect and considerable inter-patient variability in drug response, due to genetic polymorphisms of the cytochrome P450 isoezymes responsible for its metabolism to the active compound. Clopidogrel is irreversible in its action, and apart from platelet transfusion, there is no antidote.
- The third-generation thienopyridine, prasugrel, is more potent and more consistent in the antiplatelet effect it achieves when compared to clopidogrel. Prasugrel is also a pro-drug and irreversible in its action. Like clopidogrel, the time-to-peak effect can be shortened by the administration of a loading dose.
- Ticagrelor is not a thienopyridine but acts on the same platelet P_2Y_{12} ADP receptor, and like prasugrel, is more consistent and potent in its antiplatelet action. It has faster onset of antiplatelet effect than clopidogrel, but differs in its shorter duration of antiplatelet action due to reversible receptor antagonism.

Current guidelines recommend that all truly elective surgery be delayed until the indication for DAPT has passed. If surgery cannot wait that long, a decision whether surgery can be performed on DAPT needs to be made. This decision is dependent on a risk balance analysis between the consequences of excessive surgical bleeding and an individual's risk of ST. If surgery cannot be performed on DAPT, aspirin should be continued in all cases apart from where the consequences of mildly increased blood loss are unacceptable; for example, with intracranial procedures. Cessation times for the individual agents are dependent on that balance of risk.

- Traditionally, it was recommended that clopidogrel be stopped seven days prior to surgery.
- The Recovery trial identified that return of platelet reactivity on day 5 following cessation of clopidogrel was similar to day 7 post-prasugrel cessation; with return to near baseline reactivity (inhibition of platelet aggregation of ≤20%) in >75% of individuals [59].
- Inhibition of platelet activity has been shown to be similar on day 3 post-cessation of ticagrelor to day 5 post-cessation of clopidogrel [60]. However, the Food and Drug Administration (FDA) currently recommends ticagrelor be stopped five days prior to surgery.

There is now a better understanding that a single prescribed cessation time for each drug is not practical given the variations in type of surgery, bleeding, and thrombotic risk. The actual duration of antiplatelet cessation, if required, needs to be assessed individually, and therefore it may be possible to stop the second antiplatelet for a shorter time, dependent on the magnitude of the bleeding risk. This decision on cessation time needs to be taken in the setting of multidisciplinary discussion and consensus [61]. Antiplatelet drugs and regional anesthesia is discussed fully elsewhere.

Anticoagulant therapy

Guidelines for the management of antithrombotic therapy perioperatively were updated in 2012 [62]. Discontinuation of chronic oral anticoagulation will most likely be required for a few days prior to non-cardiac surgery.

All patients with mechanical heart valves requiring chronic anticoagulation are not the same. The thromboembolic risk of different types of mechanical valves and the native valve replaced varies. It is recommended currently that an assessment of the bleeding risk of surgery should be made preoperatively.

- If the bleeding risk of surgery is low, then surgery can be considered with a brief reduction in the international normalized ratio (INR) to low or subtherapeutic levels, and reinstatement of normal dose and INR range following surgery.
- For those patients undergoing more extensive surgery with a higher bleeding risk, an assessment of the thromboembolic risk of their valve needs to be made. Valves associated with a high-risk of thromboembolism include mechanical mitral and Bjork–Shiley valves. There may be additional patient risk factors for thromboembolism, including a LV ejection fraction of <30% [63].
- Where the bleeding risk of surgery is high and the thromboembolic risk is also increased, perioperative bridging with unfractionated or low-molecular weight heparin is advised [64].

In the emergency setting, vitamin K antagonist therapy can be reversed with vitamin K and prothrombin concentrate complex (PCC) [65]. Currently, there is no antidote to dabigatran although PCC has shown some promise in animal studies.

Other medications

- The European guidelines recommend that angiotensin-converting enzyme (ACE) inhibitors be continued perioperatively in stable patients, in the presence of LV dysfunction, undergoing non-cardiac surgery; however, transient discontinuation of ACE inhibitors prior to surgery should be considered in those hypertensive patients with normal LV function [2].

- Hypertensive patients stabilized on diuretic therapy should discontinue therapy on the day of surgery and recommence oral therapy when possible postoperatively. Patients with CCF maintained on diuretics should continue therapy until the day of surgery and receive intravenous therapy perioperatively until reinstigation of oral treatment is possible [2].

Mechanical therapies

Bi-ventricular pacing

CCF is a significant risk factor for MACE perioperatively and it is vital that these patients are optimally medically managed prior to surgery.

- For those patients with optimal medical management who still have New York Heart Association (NYHA) grade III or IV symptoms, an LV ejection fraction of ≤35%, and sinus rhythm with a prolonged QRS (>120 ms), ESC and AHA/ACS guidelines recommend the use of bi-ventricular pacing, otherwise known as cardiac resynchronization therapy (CRT) [66,67].
- Multiple trials have shown the benefits of CRT to patients with severe CCF and a prolonged QRS interval in terms of recurrent hospitalizations and mortality [68].
- Therefore, it seems rational to assess patients prior to elective non-cardiac surgery and refer to cardiology where CRT may be beneficial irrespective of forthcoming surgery.

Automated implantable cardiac defibrillators (AICDs) are recommended for a number of indications including structural heart disease with spontaneous sustained ventricular tachycardia, LV ejection fraction of ≤35% due to ischemic cardiomyopathy (>40 days post-MI), or non-ischemic dilated cardiomyopathy with class II or III NYHA symptoms or an LV ejection fraction of <30%, and NYHA class I symptoms in addition, in those who survive cardiac arrest. Devices that bi-ventricularly pace but also have AICD functions are often implanted. The implantation of an AICD device alone for arrhythmia cardioversion is not indicated preoperatively, given that it will require deactivation during surgery. Perioperative application of external pads to all patients with indications for an AICD or an implanted but deactivated device is advisable.

Intra-aortic balloon pump (IABP) counterpulsation device

These devices are used mainly for the treatment of cardiogenic shock in the setting of PCI or cardiac surgery. However, there are successful cases described of IABP usage in the setting of emergency or very urgent non-cardiac surgery for those patients with extremely high-risk unstable cardiac symptoms, although the reports are old. This technology is not available in every center and necessitates familiarity. It should be considered only in the extremely high-risk case where other avenues of optimization have failed.

Other comorbidities

Patients with cardiac risk factors undergoing non-cardiac surgery should have their electrolytes, fluid balance, and renal function optimized prior to surgery. Anemia is discussed further in its own chapter in this text. Glycemic control in patients with diabetes mellitus must be optimized preoperatively, and tight glucose control while avoiding episodes of hypoglycemia perioperatively is important. Likewise, respiratory function in those with respiratory disease should be maximized. Thromboembolism prophylaxis should be administered after assessment of thromboembolism risk in line with current practice.

Summary

- The take home message regarding cardiovascular assessment and optimization prior to non-cardiac surgery is to ensure the patient is at her/his peak fitness at the time of surgery, within the constraints of her/his comorbid and surgical disease.
- The literature shows there is no "one size fits all" model we can apply to either perioperative investigation or intervention to reduce cardiovascular risk. The individualization of patient assessment and care is crucial.
- Perioperative patient care would do well to learn from the critical care setting where no magic bullet therapy has been discovered for multi-organ failure, but instead, the delivery of bundles of care involving several evidence-based interventions, and attention to "small details," improves overall outcome.
- The focus of preoperative care should be medical optimization and the achievement of an individual's "best normal" results in the best possible patient outcome.
- It is particularly important to continue the patient's chronic medical therapy perioperatively.
- Ensuring a patient is fully optimized at the time of her/his surgery not only reduces perioperative risk, but if optimization can be continued past the perioperative period, there potentially can be improvement in long-term outcome.
- The perioperative time frame can be regarded as an important period of patient interaction where education and optimization potentially can result in improvements in overall health.

References

1. Fleisher LA, Beckman JA, Brown KA, et al. Focused update on perioperative beta-blockade incorporated into the ACC/AHA 2007 guidelines on Perioperative Cardiovascular Evaluation and Care for Noncardiac Surgery: report of the American College of Cardiology Foundation/American Heart Association Task Force on Practice Guidelines. *Circulation* 2009; **120**: e169–276.
2. Poldermans D, Bax JJ, Boersma E, et al. Guidelines for preoperative cardiac risk assessment and perioperative cardiac management in non-cardiac surgery. The Task Force for Preoperative Cardiac Risk Assessment and Perioperative Cardiac Management in Non-Cardiac Surgery of the European Society of Cardiology (ESC) and endorsed by the European Society of Anaesthesiology (ESA). *Eur Heart J* 2009; **22**: 2769–812.
3. Pearse RW, Moreno RP, Bauer P, et al. Mortality after surgery in Europe: a 7 day cohort study. *Lancet* 2012; **380**: 1059–65.
4. Devereaux PJ, Chan MTV, Alonso-Coello P, et al. The Vascular Events in Non-Cardiac Surgery Patient Cohort Evaluation (VISION) Study. *JAMA* 2012; **307**: 2295–304.
5. Devereaux PJ, Yang H, Yusuf S, et al. Effects of extended-release metoprolol succinate in patients undergoing non-cardiac surgery (POISE trial): a randomised controlled trial. *Lancet* 2008; **371**: 1839–47.
6. Goldman L, Caldera LDL, Nussbaum SR, et al. Multifactorial index of cardiac risk in noncardiac surgical procedures. *N Engl J Med* 1977; **297**: 845–50.

7. Lee TH, Marcantonio ER, Mangione CM, et al. Derivation and prospective validation of a simple index for prediction of cardiac risk of major noncardiac surgery. *Circulation* 1999; **100**: 1043–9.
8. Gupta PK, Gupta H, Sundaram A, et al. Development and validation of a risk calculator for prediction of cardiac risk after surgery: clinical perspective. *Circulation* 2011; **124**: 381–7.
9. Birkmeyer JD, Siewers AE, Finlayson EVA, et al. Hospital volume and surgical mortality in the United States. *N Engl J Med* 2002; **346**: 1128–37.
10. Boersma E, Kertai MD, Schouten O, et al. Perioperative cardiovascular mortality in noncardiac surgery: validation of the Lee Cardiac Risk Index. *Am J Med* 2005; **118**: 1134–41.
11. Shaw LJ, Eagle KA, Gersh BJ, et al. Meta-analysis of intravenous dipyridamole-thallium-201 imaging (1985 to 1994) and dobutamine echocardiography (1991 to 1994) for risk stratification before vascular surgery. *J Am Coll Cardiol* 1996; **27**: 787–98.
12. Hlatky MA, Boineau RE, Higginbotham MB, et al. A brief self-administered questionnaire to determine functional capacity (the Duke Activity Status Index). *Am J Cardiol* 1989; **64**: 651–4.
13. Weksler N, Klein M, Szendro G, et al. The dilemma of immediate preoperative hypertension: to treat and operate or to postpone surgery? *J Clin Anesth* 2003; **15**: 179–83.
14. Livhits M, Ko CY, Leonardi MJ, et al. Risk of surgery following recent myocardial infarction. *Ann Surg* 2011; **253**: 857–64.
15. Noordzi PG, Boersma E, Bax JJ, et al. Prognostic value of routine preoperative electrocardiography in patients undergoing noncardiac surgery. *Am J Cardiol* 2006; **97**: 1103–6.
16. Wijeysundera DN, Beattie WS, Kartouti K, et al. Association of echocardiography before major elective non-cardiac surgery with postoperative survival and length of hospital stay: a population based cohort study. *BMJ* 2011; **342**: d3695.
17. Wijeysundera DN, Beattie WS, Austin PC, et al. Non-invasive cardiac stress testing before elective major non-cardiac surgery: population based cohort study. *BMJ* 2010; **340**: b5526.
18. Mahrholdt H, Klem I, Sechtem U. Cardiovascular MRI for detection of myocardial viability and ischaemia. *Heart* 2007; **93**: 122–9.
19. Rerkpattanapipat P, Morgan TM, Neagle CM, et al. Assessment of preoperative cardiac risk with magnetic resonance imaging. *Am J Cardiol* 2002; **90**: 416–19.
20. Anderson JL, Adams CD, Antman EM, et al. 2011 ACCF/AHA focused update incorporated into the ACC/AHA 2007 guidelines for the management of patients with unstable angina/non-ST elevation myocardial infarction: a report of the American College of Cardiology Foundation/American Heart Association Task Force on Practice Guidelines. *Circulation* 2011; **123**: e426–579.
21. Howard-Alpe GM, Sear JW, Foex P. Methods of detecting atherosclerosis in non-cardiac surgical patients: the role of biochemical markers. *Br J Anaesth* 2006; **97**: 758–69.
22. Biccard BM, Naidoo P, de Vasconcellos K. What is the best pre-operative risk stratification tool for major adverse cardiac events following elective vascular surgery? A prospective observational cohort study evaluating pre-operative myocardial ischemia monitoring and biomarker analysis. *Anaesthesia* 2012; **67**: 389–95.
23. Beattie WS, Karkouti K, Tait G, et al. Use of clinically based troponin underestimates the cardiac injury in non-cardiac surgery: a single centre cohort study in 51,701 consecutive patients. *Can J Anaes* 2012; **59**: 1013–22.
24. Omland T, Sabatine MS, Jablonski KA, et al. Prognostic value of B-type natriuretic peptides in patients with coronary artery disease: the PEACE trial. *J Am Coll Cardiol.* 2007; **50**: 205–14.
25. Farzi S, Stojakovic T, Marko T, et al. Role of N-terminal pro B-type natriuretic peptide in identifying patients at high risk

for adverse outcome after emergent surgery. *Br J Anaes* 2013; **110**: 554–60.

26. Payne CJ, Gibson SC, Bryce G, et al. B-type natriuretic peptide predicts long-term survival after major non-cardiac surgery. *Br J Anaes* 2011; **107**: 144–9.

27. Deedwania PC, Carbajal EV. Medical therapy versus myocardial revascularization in chronic coronary syndrome and stable angina. *Am J Med* 2011; **124**: 681–8.

28. Eagle KA, Rihal CS, Mickel MC, et al. Cardiac risk of noncardiac surgery: influence of coronary disease and type of surgery in 3368 operations. CASS Investigators and University of Michigan Heart Care Program. Coronary Artery Surgery Study. *Circulation* 1997; **96**: 1882–7.

29. Bridgewater B, Grayson AD, Brooks N, et al. Has the publication of cardiac surgery outcome data been associated with changes in practice in northwest England: an analysis of 25,730 patients undergoing CABG surgery under 30 surgeons over eight years. *Heart* 2007; **93**: 744–8.

30. McFalls EO, Ward HB, Moritz TE, et al. Coronary-artery revascularization before elective major vascular surgery. *N Engl J Med* 2004; **351**: 2795–804.

31. Garcia S, Moritz TE, Ward HB, et al. Usefulness of revascularization of patients with multivessel coronary artery disease before elective vascular surgery for abdominal aortic and peripheral occlusive disease. *Am J Cardiol* 2008; **102**: 809–13.

32. Ward HB, Kelly RF, Thottapurathu L, et al. Coronary bypass grafting is superior to percutaneous coronary intervention in prevention of perioperative myocardial infarctions during subsequent vascular surgery. *Ann Thorac Surg* 2006; **82**: 795–801.

33. Breen P, Lee JW, Pomposelli F, et al. Timing of high-risk vascular surgery following coronary bypass surgery: a 10-year experience from an academic medical centre. *Anaesthesia* 2004; **59**: 422–7.

34. Albaladejo P, Marret E, Samama CM, et al. Non-cardiac surgery in patients with coronary artery stents: the RECO study. *Heart* 2009; **97**: 1566–72.

35. Anwarudddin S, Askari AT, Saudye H, et al. Characterization of post-opertive risk associated with prior drug-eluting stent use. *JACC Cardiovasc Interv* 2009; **2**: 542–9.

36. Tokushige A, Shiomo H, Morimoto T, et al. Incidence and outcome of surgical procedures after coronary bare-metal and drug-eluting stent implantation: a report from the CREDO-Kyoto PCI/CABG registry cohort-2. *Circ Cardiovasc Interv* 2012; **5**: 237–46.

37. Weintraub WS, Grau-Sepulveda MV, Weiss JM, et al. Prediction of long-term mortality after percutaneous coronary intervention in older adults: results from the National Cardiovascular Data registry. *Circulation* 2012; **125**: 1491–500.

38. Whitlow PL, Dimas AP, Bashore TM, et al. Relationship of extent of revascularisation with angina at one year in the Bypass Angioplasty Revascularisation Investigation (BARI). *J Am Coll Cardiol* 1999; **34**: 1750–9.

39. King SB III, Smith SC Jr, Hirshfield JW, et al. 2007 Focused update of the ACC/AHA/SCAI 2005 Guideline Update for Percutaneous Coronary Intervention: a report of the American College of Cardiology/American Heart Association Task Force on the Practice Guidelines: 2007 Writing Group to review new evidence and update the ACC/AHA/SCAI 2005 Guideline Update for Percutaneous Coronary Intervention, writing on behalf of the 2005 Writing Committee. *Circulation* 2008; **117**: 261–95.

40. Stefanini GG, Byrne RA, Serruys PW, et al. Biodegradable polymer drug-eluting stents reduce the risk of stent thrombosis at 4 years in patients undergping persutaneous coronary intervention: a pooled analysis of individual patient data from the ISAR-TEST 3, ISAR_TEST 4, and LEADERS randomized trials. *Eur Heart J* 2012; **33**: 1214–22.

41. Valgimigli M, Campo G, Monti M, et al. Short- versus long-term duration of dual-antiplatelet therapy after coronary stenting: a randomised multicenter trial. *Circulation* 2012; **125**: 2015–26.

42. Kim BK, Hong MK, Shin DH, et al. A new strategy for the discontinuation of dual antiplatelet therapy: the RESET trial (REal Safety and Efficacy of 3-month dual antiplatelet therapy following Endeavor zotarolimus-eluting stent implantation. *J Am Coll Cardiol* 2012; **60**: 1340–8.

43. Newsome LT, Weller RS, Gerancher JC, et al. Coronary artery stents: II. Perioperative considerations and management. *Anesth Analg* 2008; **107**: 570–90.

44. van Werkum JW, Heestermans AA, Zomer C, et al. Predictors of coronary artery stent thrombosis: the Dutch Stent Thrombosis Registry. *J Am Coll Cardiol* 2009; **53**: 1399–409.

45. Iakovou I, Schmidt T, Bonizzoni E, et al. Incidence, predictors, and outcome of thrombosis after successful implantation of drug-eluting stents. *JAMA* 2005; **293**: 2126–30.

46. Berger PB, Bhatt DL, Fuster V, et al. Bleeding complications with dual antiplatelet therapy among patients with stable vascular disease or risk factors for vascular disease: results from the Clopidogrel for High Atherosclerotic Risk and Ischemic Stabilization, Management, and Avoidance (CHARISMA) trial. *Circulation* 2010; **121**: 2575–83.

47. Lindenauer PK, Pekow P, Wang K, et al. Perioperative beta-blocker therapy and mortality after major noncardiac surgery. *N Eng J Med* 2005; **353**: 349–61.

48. Psaty BM, Koepsell TD, Wagner EH, et al. The relative risk of incident coronary heart disease associated with recently stopping the use of beta-lockers. *JAMA* 1990; **263**: 1653–7.

49. Teichert M, de Smet PA, Hofman A, et al. Discontinuation of beta-blockers and the risk of myocardial infarction in the elderly. *Drug Saf* 2007; **30**: 541–9.

50. Wijeysundera DN, Naik JS, Beattie WS. Alpha-2 adrenergic agonists to prevent perioperative cardiovascular complications: a meta-analysis. *Am J Med* 2003; **114**: 742–52.

51. Oliver MF, Goldman L, Julian DG, et al. Effect of mivazerol on perioperative cardiac complications during non-cardiac surgery in patients with coronary heart disease: the European Mivazerol Trial (EMIT). *Anesthesiology* 1999; **91**: 951–61.

52. ClinicalTrials.gov Identifier NCT 00860925.

53. Baigent C, Keech A, Kearney PM. Efficacy and safety of cholesterol-lowering treatment: prospective meta-analysis of data from 90 056 participants in 14 randomised trials of statins. *Lancet* 2005; **366**: 1267–78.

54. Ridker PM, Danielson E, Fonseca FA, et al. Rosuvastatin to prevent vascular events in men and women with elevated C-reactive protein. *N Eng J Med* 2008; **359**: 2195–207.

55. Smith SC Jr, Benjamin EJ, Bonow RO, et al. AHA/ACCF secondary prevention and risk reduction therapy for patients with coronary and other atherosclerotic vascular disease: 2011 update: a guideline from the American Heart Association and American College of Cardiology Foundation. *Circulation* 2011; **124**: 2458–2473.

56. Jukema JW, Cannon CP, de Craen AJ, et al. The controversies of statin therapy: weighing the evidence. *J Am Coll Cardiol* 2012; **60**: 875–81.

57. Palmer SC, Craig JC, Navaneethan SD, et al. Benefits and harms of statin therapy for persons with chronic kidney disease: a systematic review and meta-analysis. *Ann Intern Med* 2012; **157**: 263–75.

58. Le Manach Y, Godet G, Coriat P, et al. The impact of postoperative discontinuation or continuation of chronic statin therapy on cardiac outcome after major vascular surgery. *Anesth Analg* 2007; **104**: 1326–33.

59. Price MJ, Walder JS, Baker BA, et al. Recovery of platelet function after discontinuation of prasugrel or clopidogrel maintenance dosing in aspirin-treated patients with stable coronary disease: the recovery trial. *J Am Coll Cardiol* 2012; **59**: 2338–43.

60. Gurbel PA, Bliden KP, Butler K, et al. Randomized double-blind assessment of the ONSET and OFFSET of the antiplatelet effects of ticagrelor versus clopidogrel in patients with stable coronary artery disease:

the ONSET/OFFSET study. *Circulation* 2009; **120**: 2577–85.

61. Ferraris VA, Saha SP, Oestreich JH, et al. 2012 update to the Society of Thoracic Surgeons guideline on use pf antiplatelet drugs in patients having cardiac and noncardiac operations. *Ann Thorac Surg* 2012; **94**: 1761–81.
62. Douketis JD, Spyropoulos AC, Spencer FA, et al. Perioperative management of antithrombotic therapy: antithrombotic therapy and prevention of thrombosis (9th edn.): American College of Chest Physicians Evidence-Based Clinical Practice Guidelines. *Chest* 2012; **141**: e326S–50.
63. Bonow RO, Carabello B, de Leon AC, et al. ACC/AHA guidelines for the management of patients with valvular heart disease: a report of the American College of Cardiology/American Heart Association Task Force on Practice Guidelines (Committee on Management of Patients with Valvular Heart Disease). *J Am Coll Cardiol* 1998; **32**: 1486–582.
64. Douketis JD, Johnson JA, Turpie AG. Low-molecular-weight heparin as bridging anticoagulation during interruption of warfarin: assessment of a standardized periprocedural anticoagulation regimen. *Arch Intern Med* 2004; **164**: 1319–26.
65. Leissinger CA, Blatt PM, Hoots WK, et al. Role of prothrombin complex concentrates in reversing warfarin anticoagulation: a review of the literature. *Am J Hematol* 2008; **83**: 137–43.
66. Vardas PE, Auricchio A,. Blanc JJ, et al. Guidelines for cardiac pacing and cardiac resynchronization therapy: the Task Force for Cardiac Pacing and Cardiac Resynchronization Therapy of the European Society of Cardiology. Developed in collaboration with the European Heart Rhythm Association. *Eur Heart J* 2007; **28**: 2256–95.
67. Epstein AE, DiMarco JP, Ellenbogen KA, et al. ACC/AHA/HRS 2008 guidelines for device-based therapy of cardiac rhythm abnormalities: a report of the American College of Cardiology/American Heart Association Task Force on Practice Guidelines. *Circulation* 2008; **117**: 2820–40.
68. Abdulla J, Haarbo J, Køber L, et al. Impact of implantable defibrillators and resynchronization therapy on outcome in patients with left ventricular dysfunction – a meta-analysis. *Cardiology* 2006; **106**: 249–55.

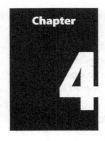

Cardiopulmonary exercise testing

M. West, L. Loughney, S. Jack, and M.P.W. Grocott

Outcome after surgery is dependent on both controllable factors, such as the medical care received before, during, and after surgery, as well as fixed factors, such as the patient's physiological ability to tolerate surgical trauma.

- It is estimated that around 234.2 million surgical procedures are undertaken annually worldwide [1]. In the U.K., more than four million surgical procedures are performed annually, 12.3% of which are performed on patients classified as "high-risk" (expected mortality of >5%). This group accounted for the majority of postoperative mortality (83.4%), and had a significantly longer hospital stay [2].
- Large audits in the U.K. reveal 30-day mortality rates of 2.1% for elective colonic cancer surgery [3], 4.1% for elective open aortic surgery [4], 1.7% for esophagectomy, 1.1% for elective gastrectomy [5], and 9.2% for emergency colorectal surgery [3].

Preoperative surgical risk assessment

Preoperative identification of patients unable to withstand trauma from major surgery should be a priority.

- Accurate risk assessment permits modification of preoperative status, optimization of intra- and postoperative management, and enhances shared decision making [6].
- Current approaches to risk prediction include clinical acumen, clinical prediction scores (e.g,. American Society of Anesthesiologists (ASA) physical score, Duke Activity Status Index (DASI), Physiological and Operative Severity Score for Enumeration of Mortality and Morbidity (POSSUM), colorectal-POSSUM) [7–9], plasma biomarkers [10], measures of cardiac function [11,12], six-minute walk tests [13], and shuttle walk tests [14–16], but their effectiveness in predicting surgical morbidity is not well established [17–19].
- Cardiopulmonary exercise testing (CPET) has been used extensively for risk assessment prior to major thoracic or abdominal surgery. While this technique needs further validation in various clinical settings, we believe it is rapidly becoming the gold-standard assessment for patients' physical fitness in the preoperative setting.

Preoperative CPET

CPET has been shown to be a well tolerated, noninvasive, cost-effective way to perform in the preoperative period prior to high-risk surgical procedures.

Anesthesia and Perioperative Care of the High-Risk Patient, Third edition, ed. Ian McConachie.
Published by Cambridge University Press.

- CPET provides a global assessment of the cardiovascular, respiratory, and skeletal-muscle systems [20].
- Despite requiring a moderate to high level of exertion, CPET is well tolerated and safe to conduct [21,22]. Variables derived from CPET include the oxygen uptake ($\dot{V}o_2$) at peak exercise ($\dot{V}o_2$ at peak), the $\dot{V}o_2$ at the anerobic threshold or at the estimated lactate threshold ($\dot{V}o_2$ at $\hat{\theta}_L$), the oxygen pulse (O_2 pulse at $\hat{\theta}_L$ and peak), and the ventilation equivalents for carbon dioxide and oxygen ($\dot{V}_E/\dot{V}co_2$ and $\dot{V}_E/\dot{V}o_2$). Some of these variables have been shown to predict morbidity and mortality in the perioperative period [23].

CPET is usually conducted on an electromagnetically braked cycle ergometer, with the patient breathing through a mouthpiece or facemask through which gas exchange is measured. The patient is continuously monitored using a continuous 12-lead electrocardiograph (ECG) and oxygen saturation (SaO_2), with periodic measurement of blood pressure. Common CPET variables and their definitions are detailed in Table 4.1.

Table 4.1. CPET variables

Lactate or anerobic threshold ($\dot{V}o_2$ at $\hat{\theta}_L$)	The exercise $\dot{V}o_2$ above which anerobic high-energy phosphate production supplements aerobic high-energy phosphate production, with consequential lowering of the cellular redox state, increase in lactate/pyruvate (L/P) ratio, and net increase in lactate production at the site of anerobiosis. Exercise above the $\hat{\theta}_L$ is reflected in the muscle effluent and central blood by an increase in lactate concentration, L/P ratio, and metabolic acidosis.
Heart rate reserve (HRR)	The difference between the predicted highest heart rate attainable during maximum exercise and the actual highest heart rate.
Maximal oxygen uptake ($\dot{V}o_{2\ max}$)	Describes the $\dot{V}o_2$ when it reaches a plateau value during a single maximum work rate test. Repeated measurements are necessary to obtain the $\dot{V}o_2$ that cannot be exceeded by the subject.
Oxygen pulse (O_2 pulse)	The oxygen uptake divided by the heart rate. Hence, this represents the amount of oxygen extracted by the tissue of the body from the O_2 carried in each stroke volume.
Oxygen uptake ($\dot{V}o_2$)	The amount of oxygen extracted from the inspired gas in a given period of time, expressed in mL or L per minute.
Peak oxygen uptake ($\dot{V}o_2$ at peak)	The highest oxygen uptake achieved during a maximum work rate test.
Work rate	The rate at which work is preformed in watts.
Ventilatory equivalents for CO_2 and O_2 ($\dot{V}_E/\dot{V}co_2$ and $\dot{V}_E/\dot{V}o_2$)	The ventilatory equivalents for CO_2 and O_2 are measurements of the ventilatory requirement for a given metabolic rate.
Minute ventilation ($\dot{V}_E$)	The volume of gas exhaled divided by the time of collection in minutes.

The test protocol normally includes four phases; an initial rest phase (approximately three minutes) is employed to establish baseline values, followed by an unloaded cycling (zero watts) phase. Following this, the incremental exercise phase begins. A ramp protocol is commonly used, during which the set work rate is increased linearly with time, with a corresponding increase in the intensity of the exercise. The ramp incremental protocol can be determined by using a formula by Wasserman and colleagues [24]:

$\dot{V}o_2$ unloaded pedaling (mL/min) = 150 + (6 × weight in kg)

$\dot{V}o_2$ at peak (mL/min) = height (cm) – age (years) × 20 (sedentary males)

$\dot{V}o_2$ at peak (mL/min) = height (cm) – age (years) × 14 (sedentary females)

Work rate increment/min = $\dot{V}o_2$ at peak – $\dot{V}o_2$ unloaded pedaling/100

The criteria for test termination differs between laboratories; in some, the test is terminated by the patient at volitional exhaustion or symptoms (e.g., shortness of breath, chest pain, etc.), while others perform a submaximal test and stop exercise when a particular criterion is met, such as an respiratory exchange ratio (RER) >1 [25].

- A valid exercise test should be between eight and 12 minutes, assuming the ramp protocol has been calculated correctly.
- Following test completion, a recovery period at low intensity exercise should be performed to maintain venous return.
- Patients should be observed throughout recovery until physiological variables, including heart rate, blood pressure, ventilation, and SaO_2, have returned close to baseline levels and any exercise induced ECG changes have resolved.
- The test should be stopped if the patient experiences any adverse symptoms [26–28], namely:

  1. angina – 2 mm ST depression if symptomatic or 4 mm if asymptomatic, or >1 mm ST elevation
  2. significant arrhythmias
  3. fall in systolic blood pressure of >20 mmHg from the highest value during the test; hypertension of >250 mmHg systolic, >120 mmHg diastolic
  4. severe desaturation: SpO_2 of $<80\%$ accompanied by limiting hypoxemia
  5. sudden pallor
  6. loss of coordination
  7. mental confusion
  8. signs of respiratory failure

The physiology behind CPET

- Energy for muscle contraction is provided by high-energy phosphate groups supplied in the form of adenosine triphosphate (ATP). ATP is supplied by the breakdown of glycogen to pyruvate, which enters the tricarboxylic acid (TCA) cycle via acetyl-coA, and breakdown of fats to produce acetyl-coA. Further processing of acetyl-coA in the TCA cycle and electron transport chain produces ATP needed for muscle contraction. If processing occurs only in the glycolytic pathway, a smaller amount of ATP is formed along with lactic acid. The extra acid produced causes an increase in $\dot{V}co_2$ by buffering of CO_2 in the blood. Controversy persists as to whether a deficiency of oxygen delivery versus oxidative capacity also contributes to the onset of lactic acid production, hence the term "anerobic threshold." It is possible that both processes, that is, the pattern of muscle fiber recruitment and a potential imbalance between oxygen supply and oxidative metabolism, contribute to the increase in lactic acid as exercise intensity increases.

- During CPET, as work rate increases, $\dot{V}o_2$ and $\dot{V}co_2$ increase linearly until exercise lactic acidosis develops. $\dot{V}co_2$ is plotted against $\dot{V}o_2$ with the former on the y-axis and the latter on the x-axis. The two variables will rise at the same rate before the lactate threshold and a best-fit line through these points will have a slope close to 1.
- At a work rate above the lactate threshold, CO_2 output increases more rapidly than O_2 uptake (slope is >1) because CO_2 generated by the bicarbonate buffering of lactic acid is added to the metabolic CO_2 production. The intercept of these two slopes is the estimated lactate or anerobic threshold ($\hat{\theta}_L$) as measured by gas exchange (Figure 4.1).
- The technique of derivation of the $\hat{\theta}_L$ is referred to as the V-slope method [24,29]. The modified V-slope method identifies the $\hat{\theta}_L$ as the tangential breakpoint in the $\dot{V}co_2$–$\dot{V}o_2$ relationship from the line of unity ("line of one") during the incremental stage of the exercise test (Figure 4.2).
- The V-slope methods depend solely on the physicochemical reaction of lactate with bicarbonate, and as such, the occurrence of the breakpoint is independent of chemoreceptor sensitivity and the ventilatory response to exercise – although the magnitude of the response is [28,29].
- The physiological basis for this variable remains controversial [30]; however, the inter-observer variability for experienced clinicians is very acceptable [31]. The $\hat{\theta}_L$ complements other very important information derived from the whole exercise test and should not be taken as a single variable in isolation.

For more detailed descriptions of CPET protocols and physiology, the reader is directed to the American Thoracic Society/American College of Chest Physicians statement on CPET [21] and *Principles of Exercise Testing* by Wasserman and colleagues [24].

CPET in the high-risk surgical patients

Almost two decades ago, Older identified an association between low physical fitness determined by objective CPET, and poor patient outcome following non-cardiopulmonary surgery [32]. CPET-derived variables have increasingly been adopted as the objective measure of fitness prior to surgery, particularly within the National Health Service (NHS) in the U.K. [33]. CPET is now used to inform operative decisions, for choice of peri- and intraoperative management, as well as to inform discussions regarding operative risk. A large number of studies have addressed the association between CPET-derived variables with perioperative risk and outcomes in a variety of clinical contexts. This section will provide the reader with a review of current literature pertaining to the value of CPET in this context.

Vascular surgery

A recent systematic review [34] assesses the role of CPET in patients with abdominal aortic aneurysm (AAA) or peripheral vascular disease requiring surgery. The review concludes

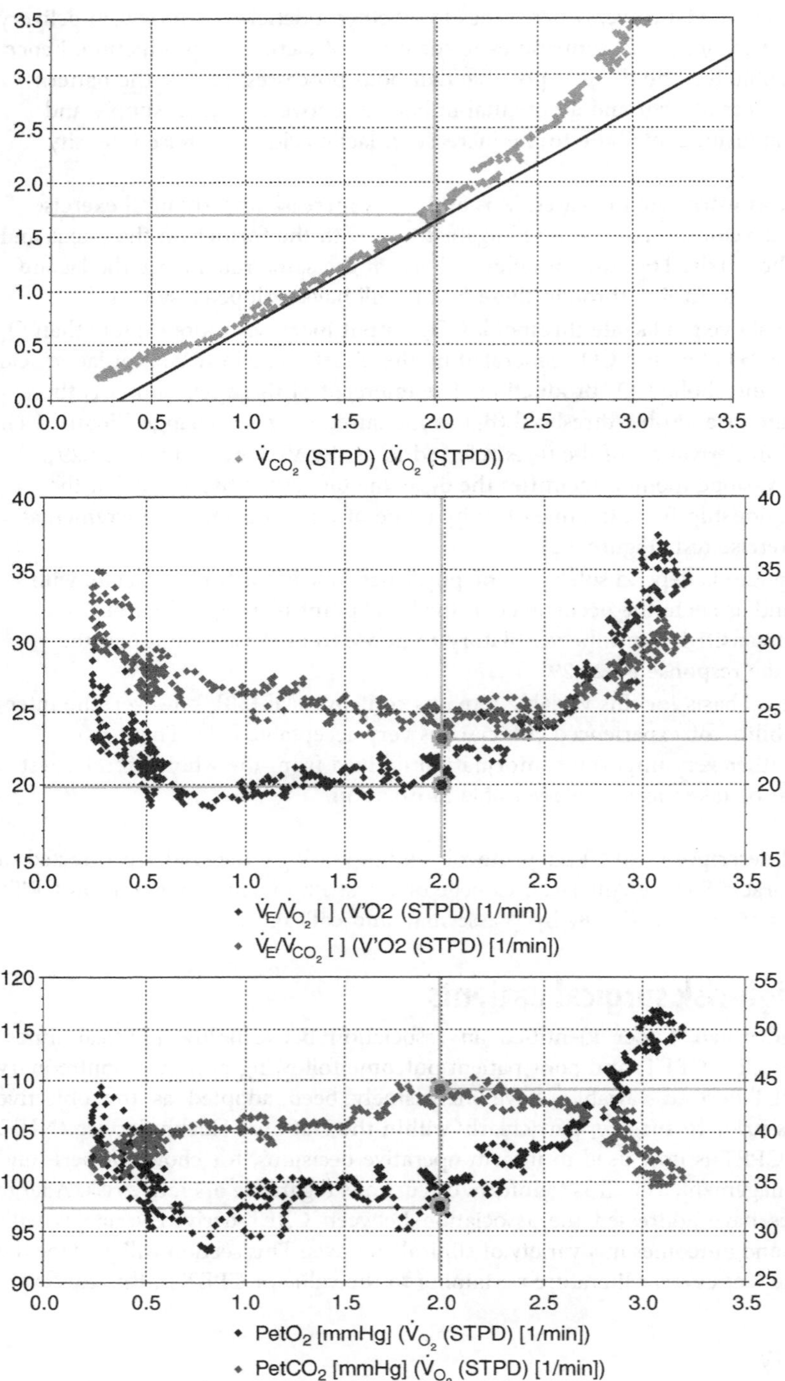

Figure 4.1. Estimated lactate or anerobic threshold ($\hat{\theta}_L$) as measured by gas exchange.

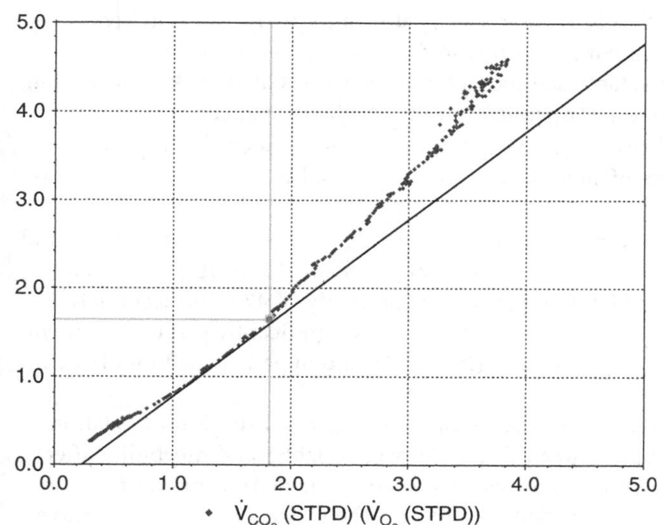

Figure 4.2. Derivation of the $\hat{\theta}_L$ by the V-slope method.

(albeit with major limitations) that paucity of robust data precludes routine adoption of CPET and that its use should be restricted to clinical trials and experimental registries. However, we believe that the evidence published to date suggests that CPET is a valuable prognostic assessment in AAA surgery, and as such, merits consideration as a preoperative investigation.

- Young et al. [34] reviewed six studies [16,35–39] with the largest three all reporting that CPET was a useful predictor of outcome in patients undergoing AAA repair.
- Carlisle et al. [37] retrospectively studied the association between four CPET markers ($\dot{V}O_2$ at peak, $\dot{V}O_2$ at $\hat{\theta}_L$, $\dot{V}_E/\dot{V}CO_2$ and $\dot{V}_E/\dot{V}O_2$, four other risk stratification methods [revised Cardiac Risk Index (RCRI), POSSUM, Simplified Acute Physiology Score (SAPS) II, and the Acute Physiology And Chronic Health Evaluation (APACHE) II], and all-cause mortality following AAA repair. Of the 130 patients studied, a total of 29 (22.3%) died by the time of their last follow-up, 14 (10.8%) doing so in hospital within 30 days of surgery. All CPET variables correlated with mid-term survival, as did the other four risk stratification methods, although to a lesser degree. The $\dot{V}_E/\dot{V}CO_2$ had the strongest association with mortality rate at 30 days and at mid-term (the hazard ratio for mortality was 1.14 [95% CI (CI_{95}), 1.08–1.20; $P<0.001$]). A $\dot{V}_E/\dot{V}CO_2$ value of ≥ 42 and RCRI of >1 were found to be the optimal thresholds in predicting increased risk of mortality.
- Very recent publications by Hartley et al. [40], Prentis et al. [41], and Thompson et al. [38] agree that a low $\dot{V}O_2$ at $\hat{\theta}_L$ is associated with postoperative complications, prolonged length of hospital stay, prolonged length of critical care stay, and early death following AAA surgery.

Major intra-abdominal surgery

Several studies have addressed the utility of CPET prior to major intra-abdominal surgery:

- Older and colleagues [42] illustrated that a $\dot{V}O_2$ at $\hat{\theta}_L$ of <11 mL/kg/min in elderly patients prior to major surgery was associated with increased cardiovascular mortality.

Furthermore, in patients with a low value of $\dot{V}o_2$ at $\hat{\theta}_L$ and preoperative ischemia, the mortality rate was 42%, in comparison with 4% in patients not meeting these criteria. This seminal paper established the first link between CPET, risk stratification, and the provision of increased perioperative care for high-risk patients.

- In a later study and clinical review [23,32], Older et al. investigated the impact of triaging patients on the basis of such data, with no recorded mortality in the patients triaged to ward care.
- Assessing 843 patients undergoing major colorectal surgery, radical nephrectomy, and cystectomy, Wilson et al. [25] concluded that a $\dot{V}o_2$ at $\hat{\theta}_L$ of ≤10.9 mL/kg/min/ and a $\dot{V}_E/\dot{V}co_2$ of ≥34 had a sensitivity of 88% and a specificity of 47% for accurately predicting in-hospital mortality. Survival at 90 days was significantly greater in patients with an $\hat{\theta}_L$ of ≥11 (P=0.034), $\dot{V}_E/\dot{V}co_2$ ≤34 (P=0.021), and in patients without ischemic heart disease (P=0.02).
- Snowden et al. [19] also evaluated the use of CPET in a general surgical population. They reported the relationship between CPET-derived variables and morbidity after major intra-abdominal surgery and showed that a $\dot{V}o_2$ at $\hat{\theta}_L$ of 10.1 mL/kg/min was accurate (sensitivity – 88% and specificity – 79%) for the prediction of postoperative complications. In a follow-up study [43], they investigated the relationship between cardiorespiratory fitness and age in the context of postoperative mortality and morbidity in older people undergoing hepatobiliary surgery. Their sample included 389 adults. $\dot{V}o_2$ at $\hat{\theta}_L$ was the most significant independent predictor for postoperative mortality (P=0.003). Of the 4.6% of patients who died during their in-hospital stay, age was not found to be a significant predictor.
- In a smaller study of 32 patients undergoing major intra-abdominal surgery, Hightower et al. [7] reported that $\dot{V}o_2$ at $\hat{\theta}_L$ (<75% of the predicted value based on age, weight, and height) accurately identified those at increased risk of complications (area under the curve [AUC] 0.72; sensitivity 88%; specificity 79%; P=0.016).
- Studies undertaken by Snowden and Hightower and their colleagues [7,43] had clinicians blinded to the CPET results, ensuring that these did not influence patient care or data collection based on the CPET results. This represents a more accurate reflection of the true magnitude of association between CPET variables and outcome.
- Other recently published CPET studies performed by Junjeo et al. [44], Otto et al. [45], Ausania et al. [46], and Chandrabalan et al. [47] evaluate the utility of CPET in predicting outcome following major high-risk surgery. (The reader is directed to the individual publications.)
- Very recently, Colson and colleagues [48] undertook a review of 1725 patients referred for CPET who subsequently underwent major surgery. Thirty-six percent died within five years. Death was associated with gender, type of surgery (worst for upper gastrointestinal (GI) and best for vascular surgery), and forced vital capacity.
- Additionally, very recently, Lai et al. [49] concluded that patients' inability to perform CPET is associated with inferior outcomes after major colorectal surgery (significantly higher length of hospital stay and mortality at two years in the unable to perform CPET group).

In conclusion, all studies presented here agree that selected CPET variables have a predicative value in determining postoperative complications and length of hospital stay across a range of intra-abdominal surgical procedures.

Upper gastrointestinal surgery

- In 1994, Nagamatsu et al. investigated the association between CPET-derived variables and outcome following upper GI surgery [50]. They analyzed data from 52 patients who had a right thoracolaparotomy for thoracic esophageal cancer, and observed significant differences in $\dot{V}o_{2\ max}$ and $\dot{V}o_2$ at $\hat{\theta}_L$ (both normalized to body surface area) between patients with and without postoperative cardiopulmonary complications.
- In a follow-up study, they retrospectively analyzed data from 91 patients (mean age 59 years) who had undergone an esophagectomy with three-field lymphadenectomy for squamous cell carcinoma and preoperative CPET [50]. Consistent with their original study, $\dot{V}o_{2\ max}$ values (normalized to body surface area) were significantly lower in the cohort of patients that experienced cardiopulmonary complications than in those without complications ($P<0.001$). However, no association was observed between complications and $\dot{V}o_2$ at $\hat{\theta}_L$.
- Consistent with previous CPET studies in patients undergoing upper GI surgery, Forshaw et al. [51] did not find $\hat{\theta}_L$ to differ between those with and without cardiopulmonary complications.

Bariatric surgery

- The association between CPET variables and outcome following bariatric surgery was investigated in 109 obese patients (mean Body Mass Index [BMI] 48.1 kg/m^2) undergoing laparoscopic Roux-en-Y gastric bypass surgery [52]. Postoperative complications and length of hospital stay were significantly higher for the first tertile (threshold $\dot{V}o_2$ at peak value of 15.8 mL/kg/min; sensitivity of 75%; specificity of 73.3%). These results indicate that for a morbidly obese population having bariatric surgery, a $\dot{V}o_2$ at peak of ≤15.8 mL/kg/min has a reasonable capacity to predict those at increased risk of postoperative complications and hospital stay.
- In a recent paper published by Hennis et al. [53], $\dot{V}o_2$ at $\hat{\theta}_L$ was lower in patients with postoperative complications than in those without (9.9 [1.5] versus 11.1 [1.7] mL/kg/min, $P=0.049$) and in patients with a length of stay of >3 days compared with ≤3 days (10.4 [1.4] versus 11.3 [1.8] mL/kg/min, $P=0.023$). Receiver operating characteristic (ROC) curve analysis identified $\dot{V}o_2$ at $\hat{\theta}_L$ as a significant predictor of length of stay of more than three days (area under the curve [AUC] 0.640, $P=0.030$). They conclude that $\dot{V}o_2$ at $\hat{\theta}_L$ predicts length of stay after gastric bypass surgery.

Transplant surgery

- In a study performed by Epstein et al. [54] in 2004, symptom-limited cardiopulmonary exercise testing, conducted an average of approximately 15 months before surgery, was found to be associated with short-term outcome after hepatic transplantation. Specifically, a reduced peak $\dot{V}o_2$ (% predicted) and reduced $\dot{V}o_2$ at $\hat{\theta}_L$ were associated with increased mortality during the first 100 days after hepatic transplantation.
- Very recently, Snowden et al. [55] assessed the feasibility of preoperative submaximal CPET in determining the cardiopulmonary reserve in patients being assessed for liver transplantation and its potential for predicting 90-day post-transplant survival. Sixty of the 182 patients (33%) underwent liver transplantation, and the mortality rate was 10% (6/60). The mean $\dot{V}o_2$ at $\hat{\theta}_L$ value was significantly higher for survivors versus

non-survivors (12.0 ± 2.4 versus 8.4 ± 1.3 mL/kg/min, P<0.001). Logistic regression revealed that $\dot{V}O_2$ at $\hat{\theta}_L$, donor age, blood transfusions, and fresh frozen plasma transfusions were significant univariate predictors of outcomes. In a multivariate analysis, only $\dot{V}O_2$ at $\hat{\theta}_L$ was retained as a significant predictor of mortality. An ROC curve analysis demonstrated sensitivity and specificity of 90.7% and 83.3%, respectively, with good model accuracy (CI_{95} 0.82–0.97, P=0.001). The optimal $\dot{V}O_2$ at $\hat{\theta}_L$ level for survival was defined as being greater than 9 mL/kgmin.

Prehabilitation in the high-risk surgical patient

Prehabilitation is defined as "the process of enhancing the functional capacity of the individual to enable him or her to withstand a stressful event" [56]. Prehabilitation may be used as an optimal time to exercise train an unconditioned individual for an upcoming stressor such as surgery [57].

- As discussed in the previous sections, low levels of physical fitness are associated with poor outcome; less fit patients have a greater risk of complications and death [7,19,25,58,59].
- There is convincing evidence that prehabilitation can improve physical fitness variables. However, a prehabilitation program, in the form of an exercise intervention, may also improve emotional well-being. Preparing for major surgery can cause unanticipated fear, anxiety, and psychological stresses. Burke et al. recently demonstrated that a six-week prehabilitation exercise program following neoadjuvant chemoradiotherapy prior to surgery promoted positive changes in rectal cancer patients' behaviors and helped them view their lives in a way that was fuller, richer, and more meaningful [60].
- The duration of any prehabilitation program is dependent on the time frame from diagnosis to surgery. However, significant improvements in physical fitness can be achieved in a short period of time [61].

The next section will give an overview of the prehabilitation literature to date prior to high-risk procedures.

Prehabilitation in vascular surgery

Patients awaiting AAA surgery represent a high-risk group. Physical fitness levels in this patient population are poor as a consequence of comorbid disease processes, sedentary lifestyle, and age.

- Kothmann et al. [62] studied the effects of a short-term exercise program in AAA patients awaiting surgical repair (exercise group [EG; n=20] and control group [CG; n=10]). This pilot study illustrated that physical fitness increased by 10% in the EG compared to the CG (P=0.007).
- Myers et al. [63] combined aerobic endurance and resistance training protocol and undertook a randomized controlled trial (RCT) in AAA patients over a one-year follow-up period (n=108 recruited, n=57 follow-up data). Following one-year follow up, the EG expended an average 2269 calories (kcal) per week and increased exercise capacity.
- More recently, Tew et al. [64] examined the effects of a 12-week exercise program in patients with small AAA disease (EG, n=14; CG, n=14). The exercise program was based in an exercise suite in the university and patients undertook

aerobic endurance exercise of moderate intensity. There was a significant increase in $\dot{V}O_2$ at $\hat{\theta}_L$ in the EG (P=0.016).

- All three studies report that moderate aerobic exercise training is feasible in this patient group and that results are encouraging. Exercise training prior to aortic surgery may have potential improvements in surgical outcomes.

Prehabilitation in colorectal surgery

- Kim et al. [65] undertook a pilot study in colorectal cancer patients awaiting surgery to assess the feasibility of a prehabilitation program (EG, n=14; CG, n=7). The exercise program took place in the patients' homes over a four-week period. The program was of a moderate intensity, based on heart rate reserve, and patients were asked to exercise for 20 to 30 minutes every day. This program found that peak power output was the only measure responsive to maximal exercise and heart rate and oxygen uptake were responsive to submaximal exercise. However, there was a lack of change in $\dot{V}O_{2\ max}$ in the EG even with a 74% adherence rate.
- Carli et al. [66] then compared the extent to which an in-hospital prehabilitation program (n=58) optimized recovery of functional walking capacity following surgery compared to a home-based walking program (n=54). There were no differences between the groups; however, there was an unexpected benefit in the CG with an increase in walking and breathing exercises albeit with low adherence rates.
- The same group then investigated the extent to which physical function (as measured by Six-Minute Walk Test) could have been improved with a prehabilitation program [67]. The change in physical function between pre- and postsurgery was explored in 95 patients scheduled for colorectal surgery, who completed the prehabilitation program (over a median of 38 days), and 75 patients who were also evaluated postoperatively (mean nine weeks). They concluded that during the prehabilitation program, 33% improved their physical function, 38% stayed within 20 meters of their baseline score, and 29% deteriorated. In the postoperative phase, the patients who had improved were also more likely to have recovered to their baseline walking capacity (77% versus 59% and 32%; P=0.0007). Patients who deteriorated were at greater risk of complications requiring reoperation and/or intensive care management.
- In 2013, Li et al. [68] initiated a trimodal prehabilitation intervention in colorectal cancer patients, which incorporated nutritional counseling, protein supplementation, and anxiety reduction (EG, n=42; CG, n=45). This four-week program improved functional walking capacity and was associated with better postoperative recovery.

Prehabilitation in lung surgery

- Lung resection is the treatment pathway for non-small cell lung cancer (NSCLC), selected cases of oligometastic disease (sarcoma, colorectal cancer, melanoma), and some non-malignant lesions [69].
- Complications following resection are significant and depend on the patients' cardiopulmonary reserves, existing comorbidities, and the extent of the surgery.
- Bobbio et al. [70] investigated the effect of a four-week prehabilitation program on pulmonary function and exercise performance in chronic obstructive pulmonary disease (COPD) patients undergoing lung resection for NSCLC (n=12). Patients were taught

physical modality therapy, incentive spirometry exercises, aerobic exercise on a cycle ergometer, stretching, and muscle strengthening exercises. They found a significant increase in $\dot{V}O_2$ at $\hat{\theta}_L$, $\dot{V}O_{2\ max}$, and O_2 pulse.

- Jones and colleagues [69] were the first to exercise NSCLC patients undergoing surgical resection. Patients (n=25) exercised for five consecutive days per week for four to six weeks prior to surgery. This program was individually tailored and increased in time and intensity over the four to six-week period. This resulted in an increase of $\dot{V}O_2$ at peak by 14.6% and an increase in six-minute walk distance by 9% with an adherence rate of 72%.
- Adjuvant chemotherapy is now standard care after surgical resection and recent trials reported that 5%–24% of patients received no chemotherapy and only 57%–69% completed planned therapy [71]. Prehabilitation may play a role in getting patients physiologically prepared for the adjuvant setting.

Discussion

Literature presented in this chapter illustrates the reliability and association of CPET variables with outcome following major surgery. CPET has the utility of identifying high-risk surgical patients; however, the optimal predictor appears to differ between surgery types, with $\dot{V}O_2$ at $\hat{\theta}_L$ shown to be the best indicator for major intra-abdominal surgery, and $\dot{V}_E/\dot{V}_{CO2}$ for AAA repair surgery [19,25,37]. Furthermore, it appears that the role of CPET is of less clear value in upper GI surgery. The evidence supporting preoperative CPET as a useful test to aid the patient's and the clinician's decisions in relation to surgical risk is, at present, incomplete. The literature comprises a number of small- and medium-sized studies on a limited range of surgical patients. A significant weakness in most of the included studies is the problem of "confounding by indication" due to lack of clinician blinding [72]. The effect of this will be to reduce the strength of association between predictor variable (CPET) and outcome, in relation to the true association. Variation in the type and strength of the association between CPET variables and outcome in different types of surgery is likely to be due to variation in the relative importance of different factors predisposing to adverse outcome – the relative contribution of surgical technique, perioperative care, and patient physiological responses – which are likely to vary between different surgical procedures.

Furthermore, the current literature relating CPET variables to outcome is inconsistent in methods of analysis and presentation of data. This precludes firm conclusions with respect to choice of variable and optimal cut points for identifying high-risk patients for specific procedures; however, several studies identified that CPET variables could be used in conjunction with other non-CPET markers (RCRI, Veterans Specific Activity Questionnaire (VSAQ), POSSUM) to enhance our capacity to predict perioperative risk.

Prehabilitation also requires further research, due to the lack of robust RCTs. The ultimate aim is to tailor an exercise program of the correct intensity, mode, and frequency to suit an individual patient cohort. Although in-hospital prehabilitation programs may illustrate significant results, they have practical constraints. The debate around adherence and the use of an in-hospital or home-based exercise program to improve physical fitness between the time of diagnosis and surgery is of paramount importance.

Together, both CPET and prehabilitation potentially could represent an opportunity to maximize our ability to identify high-risk patients prior to surgery and intervene in a timely fashion prior to a major surgical event; however, adequately powered, blinded, randomized controlled studies need to be conducted to further clarify their respective roles.

Key points for clinical practice

- Risk prediction from CPET should always be evaluated in the context of the overall clinical picture.
- CPET can be used for risk stratification, perioperative patient counseling, and management.
- Specific CPET-derived variables seem to have particular predictive value for specific surgical types.
- Future studies should endeavor to use more robust study designs (blinded studies with an appropriate sample size), ROC curve validations, and statistical methods that properly evaluate the predictive capacity of CPET variables.

References

1. Weiser TG, Regenbogen SE, Thompson KD, et al. An estimation of the global volume of surgery: a modelling strategy based on available data. *Lancet* 2008; **372**: 139–44.
2. Pearse RM, Harrison DA, James P, et al. Identification and characterisation of the high-risk surgical population in the United Kingdom. *Crit Care* 2006; **10**: R81.
3. Association of Coloproctology of Great Britain and Ireland. *National Bowel Cancer Audit Annual Report*. 2013.
4. Royal College of Surgeons England. *Report on Surgical Outcomes Consultant-level statistics*. National Vascular Registry 2013; 8.
5. Royal College of Surgeons England. *National Oesophagogastric Cancer Audit*. 2013.
6. Barry MJ, Edgman-Levitan S. Shared decision making – pinnacle of patient-centered care. *N Eng J Med* 2012; **366**: 780–1.
7. Hightower CE, Riedel BJ, Feig BW, et al. A pilot study evaluating predictors of postoperative outcomes after major abdominal surgery: physiological capacity compared with the ASA physical status classification system. *Br J Anaesth* 2010; **104**: 465–71.
8. Menon KV, Farouk R. An analysis of the accuracy of P-POSSUM scoring for mortality risk assessment after surgery for colorectal cancer. *Colorectal Dis* 2002; **4**: 197–200.
9. Tekkis PP, Prytherch DR, Kocher HM, et al. Development of a dedicated risk-adjustment scoring system for colorectal surgery (colorectal POSSUM). *Br J Surg* 2004; **91**: 1174–82.
10. Edwards M, Whittle J, Ackland GL. Biomarkers to guide perioperative management. *Postgrad Med J* 2011; **87**: 542–9.
11. Baron J, Mundler O, Bertrand M, et al. Dipyridamole-thallium scintigraphy and gated radionuclide angiography to assess cardiac risk before abdominal aortic surgery. *N Eng J Med* 1994; **330**: 663–9.
12. Halm EA, Browner WS, Tubau JF, et al. Echocardiography for assessing cardiac risk in patients having noncardiac surgery. *Ann Intern Med* 1996; **125**: 433–41.
13. Lee L, Schwartzman K, Carli F, et al. The association of the distance walked in 6 min with pre-operative peak oxygen consumption and complications 1 month after colorectal resection. *Anaesthesia* 2013; **68**: 811–16.
14. Murray P, Whiting P, Hutchinson SP, et al. Preoperative shuttle walking testing and outcome after oesophagogastrectomy. *Br J Anaesth* 2007; **99**: 809–11.
15. Singh S, Morgan M, Hardman A. Comparison of oxygen uptake during a conventional treadmill test and the shuttle walking test in chronic airflow limitation. *Eur Respir J* 1994; **7**: 2016–20.

16. Struthers R, Erasmus P, Holmes K, et al. Assessing fitness for surgery: a comparison of questionnaire, incremental shuttle walk, and cardiopulmonary exercise testing in general surgical patients. *Br J Aanaesth* 2008; **101**: 774–80.

17. Kertai MD, Klein J, Bax JJ, et al. Predicting perioperative cardiac risk. *Prog Cardiovasc Dis* 2005; **47**: 240–57.

18. Schouten O, Bax JJ, Poldermans D. Assessment of cardiac risk before non-cardiac general surgery. *Heart* 2006; **92**: 1866–72.

19. Snowden CP, Prentis JM, Anderson HL, et al. Submaximal cardiopulmonary exercise testing predicts complications and hospital length of stay in patients undergoing major elective surgery. *Ann Surg* 2010; **251**: 535–41.

20. Ridgway ZA, Howell SJ. Cardiopulmonary exercise testing: a review of methods and applications in surgical patients. *Eur J Anaesthesiol* 2010; **27**: 858–65.

21. Weisman IM, Marciniuk D, Martinez FJ, et al. ATS/ACCP Statement on cardiopulmonary exercise testing. *Am J Respir Crit Care Med* 2003; **167**: 211–77.

22. Doherty AFO, West M, Jack S, et al. Preoperative aerobic exercise training in elective intra-cavity surgery: a systematic review. *Br J Anaesth* 2013; **110**: 679–89.

23. Stringer W, Casaburi R, Older P. Cardiopulmonary exercise testing: does it improve perioperative care and outcome? *Curr Opin Anaesthesiol* 2012; **25**: 178–84.

24. Wasserman K, Hansen JE, Sue DY, et al. *Principles of Exercise Testing and Interpretation: Pathophysiology and Clinical Applications*. 4th edn. Baltimore, MD: Lippincott Williams & Wilkins, 2005; 1–180.

25. Wilson RJT, Davies S, Yates D, et al. Impaired functional capacity is associated with all-cause mortality after major elective intra-abdominal surgery. *Br J Anaesth* 2010; **105**: 297–303.

26. Palange P, Ward SA, Carlsen KH, et al. Recommendations on the use of exercise testing in clinical practice. *Eur Respir J* 2007; **29**: 185–209.

27. Fleisher LA, Beckman JA, Brown K, et al. ACC/AHA 2007 guidelines on perioperative cardiovascular evaluation and care for noncardiac surgery: a report of the American College of Cardiology/American Heart Association Task Force on Practice Guidelines. *J Am Coll Cardiol* 2007; **116**: e418–99.

28. William B, Wasserman K, Whipp J. A new method for detecting anaerobic threshold by gas exchange. *J Appl Physiol* 1986; **60**: 2020–7.

29. Sue D, Wasserman K, Moricca R, et al. Metabolic acidosis during exercise in patients with chronic obstructive pulmonary disease. Use of the V-slope method for anaerobic threshold determination. *Chest* 1988; **94**: 931–8.

30. Hopker JG, Jobson S, Pandit JJ. Controversies in the physiological basis of the "anaerobic threshold" and their implications for clinical cardiopulmonary exercise testing. *Anaesthesia* 2011; **66**: 111–23.

31. Sinclair RCF, Danjoux GR, Goodridge V, et al. Determination of the anaerobic threshold in the pre-operative assessment clinic: inter-observer measurement error. *Anaesthesia* 2009; **64**: 1192–5.

32. Older P, Hall A, Hader R. Cardiopulmonary exercise testing as a screening test for perioperative management of major surgery in the elderly. *Chest* 1999; **116**: 355–62.

33. Simpson JC, Sutton H, Grocott MPW. Cardiopulmonary exercise testing – a survey of current use in England. *J Intesive Care Soc* 2009; **10**: 275–8.

34. Young EL, Karthikesalingam A, Huddart S, et al. A systematic review of the role of cardiopulmonary exercise testing in vascular surgery. *Eur J Vasc Endovasc Surg* 2012; **44**: 64–71.

35. Nugent a M, Riley M, Megarry J, et al. Cardiopulmonary exercise testing in the pre-operative assessment of patients for repair of abdominal aortic aneurysm. *Irish J Med Sci* 1998; **167**: 238–41.

36. Kothmann E, Danjoux G, Owen SJ, et al. Reliability of the anaerobic threshold in

cardiopulmonary exercise testing of patients with abdominal aortic aneurysms. *Anaesthesia* 2009; **64**: 9–13.

37. Carlisle J, Swart M. Mid-term survival after abdominal aortic aneurysm surgery predicted by cardiopulmonary exercise testing. *Br J Surg* 2007; **94**: 966–9.
38. Thompson A, Peters N, Lovegrove R, et al. Cardiopulmonary exercise testing provides a predictive tool for early and late outcomes in abdominal aortic aneurysm patients. *Ann R Coll Surg Engl* 2011; **93**: 474–81.
39. McEnrow G, Wilson R. Use of cardiopulmonary exercise (CPX) testing to assess patients' suitability for elective aortic aneurysm surgery. *Anaesthesia* 2006; **61**: 415–17.
40. Hartley R, Pichel C, Grant SW, et al. Preoperative cardiopulmonary exercise testing and risk of early mortality following abdominal aortic aneurysm repair. *Br J Surg* 2012; **99**: 1539–46.
41. Prentis JM, Trenell MI, Jones DJ, et al. Submaximal exercise testing predicts perioperative hospitalization after aortic aneurysm repair. *J Vasc Surg* 2012; **56**: 1564–70.
42. Older P, Smith R, Hone R. Preoperative evaluation of cardiac failure and ischemia in elderly patients by cardiopulmonary exercise testing. *Chest* 1993; **104**: 701–4.
43. Snowden CP, Prentis J, Jacques B, et al. Cardiorespiratory fitness predicts mortality and hospital length of stay after major elective surgery in older people. *Ann Surg* 2013; **257**: 999–1004.
44. Junejo M, Mason JM, Sheen J, et al. Cardiopulmonary exercise testing for preoperative risk assessment before hepatic resection. *Br J Surg* 2012; **99**: 1097–104.
45. Otto JM, O'Doherty F, Hennis PJ, et al. Preoperative exercise capacity in adult inflammatory bowel disease sufferers, determined by cardiopulmonary exercise testing. *Int J Colorectal Dis* 2012; **27**: 1485–91.
46. Ausania F, Snowden CP, Prentis JM, et al. Effects of low cardiopulmonary reserve on pancreatic leak following pancreaticoduodenectomy. *Br J Surg* 2012; **99**: 1290–4.
47. Chandrabalan VV, McMillan DC, Carter R, et al. Pre-operative cardiopulmonary exercise testing predicts adverse post-operative events and non-progression to adjuvant therapy after major pancreatic surgery. *HPB (Oxford)* 2013; **15**: 899–907.
48. Colson M, Baglin J, Bolsin S, et al. Cardiopulmonary exercise testing predicts 5 yr survival after major surgery. *Br J Anaesth* 2012; **109**: 735–41.
49. Lai CW, Minto G, Challand CP, et al. Patients' inability to perform a preoperative cardiopulmonary exercise test or demonstrate an anaerobic threshold is associated with inferior outcomes after major colorectal surgery. *Br J Anaesth* 2013; **111**: 607–11.
50. Nagamatsu Y, Shima I, Yamana H, et al. Preoperative evaluation of cardiopulmonary reserve with the use of expired gas analysis during exercise testing in patients with squamous cell carcinoma of the thoracic esophagus. *J Thorac Cardiovasc Surg* 2001; **121**: 1064–8.
51. Forshaw MJ, Strauss DC, Davies AR, et al. Is cardiopulmonary exercise testing a useful test before esophagectomy? *Ann Thorac Surg* 2008; **85**: 294–9.
52. McCullough P, Gallagher MJ, Dejong AT, et al. Cardiorespiratory fitness and short-term complications after bariatric surgery. *Chest* 2006; **130**: 517–25.
53. Hennis PJ, Meale PM, Hurst R, et al. Cardiopulmonary exercise testing predicts postoperative outcome in patients undergoing gastric bypass surgery. *Br J Anaesth* 2012; **109**: 566–71.
54. Epstein SK, Freeman RB, Khayat A, et al. Aerobic capacity is associated with 100-day outcome after hepatic transplantation. *Liver Transpl* 2004; **10**: 418–24.
55. Prentis J, Manas D, Trenell M. Submaximal cardiopulmonary exercise testing predicts 90-day survival after liver transplantation. *Transplantation* 2012; **18**: 152–9.
56. Ditmyer N, Topp R, Pifer M. Prehabilitation in preparation

for orthopaedic surgery. *Orthop Nurs* 2002;**21**: 43–51.

57. Silver JK, Baima J. Cancer prehabilitation: an opportunity to decrease treatment-related morbidity, increase cancer treatment options, and improve physical and psychological health outcomes. *Am J Phys Med Rehabil* 2013; **92**: 715–27.

58. Hennis PJ, Meale PM, Grocott MPW. Cardiopulmonary exercise testing for the evaluation of perioperative risk in non-cardiopulmonary surgery. *Postgrad Med J* 2011; **87**: 550–7.

59. West M, Jack S, Grocott MPW. Perioperative cardiopulmonary exercise testing in the elderly. Best practice and research. *Clin Anaesthesiol* 2011; **25**: 427–37.

60. Burke SM, Brunet J, Sabiston CM, et al. Patients' perceptions of quality of life during active treatment for locally advanced rectal cancer: the importance of preoperative exercise. *Support Care Cancer* 2013; **21**: 3345–53.

61. Macfarlane DJ, Taylor LH, Cuddihy TF. Very short intermittent vs continuous bouts of activity in sedentary adults. *Prevent Med* 2006; **43**: 332–6.

62. Kothmann E, Batterham M, Owen SJ, et al. Effect of short-term exercise training on aerobic fitness in patients with abdominal aortic aneurysms: a pilot study. *Br J Anaesth* 2009; **103**: 505–10.

63. Myers JN, White JJ, Narasimhan B, et al. Effects of exercise training in patients with abdominal aortic aneurysm: preliminary results from a randomized trial. *J Cardiopulm Rehabil Prev* 2010; **30**: 374–83.

64. Tew G, Moss J, Crank H, et al. Endurance exercise training in patients with small abdominal aortic aneurysm: a randomized controlled pilot study. *Arch Phys Med Rehabil* 2012; **93**: 2148–53.

65. Kim DJ, Mayo NE, Carli F, et al. Responsive measures to prehabilitation in patients undergoing bowel resection surgery. *Tohoku J Exp Med* 2009; **217**: 109–15.

66. Carli F, Charlebois P, Stein B, et al. Randomized clinical trial of prehabilitation in colorectal surgery. *Br J Surg* 2010; **97**: 1187–97.

67. Mayo NE, Feldman L, Scott S, et al. Impact of preoperative change in physical function on postoperative recovery: argument supporting prehabilitation for colorectal surgery. *Surgery* 2011; **150**: 505–14.

68. Li C, Carli F, Lee L, et al. Impact of a trimodal prehabilitation program on functional recovery after colorectal cancer surgery: a pilot study. *Surg Endosc* 2013; **27**: 1072–82.

69. Jones LW, Peddle CJ, Eves ND, et al. Effects of presurgical exercise training on cardiorespiratory fitness among patients undergoing thoracic surgery for malignant lung lesions. *Cancer* 2007; **110**: 590–8.

70. Bobbio A, Chetta A, Ampollini L, et al. Preoperative pulmonary rehabilitation in patients undergoing lung resection for non-small cell lung cancer. *Eur J Cardiothorac Surg* 2008; **33**: 95–8.

71. Alam N, Shepherd F, Winton T, et al. Compliance with post-operative adjuvant chemotherapy in non-small cell lung cancer. An analysis of National Cancer Institute of Canada and intergroup trial JBR.10 and a review of the literature. *Lung Cancer* 2005; **47**: 385–94.

72. Grocott MPW, Pearse RM. Prognostic studies of perioperative risk: robust methodology is needed. *Br J Anaesth* 2010; **105**: 243–5.

Perioperative cardiovascular medication management

C. Railton

Perioperative medication management remains one of the most problematic and controversial areas of perioperative medicine. The area is filled with recommendations based on expert opinion and information based on flawed clinical studies. The integrity of some of the data used to develop guidelines has been questioned [1,2].

The American College of Cardiology/American Heart Association (ACC/AHA) Guidelines [3] have not been updated since 2007, but supplemental information on β-blockade [4] was released in 2009. The European Society of Cardiology (ESC) published similar guidelines in 2009 [5]. However, the validity of ESC guidelines has been questioned because of concerns of bias [6]. The most recent literature has focused largely on the area of perioperative β-blockade. A systematic review of guidelines for perioperative medications was published in 2011 [7].

- The goal of the perioperative physician should be to continue or start beneficial medications and hold or stop harmful medications.
- Traditionally, all medications were held at the time of anesthesia and surgery for fear that blunting natural physiological reflexes would result in catastrophe for the patient.
- However, during the early 1980s, practice changed where most cardiovascular medications were continued at the time of surgery to improve cardiovascular stress tolerance [8].
- The change in practice was not dictated by clinical research, but largely by opinion.
- Most physicians still use opinion to guide therapy, given the quality of information available.

The information that follows is not an exhaustive review of the literature but more of a highlight of important papers and a practical approach to making sense of a controversial area of perioperative medicine.

β-blockade

Despite being one of the most researched areas of perioperative medication management, the answer to the question of whether perioperative β-blockade is beneficial still remains elusive. How to manage this class of medications perioperatively is even more confusing.

- Randomized studies of perioperative β-blockade have been done in the past using atenolol, bisoprolol, metoprolol, and propranolol. The 2009 ACC/AHA 4 supplement fully discusses these trials and relevant issues and provides a comprehensive literature review up to that time.

Anesthesia and Perioperative Care of the High-Risk Patient, Third edition, ed. Ian McConachie. Published by Cambridge University Press.

- All of these studies showed cardio-protective effects of β-blockade.
- Cardiac events can be prevented but seemingly at the cost of increased rates of perioperative hypotension and cerebrovascular events and mortality [9,10].
- No recent meta-analysis examining all the trials has been published – it is not clear if the results can or should be meta-analyzed due to differences in studies.
- All of the largest trials have been strongly criticized for a variety of reasons and have resulted in a less clear treatment plan for the attending physician.

Multiple factors affect postoperative outcomes related to β-blockade:

- Redelmeier et al. argued that the half-life of the β-blocker used determines the effectiveness in the prevention of postoperative myocardial infarction (MI) [11]. Redelmeier et al. compared over 37 000 patients, taking metoprolol (half-life 3 h) and atenolol (half-life 9 h) at the time of surgery. They found that patients on atenolol, the longer half-life drug, had fewer myocardial events than the patients taking metoprolol (atenolol 2.5% versus metoprolol 3.5%, $P<0.001$) [11].
- Wallace et al. conducted a similar study in an American Veterans Affairs database of 38 800 patients and found that atenolol afforded better postoperative mortality protection than metoprolol (atenolol 1% versus metoprolol 3%, $P<0.0008$) [12].
- Feringa et al. [13] have shown a dose–response effect in 272 vascular surgery patients in cardio-protection as assessed by serial troponin-T measurements and long-term outcome. The most common β-blocker used in the study was bisoprolol (67%, half-life 9–12 h), although atenolol (5%, half-life 9 h) and metoprolol (15%, half-life 3–4.5 h) were also included.
- Meta-analysis of major trials failed to show a clinical benefit of β-blockers [14,15].
- However, a reanalysis of largely the same data from a pharmacogenetic approach that accounted for variations in β-blocker pharmacology showed that not all β-blockers have similar effects and there was great heterogeneity between studies [16]. β-blockers cleared by cytochrome 2D6 (metoprolol) failed to show a clinical benefit.
- Anemia has also been implicated to play a role in adverse outcomes associated with β-blockade [17]. Chronically, β-blocked patients were less tolerant of acute development of anemia.
- Angeli et al. found that only the highest-risk surgical procedure patients benefited from perioperative β-blockade [18].
- Perioperative hypotension has been strongly implicated in adverse outcomes [4,19].

The earliest papers in the area of β-blockade focused largely on the benefits heart rate control had on coronary perfusion and cardiac ischemia. β-blockade can be successfully used to prevent cardiac ischemia by rate control as assessed by Holter monitoring [14]. Early ideas on the benefits of heart rate control have been confirmed by meta-analysis of more recent trials, showing that fewer cardiac events occurred in the better rate-controlled patients [20].

β-blockers cannot be stopped abruptly because a withdrawal syndrome results, predisposing patients to increased rates of myocardial infarction (MI) and stroke [21–23]. This was discovered largely in the early 1970s, when patients, awaiting surgery, had adverse events after their β-blockers were held. Reluctance of physicians to continue β-blockers in a hypotensive postoperative patient places the patient at risk of withdrawal syndrome and at increased risk of MI or worse. It has also been found recently that up to 20% of patients on chronic β-blockade are subtherapeutic on presentation for surgery with current management advice, suggesting that up to 20% of patients may be actively undergoing β-blocker withdrawal at the time of surgery [24].

Further, recent meta-analysis omitting major studies that have either been discredited or are under suspicion suggests that the use of perioperative β-blockers may increase overall mortality (largely from side effects and hypotension), despite myocardial protection [25].

In summary, the data regarding perioperative β-blockade remains controversial.

The current recommendation regarding β-blocker therapy is that only patients with stable coronary artery disease (CAD) and high-risk patients are likely to benefit from therapy [4,10]. The most recent guidelines regarding perioperative β-blockade have been revised to reflect this opinion [4].

- The general recommendation in the guidelines is to continue β-blocker therapy in patients already taking β-blockers.
- Patients should be risk stratified and therapy started in patients with multiple risk factors or documented as stable CAD.
- If a patient has demonstrated ischemia on preoperative testing or multiple risk factors for cardiac ischemia, consider starting a β-blocker.
- It seems likely that only the highest-risk patients will receive the most benefit, especially in large surgeries.
- Heart rate control and the maintenance thereof is the most beneficial effect of β-blockers in the perioperative setting.
- The choice of β-blocker and how it is dosed matters. The effects do not appear equal across all members of the class of medications. Longer half-life β-blockers may possibly provide more benefit to patients. It is unclear from the available information if β-selectivity matters. Above all, for patients chronically taking β-blockers, do not stop them abruptly in the perioperative period because of the risk of developing adverse events due to β-blocker withdrawal syndrome.
- If required, β-blockers should be started weeks before surgery and titrated to heart rate and blood pressure targets to avoid risks associated with hypotension.
- Recommendations and guidelines may continue to be revised as further information becomes available.

Renin–angiotensin blockade

In contrast to β-blockade, this is an area of perioperative medication management where little is known and no large randomized control trials (RCTs) have been published. It was established over thirty years ago that the renin–angiotensin system (RAS) plays an important role in blood pressure management during anesthesia.

Blockade of the RAS by angiotensin-converting enzyme (ACE) inhibitors or angiotensin receptor blocking (ARB) agents is associated with intraoperative hypotension [26,27]. Intraoperative hypotension associated with ACE inhibitor use was the subject of a recent Anesthesia Safety Patient Foundation article [28].

Use of medications that block the RAS may be associated with more severe disease states. A recent study found that RAS-blocked patients had higher Euro-SCORE and Acute Physiology and Chronic Health Evaluation (APACHE) II scores compared to unblocked patients ($P<0.001$) [29]. Recent consensus guidelines showed a majority of perioperative experts believe that these classes of medications should be held perioperatively [7].

However, other physicians have countered that the beneficial effects of after-load reduction, cardiac remodeling, and possible antioxidant effects of ACE inhibitors and ARBs justifies their continuation at the time of surgery. There is considerable disagreement among physicians with respect to perioperative management of RAS-blocking agents and whether they should be held at the time of surgery.

A few published retrospective studies examining the effects of ACE inhibitors on postoperative outcome exist:

- Sear et al. [30] used registry data to study the effects of intercurrent medical therapy on cardiac death rates in elective and emergency surgery patients. Only eight deceased patients taking ACE inhibitors were identified, and due to small numbers and problems with matching, only simple odds ratios (ORs) could be calculated. The OR for increased risk of death for ACE-exposed patients undergoing elective surgery was 0.19 but not statistically significant. Sear et al. reported increased mortality risk for emergency surgery of 1.18 ($P=0.0032$) but the 95% confidence interval (CI_{95}) could not be calculated.
- Kurzencwyg et al. [31] used hospital computing systems to study emergency and elective abdominal aortic aneurysm (AAA) patients exposed to many classes of medications. They examined 223 consecutive cases and identified 24 deaths (11 elective repair and 13 emergency repair for ruptured aneurysm). Kurzencwyg et al. reported that ACE inhibitor exposure showed a statistically non-significant trend toward protection (OR 0.09, CI_{95} 0.01–1.31, $P=0.08$). However, comparing emergency and elective AAA does not seem reasonable due to mortality rates. The surgical factors in emergency AAA repair likely dominated medical factors.
- Railton et al. [32] reported on 874 elective AAA repair patients at two hospitals. ACE/ARB-exposed patients were at higher risk of death within 30 days of surgery. The crude mortality rate in RAS-blocked patients was 5.8% (21/359) versus 1.9% (10/524) in unexposed patients (OR 3.2, CI_{95} 1.5–6.7, $P<0.001$). Propensity score matching was used to identify 261 matched pairs with a 30-day mortality rate of 6.1% (16/261) in the RAS-blocked group versus 1.5% (4/261) in the unblocked patients with an estimated OR for increased mortality of 5 (CI_{95} 1.5–6.7, $P=0.008$).
- Micelli et al. reported on a series of 10 023 patients undergoing coronary artery bypass [33]. Propensity matching was used to identify 3052 ACE-exposed patients and matched controls. Micelli et al. found an increased risk of death in RAS-blocked patients (OR 2.00, CI_{95} 1.17–3.42, $P=0.013$). Multivariate analysis of the dataset showed preoperative ACE inhibitor treatment was an independent predictor of mortality ($P=0.04$), postoperative renal failure ($P=0.0002$), use of inotropic drugs ($P=0.0001$), and atrial fibrillation (AF) ($P=0.0001$).
- In a similar study on heart surgery patients (bypass and valve), Rader et al. did not find that postoperative AF was associated with RAS blockade [34]. However, Rader et al.'s (34) finding of increased rates of postoperative renal failure in RAS-blocked patients has been observed in other studies [35,36].
- Drenger et al. [29] reported on a series of prospectively enrolled patients (4224) undergoing coronary artery bypass surgery, in which the perioperative management of ACE inhibitors was studied. They examined four possible management strategies of perioperative RAS blockade. Postoperative continuation of an ACE inhibitor versus postoperative withdrawal of the ACE inhibitor was associated with decreased risk of

adverse outcomes (combined endpoint: in hospital mortality, cardiac, renal, and central nervous system complications) (OR 0.50, CI_{95} 0.38–0.66, P<0.001).

- Turan et al. found that holding ACE inhibitors for a single dosing interval prior to surgery and restarting RAS blockade postoperatively was not associated with adverse outcomes [37].

Corait [38] has argued that the beneficial effects of renin–angiotensin blockade persist beyond the time when the medication is held. Comfère et al. [39] have shown that holding ACE inhibitors and ARB agents on the morning of surgery reduces the incidence of hypotension on the induction of anesthesia. The active metabolites of ACE inhibitors and ARBs can have very long half-lives and may persist in patients systems for days. Goldstein and Amar's [40] recommendation seems to be prudent, which is to hold the medication for one dosage interval prior to surgery. This approach would at least reduce the amount of hypotension following the induction of anesthesia, as reported by Comfère et al. [39], and not increase perioperative risk [37].

In summary, little is known about the benefits or risks associated with the continuation or stopping of ACE inhibitors and ARBs in the perioperative period. One should consider the following when making a decision regarding the management of ACE inhibitors and ARBs:

- Patients under anesthesia are heavily dependent on the renin–angiotensin system for the maintenance of blood pressure and volume regulation.
- RAS blockade may be an independent risk factor for death within 30 days of surgery in high-risk patients (cardiac and major vascular).
- Exposure to ACE inhibitors and ARB agents is associated with hypotension following the induction of anesthesia.
- Holding a RAS-blocking medication for one dosing interval prior to surgery is associated with a reduction in the frequency of hypotension during anesthesia, and no postoperative adverse events appear to occur if the RAS-blocking medication is restarted postoperatively.
- Failure to restart the RAS blockade following surgery may be associated with worse postoperative outcomes.

Calcium channel blockers

In contrast to the first two classes of medications examined, the perioperative use of calcium channel blockers (CCB) is less controversial. Very little new literature has been published in the last five years. Only a few of the papers on perioperative use of CCB have examined outcomes. In theory, the decrease in systemic vascular resistance (SVR), negative chronotropic effects, and prolongation of sinoatrial and atrioventricular (A-V) node conduction would appear to be very dangerous when anesthetic agents are present. There have been case reports of intraoperative hypotension and sudden death. However, to date, no study has found any increased risk due to perioperative CCB exposure.

It has been shown that pretreatment with CCB prior to the induction of anesthesia does result in a lower mean arterial pressure and less SVR in cardiac surgery patients [41]. A potentiation of A-V nodal block has been reported when inhalational anesthetics are used in patients chronically treated with CCB [42]. However, the acute administration of CCB under anesthesia has been reported to result in hypotension [43]. CCB may also interact with non-depolarizing and polarizing neuromuscular blocking agents resulting in prolonged neuromuscular blockade [44].

The studies of CCB and anesthesia have been fairly small. Meta-analysis has been used to examine if there are any beneficial effects of perioperative use of CCB. Wijeysundera et al. studied both non-cardiac [45] and cardiac surgery patients [46].

- In non-cardiac surgery, patients exposed had a decrease in cardiac ischemia (relative risk [RR] 0.49, CI_{95} 0.30–0.80, P=0.004), and a trend toward the reduction of MI (RR 0.25, CI_{95} 0.05–1.18, P=0.08), and a possible reduction in mortality (RR 0.40, CI_{95} 0.14–1.16, P=0.09).
- In cardiac surgery, patients perioperative exposure to CCB reduced MI (OR 0.58, CI_{95} 0.37–0.91; P=0.02), and ischemia (OR 0.53, CI_{95} 0.39–0.72; $P<0.001$). Despite the reductions in MI and ischemia, no decrease in mortality was observed.

Regardless of the theoretical risks and possible interactions with medications commonly used in anesthesia, there appears to be some reduction of postoperative adverse events in patients treated with CCB. However, given the large sample sizes needed to show effect, it seems likely the benefit derived by individual patients is small. It seems limited benefit would result from starting a patient perioperatively on CCB.

In summary, the following should be considered when deciding to treat a patient on CCB perioperatively:

- CCB does interact with inhaled anesthetic agents and neuromuscular blocking agents used in anesthesia.
- Patients chronically treated with CCB do show decreases in SVR and mean arterial pressure compared to controls.
- No harm has been reported in large studies of perioperative use of CCB.
- Meta-analysis has shown some benefit toward reduction of ischemia, arrhythmias, MI, but not mortality.
- The expected risks or benefits are small due to the large numbers of patients that need to be treated to show effects.
- It seems reasonable continue patients chronically taking CCB but not to start patients acutely in the perioperative period.

HMG CoA reductase inhibitors

HMG (3-hydroxy-3-methyl-glutaryl) CoA reductase inhibitors, more commonly known as statins, have been examined for beneficial perioperative effects. The mechanism of any potential beneficial effects is not understood. The inhibition of cholesterol synthesis in the liver does not seem to be the likely mechanism. It has been suggested the pleotropic effects on inflammation, plaque stabilization, and platelet aggregation are the most likely explanation of the suggested possible benefits [47].

There has been much controversy in this area due to questions arising regarding integrity of some of the major studies in the area. Recent Cochrane systematic reviews have been published on statin use in a cardiac surgery population [48] and non-cardiac surgery population [49]. Systematic reviews have also been published by Chan et al. [50] and Chopra et al. [51]. The total number of patients in RCTs published remains small, less than 3000 cases. This becomes especially true when the largest, most controversial studies are removed from consideration, resulting in an inability to draw conclusions about relatively rare events in a small sample size [49].

In summary, the available information appears to point toward perioperative statin use being of some benefit in high-risk patients. The following issues should be considered when making a decision for the management of HMG CoA reductase inhibitors:

- Available evidence points toward improved postoperative cardiac outcomes with perioperative statin use.
- Until more information is available, it seems reasonable to maintain patients already taking a statin on their HMG CoA reductase inhibitor and to restart the medication following surgery.
- At this time, one meta-analysis points toward the benefit of starting statin-naïve patients on statin therapy [48]. However, when the controversial studies are removed from the database, the results are inconclusive [49].

Nitrates

The perioperative use of nitrates for the treatment of angina has raised concerns among some physicians that the use of such medications may lead to endothelial cell dysfunction and possibly worse postoperative outcomes. Despite obvious concerns that nitrates may predispose a patient toward developing postoperative complications, very little information is available.

- Sear et al. found that nitrate exposure after adjustment for the effects of age, cardiac disease, and medication exposure were at increased risk of death (corrected OR 4.79, CI_{95} 1.00–22.72, P=0.049) [30]. Nitrate exposure in emergency surgical patients was not associated with worse outcomes in the same study.

The simple approach for the perioperative management of nitrates in high-risk patients would be to advise the patient to use the medications as needed but to otherwise minimize use. No guidelines have been published.

α_2-adrenoreceptor agonists

Interest in the perioperative use of α_2-adrenoreceptor agonists has been increasing. This class of medications reduces sympathetic outflow, causing a reduction in norepinephrine levels and heart rate. Additionally, these agents can provide anxiolysis, analgesia, antiemesis, and antisialogogic actions. The initial goal of perioperative use was pain reduction, but possible cardioprotection is now suggested as the main clinical benefit of this class of medication.

- A 2009 Cochrane review described the quality of available studies as poor, but found reduced mortality (RR 0.66, CI_{95} 0.44–0.98, P=0.04), fewer episodes of myocardial ischemia (RR 0.68, CI_{95} 0.57–0.81, P<0.0001), but at the cost of hypotension (RR 1.32, CI_{95} 1.07–1.62, P=0.009) and bradycardia (RR 1.66, CI_{95} 1.14–2.41, P=0.008). The largest benefit appeared to occur in vascular surgery cases [52].
- The POISE-2 Trial found that low-dose clonidine did not prevent myocardial infarction (OR 1.11, CI_{95} 0.95–1.30, P=0.18), hypotension was more prevalent in clonidine exposed patients (OR 1.32, CI_{95} 1.24–1.40, P<0.001) and the rate of non-fatal cardiac arrest was increased (OR 3.20, C95 1.17–8.73, P=0.02 [53].

The results of the Perioperative Ischemic Events (POISE-2) Trial seem to cast a shadow over these potentially promising medications. No advice on how to manage these medications can be given. There is an associated withdrawal syndrome when this type of medication is stopped abruptly.

Selective serotonin reuptake inhibitors

Selective serotonin reuptake inhibitors (SSRIs) have recently been identified as a possible factor causing increased perioperative bleeding risk. The mechanism of the increased bleeding is proposed to be inhibition of uptake of serotonin by platelets causing platelet dysfunction.

- There has been a wide range of results from no increased risk to over a four-fold increased risk in cosmetic breast surgery patients [54].
- Using data collected on multiple types of surgery from 375 hospitals (530 000 patients), Auerback et al. showed that SSRIs may be linked with increased perioperative mortality (adjusted OR 1.20, CI_{95} 1.07–1.36), increased bleeding (adjusted OR 1.09, CI_{95} 1.04–1.15), and postoperative readmission before 30 days (adjusted OR 1.22, CI_{95} 1.18–1.26) [55].

No guidelines for SSRI management exist and abruptly stopping SSRIs can cause a withdrawal syndrome. Psychiatric complications may occur if the medication is stopped. At therapeutic drug levels, there is likely enough SSRI in a patient's blood to cause platelet dysfunction in any transfused platelets that might be administered to the patient. There appears to be no clear solution to the management of this class of medication. The best approach may be to look at the bleeding and mortality risk of the planned procedure and then make clinical decisions.

System design and safety

The medical system is seeing an increased emphasis on improving quality and safety of care. The overall design of a management plan and the process of how the care is implemented play an important role in achieving improved quality and patient safety. The recording of preoperative medication histories is known to have many problems [56]. The complex perioperative environment can make the design and implementation of quality and improvement processes difficult [57]. The preoperative use of medication reconciliation has been demonstrated to improve perioperative quality of care and patient safety:

- Hale et al. showed how medication reconciliation can reduce omissions of medications: 11 of 887 (1.2%) intervention orders compared with 383 of 1217 (31.5%) control ($P<0.001$); fewer prescribing errors (2 in 857 [0.2%] intervention orders compared with 51 in 807 [6.3%] control [$P<0.001$]) [58].
- The ability of patients to comply with perioperative medication management decisions is also improved by the medication reconciliation process [59].

Summary

The perioperative medication management is difficult and often an area of disagreement between anesthesiologists, surgeons, and internal medicine specialists. Trying to keep abreast of the latest information is challenging. Trying to use an evidence-based approach is especially difficult when the quality of evidence is poor or where little evidence is available to guide decision making.

References

1. Chopra V, Eagle KA. Perioperative mischief: the price of academic misconduct. *Am J Med* 2012; **125**: 953–5.
2. Poldermans D. Scientific fraud or a rush to judgment? *Am J Med* 2013; **126**: e5–6.
3. Fleisher LA, Beckman JA, Brown KA, et al. ACC/AHA 2006 Guideline update on perioperative cardiovascular evaluation for noncardiac surgery: focused update on perioperative beta-blocker therapy – a report of the American College of Cardiology/American Heart Association Task Force on Practice Guidelines (Writing Committee to Update the 2002 Guidelines on Perioperative Cardiovascular Evaluation for Noncardiac Surgery). *Circulation* 2007; **116**: e418–500.
4. Fleischmann KE, Beckman JA, Buller CE, et al. ACCF/AHA Focused update on perioperative beta blockade: a report of the American College of Cardiology Foundation/American Heart Association Task Force on Practice Guidelines. *Circulation* 2009; **120**: 2123–51.
5. Poldermans D, Bax JJ, Boersma E, et al. Guidelines for pre-operative cardiac risk assessment and perioperative cardiac management in non-cardiac surgery. *Eur Heart J* 2009; **30**: 2769–812.
6. Foex P, Sear JW. Guidelines for preoperative cardiac assessment. *Br J Anaesth* 2012; **108**: 525.
7. Castanheira L, Fresco P, Macedo AF. Guidelines for the management of chronic medication in the perioperative period: systematic review and formal consensus. *J Clin Pharm Ther* 2011; **36**: 446–67.
8. Kim Y, Danchak M, Macnamara TE. Drug interaction and anesthesia. *Clin Ther* 1987; **9**: 342–3.
9. Devereaux PJ, Yang H, Yusuf S, et al. Effects of extended release metoprolol succinate in patients undergoing non-cardiac surgery (POISE trial): a randomized controlled trial. *Lancet* 2008; **371**: 1839–47.
10. Holt NF. Perioperative cardiac risk reduction. *Am Fam Physician* 2012; **85**: 239–46.
11. Redelmeier D, Scales D, Kopp A. Beta blockers for elective surgery in elderly patients: population based retrospective cohort study. *BMJ* 2005; **331**: 932–8.
12. Wallace AW, Au S, Cason BA. Perioperative β-blockade: atenolol is associated with reduced mortality when compared to metoprolol. *Anesthesiology* 2011; **114**: 824–36.
13. Feringa HH, Bax JJ, Boersma E, et al. High-dose beta-blockers and tight heart rate control reduce myocardial ischemia and troponin T release in vascular surgery patients. *Circulation* 2006; **114**: I344–9.
14. Stone J, Foëx P, Sear JW, et al. Myocardial ischemia in untreated hypertensive patients: effects of a single small dose of beta-adrenergic blocking agent. *Anesthesiology* 1988; **68**: 495–500.
15. Bangalore S, Wetterslev J, Pranesh S, et al. Perioperative beta blockers in patients having non-cardiac surgery: a meta-analysis. *Lancet* 2008; **372**: 1962–76.
16. Badgett RG, Lawrence VA, Cohn SL. Variations in pharmacology of beta-blockers may contribute to heterogeneous results in trials of perioperative beta-blockade. *Anesthesiology* 2010; **113**: 585–92.
17. Beattie WS, Wijeysundera DN, Karkouti K, et al. Acute surgical anemia influences the cardioprotective effects of beta-blockade: a single-center, propensity-matched cohort study. *Anesthesiology* 2010; **112**: 25–33.
18. Angeli F, Verdecchia P, Karthikeyan G, et al. Beta-blockers and risk of all-cause mortality in non-cardiac surgery. *Ther Adv Cardiovasc Dis* 2010; **4**: 109–18.
19. Leslie K, Myles P, Devereaux P, et al. Neuraxial block, death and serious cardiovascular morbidity in the POISE trial. *Br J Anaesth* 2013; **111**: 382–90.
20. Beattie WS, Wijeysundera DN, Karkouti K, et al. Does tight heart rate control improve beta-blocker efficacy? An updated analysis

of the noncardiac surgical randomized trials. *Anesth Analg* 2008; **106**: 1039–48.

21. Shammash JB, Trost JC, Gold JM, et al. Perioperative beta-blocker withdrawal and mortality in vascular surgery patients. *Am Heart J* 2001; **141**: 148–53.

22. Ponten J, Biber B, Bjurö T, et al. Beta-receptor blocker withdrawal. A preoperative problem in general surgery. *Acta Anaesthesiol Scand Supp* 1982; **76**: 32–7.

23. Psaty BM, Koepsell TD, Wagner EH, et al. The relative risk of incident coronary heart disease associated with recently stopping the use of beta-blockers. *JAMA* 1990; **263**: 1653–7.

24. Schonberger RB, Lukens CL, Turkoglu OD, et al. Beta-blocker withdrawal among patients presenting for surgery from home. *J Cardiothorac Vasc Anesth* 2012; **26**: 1029–33.

25. Bouri S, Shun-Shin MJ, Cole GD, et al. Meta-analysis of secure randomised controlled trials of β-blockade to prevent perioperative death in non-cardiac surgery. *Heart*. 2013 [Epub ahead of print].

26. Colson P, Ryckwaert F, Coriat P. Renin angiotensin system antagonists and anesthesia. *Anesth Analg* 1999; **89**:1143–55.

27. Brabant S, Bertrand M, Eyraud D, et al. The hemodynamic effects of anesthetic induction in vascular surgery patients chronically treated with angiotensin II receptor antagonists. *Anesth Analg* 1999; **88**: 1388–92.

28. Shear T, Greenberg S. Vasoplegic syndrome and renin-angiotensin system antagonists. *APSF Newsletter*, 2012; **27**.

29. Drenger B, Fontes ML, Miao Y, et al. Patterns of use of perioperative angiotensin-converting enzyme inhibitors in coronary artery bypass graft surgery with cardiopulmonary bypass – effects on in-hospital morbidity and mortality. *Circulation* 2012; **126**: 261–9.

30. Sear J, Howell SJ, Sear YM, et al. Intercurrent drug therapy and perioperative cardiovascular mortality in elective and urgent/emergent surgical patients. *Br J Anaesth* 2001; **86**: 506–12.

31. Kurzencwyg D, Filion KB, Pilote L, et al. Cardiac medical therapy among patients undergoing abdominal aortic aneurysm repair. *Ann Vasc Surg* 2006; **20**: 569–76.

32. Railton CJ, Wolpin J, Lam-McCulloch J, et al. Renin-angiotensin blockade is associated with increased mortality after vascular surgery. *Can J Anesth* 2010; **57**: 736–44.

33. Miceli A, Capoun R, Fino C, et al. Effects of angiotensin-converting enzyme inhibitor therapy on clinical outcome in patients undergoing coronary bypass grafting. *J Am Coll Cardiol* 2009; **54**: 1778–84.

34. Rader F, Van Wagoner DR, Gillinov AM, et al. Preoperative angiotensin-blocking drug therapy is not associated with atrial fibrillation after cardiac surgery. *Am Heart J* 2010; **160**: 329–36.

35. Arora P, Rajagopalam S, Ranjan R, et al. Preoperative use of angiotensin-converting enzyme inhibitors/angiotensin receptor blockers is associated with increased risk for acute kidney injury after cardiovascular surgery. *Clin J Am Soc Nephrol* 2008; **3**: 1266–73.

36. Che M, Li Y, Liang X, et al. Prevalence of acute kidney injury following cardiac surgery and related risk factors in Chinese patients. *Nephron Clin Pract* 2011; **117**: 305–11.

37. Turan A, You J, Shiba A, et al. Angiotensin converting enzyme inhibitors are not associated with respiratory complications or mortality after noncardiac surgery. *Anesthesiology* 2012; **114**: 552–660.

38. Corait P. Interactions between inhibitors of the renin angiotensin system and anesthesia, European Society of Anesthesiologists, Refresher Courses, Gothenburg, Apr 7, 2001.

39. Comfère T, Sprung J, Kumar MM, et al. Angiotensin system inhibitors in a general surgical population. *Anesth Analg* 2005; **100**: 636–44.

40. Goldstein S, Amar D. Pharmacotherapeutic considerations in Anesthesia. *Heart Dis* 2003; **5**: 34–48.

41. Hess W, Meyer C. Haemodynamic effects of nifedipine in patients undergoing

coronary artery bypass. *Acta Anaesthesiol Scand* 1986; **30**: 614–19.

42. Kates RA, Kaplan JA, Guyton RA, et al. Hemodynamic interactions of verapamil and isoflurane. *Anesthesiology* 1983; **59**: 132–8.

43. Schulte-Sasse U, Hess W, Markschies-Hornung A, et al. Combined effects of halothane anesthesia and verapamil on systemic hemodynamics and left ventricular myocardial contractility in patients with ischemic heart disease. *Anesth Analg* 1984; **63**: 791–8.

44. Bikhazi GB, Leung I, Flores C, et al. Potentiation of neuromuscular blocking agents by calcium channel blockers in rats. *Anesth Analg* 1988; **67**: 1–8.

45. Wiejeysundera DN, Beattie WS. Calcium channel blockers for reducing cardiac morbidity after noncardiac surgery: a meta-analysis. *Anesth Analg* 2003; **97**: 634–41.

46. Wijeysundera DN, Beattie WS, Rao V, et al. Calcium antagonists reduce cardiovascular complications after cardiac surgery: a meta-analysis. *J Am Coll Cardiol* 2003; **41**: 1496–505.

47. Wang CY, Liu PY, Liao JK. Pleiotropic effects of statin therapy: molecular mechanisms and clinical results. *Trends Mol Med* 2008; **14**: 37–44.

48. Liakopoulos OJ, Kuhn EW, Slottosch I, et al. Preoperative statin therapy for patients undergoing cardiac surgery. *Cochrane Database Syst Rev* 2012; **4**: CD008493.

49. Sanders RD, Nicholson A, Lewis SR, et al. Perioperative statin therapy for improving outcomes during and after noncardiac vascular surgery. *Cochrane Database Syst Rev* 2013; **7**: CD009971.

50. Chan WW, Wong GT, Irwin MG. Perioperative statin therapy. *Expert Opin Pharmacother* 2013; **14**: 832–42.

51. Chopra V, Wesorick DH, Sussman JB, et al. Effect of perioperative statins on death, myocardial infarction, atrial fibrillation and length of stay: a systematic review and meta-analysis. *Arch Surg* 2012; **147**: 181–9.

52. Wijeysundera DN, Bender JS, Beattie WS. Alpha-2 adrenergic agonists for the prevention of cardiac complications among patients undergoing surgery. *Cochrane Database Syst Rev* 2009; **4**: CD004126.

53. Devereaux PJ, Sessler DI, Leslie K, et al. Clonidine in patients undergoing non-cardiac surgery. *N Engl J Med* 2014; **370**: 1504–13.

54. Basile FV, Basile AR, Basile VV, et al. Use of selective serotonin reuptake inhibitors, antidepressants, and bleeding risk in breast cosmetic surgery. *Anesthetic Plast Surg* 2013; **37**: 561–6.

55. Auerbach AD, Vittinghoff E, Maselli J, et al. Perioperative use of selective serotonin reuptake inhibitors and risks for adverse outcomes of surgery. *JAMA* 2013; **173**: 1075–81.

56. Burda SA, Hobson D, Pronovost PJ. What is the patient really taking? Discrepancies between surgery and anesthesiology preoperative medication histories. *Qual Saf Health Care* 2005; **14**: 414–16.

57. Stratman RC, Wall MH. Implementation of a comprehensive drug safety program in the perioperative setting. *Int Anesthesiol Clin* 2011; **51**: 13–30.

58. Hale AR, Coombes ID, Stokes J, et al. Perioperative medication management expanding the role of the preadmission clinic pharmacist in a single centre randomized controlled trial of collaborative prescribing. *BMJ Open* 2013; **3**: e003027.

59. Roure Nuez C, González Navarro M, González Valdivieso J, et al. Effectiveness of a perioperative chronic medication reconciliation program in patients scheduled for elective surgery. *Med Clin (Barc)* 2012; **139**: 662–7.

Chapter 6

Perioperative optimization

I. McConachie

Perioperative optimization means different things to different people:

- It can refer to just medical optimization of comorbidities (e.g., appropriate control of blood pressure).
- It can refer to enhanced recovery after surgery (ERAS) protocols (see chapter on gastrointestinal [GI] surgery).
- It can refer to fluid-loading strategies while monitoring cardiac index (CI) – the cardiac output (CO) indexed to body surface area – or stroke volume, so as to optimize stroke volume intraoperatively.
- The original meaning (and still probably the most controversial) is the reference to Shoemaker's oxygen transport supranormal goals – mainly of CI, global oxygen delivery (DO_2), and oxygen consumption (VO_2).

All are important but it is the last meaning given here that this chapter will discuss. Later authors also used the term goal-directed therapy (GDT) to include the latter two definitions. "Perioperative" in this context usually refers to the intra- and postoperative period. Some authors have applied the approaches discussed later to the patient preoperatively, but this fell out of favor – for logistical reasons, if nothing else.

Oxygen transport

> Oxygen lack not only stops the machine but wrecks the machinery.
>
> J.S. Haldane (1860–1936)

DO_2 is the oxygen content of the arterial blood (CaO_2) multiplied by the blood flow or CO, as discussed in the chapter on anemia. Thus:

$$DO_2 = CO \times CaO_2$$
$$\text{i.e., } DO_2 = CO \times Hb \times SaO_2 \times 1.34$$

Normal DO_2, assuming 100% arterial oxygen saturation (SaO_2) therefore is:

$$5 \times 150 \times 1.34$$
$$= 5 \times 200$$
$$= \text{approx } 1000 \text{ mL/min}$$

Anesthesia and Perioperative Care of the High-Risk Patient, Third edition, ed. Ian McConachie. Published by Cambridge University Press.

If CI is used, the resultant DO_2 is also indexed to body surface area.

i.e., DO_2 = approx. 600 mL/min/m^2.

Adequate DO_2 is achieved by attention to cardiac function, hemoglobin (Hb), and oxygenation. Normal mixed venous oxyhemoglobin saturation (SVO_2) is 75% (68%–77%), and therefore venous oxygen content (CvO_2) is 150 mL. Oxygen consumption (VO_2) of the whole body (indexed) is therefore:

$VO_2 = CI \times (CaO_2 - CvO_2)$

= approx 150 mL/min/m^2

Shoemaker's supranormal goals

The team led by W.C. Shoemaker (a surgeon initially but a founding father of Critical Care and first editor of the journal *Critical Care Medicine*) identified values of CI, DO_2 and VO_2, and blood volume, retrospectively associated with increased survival of trauma and high-risk surgical patients [1]. These flow-related values were found to be more predictive of mortality compared to conventional vital signs such as blood pressure and heart rate.

Further non-randomized trials by the same group confirmed that these higher values in surviving patients were associated with improved survival. They proposed that if patients could achieve these goals prospectively with the administration of intravenous fluids and/or positive inotropes, outcome and survival may be improved.

The goals were:

$CI > 4.5$ L/min/m^2
$DO_2 > 600$ mL/min/m^2
$VO_2 > 170$ mL/min/m^2

Shoemaker's group reported several non-randomized studies looking at these physiological values associated with increased chance of survival and the effect of achieving these goals prospectively on patient outcome. For the prospective studies, they advocated additional goals of a normal blood pressure and a blood volume estimated as >500 mL greater than normal, as long as pulmonary capillary wedge pressure was not >20 mmHg; that is, patients were adequately fluid loaded without being overloaded.

Arguably, his most influential study [2] was a randomized trial published in 1988, which showed an impressive reduction in mortality from 33% in the control group to 4% in the treatment group, and a significant reduction in organ failures especially renal failure. This study was criticized for low patient numbers, poor randomization details and details of management of the control groups, and concern was expressed at the seemingly high mortality in the control group. Indeed, there was some difficulty in getting the study published. Nevertheless, the study was hugely influential (and controversial, even divisive) and prompted further studies from many institutions. Similar protocols were eagerly adopted by many intensive care units (ICUs) and many practitioners (including the author) have recollections in the late 1980s and early 1990s of calculating DO_2 and VO_2 from CI measurements from a pulmonary artery catheter (PAC) and oxygen content from a co-oximeter. Why did we stop? This will be addressed later.

A key concept at the time was that of "oxygen supply dependency" or that the patient's VO_2 was directly linked to the available DO_2 – such that increasing the patient's DO_2 would be expected to promote an increase in VO_2. Later opinion would be that much of this evidence came from "mathematical coupling" (the same variables involved in measuring both DO_2 and VO_2). In addition, the importance of VO_2 as a goal was challenged by observations that sedation [3] and patient temperature [4] directly influenced the patient's VO_2. Thus, later studies, such as by Boyd et al. [5], did not include VO_2 as one of their optimal goals. The emphasis turned to optimizing flow to the tissues.

What is a high-risk patient?

It is perhaps interesting to review the criteria for being considered high-risk. Shoemaker, in his original papers, defined what he considered to be high-risk surgical patients [2]. Many studies have used these criteria:

Previous severe cardiorespiratory illness, e.g., acute myocardial infarction or chronic obstructive airways disease
Extensive ablative surgery planned for malignancy, e.g., gastrectomy, esophagectomy, or surgery of >6 h
Multiple trauma, e.g., more than three organ injury, more than two systems or opening two body cavities
Massive acute hemorrhage, e.g., more than eight units
Age >70 years and limited physiological reserve of one or more organs
Septicemia (positive blood cultures or septic focus), WCC >13, pyrexia to 38.3 °C for 48 h
Respiratory failure (PaO_2 <8 kPa on an FiO_2 >0.4 or mechanical ventilation >48 h)
Acute abdominal catastrophe with hemodynamic instability, e.g., pancreatitis, perforated viscus, peritonitis, GI bleed
Acute renal failure: urea >20 mmol/L, creatinine >260 mmol/L
Late-stage vascular disease involving aortic disease
Shock, e.g., MAP < 60 mmHg, CVP <15 cm H_2O, urine output < 20 mL/h

There are many definitions of "high-risk" but few would argue that these are challenging patients indeed!

Normal may not be enough

Thus, the initial proposed concept was that "normal" physiological values in the postoperative period somehow are not sufficient for an optimal outcome. Why might normal not be enough?

Reduced organ reserve

- Invasive monitoring of elderly surgical patients reveals a high incidence of "hidden" abnormalities reflecting their reduced physiological reserve – even in patients "cleared" for surgery [6]. This has been known for many decades.

- Also known for many decades is that patients who fail to maintain CO postoperatively have poor outcome [7].
- There may be interesting parallels with patients with multiple trauma. One study in the elderly [8] emphasized the importance of early detection of cardiac dysfunction by invasive monitoring using a pulmonary artery catheter. Delays in monitoring cardiac output, and therefore delays in administering inotropic therapy, were associated with very low survival rates compared to similar patients with early monitoring, who had low COs that were detected and inotropic support provided. The message is clear: elderly trauma patients may have dangerously low CO unrecognized by noninvasive monitoring. If this is left untreated, cardiogenic shock and organ failure may supervene. Further studies on younger trauma patients have shown similar results with comparable conclusions [9].

The wound as an organ

- A wound is metabolically active with a resultant requirement for increased VO_2 and glucose oxidation – the concept of "the wound as an organ." In addition to the local reasons for increased metabolic demands, there are systemic inflammatory and catabolic causes of increased metabolic demand requiring an increased CO compared to normal. This may imply a need for increased CO and DO_2 in trauma and high-risk surgical patients.
- Animal studies clearly support this concept, showing that an injured leg has considerably increased blood flow, VO_2, and glucose oxidation compared to noninjured legs in the same animal.
- Thus, in metabolic terms, having major abdominal surgery may be the same as having a second liver grafted onto the body.

Intraoperative oxygen debt

- Even when DO_2 is well maintained, VO_2 falls under anesthesia. Anesthesia reduces metabolic rate and oxygen demand but tissue oxygen extraction may be reduced (especially in the presence of sepsis) and microcirculatory organ blood flow may be altered. Anesthetic cardiac depression, failure to maintain adequate fluid levels during surgery, and perhaps hypothermia also potentiate an oxygen supply demand imbalance at the tissue level.
- An oxygen debt may develop, especially if there are falls in CO and/or DO_2 below a critical level [10]. Worryingly, the reduction of tissue oxygen extraction under anesthesia may decrease the threshold for oxygen deliveryDO_2 to be "critical" [11]; that is, lesser degrees of fall in CO and DO_2 may result in tissue hypoxia. This has obvious implications for anesthesia of the critically ill or shocked patient, in whom maintenance of CO and DO_2 are crucial.
- It is well recognized that surgical patients develop an intraoperative "oxygen debt." Patients who rapidly reverse their oxygen debt have a good outcome, but slow oxygen debt resolution is associated with increased risk of postoperative organ failure, and very slow or incomplete resolution is associated with an increased risk of debt [12,13].
- It is postulated therefore that achieving supranormal oxygen transport goals intraoperatively may limit this oxygen debt and promote its early reversal.

Limitations of concept

- The main flaw in the whole concept is that global measurements of CO and DO_2 take little notice of regional disturbances in organ flow and/or microcirculatory disturbances.
- The best evidence for a beneficial therapeutic effect of maximizing oxygen transport is from studies where therapy was initiated very early in the presence of tissue hypoperfusion, that is, pre- or intraoperatively in high-risk surgical patients [3], and before organ dysfunction has developed.
- GDT is too late to be effective once organ failure has occurred. Dead cells do not recover, no matter how much oxygen is supplied to them! Shoemaker said in his lectures "Pay me now or pay me later–but if you pay me later you don't get your money's worth"–referring to a reluctance by some to spend money on insertion of a PAC early versus the increased costs (and poor outcomes) of admitting patients to ICU with established organ failure that might have been preventable.

Responses within a patient population

Within a patient population there will be four groups of patients:

- Spontaneous achievement of goals as part of physiological responses to surgery. This is a confounding factor in some studies; that is, some patients in the control study group will spontaneously achieve study goals.
- Goals achieved with fluids only: these patients intuitively should achieve a good result compared to those patients who require inotropic support to achieve their goals as it implies a well-functioning myocardium able to meet the oxygen demands following surgery.
- Goals requiring inotropic support: conversely, the need for inotropic support implies lack of myocardial reserve to be able to easily meet the oxygen demands following surgery.
- Goals not achieved: this could be because of poor application of the protocol, that is, too little fluid or too little vasoactive support, or because the patient does not respond to the therapy. Either way, the potential benefit of the protocol is lessened and outcome may be poor. Excessive use of inotropes may promote myocardial ischemia.

Supranormal goals and myocardial ischemia

- It now seems that this approach may be detrimental in some groups of patients, such as the elderly in whom attempts to aggressively raise CI with positive inotropic drugs may result in tachycardia, promoting myocardial ischemia [14].
- A thought-provoking review points out that there are conflicting priorities in managing surgical patients at risk of myocardial ischemia and those in whom the cardiac output and oxygen delivery need to be increased [15]. Both are at risk of an adverse outcome, but the approach is different and identification of the group to which patients belong is important.
- Thus, this approach cannot be recommended universally but there may be benefits in specific groups, such as high-risk surgical patients, when applied perioperatively.

The literature on supranormal goals

It is over 30 years since the original Shoemaker studies. There are now many studies that have been published, addressing supranormal goals in surgical patients (and others in general critically ill and trauma patients). There is perhaps little merit in listing them all here. For a more exhaustive discussion of these studies, the reader is directed to the various reviews and meta-analyses already published [16–22]. Four recent reviews and meta-analyses are of particular interest:

- In 2011, Hamilton reviewed the optimization literature [19], concluding that, overall, GDT reduced both mortality and complication rates. The most significant improvements in mortality were seen in the early studies and in patients at highest risk of death (as stratified by predicted control group mortalities). Complications were reduced in all patients.
- A meta-analysis of five studies of hemodynamic optimization cardiac surgery patients showed an overall beneficial effect on complication rates and postoperative length of hospital stay – but not on overall mortality [20]. The lack of effect on mortality is perhaps not surprising given the overall low mortality in cardiac surgery patients – two studies reported no mortality!
- In surgical patients, another recent meta-analysis recommends more widespread use of early GDT after finding that it significantly reduces the incidence of surgical infections [21].
- A recent systematic review is the most scientifically rigorous examination in the literature [22]. The overall conclusion was that perioperative optimization overall did not result in a significant decrease in mortality but did lead to a reduction in the rate of postoperative complications and postoperative length of stay (on average, one day less). Further analysis showed that smaller studies tended to show reduced mortality and that well-controlled studies where specific goals were defined for both groups, but with lesser values as goals in the control group (i.e., "normal" as opposed to "supranormal"), found no reductions in mortality.

With regard to postoperative organ failure specifically, many studies have included organ failure incidences as part of their outcome criteria. Two meta-analyses have particularly examined the effect of perioperative optimization on organ failures.

- In the first [23], the use of perioperative optimization was associated with a significant reduction in the incidence of major GI complications – ascribed by the authors as being due to organ protection in the increased flow group.
- Perioperative optimization using fluids and inotropes was associated in the more recent meta-analysis with a reduction in the incidence of renal dysfunction and need for renal replacement therapy [24].

The pulmonary artery catheter

- Perioperative optimization of cardiac function and oxygen transport obviously will require invasive monitoring of cardiac function – commonly with the aid of a PAC in early studies.
- The discussion over the appropriateness of perioperative optimization via supranormal goals in the 1990s became only a part of the discussion on the use of the PAC.

- Perioperative use of the PAC is controversial, with studies casting doubt on the role of the PAC in elective high-risk surgery. For example, there is no benefit from the pulmonary artery flotation catheter (PAFC) for routine coronary artery bypass grafting (CABG) surgery [25]. Even in ICU patients, there is no convincing evidence of benefit (but no convincing evidence of harm either) arising from the use of the PAFC [26]. The American Society of Anesthesiologists (ASA) has published guidelines for its perioperative use [27].
- More recent studies have utilized other methods of measuring CI and stroke volume, for example, by such as arterial pressure pulse analysis, lithium dilution, and esophageal Doppler. For example, a recent study [28] utilized radial arterial pulse contour analysis as their guide for therapy and showed a reduction in the complication rates in the treatment group.

Tailored fluid therapy

The administration of intravenous (IV) fluids titrated to optimize stroke volume using the esophageal Doppler monitor has been shown to shorten postoperative length of stay, and reduce complications and overall morbidity in several studies of surgical patients [29–31]. Stroke volume and flow are maximized while also avoiding fluid overload with its potential detrimental effects (see the chapter on GI surgery). The administration of IV fluids needs to be not too much and not too little but just right – the Goldilocks approach.

Choice of inotrope: dopexamine

- Many early studies were peformed using dobutamine as the standard positive inotropic drug. Epinephrine has also been used.
- Dopexamine is a positive inotropic drug with significant β_2-agonist activity as well as β_1- and dopaminergic receptor activity, which has been used in many countries worldwide. It might be predicted that dopexamine would improve splanchnic blood flow, but evidence is mainly from animal studies.
- Boyd [5], in his study on perioperative optimization, showed improvements in survival in the high-oxygen delivery group. It was later suggested that the improvement may have been related to the choice of inotrope – dopexamine – rather than the cardiac output achieved in the patients.
- Catecholamines may have differing effects on inflammation, such as β_1 stimulation may be proinflammatory while α_1 and β_2 stimulation may be anti-inflammatory. This adds a whole new dimension to a debate on choice of inotropic drug! The most interesting aspect of dopexamine and the most controversial is the suggestion that dopexamine may have specific anti-inflammatory properties [32]. Animal studies clearly show [33] that dopexamine reduces the inflammatory response in a laparotomy/endotoxin model without changing hemodynamics or regional blood flow.
- Wilson et al.'s study [34] included three groups – a control group managed conventionally and two other groups who were admitted preoperatively to ICU and given GDT with either epinephrine or dopexamine. Both the treatment groups had significantly improved survival rate; however, only the dopexamine group saw a significant reduction in morbidity. This is particularly interesting because the dopexamine-treated group did not see an increase in CI by as much as the

epinephrine-treated group. The reduced morbidity was due to a reduction in sepsis and acute respiratory distress syndrome (ARDS).

- However, a follow-up study from the same group found no apparent benefit from dopexamine in surgical patients [35] (although perhaps there was a benefit in both groups from volume loading).
- This echoed a multicenter European study, which also failed to find any benefit from the routine perioperative use of dopexamine in elective surgery [36]. However, the authors suggested, based on subgroup analysis and stratification according to the number of risk factors, that dopexamine should be tested further in patients at higher risk of complications or undergoing emergency surgery. This supports Shoemaker's contention that benefits will only be seen when the patients are sick enough and/or the control group have a high enough mortality to enable a benefit to be shown [18].
- Further disappointment from the use of dopexamine came from a study [37] that found no extra benefit from dopexamine when IV fluids were given to optimize stroke volume. No differences were seen in mortality or morbidity – but the dopexamine group tolerated enteral diet sooner.

Optimization in critical illness

- Results of studies of supranormal goals in the general ICU population – chiefly patients with sepsis – have been even more mixed. Arguably, this approach is less likely to be effective in patients with established organ failure; that is, in many ICU patients mortality may not be improved [14,38].
- Conversely, an important study by Rivers et al. [39] studied the early implementation of GDT titrated to SVO_2 and serum lactate values – flow dependent physiological variables. Crucially, the patients were identified and enrolled in the study on admission to the emergency room, very early in the course of their illness and before the onset of organ failures. The patients were treated with blood transfusion, fluids, and positive inotropic drugs to achieve their goals. Early interventions in these patients resulted in a significant improvement in mortality and fewer organ failures. There are interesting parallels between this study and the previously mentioned studies on trauma patients [8,9].
- This approach has been validated in a larger multicenter study from China [40], which essentially replicated the findings of Rivers et al.
- Again, the message is: early detection and intervention is important in optimizing outcome.

Optimization in trauma

- Bishop et al. showed that reaching supranormal circulatory values, especially within 24 h of injury, improved survival and reduced organ failures in severely traumatized patients [41].
- A study of injured patients with shock found no difference in overall survival between those resuscitated to "normal" hemodynamic values (including CO) and those resuscitated to "supranormal" values (including increased CO and DO_2) [42]. Interestingly, many of the young trauma patients in the "normal" group spontaneously

achieved the goals of the "supranormal" study group. Achievement of these supranormal goals, in whichever patient group, was associated with improved survival.

- Durham et al. [43] also found that resuscitation of trauma patients according to oxygen transport principles did not influence outcome. Again, the achievement of supranormal oxygen transport values in young patients was an important predictor of survival. This suggest that, in trauma patients, oxygen transport physiological variables may be more important as predictors of outcome than goals of resuscitation.
- The administration of large volumes of crystalloid to multiple trauma patients in an attempt to boost oxygen transport goals was found, in a retrospective study, to increase the incidence of abdominal compartment syndrome, impair indices of splanchnic perfusion, and increase mortality [44].

Perioperative optimization or perioperative optimism? Why are we not all doing this to all our surgical patients?

A survey of the ASA and European Society of Anesthesiology (ESA) members [45] revealed that only 34% monitored CO during high-risk surgery. Clearly, the profession remains unconvinced. There are several reasons why this approach has not been more widely adopted.

Early studies were often flawed

- Many of the early studies were arguably flawed: retrospective, poor, or no blinding, lack of a protocol to control therapy in control groups, and small sample sizes.
- In some studies the therapeutic goals were not always reached in the treatment group (see earlier discussion for reasons why goals may not have been attained). In addition, some patients in control groups spontaneously achieved the "goals" (also see earlier).
- Skepticism was expressed because of seemingly inappropriately high mortality in control groups.

The world has changed

- More modern reasons for skepticism over the early trial is that studies performed 20 to 30 years ago do not reflect current practice with the recent growth in laparoscopic minimally invasive surgery, improvements in anesthetic drugs, and techniques and growth of acute pain services with improvements in postoperative pain relief. Compared to 20 to 30 years ago, it is now routine to try to identify (although not always successfully) high-risk patients, to monitor them postoperatively in high care areas, and to pay close attention to fluid balance with increasing recognition of the dangers in GI surgery, for example, of fluid overload – a polite term for drowning.
- Thus studies from the 1980s and 1990s are not necessarily reflective of current practice and their results not able to be replicated, as "usual care" has evolved greatly.

Trials were often not comparable

- Different trials would have various case mixes with different surgeries being performed within and between studies, patients had differing comorbidities, and the surgeries would have different expected mortality outcomes.

- Trials included patients with and without cancer – cancer surgery, with its variable prognosis depending on cancer type and progression, adds another prognostic variable into the mix.
- The technique of CO or CI measurement varied – in the early days it was usually a PAC, with later studies measuring CO with less invasive techniques.
- Goals varied and included CO, DO_2, and stroke volume. Primary outcomes were also different – usually involving mortality and organ failures but also length of hospital stay and infectious complications.
- Studies of patients who would not be predicted to have a reasonably high baseline mortality for the proposed surgery are unlikely to show a statistically significant difference in outcomes – the vast majority of patients in both groups will do well.

Why do all studies not show benefit?

- Although initial studies of perioperative optimization were promising, others attempted to apply these goals in other groups of patients with less success. Why should this be so?
- Firstly, neither Shoemaker nor anyone else ever said that this approach was appropriate for all surgical patients (or indeed all ICU patients), or that adoption of these goals as a therapeutic strategy guaranteed survival.
- An alternative question could be why does this approach not benefit all patients? For benefit to be seen, optimization must be performed in very high-risk patients with a reasonably high expected baseline mortality, or one will not see differences in outcome – the vast majority of patients in both groups will do well.
- Indeed, patients who are identified as being very fit aerobically may actually do worse with GDT! An interesting study [46] was performed on patients undergoing major surgery who assessed as either aerobically fit or unfit, based on cardiopulmonary exercise testing (CPET). The authors' hypothesis was that goal-directed fluid therapy to optimize stroke volume would improve outcomes in the unfit patients but not benefit the fit patients. Surprisingly, they found that the fit patients who received GDT actually had a worse outcome – an increased length of hospital stay compared to the fit patients who received control therapy. Perhaps the extra fluid that the GDT patients received (but may not have needed) in the fit patients increased complications.
- High-risk patients undergoing brief or minor surgery may also not benefit – because of a lesser magnitude of oxygen debt. Studies of patients who would not be predicted to have a reasonably high baseline mortality for the proposed surgery are unlikely to show a statistically significant difference in outcomes.
- The best evidence for a beneficial therapeutic effect of maximizing oxygen transport is from studies where therapy was initiated very early in the presence of tissue hypoperfusion, that is, preoperatively in high-risk surgical patients [5].

Bringing it all together

The crucial message is that high-risk surgical patients may have reduced cardiac reserves, especially in the elderly, suffer occult tissue hypoperfusion with a developing oxygen debt postoperatively, proceed to multiple organ failure if there is no intervention to reverse the tissue hypoperfusion, and have a higher mortality than patients who do have sufficient reserves to reverse their oxygen debt and prevent serious tissue hypoxia.

A key issue may be timing – improvements in outcome may be seen when patients are treated early to achieve optimal goals before the development of organ failure, and when therapy produces differences in oxygen delivery between the control and protocol groups. One conclusion from this discussion is clear, when the patients are not "high-risk" and the expected mortality from surgery is low, there will be little benefit from perioperative optimization.

The concepts discussed in this chapter have relevance to an overall approach to the high-risk surgical patient and tie in to concepts explored in other chapters in this text.

For example:

- CPET – detect reduced cardiopulmonary reserve. Some studies [37] have used CPET criteria to identify patients who will receive GDT
- elderly patient with reduced organ reserves and muscle wasting (sarcopenia)
- prehabilitation and exercise to improve aerobic capacity and muscle function
- identification of cardiac and respiratory pathology
- optimization of cardiac and respiratory function
- improvement in oxygen carrying capacity by treatment of anemia
- undetected oxygen debt and inadequate organ blood flow,which results in postoperative deterioration
- prevention of decreases in respiratory function by adequate analgesia and regional anesthesia, for example.
- Avoidance of intraoperative hypothermia, which potentially increases oxygen debt, and postoperative shivering, which increases oxygen demand
- ERAS protocols for GI surgery, which include optimizing fluid loading to maintain stroke volume

The future?

There may still be a place for perioperative optimization but timing is crucial. The very high-risk patient undergoing major surgery may benefit, but fluid loading and/or use of inotropic support must be commenced intraoperatively and goals achieved without promoting fluid overload or myocardial ischemia. It will be important to identify appropriately patients at high risk of death. This is a relatively small group of patients – Pearse et al. showed [47] that the vast majority of all postoperative deaths come from a small group of patients who are identifiable preoperatively as being very high-risk. Perhaps CPET may help guide those patients who would benefit from perioperative optimization. It is also important to identify those patients unlikely to benefit from this approach – low-risk patients having low-risk surgery and the physically fit patient [46].

A global approach to treating all patients the same (as advocated in the original Shoemaker studies) has been (and should be) replaced by a more individualized approach based on age, physiology, and titrated therapy.

National organizations, for example in the U.K., are advocating individualized goal-directed fluid strategies [48]. The widespread adoption of ERAS protocols and their inclusion of goal-directed fluid therapy may therefore encourage a resurgence of interest in perioperative optimization. In truth, it has never completely gone away.

References

1. Shoemaker WC. Relation of oxygen transport patterns to the pathophysiology and therapy of shock states. *Intensive Care Med* 1987; **13**: 230–43.
2. Shoemaker WC, Appel PL, Kram HB, et al. Prospective trial of supranormal values of survivors as therapeutic goals in high-risk surgical patients. *Chest* 1988; **94**: 1176–86.
3. Boyd O, Grounds RM, Bennett ED. The dependency of oxygen consumption on oxygen delivery in critically ill postoperative patients is mimicked by variations in sedation. *Chest* 1992; **101**: 1619–24.
4. McConachie I, Edwards JD, Nightingale P, et al. The relationship between central temperature and oxygen consumption in critically ill patients. *Intensive Care Med* 1990; **16**: S57.
5. Boyd O, Grounds RM, Bennett ED. A randomized clinical trial of the effect of deliberate perioperative increase of oxygen delivery on mortality in high-risk surgical patients. *JAMA* 1993; **270**: 2699–707.
6. Del Guercio LRN, Cohn JD. Monitoring operative risk in the elderly. *JAMA* 1980; **297**: 845–50.
7. Boyd AD, Tremblay RE, Spencer FC, et al. Estimation of cardiac output soon after intracardiac surgery with cardio pulmonary bypass. *Ann Surg* 1959; **150**: 613–25.
8. Scalea TM, Simon HM, Duncan AO, et al. Geriatric blunt multiple trauma: improved survival with early invasive monitoring. *J Trauma* 1990; **30**: 129–34.
9. Abou-Khalil B, Scalea TM, Trooskin SZ, et al. Hemodynamic responses to shock in young trauma patients: need for invasive monitoring. *Crit Care Med* 1994; **22**: 633–9.
10. Lugo G, Arizpe D, Dominguez G. Relationship between oxygen consumption and oxygen delivery during anesthesia in high-risk surgical patients. *Crit Care Med* 1993; **21**: 64–9.
11. Van der Linden P,. Schmartz D, Gilbart E, et al. Effects of propofol, etomidate, and pentobarbital on critical oxygen delivery. *Crit Care Med* 2000; **28**: 2492–9.
12. Shoemaker WC, Appel PL, Kram HB. Role of oxygen debt in the development of organ failure sepsis, and death in high-risk surgical patients. *Chest* 1992; **102**: 208–15.
13. Hess W, Frank C, Hornburg B. Prolonged oxygen debt after abdominal aortic surgery. *J Cardiothorac Vasc Anesth* 1997; **11**: 149–54.
14. Hayes MA, Timmins AC, Yau EH, et al. Elevation of systemic oxygen delivery in the treatment of critically ill patients. *N Engl J Med* 1994; **330**: 1717–22.
15. Juste RN, Lawson AD, Soni N. Minimising cardiac anaesthetic risk: the tortoise or the hare? *Anaesthesia* 1996; **51**: 255–62.
16. Boyd O, Bennett ED.Enhancement of perioperative tissue perfusion as a therapeutic strategy for major surgery. *New Horizons* 1996; **4**: 453–65.
17. Heyland DK, Cook DJ, King D, et al. Maximizing oxygen delivery in critically ill patients: a methodologic appraisal of the evidence. *Crit Care Med* 1996; **24**: 517–24.
18. Kern JW, Shoemaker WC. Meta-analysis of hemodynamic optimization in high-risk patients. *Crit Care Med* 2002; **30**: 1686–92.
19. Hamilton MA, Cecconi M, Rhodes A. A systematic review and meta-analysis on the use of preemptive hemodynamic intervention to improve postoperative outcomes in moderate and high-risk surgical patients. *Anesth Analg* 2011; **112**: 1392–402.
20. Aya HD, Cecconi M, Hamilton M, et al. Goal-directed therapy in cardiac surgery: a systematic review and meta-analysis. *Br J Anaesth* 2013; **110**: 510–17.
21. Dalfino L, Giglio MT, Puntillo F, et al. Haemodynamic goal-directed therapy and postoperative infections: earlier is better. A systematic review and meta-analysis. *Crit Care* 2011; **15**: R154.
22. Grocott MP, Dushianthan A, Hamilton MA, et al. Perioperative increase in global blood flow to explicit defined goals and outcomes after surgery: a Cochrane Systematic Review. *Br J Anaesth* 2013; **111**: 535–48.

23. Giglio MT, Marucci M, Testini M, et al. Goal-directed haemodynamic therapy and gastrointestinal complications in major surgery: a meta-analysis of randomized controlled trials. *Br J Anaesth* 2009; **103**: 637–46.

24. Brienza N, Giglio MT, Marucci M, et al. Does perioperative hemodynamic optimization protect renal function in surgical patients? A meta-analytic study. *Crit Care Med* 2009; **37**: 2079–90.

25. Tuman KJ, McCarthy RJ, Spiess BD, et al. Effect of pulmonary artery catheterization on outcome in patients undergoing coronary artery surgery. *Anesthesiology* 1989; **70**: 199–206.

26. Harvey S, Harrison DA, Singer M, et al. Assessment of the clinical effectiveness of pulmonary artery catheters in management of patients in intensive care (PAC-Man): a randomised controlled trial. *Lancet* 2005; **366**: 472–7.

27. American Society of Anesthesiologists Task Force on Pulmonary Artery Catheterization. Practice guidelines for pulmonary artery catheterization: an updated report by the American Society of Anesthesiologists Task Force on Pulmonary Artery Catheterization. *Anesthesiology* 2003; **99**: 988–1014.

28. Salzwedel C, Puig J, Carstens A, et al. Perioperative goal-directed hemodynamic therapy based on radial arterial pulse pressure variation and continuous cardiac index trending reduces postoperative complications after major abdominal surgery: a multi-center, prospective, randomized study. *Crit Care* 2013; **17**: R191.

29. Mythen MG, Webb AR. Perioperative plasma volume expansion reduces the incidence of gut mucosal hypoperfusion during cardiac surgery. *Arch Surg* 1995; **130**: 423–9.

30. Sinclair S, James S, Singer M. Intraoperative intravascular volume optimisation and length of hospital stay after repair of proximal femoral fracture: randomised controlled trial. *BMJ* 1997; **315**: 909–12.

31. Noblett SE, Snowden CP, Shenton BK, et al. Randomized clinical trial assessing the effect of Doppler-optimized fluid management on outcome after elective colorectal resection. *Br J Surg* 2006; **93**: 1069–76.

32. Hollenberg SM. Dopexamine: immunomodulatory, hemodynamic, or both? *Crit Care* 2013; **17**: 143.

33. Bangash MN, Patel NS, Benetti E, et al. Dopexamine can attenuate the inflammatory response and protect against organ injury in the absence of significant effects on hemodynamics or regional microvascular flow. *Crit Care* 2013; **17**: R57.

34. Wilson J, Woods I, Fawcett J, et al. Reducing the risk of major elective surgery: randomised controlled trial of preoperative optimisation of oxygen delivery. *BMJ* 1999; **318**: 1099–103.

35. Stone MD, Wilson RJ, Cross J, et al. Effect of adding dopexamine to intraoperative volume expansion in patients undergoing major elective abdominal surgery. *Br J Anaesth* 2003; **91**: 619–24.

36. Takala J, Meier-Hellmann A, Eddleston J, et al. Effect of dopexamine on outcome after major abdominal surgery: a prospective, randomized, controlled multicenter study. European Multicenter Study Group on Dopexamine in Major Abdominal Surgery. *Crit Care Med* 2000; **28**: 3417–23.

37. Davies SJ, Yates D, Wilson RJ. Dopexamine has no additional benefit in high-risk patients receiving goal-directed fluid therapy undergoing major abdominal surgery. *Anesth Analg* 2011; **112**: 130–8.

38. Gattinoni L, Brazzi L, Pelosi P, et al. A trial of goal-oriented hemodynamic therapy in critically ill patients. SvO_2 Collaborative Group. *N Engl J Med* 1995; **333**: 1025–32.

39. Rivers E, Nguyen B, Havstad S, et al. Early goal-directed therapy in the treatment of severe sepsis and septic shock. *N Engl J Med* 2001; **345**: 1368–77.

40. Early Goal-Directed Therapy Collaborative Group of Zhejiang Province. The effect of early goal-directed therapy on treatment of

critical patients with severe sepsis/septic shock: a multi-center, prospective, randomized, controlled study. *[Article in Chinese] Zhongguo Wei Zhong Bing Ji Jiu Yi Xue* 2010; **22**: 331–4.

41. Bishop MH, Shoemaker WC, Appel PL, et al. Relationship between supranormal circulatory values, time delays, and outcome in severely traumatized patients. *Crit Care Med* 1993; **21**: 56–63.
42. Velmahos GC, Demetriades D, Shoemaker WC, et al. Endpoints of resuscitation of critically injured patients: normal or supranormal? A prospective randomized trial. *Ann Surg* 2000; **232**: 409–18.
43. Durham R, Neunaber K, Mazuski J, et al. The use of oxygen consumption and delivery as endpoints for resuscitation in critically ill patients. *J Trauma* 1996; **41**: 32–40.
44. Balogh Z, McKinley BA, Cocanour CS, et al. Supranormal trauma resuscitation causes more cases of abdominal compartment syndrome. *Arch Surg* 2003; **138**: 637–42.
45. Cannesson M, Pestel G, Ricks C, et al. Hemodynamic monitoring and management in patients undergoing high risk surgery: a survey among North American and European anesthesiologists. *Crit Care* 2011; **15**: R197.
46. Challand C, Struthers R, Sneyd JR, et al. Randomized controlled trial of intraoperative goal-directed fluid therapy in aerobically fit and unfit patients having major colorectal surgery. *Br J Anaesth* 2012; **108**: 53–62.
47. Pearse RM, Harrison DA, James P, et al. Identification and characterisation of the high-risk surgical population in the United Kingdom. *Crit Care* 2006; **10**: R81.
48. Intraoperative fluid management. Available from: http://iofm.innovation.nhs.uk/pg/dashboard (Accessed December 5, 2013.)

Chapter 7

Respiratory risk and assessment

J. Cooke, A. Schlachter, and M. Yoder

Postoperative pulmonary complications are highly important considerations that can impact evaluation for surgery and anesthesia. While the incidence of such complications is widely reported, ranging from 5% to 70%, their morbidity can be profound and hospital length of stay significantly increased. In fact, the severity can be such that pulmonary complications result in about one quarter of all deaths occurring within six days of surgery. While more intuitively considered to be prevalent in thoracic operations (particularly lung resection), postoperative pulmonary complications can occur commonly in non-thoracic procedures as well. Defining such complications can be difficult, however; postoperative pulmonary complications can be as mild as a dry cough and dyspnea to as severe as respiratory failure requiring new or prolonged mechanical ventilation. Imperative in attempting to minimize postoperative pulmonary complications is being able to identify at-risk patients and aim to minimize risk in the pre-, intra-, and postoperative time frames. This review intends to discuss these aforementioned topics briefly as well as the rationale and data behind the current approach to perioperative respiratory risk and assessment.

Perioperative pulmonary physiology

Normal pulmonary physiology is subjected to significant changes both due to general anesthesia (GA) and during the postoperative phase.

GA and neuromuscular blockade can lead to significant derangements in pulmonary physiology and, additionally, patients cannot mount a normal physiological response to either hypoxemia or hypercapnia while under the effects of these agents.

- Both anesthetic agents and neuromuscular blockers lead to diaphragm and chest wall relaxation. This leads to a marked reduction in functional residual capacity and thoracic volume.
- Decreases in lung volume tend to cause atelectasis in dependent lung regions and this can persist for up to 24 hours in approximately half of patients.
- Prolonged atelectasis will lead to ventilation–perfusion (V/Q) mismatching and shunting, which in turn can cause hypoxemia.
- As stated earlier, significant decreases in the vital capacity and functional residual capacity occur in thoracic and upper abdominal surgery and usually persist into the early postoperative phase.

Anesthesia and Perioperative Care of the High-Risk Patient, Third edition, ed. Ian McConachie.
Published by Cambridge University Press.

- These changes occur due to contributions from diaphragmatic dysfunction, postoperative pain, and splinting.
- A complex interplay of reflex mechanisms from sympathetic, vagal, and splanchnic receptors is postulated to decrease output to phrenic nerves following upper abdominal surgery. This can cause patients to rely on accessory muscles of respiration more so than usual. This reflex inhibition is attenuated with the use of epidural anesthesia (EA), however.
- Patients tend to be capable of maintaining minute ventilation; however, as tidal volume decreases, this must be accomplished by increasing respiratory rate.
- Such a respiratory pattern, particularly when paired with residual medication effects of anesthesia and narcotics for pain control, leads to impaired cough and thereby mucociliary clearance and ultimately an increased risk of postoperative pneumonia.

Patient- and procedure-related risk factors

An individual patient's risk of sustaining a postoperative complication derives from the interaction between characteristics of the patient (medical conditions, general health status) and features of the planned procedure (anesthesia and surgical technique). Some of these factors are modifiable, or their impact can at least be minimized by preoperative identification and perioperative intervention.

Patient-related risk factors

- Age appears to be an independent risk factor for postoperative pulmonary complications [1]. This conclusion is controversial, as several studies have shown that age is not a predictor for postoperative pulmonary complications. Importantly, acceptable operative mortality rates can be achieved in older patients [2]. As age is obviously a non-modifiable risk factor, and the potential risk of complications does not invariably translate into increased mortality, surgery should not be declined solely on the basis of advanced age.
- Obesity (i.e., Body Mass Index [BMI] $\geq$30 kg/m^2) causes a reduction in lung volume, ventilation–perfusion mismatch, and relative hypoxemia, which are accentuated after surgery. Obese patients may present difficulties with endotracheal intubation. In severe cases, obesity is associated with pulmonary hypertension, cor pulmonale, and hypercapnic respiratory failure (Pickwickian syndrome). Although some studies suggest that obesity increases the risk of postoperative pulmonary complications, others suggest that obesity is not an independent risk factor. Data suggest risk is not increased with abdominal or peripheral procedures [3], and specifically with laparoscopic cholecystectomy [4], hip fracture surgery [5], and laparoscopic colectomy [6]. Risk was increased with lobectomy for lung cancer [7], and among patients with BMI $\geq$35 undergoing cardiac surgery [8].
- General health status: measures such as the American Society of Anesthesiologists (ASA) classification and the Goldman Cardiac Risk Index (CRI) are useful for risk stratification. Dependent functional status, low albumin, and weight loss are specific and independent risk factors for complications [1,9,10].

- Smoking: patients who currently smoke have a two-fold increased risk of postoperative complications, even in the absence of chronic obstructive pulmonary disease (COPD). The risk is highest in patients who smoked within the previous two months. Patients who have quit smoking for more than six months have a risk similar to those who do not smoke, although the risk of postoperative pneumonia appears to remain elevated up to one year after smoking cessation [1].
- Neurological impairment: patients with impaired sensorium or residual deficits from a previous stroke have an increased risk of postoperative pneumonia and respiratory failure [1].
- Immunosuppression: chronic steroid use, daily use of alcohol within two weeks of surgery, and insulin-treated diabetes are associated with an increased risk of postoperative pulmonary complications [1].

Specific diseases

- COPD: patients with severe COPD (forced expiratory volume in one second [FEV_1] <40% predicted) are six times more likely to have major postoperative complications, and an FEV_1 <60% predicted was found to be an independent predictor of increased mortality in patients undergoing coronary artery bypass graft (CABG) procedures [11]. Despite the increased risk, a prohibitive level of pulmonary function for an absolute contraindication is not apparent. Preoperative evaluation should be aimed at diagnosing patients with suspected COPD and instituting appropriate therapy based on disease severity. Surgery should be delayed in patients having an acute exacerbation of COPD.
- Asthma: well-controlled asthma does not appear to pose an increased risk of complications, but suboptimal control is associated with an increased risk of bronchospasm, hypoxemia, hypercapnia, inadequate cough, atelectasis, and pulmonary infection [12].
- Pulmonary hypertension: patients with pulmonary hypertension have an increased risk of congestive heart failure, hemodynamic instability, sepsis, and respiratory failure, and have higher intensive care unit (ICU) and hospital length of stay and mortality with both cardiac and non-cardiac surgery [13,14]. Patients with a history of pulmonary embolism (PE), obstructive sleep apnea (OSA), chronic kidney disease (CKD), or coronary artery disease (CAD); New York Heart Association (NYHA) class 2 or above; right axis deviation or right ventricular (RV) hypertrophy on the electrocardiograph (ECG); or unfavorable hemodynamic parameters (including RV systolic pressure of >70 mmHg, right atrial (RAt) dilation, decreased left ventricular (LV) ejection fraction) are at particularly high-risk of complications. Surgery should generally be avoided in patients with evidence of RV failure (elevated RAt pressure or decreased cardiac output [CO]) [15].
- Interstitial lung disease: patients with pulmonary fibrosis are at risk for acute exacerbation following lung surgery. Several scoring systems may be useful to predict increased risk [16,17], and independent risk factors include low forced vital capacity, low diffusing capacity, ongoing exacerbation at the time of surgery, a larger extent of resection, and a greater degree of radiographic fibrosis [18,19].
- OSA: this is discussed fully elsewhere in this text.

Procedure-related risk factors

- Surgical site: the incidence of postoperative pulmonary complications is inversely related to the distance of the surgical incision from the diaphragm. Upper abdominal surgery complication rates range from 17% to 76%, while the rate is 0%–5% for lower abdominal procedures. Thoracic surgery runs a risk of 19%–59%, and the highest risk procedure is abdominal aortic aneurysm (AAA) repair [1].
- Duration of surgery: patients undergoing procedures lasting longer than three to four hours have a higher incidence rate of pulmonary complications (40%) compared with those undergoing operations lasting less than two hours (8%).
- Type of anesthesia: data are inconsistent about whether the pulmonary complication rate is lower with spinal anesthesia (SpA) or EA compared with GA, although a majority of studies suggest such. This is discussed further in its own chapter.
- Minimally invasive surgery, laparoscopic abdominal surgery, particularly cholecystectomy, is associated with fewer postoperative pulmonary abnormalities and a shorter hospital stay [20]. Video-assisted thoracoscopic surgery uses smaller incisions without separation of the ribs, thereby reducing postoperative pain and leading to earlier ambulation, reduced pulmonary complications, and shorter hospital length of stay.

Preoperative pulmonary risk assessment

Owing to the impact of postoperative pulmonary complications, attention should be devoted to ensuring ample time is spent in assessing an individual patient's risk. A complete and thorough history and physical examination should be performed to assess risk factors that may lead to postoperative pulmonary complications. Particular interest should be paid to assessing for the presence of COPD by history of smoking or symptoms of poor exercise tolerance, dyspnea, or cough. Physical examination findings of poor air movement, wheezes, or prolonged expiratory phase should further prompt suspicion.

Pulmonary function tests

Several studies have looked at the use of preoperative pulmonary function tests (PFTs) in risk stratifying patients not undergoing lung resection. In 1999, a review of the evidence suggested that there appears to be no predictive value of PFTs in such patients [21]. Therefore, the current recommendation in non-resectional surgery is to obtain preoperative PFTs only in patients with signs or symptoms that would otherwise prompt such testing.

Arterial blood gases

Although fewer individual studies have looked at the prognostic potential for arterial blood gases, the most comprehensive systematic review done to date suggests hypercapnia is not associated independently with increased postoperative pulmonary risk [22]. The underlying disease (most often COPD), rather than hypercapnia per se, is likely responsible for the increased risk.

Chest X-rays

Chest X-rays (CXRs) are ordered fairly commonly in preoperative practice; however, studies have failed to show any benefit to this as a risk-stratifying tool.

A systematic review looking at 14 studies addressing the utility of preoperative CXRs was published in 2005 and it was shown that only 10% of CXRs obtained led to a change in patient management. The abnormalities detected on CXRs tended to reflect known, chronic disease processes in patients with increased age and more baseline risk factors for cardiopulmonary disease. Not surprisingly, there was no significant difference in postoperative pulmonary complications between patients who had a preoperative CXR (12.8%) and those who did not (16%) [23]. Preoperative CXRs are not recommended except in those patients with significant risk factors for pulmonary disease.

To assist in risk stratification for postoperative pulmonary complications, multiple scoring systems have been devised over the years, all of which have potential limitations.

Postoperative pneumonia and respiratory failure risk index

- In a large, multi-center, observational trial, Arozullah et al. created and validated scoring systems to predict the risk of postoperative pneumonia and respiratory failure, respectively [1,24]. The respiratory failure model was subsequently revised [25]. The indices incorporate procedure- and patient-related factors, including general health status, degrees of immunosuppression and neurological impairment, presence of pre-existing lung disease, and overall fluid status. Points are assigned to each risk factor and the total number of points is used to stratify patients into five risk classes (1–5, from lowest to highest risk). Although these indices were developed using a massive database of patients (almost 200 000), they were derived from Veterans Affairs Medical Center data and thus may not be as valid in women and younger patients.
- A similar clinical risk score was developed and validated by Kinlin et al. more recently for predicting the likelihood of pneumonia after coronary artery bypass surgery. Aside from the procedure being specified, this model was also different from the one derived by Arozullah et al., in that the population had a much higher proportion of women (30%) [26].
- While the prior-mentioned indices looked at the risk of postoperative pnueumonia, Kor et al. created and developed a model to predict postoperative lung injury. In this model, the risk factors most predictive of developing acute lung injury (ALI) or acute respiratory distress syndrome (ARDS) were high-risk vascular, cardiac, or thoracic surgeries and the presence of diabetes, COPD, gastroesophageal reflux disease, and a history of alcohol abuse [27].

Pulmonary risk index/cardiopulmonary risk index

A combined cardiopulmonary risk index has been proposed by adding pulmonary risk factors to the existing Goldman CRI. These risk factors are:

- obesity (BMI >27)
- cigarette smoking within eight weeks of surgery
- productive cough within five days of surgery
- diffuse wheezing within five days of surgery
- FEV_1/forced vital capacity (FVC) ratio of <70% and $PaCO_2$ >45 mmHg

It has been proposed that patients with a combined score of >4 (out of 10) are 17 times more likely to develop a postoperative pulmonary complication following thoracic surgery.

However, a prospective validation study done by Melendez and Carlon showed that, except for a very high positive predictive value in patients undergoing lobectomy, this index had significant limitations [28].

ASA classification

This method of risk stratification is based on straightforward clinical characteristics and is simple to score. Patients are placed into five classes (I–V) with increasing level of severity and therefore presumed postoperative morbidity. This tool has not been validated with respect to predicting postoperative pulmonary complications but nonetheless is used due to its ease and rationality.

Physiologic and Operative Severity Score for Enumeration of Mortality and Morbidity (POSSUM)

This score incorporates 12 patient-specific variables and can stratify risk among patients undergoing a particular type of operation [29]. It has been used to assess outcomes among patients undergoing general surgery, ruptured abdominal aorta repair, vascular surgery, and lung resection for lung cancer. Additional procedure-related variables are needed to enable comparison between low- and high-risk operations.

Resection surgery

Surgical resection remains the mainstay of potentially curative therapy for patients diagnosed with localized non-small cell lung cancer (NSCLC). Given the high association of lung cancer with tobacco abuse, many patients have concomitant obstructive pulmonary disease and/or emphysema. Lung resection surgery for cancer first began in 1933 after Graham and Singer performed the first pneumonectomy. Today, five-year survival for early stage complete resection approaches 70%. Contrasting with the dismal five-year overall survival in lung cancer, at 14%, resection surgery has a significant therapeutic potential, and therefore should not be unjustifiably prohibited in patients with comorbid pulmonary disease. Preoperative assessment helps to identify patients at greatest risk for postoperative complications and those for whom nonsurgical options may be preferred.

Operative mortality varies according to surgical procedure and is associated with significant risk factors.

- Current mortality rates in general thoracic surgical databases estimate a 1.6%–2.3% risk after lobectomy and 3.7%–6.7% risk after pneumonectomy, which are seemingly lower than previous estimates [30].
- The significant predictors of mortality identified were aged >60 years, larger resections, chronic cardiac or pulmonary disease, and reduced preoperative FEV_1 [31].

The American College of Chest Physicians (ACCP), British Thoracic Society, and Society of Cardiothoracic Surgeons of Great Britain and Ireland all provide guidelines on the sequential testing of cardiac and pulmonary function as well as exercise capacity as part of the preoperative evaluation prior to lung resection.

- The ACCP recommends that all patients undergoing evaluation for curative lung cancer resection surgery be evaluated by a multidisciplinary team including a thoracic surgeon, medical oncologist, radiation oncologist, and pulmonologist.

- Testing includes noninvasive and invasive cardiac testing, spirometry, and estimation of postoperative lung function, as well as exercise tolerance testing.

Patients with lung cancer often are predisposed to atherosclerotic cardiovascular disease owing to tobacco abuse, including coronary artery disease, which has an approximate prevalence of 11%–17% [32,33].

- This underlying prevalence lends risk to major perioperative complications including myocardial infarction (MI), cardiogenic pulmonary edema, dysrhythmias, and cardiac-related death.
- As a result, the American Heart Association/American College of Cardiology (AHA/ACC) and the European Society of Cardiology/European Society of Anesthesiology (ESC/ESA) recommend cardiac risk scoring systems as a screening modality to identify patients in need of specialized cardiac testing prior to resection.
- A validated scoring system for thoracic patients called the Thoracic Revised CRI (ThRCRI) was derived from an initial mixed surgical population scoring system after recalibration for a lung resection cohort [34].
- Patients with ThRCRI scores of ≥ 2 or those presenting with new cardiac conditions or significant functional disability should proceed with cardiac consultation and evaluation (Figure 7.1).
- In terms of invasive cardiac interventions, there has been no significant benefit shown for patients who underwent procedures specifically for surgery, prophylactic coronary revascularization, for instance. Rather, cardiac interventions should only be performed when deemed necessary, regardless of lung resection surgery. Further details on cardiac assessment are covered in a specific chapter elsewhere in this text.

Preoperative lung function

The ACCP has revised its guidelines for the pulmonary evaluation prior to lung cancer resection surgery. Patients who have a positive low-risk or negative cardiac screen should proceed to pulmonary function testing, including spirometry and gas diffusion testing using diffusion capacity of the lung for carbon monoxide (DLCO).

- Several studies point to FEV_1 as an independent predictor of postoperative morbidity, mortality, and functional disability.
- Berry et al. showed that a preoperative FEV_1 of <30% had an incidence of respiratory complications as high as 43%; in contrast, those patients with FEV_1 of >60% had a reduced rate of 12% [35].
- Other work by Ferguson et al. calculated an odds ratio (OR) for pulmonary morbidity of 1.1 for every 10% decrease in FEV_1 and an OR of 1.13 for every 10% decrease for cardiovascular complications [36].
- Multiple statistical models have confirmed an ideal cutoff value of 60% predicted FEV_1 for predicting pulmonary complications.

Measuring diffusion capacity is a noninvasive method to assess the pulmonary circulation. Findings are meant to reflect the volume of the pulmonary capillary bed and have been reported to be an accurate marker for operative risk.

- Studies have shown DLCO reductions of <60% have been associated with 25% mortality and 40% pulmonary morbidity, and supportive literature confirms the DLCO and

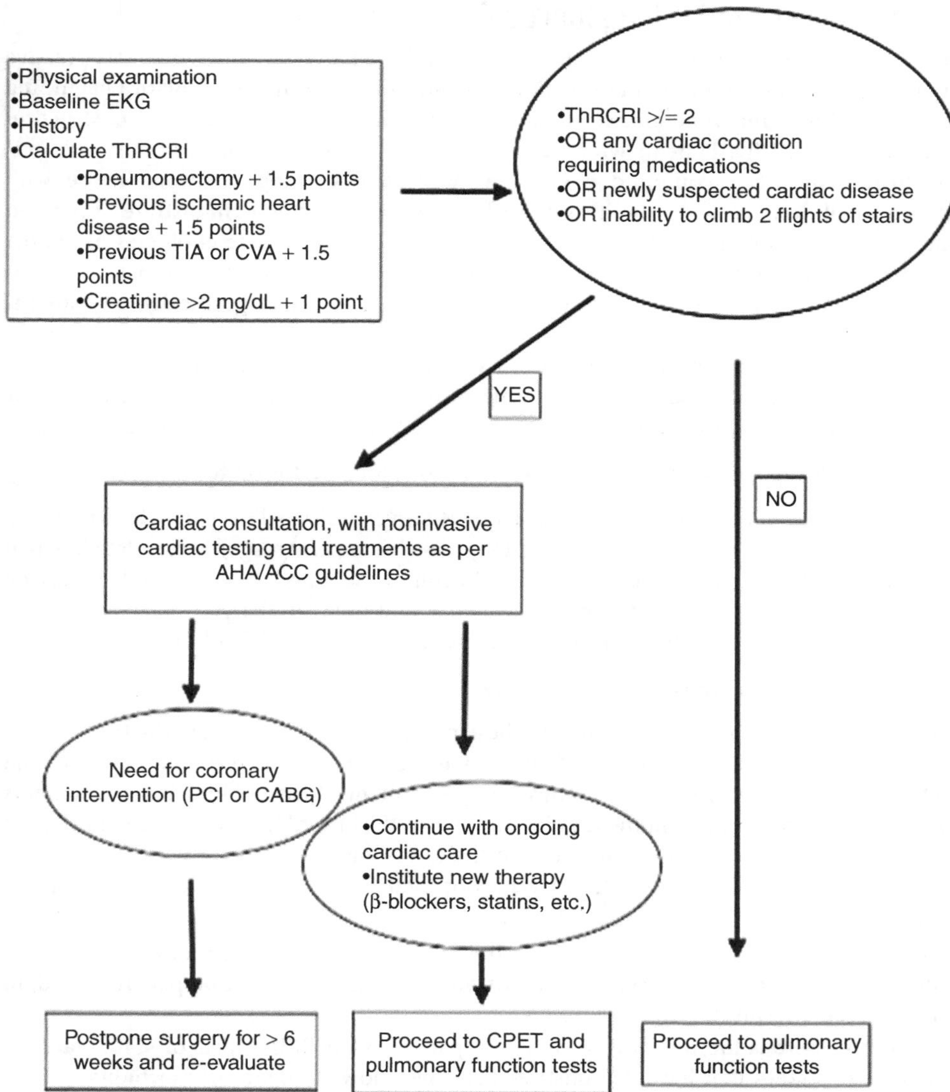
•Physical examination
•Baseline EKG
•History
•Calculate ThRCRI
•Pneumonectomy + 1.5 points
•Previous ischemic heart disease + 1.5 points
•Previous TIA or CVA + 1.5 points
•Creatinine >2 mg/dL + 1 point
•ThRCRI >/= 2
•OR any cardiac condition requiring medications
•OR newly suspected cardiac disease
•OR inability to climb 2 flights of stairs
YES
NO
Cardiac consultation, with noninvasive cardiac testing and treatments as per AHA/ACC guidelines
Need for coronary intervention (PCI or CABG)
•Continue with ongoing cardiac care
•Institute new therapy (β-blockers, statins, etc.)
Postpone surgery for > 6 weeks and re-evaluate
Proceed to CPET and pulmonary function tests
Proceed to pulmonary function tests

Figure 7.1. Cardiac screening using the ThRCRI.

predicted postoperative (PPO) DLCO value, like FEV_1 and PPO FEV_1, to be predictive of pulmonary complications following lung resection [37,38].

- Previously, DLCO testing was recommended only in those patients with reduced FEV_1; however, the correlation between FEV_1 and DLCO is poor, with several cohort studies showing an association between a reduced PPO DLCO despite normal FEV_1 values.
- Therefore, guidelines have been revised to recommend DLCO testing in all patients undergoing lung resection preoperative evaluation. In addition to preoperative risk stratification, DLCO and PPO DLCO values are useful tools for predicting postoperative quality of life and long-term survival.

Predicted postoperative lung function

For all patients with lung cancer being evaluated for lung resection, both preoperative lung function as well as PPO lung function evaluation is recommended. Before beginning to evaluate PPO lung function, it is essential to note that not all airflow obstruction is secondary to COPD. Patients who are debilitated or otherwise weak may have suboptimal effort, which can confound baseline as well as PPO lung function. Those with endobronchial lesions with significant airflow limitation may demonstrate improved airflow following surgery. Although it is important to consider these etiologies of abnormal preoperative or baseline pulmonary function, there is a paucity of data in these subgroups, and therefore PPO pulmonary function is focused specifically on patients with COPD.

The same equations are used for PPO FEV_1 and DLCO; however, the equation differs between those patients undergoing pneumonectomy and those undergoing lobectomy. For pneumonectomy cases, the perfusion method is widely used with the following formula:

$$\text{PPO FEV}_1 = \text{preoperative FEV}_1 \times (1 - \text{fraction of total lung perfusion for the resected lung})$$

Perfusion mapping is accomplished via a quantitative radionuclide study in which the relative perfusion for each area of the lung (expressed as a percentage) is calculated, which as seen above, is subtracted from the total perfusion of the lung. Other methods involving computed tomography (CT) scanning are available and used similarly.

For lobectomy cases, a different method is usually chosen for PPO lung function:

$$\text{PPO FEV}_1 = \text{preoperative FEV}_1 \times (1 - y/z)$$

As in the pneumonectomy equation, the best preoperative post-bronchodilator FEV_1 is used; y and z refer to the number of functional segments being removed (y) and total functional segments (z). In total, the lungs have 19 segments; the right lung has 10 segments (three in the upper lobe, two in the middle, and five in the lower lobe) while the left lung has nine segments (five in the upper and four in the lower lobe).

Historically, PPO FEV_1 and DLCO values of >40% were considered average risk for operative mortality.

- It was thought that values of <40% not only increased mortality but also markedly decreased functional capacity, with the concern that the post-resection patient would, in essence, be a respiratory invalid.
- However, there is limited data on how well patients with PPO values of <40% fare. There are studies that have demonstrated relatively low incidence of morbidity (15%–25%) and mortality (1%–15%) in patients with severe airflow limitation with FEV_1 ranging from 26% to 45% predicted [39–41].
- These patients, who were below previously recommended FEV_1 cutoff values, suggest that surgery can be safely performed in a select group of patients with advanced lung disease.
- Martin-Ucar et al. evaluated the five-year survival for patients with stage 1 upper-lobe disease and advanced airflow obstruction (mean FEV_1 34%). While the survival rate was modestly reduced at 35% after lobectomy at five years, this exceeded expected survival if no resection had been performed [40].
- Lastly, patients with advanced upper-lobe bullous disease may, in fact, benefit from lung resection surgery, as in addition to excision of neoplasm, there is an effective lung

volume reduction, which improves the elastic recoil and possibly obstructive deficit that were present preoperatively.

- In these patients with marginal preoperative or PPO lung function, further risk stratification can be achieved with exercise testing.

Exercise testing

Cardiopulmonary exercise testing (CPET) is an advanced physiological technique of testing, which is discussed fully elsewhere in this text. Maximal oxygen consumption ($VO_{2\ max}$) can be measured and utilized in the preoperative risk assessment. Several American and European trials have correlated VO_2 measurements with postoperative outcomes for pulmonary resection surgery.

- Benzo et al. found a statistically significant decrease in $VO_{2\ max}$ in those patients who developed postoperative pulmonary complications, and concluded that CPET testing can be a useful diagnostic tool in preoperative assessment [42].
- Others found that a $VO_{2\ max}$ of 10–15 mL/kg/min or 35%–75% predicted correlated with a significant increase in postoperative death. Those with $VO_{2\ max}$ of >20 mL/kg/min were deemed safe for all forms of resection, including even pneumonectomy [43,44].

Stair climbing or shuttle walk testing is a cost-effective alternative to assess exercise tolerance. The exercise involved, for example stair climbing, is a widely used form of exercise and also provides a more goal-oriented approach to exercise compared to continuous cycling, as patients can follow their progress easily and work toward a set goal.

- When compared to preoperative FEV_1 measurements, climbing three flights of stairs correlated well with an FEV_1 of >1.7 L and five flights an FEV_1 of >2.0 L [45].
- In a major series of 640 patients who underwent lobectomy or pneumonectomy, an ability to climb 12 m or greater served as an important marker for risk of postoperative morbidity or mortality. Those patients who failed to meet 12 m on preoperative stair climbing were found to have a 2.5 times increased risk of morbidity and 13 times higher risk of death. Importantly, in the group who could climb >22 m, despite poor PPO FEV_1 and DLCO values, no increased mortality risk was observed [46].

Functional algorithm

In the ACCP latest guideline statement, a functional algorithm (Figure 7.2) was offered as a means of incorporating the cardiac, pulmonary function testing, and exercise variables in assessing preoperative risk prior to lung resection surgery. All patients should begin an evaluation with an assessment of cardiac risk. Those with low or negative cardiac evaluations may proceed to pulmonary function testing and PPO assessments. Depending on PPO function, either CPET or surrogate exercise testing is then performed. The algorithm places patients in low-, moderate-, or high-risk groups. Those deemed low risk are estimated to have a mortality risk of <1%, and those in the high-risk group with mortality assessments, >10%. The mortality associated with moderate-risk patients depends on the surgical procedure planned along with the specifics of preoperative testing, including exercise testing and PPO lung function.

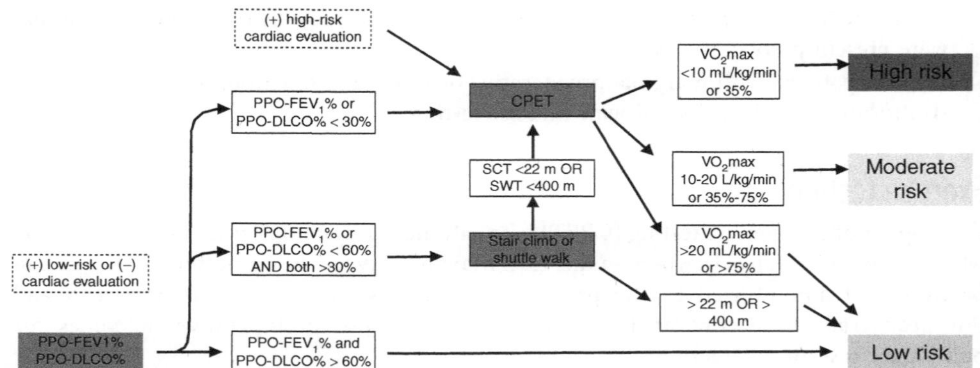

Figure 7.2. Preoperative assessment algorithm for resection surgery. Patients begin testing with cardiac evaluations; those negative or low-risk proceed with pulmonary function testing and calculation of PPO function. Lastly, depending on PPO lung function, exercise testing, either low-technology such as stair climbing or formal CPET, can be performed. SCT=stair climb testing, SWT=shuttle walk test.

Cardiac surgery

While preoperative pulmonary function assessment has been shown, in part, to accurately approximate morbidity and mortality following resection surgery, its role in other subgroups of surgical patients remains less clear. In open-heart surgery, atelectasis (specifically of the left lower lobe) has been the leading postoperative complication. This has been reported in up to 90% of patients and can contribute to postoperative complications. The atelectasis can be associated with phrenic nerve injury, bypass time, temperature of the cardioplegia solution, and the surgical approach.

Following bypass surgery, the overall incidence of pulmonary complications approximates 7.5%.

- Patients with abnormal pulmonary function tests were more likely to suffer prolonged mechanical ventilation and were at higher risk for postoperative pneumonia.
- Fuster et al. evaluated 1412 patients with pulmonary function testing prior to bypass grafting. Thirty-nine percent of patients had abnormal testing, the majority of whom were obstructive. In those patients, increased in-hospital mortality was higher, with the highest risk associated with the lowest FEV_1 values [11].

With the advent of less invasive percutaneous valve replacement, higher-risk patients are undergoing valve repair or replacement, and further study to evaluate risk factors among this subgroup of patients is indicated.

Bariatric surgery

Obesity continues to plague the modernized world and is considered to be one of the newest and most serious public health risks. Given the impact of obesity on the chest wall, diaphragm, and respiratory muscle function, it is not surprising that bariatric patients have altered pulmonary function testing.

- The most common abnormal findings on preoperative pulmonary testing in the bariatric population include restrictive ventilatory defects, specifically decreased residual volume, functional residual capacity (FRC), and total lung capacity (TLC); and decreased maximal voluntary ventilation.

- Bariatric patients are also at increased risk for sleep disordered breathing, specifically OSA and obesity-related hypoventilation.
- Hamoui et al. evaluated 146 patients who underwent PFTs prior to open bariatric surgery, and compared the characteristics between the groups with and without postoperative complications. The patients with complications weighed more, were older, and had lower values of TLC, FVC, and FEV_1. It was suggested by these findings that preoperative PFTs aid in prediction of postoperative complications [47].

Investigations are underway to assess for preoperative sleep apnea and hypoventilation syndromes as part of preoperative evaluation, but presently there is no evidence base for preoperative polysomnography in the bariatric population.

Preparation for surgery

Along with careful risk stratification, appropriate preparation for planned surgery should be undertaken in order to attempt to minimize postoperative pulmonary complications. A number of the relevant aspects of preparation are discussed as follows.

Smoking cessation

- As previously discussed, smoking appears to be an independent risk factor for postoperative pulmonary complications. However, abrupt cessation in the immediate preoperative period has been postulated to be potentially harmful. In theory, cough may become inhibited, thereby leading to retention of secretions and small airway obstruction once the irritant effects of cigarettes are removed. Owing to these concerns, a longer duration of smoking cessation prior to surgery had been advocated in the past.
- The theoretical concerns stated here have been demonstrated in only one study, by Warner et al. in 1989, as current smokers developed postoperative pulmonary complications at a rate significantly lower than those who had stopped smoking within eight weeks of surgery (33% versus 57%, respectively) [48].
- However, a systematic review of 12 studies on this topic showed that the study by Warner et al. was the only one to demonstrate increased risk in patients who quit smoking within two months of surgery. Conclusions from this review suggest that patients should be counseled on smoking cessation in the preoperative period, regardless of the interval prior to surgery [49].
- Therefore, when possible, smoking cessation should be strongly encouraged in individuals undergoing surgery, regardless of the time remaining before surgery. Aggressive use of counseling, nicotine replacement, or pharmacological therapy should be considered for these individuals.

COPD

- Optimizing baseline function is crucial in the preoperative period for patients with COPD. This includes continuing long-acting bronchodilator and inhaled corticosteroid regimens, smoking cessation, and possibly chest physical therapy in the appropriate patients.

- Patients with functional limitation, persistent wheezing, and severe airflow limitation due to COPD should be treated with perioperative steroids prior to surgery.
- Preoperative steroids in COPD have been studied most extensively in patients undergoing CABG, although only in trials with relatively small sample sizes. One such study randomized patients in this population to prednisolone 20 mg/d for 10 days preoperatively, continuing until hospital discharge, or placebo, and showed that the preoperative steroid group had significantly fewer pulmonary complications as well as decreased ICU and hospital length of stay [50]. A similar study done by Starobin et al. did not show a decrease in postoperative pulmonary complications but did show a reduced ICU length of stay in patients treated with preoperative steroids. It should be noted, however, that the treatment group in this study received only one dose of long-acting corticosteroids preoperatively [51].

Asthma

- As for COPD, asthma control should be optimized by continuing maintenance therapies in patients preparing for surgery.
- A small trial of patients with asthma with persistent symptoms and FEV_1 and peak flow rate of <80% predicted were randomized to groups: methylprednisolone 40 mg IV with a short-acting β-agonist (SABA) for five days, SABA pretreatment for five days, or SABA before induction of anesthesia. This study showed a dramatic reduction in wheezing for patients pretreated with steroids [52].
- Steroids have been shown to be safe and well tolerated when given to asthmatics perioperatively and do not appear to increase the risk of death, infections, or adrenal insufficiency [53]. Patients who have received steroids for more than three weeks in the preceding six months, however, are at risk of adrenal insufficiency and should receive stress-dose steroids in the perioperative period.

Preoperative antibiotics

- No studies have suggested that prophylactic antibiotics are beneficial in preventing postoperative pulmonary complications, and thus their administration is not recommended.
- Antibiotics remain appropriate for treatment in patients with clinically apparent respiratory infections, and when feasible elective surgery should be delayed until after resolution of infection.

Inspiratory muscle training

- Some of the strongest data for reducing postoperative pulmonary complications comes from a study by Hulzebos et al., in which the intervention was preoperative inspiratory muscle training (IMT) consisting of incentive spirometry, education in active cycle of breathing, and forced expiration techniques [54]. In this randomized trial of 279 patients undergoing CABG, those receiving IMT daily for at least two weeks prior to surgery had a postoperative pulmonary complication rate of 18% compared to 35% in the control group. This result was supported by a similar, albeit smaller (20 patients total), randomized trial, looking at the efficacy of IMT in patients undergoing AAA repair [55].

- Studies have not demonstrated reduction in postoperative pulmonary complications using IMT in lower-risk procedures, but this intervention may be considered in patients judged to be high-risk, based on other factors.
- When employed, thorough patient education well prior to surgery (ideally greater than two weeks) is recommended to maximize the utility of IMT.

Pulmonary rehabilitation

- Pulmonary rehabilitation (PR) has been shown by multiple studies to improve function in patients who previously did not fulfill criteria for lung resection.
- A retrospective review of patients with COPD undergoing lobectomy performed in Japan compared 22 patients who underwent preoperative PR with 60 historic controls. The PR group had a statistically significant decrease in postoperative pulmonary complications and hospital length of stay, as well as a statistically significant increase in FEV_1 from baseline compared with controls [56].
- A recent retrospective study looked at 100 similarly matched patients, 63 of whom underwent preoperative PR, also showed a statistically significant decrease in postoperative pulmonary complications (6.4%) compared with the control group (24.3%). The study population consisted of patients undergoing esophagectomy for esophageal cancer [57].
- Bobbio et al. demonstrated that brief, intense pulmonary rehabilitation prior to lobectomy could significantly improve exercise tolerance ($VO_{2\ max}$) [58]. These results were corroborated by a slightly larger study by Stefanelli et al., where similar high-intensity training in a similar comparable population led to improved $VO_{2\ max}$ preoperatively and two months postoperatively [59].

Intraoperative strategies

Specific interventions that can reduce the risk of postoperative complications include the following:

- Type of anesthesia: SpA or EA in combination with GA is associated with less postoperative respiratory depression, but there is no difference in the incidence of postoperative pneumonia than GA alone. Adjunctive neuraxial anesthesia should therefore be considered for high-risk patients. SpA is contraindicated in patients with pulmonary hypertension, due to its more rapid onset and attendant risk of hemodynamic instability as compared to EA. Depending on the type and duration of surgery, endotracheal intubation and mechanical ventilation may be preferable because of the ability to monitor and control respiratory parameters better.
- Type of neuromuscular blockade: intermediate- and shorter-acting agents (e.g., vecuronium, rocuronium) are preferred, because residual neuromuscular blockade from longer-acting agents may contribute to pulmonary complications.
- Duration and type of surgery: when available, a less ambitious, shorter procedure should be considered in extremely high-risk patients, as the duration of the surgical procedure influences the rate of postoperative complications. Because upper abdominal and thoracic operations carry the greatest risk, a percutaneous (laparoscopic) procedure should be substituted for an open procedure, if possible.

- Ventilatory strategy: in patients with COPD undergoing lung resection via thoracotomy, the use of high-frequency percussive ventilation for the non-dependent lung (the lung on which the surgeon was operating) resulted in improved sputum clearance following surgery and a shorter duration of hospitalization compared to intraoperative continuous positive airway pressure (CPAP) [60]. Low tidal volume ventilation and recruitment maneuvers are discussed in the chapter on intraoperative ventilatory management.
- Fluid management: a more positive fluid balance (>5 mL/kg/hr) intraoperatively was associated with an increased risk of acute exacerbation in patients with idiopathic pulmonary fibrosis who underwent resection for lung cancer [61]. Similar findings were noted among patients undergoing spine surgery [62]. The opposite was shown in a study of patients undergoing laparoscopic cholecystectomy, however [63]. These discordant findings suggest that a liberal fluid management strategy may be acceptable for minor surgical procedures.
- Blood transfusion: the adjusted risk of postoperative pulmonary complications increases incrementally with each unit of packed red blood cells transfused intraoperatively [64].
- Pulmonary hypertension: inhaled nitric oxide, inhaled or IV prostacyclins, IV sildenafil, and milrinone may all be useful to decrease pulmonary vascular resistance. Dobutamine is often used in the event of systemic hypotension, with norepinephrine or vasopressin added should hypotension persist. Extracorporeal membrane oxygenation (ECMO) may be required for the management of pulmonary hypertensive crisis [65].

Postoperative strategies

Lung expansion and airway clearance maneuvers

Lung expansion maneuvers include deep breathing exercises, incentive spirometry devices, percussion (flutter valves), postural drainage, cough-assist devices, suctioning, early mobilization, and CPAP or nasal intermittent positive pressure ventilation.

- Incentive spirometry is the most-utilized modality of lung expansion, although meta-analysis of five trials has not shown any clear benefit following either abdominal or cardiac surgery [66]. Comparisons between different modalities of lung expansion have not demonstrated the superiority of any individual method. Incentive spirometry is by far the least expensive, but requires patient adherence and effort, which may account for its lack of significant effect in many of the analyzed trials.
- Some studies suggest CPAP is the most efficacious lung expansion maneuver, owing in part perhaps to the lack of patient cooperation or effort. However, the cost and risk of adverse effects preclude its immediate use on all patients. The use of CPAP has been shown to decrease postoperative complications in patients following cardiac or lung resection surgery [67,68].

For most patients, lung expansion maneuvers aside from early mobilization may not need to be employed. For those at high-risk for complications, some modality of therapy should be offered, with the selection focused on cost, availability, and institutional expertise. CPAP should be considered for high-risk patients, particularly those whose effort or cooperation may be suboptimal.

Other postoperative strategies

- Pain control: adequate pain control in the postoperative setting can be both helpful and potentially harmful: controlling pain helps minimize complications by aiding in early mobilization and lung expansion maneuvers, but heavy narcotic use potentially can lead to over-sedation with associated hypoventilation, risk of aspiration, and exacerbation of OSA. Postoperative analgesia is further discussed in its own chapter.
- Fast-track protocols. Fast-track protocols are evidence-based workflows designed to standardize medical care and improve outcomes while remaining conscious of healthcare costs. Fast-track protocols have been applied primarily in the field of colorectal surgery and employ evidence-based practices in perioperative care. In particular, the mainstay of postoperative strategies in the fast-track protocols involves the aforementioned early mobilization and pain control efforts.
- Nasogastric (NG) decompression: the routine use of NG tubes until the return of normal bowel function in the setting of abdominal surgery has been associated with higher risks of aspiration and atelectasis when compared with the selective use of these enteric tubes. Use should be limited to patients with postoperative intolerance to oral intake, nausea/vomiting, or symptomatic ileus with abdominal distension, in whom NG decompression is associated with shorter time to return of normal oral intake with no increased risk of aspiration.
- Glycemic control: optimal glucose targeting has been a subject of significant debate in inpatient, outpatient, and critical care settings. With regard to postoperative pulmonary complications, the role of blood glucose control remains unclear.
- Total parenteral nutrition (TPN): similar to glucose control, the impact of the type and amount of nutritional support in postoperative pulmonary complications is unclear, although it is known that poor nutritional status increases postoperative risk. TPN provides no added benefit to enteral feeding except perhaps in a select group of highly malnourished patients or when enteral feeding is likely to be prohibited for a prolonged time (>14 days) [69].
- CPAP: with the ever-increasing incidence of obesity and improved awareness of OSA, the use of postoperative CPAP to reduce pulmonary risk has been entertained. CPAP therapy has the possibility of reducing the risk of apnea or hypoventilation associated with narcotic use, and as mentioned earlier, is also an effective tool for lung re-expansion. More randomized control trials (RCTs) are needed to look at the effect of empiric CPAP therapy in patients undergoing bariatric surgery or those with suspected OSA. One study of 1095 patients undergoing bariatric Roux-en-Y surgery demonstrated no negative impact of withholding CPAP therapy from patients with known OSA who were treated with CPAP preoperatively, although all patients in this study were closely monitored, received aggressive incentive spirometry, and early ambulation was encouraged [70].
- Prevention of thromboembolism: although not technically considered a postoperative pulmonary complication, venous thromboembolitic disease (VTE) is an ever-present threat to patients, with the postoperative state and immobility being the main contributing risk factors. The risk of deep vein thrombosis (DVT) and pulmonary embolism are influenced by patient- and procedure-related factors. The ACCP recently updated their recommendations for prevention of VTE in surgical patients [71].

References

1. Arozullah AM, Conde MV, Lawrence VA. Preoperative evaluation for postoperative pulmonary complications. *Med Clin North Am* 2003; **87**: 153–73.
2. Djokovic JL, Hedley-Whyte J. Prediction of outcome of surgery and anesthesia in patients over 80. *JAMA* 1979; **242**: 2301–6.
3. Smetana GW. Preoperative pulmonary evaluation. *N Engl J Med* 1999; **340**: 937–44.
4. Phillips EH, Carroll BJ, Fallas MJ, et al. Comparison of laparoscopic cholecystectomy in obese and non-obese patients. *Am Surg* 1994; **60**: 316–21.
5. Batsis JA, Huddleston JM, Melton LJ, et al. Body mass index (BMI) and risk of noncardiac postoperative medical complications in elderly hip fracture patients: a population-based study. *J Hosp Med* 2009; **4**: E1–9.
6. Mustain WC, Davenport DL, Hourigan JS, et al. Obesity and laparoscopic colectomy: outcomes from the ACS-NSQIP database. *Dis Colon Rectum* 2012; **55**: 429–35.
7. Launer H, Nguyen DV, Cooke DT. National perioperative outcomes of pulmonary lobectomy for cancer in the obese patient: a propensity score matched analysis. *J Thorac Cardiovasc Surg* 2013; **145**: 1312–18.
8. Demir A, Aydınlı B, Güçlü ÇY, et al. Obesity and postoperative early complications in open heart surgery. *J Anesth* 2012; **26**: 702–10.
9. Qaseem A, Snow V, Fitterman N, et al: Clinical Efficacy Assessment Subcommittee of the American College of Physicians. Risk assessment for and strategies to reduce perioperative pulmonary complications for patients undergoing noncardiothoracic surgery: a guideline from the American College of Physicians. *Ann Intern Med* 2006; **144**: 575–80.
10. Smetana GW, Lawrence VA, Cornell JE, et al. Preoperative pulmonary risk stratification for noncardiothoracic surgery: systematic review for the American College of Physicians. *Ann Intern Med* 2006; **144**: 581–95.
11. Fuster RG, Argudo JA, Albarova OG, et al. Prognostic value of chronic obstructive pulmonary disease in coronary artery bypass grafting. *Eur J Cardiothorac Surg* 2006; **29**: 202–9.
12. National Asthma Education and Prevention Program (NAEPP) Coordinating Committee. Expert Panel Report 3: *Guidelines for the Diagnosis and Management of Asthma*. Bethesda, MD: National Heart, Lung, and Blood Institute, 2007.
13. Ramakrishna G, Sprung J, Ravi BS, et al. Impact of pulmonary hypertension on the outcomes of noncardiac surgery: predictors of perioperative morbidity and mortality. *J Am Coll Cardiol* 2005; **45**: 1691–9.
14. Kaw R, Pasupuleti V, Deshpande A, et al. Pulmonary hypertension: an important predictor of outcomes in patients undergoing non-cardiac surgery. *Respir Med* 2011; **105**: 619–24.
15. Minai OA, Yared JP, Kaw R, et al. Perioperative risk and management in patients with pulmonary hypertension. *Chest* 2013; **144**: 329–40.
16 Kumar P, Goldstraw P, Yamada K, et al. Pulmonary fibrosis and lung cancer: risk and benefit analysis of pulmonary resection. *J Thorac Cardiovasc Surg* 2003; **125**: 1321–7.
17. Fibla JJ, Brunelli A, Cassivi SD, et al. Aggregate risk score for predicting mortality after surgical lung biopsy for interstitial lung disease. *Interact Cardiovasc Thorac Surg* 2012; **15**: 276–9.
18. Ghatol A, Ruhl AP, Danoff SK. Exacerbations in idiopathic pulmonary fibrosis triggered by pulmonary and nonpulmonary surgery: a case series and comprehensive review of the literature. *Lung* 2012; **190**: 373–80.
19. Suzuki H, Sekine Y, Yoshida S, et al. Risk of acute exacerbation of interstitial pneumonia after pulmonary resection for lung cancer in patients with idiopathic pulmonary fibrosis based on preoperative high-resolution computed tomography. *Surg Today* 2011; **41**: 914–21.

20. Torrington KG, Bilello JF, Hopkins TK, et al. Postoperative pulmonary changes after laparoscopic cholecystectomy. *South Med J* 1996; **89**: 675.

21. Lawrence VA, Page CP, Harris GD. Preoperative spirometry before abdominal operations. A critical appraisal of its predictive value. *Arch Intern Med* 1989; **149**: 280–5.

22. Fisher BW, Majumdar SR, McAlister FA. Predicting pulmonary complications after nonthoracic surgery: a systematic review of blinded studies. *Am J Med* 2002; **112**: 219–25.

23. Joo HS, Wong J, Naik VN, et al. The value of screening preoperative chest x-rays: a systematic review. *Can J Anaesth* 2005; **52**: 568–74.

24. Arozullah AM, Khuri SF, Henderson WG, et al. Development and validation of a multifactorial risk index for predicting postoperative pneumonia after major noncardiac surgery. *Ann Intern Med* 2001; **135**: 847–57.

25. Johnson RG, Arozullah AM, Neumayer L, et al. Multivariable predictors of postoperative respiratory failure after general and vascular surgery: results from the patient safety in surgery study. *J Am Coll Surg* 2007; **204**: 1188–198.

26. Kinlin LM, Kirchner C, Zhang H, et al. Derivation and validation of a clinical prediction rule for nosocomial pneumonia after coronary artery bypass graft surgery. *Clin Infect Dis* 2010; **50**: 493–501.

27. Kor DJ, Warner DO, Alsara A, et al. Derivation and diagnostic accuracy of the surgical lung injury prediction model. *Anesthesiology* 2011; **115**: 117–28.

28. Melendez JA, Carlon VA. Cardiopulmonary risk index does not predict complications after thoracic surgery. *Chest* 1998; **114**: 69–75.

29. Neary WD, Heather BP, Earnshaw JJ. The physiological and operative severity score for the enmeration of mortality and morbidity (POSSUM). *Br J Surg* 2003; **90**: 157–65.

30. Little AG, Rusch VW, Bonner JA, et al. Patterns of surgical care of lung cancer patients. *Ann Thorac Surg* 2005; **80**: 2051–6.

31. Romano PS, Mark DH. Patient and hospital characteristics related to in-hospital mortality after lung cancer resection. *Chest* 1992; **101**: 1332–7.

32. Brunelli A, Varela G, Salati M, et al. Recalibration of the revised cardiac risk index in lung resection candidates. *Ann Thorac Surg* 2010; **90**: 199–203.

33. Brunelli A, Cassivi SD, Fibla J, et al. External validation of the recalibrated thoracic revised cardiac risk index for predicting the risk of major cardiac complications after lung resection. *Ann Thorac Surg* 2011; **92**: 445–8.

34. Ferguson MK, Celauro AD, Vigneswaran WT. Validation of a modified scoring system for cardiovascular risk associated with major lung resection. *Eur J Cardiothorac Surg* 2012; **41**: 598–602.

35. Berry MF, Villamizar-Ortiz NR, Tong BC, et al. Pulmonary function tests do not predict pulmonary complications after thoracoscopic lobectomy. *Ann Thorac Surg* 2010; **89**: 1044–51.

36. Ferguson MK, Siddique J, Karrison T. Modeling major lung resection outcomes using classification trees and multiple imputation techniques. *Eur J Cardiothorac Surg* 2008; **34**: 1085–9.

37. Brunelli A, Refai MA, Salati M, et al. Carbon monoxide lung diffusion capacity improves risk stratification in patients without airflow limitation: evidence for systematic measurement before lung resection. *Eur J Cardiothorac Surg* 2006; **29**: 567–70.

38. Ferguson MK, Vigneswaran WT. Diffusing capacity predicts morbidity after lung resection in patients without obstructive lung disease. *Ann Thorac Surg* 2008; **85**: 1158–64.

39. Linden PA, Bueno R, Colson YL, et al. Lung resection in patients with preoperative FEV1 <35% predicted. *Chest* 2005; **127**: 1984–90.

40. Martin-Ucar AE, Fareed KR, Nakas A, et al. Is the initial feasibility of lobectomy for stage I non-small cell lung cancer in severe

heterogeneous emphysema justified by long-term survival? *Thorax* 2007: **62**: 577–80.

41. Lau KK, Martin-Ucar AE, Nakas A, et al. Lung cancer surgery in the breathless patient–the benefits of avoiding the gold standard. *Eur J Cardiothorac Surg* 2010; **38**: 6–13.
42. Benzo R, Kelley GA, Recchi L, et al. Complications of lung resection and exercise capacity: a meta-analysis. *Respir Med* 2007; **101**: 1790–7.
43. Bechard D, Westein L. Assessment of exercise oxygen consumption as preoperative criterion for lung resection. *Ann Thorac Surg* 1987; **44**: 344–9.
44. Olsen GN, Weiman DS, Bolton JW, et al. Submaximal invasive exercise testing and quantitative lung scanning in the evaluation for tolerance of lung resection. *Chest* 1989; **95**: 267–73.
45. Bolton JW, Weiman DS, Haynes JL, et al. Stair climbing as an indicator of pulmonary function. *Chest* 1987; **92**: 783–8.
46. Brunelli A, Refai M, Xiumé F, et al. Performance at symptom-limited stair-climbing test is associated with increased cardiopulmonary complications, mortality, and costs after major lung resection. *Ann Thorac Surg* 2008; **86**: 240–7.
47. Hamoui N, Anthone G, Crookes PF. The value of pulmonary function testing prior to bariatric surgery. *Obes Surg* 2006; **16**: 1570–3.
48. Warner MA, Offord KP, Warner ME, et al. Role of preoperative cessation of smoking and other factors in postoperative pulmonary complications: a blinded prospective study of coronary artery bypass patients. *Mayo Clin Proc* 1989; **64**: 609–16.
49. Theadom A, Cropley M. Effects of preoperative smoking cessation on the incidence and risk of intraoperative and postoperative complications in adult smokers: a systematic review. *Tob Control* 2006; **15**: 352–8.
50. Bingol H, Cingoz F, Balkan A, et al. The effect of oral prednisolone with chronic obstructive pulmonary disease undergoing coronary artery bypass surgery. *J Card Surg* 2005; **20**: 252–6.
51. Starobin D, Kramer MR, Garty M, et al. Morbidity associated with systemic corticosteroid preparation for coronary artery bypass grafting in patients with chronic obstructive pulmonary disease: a case control study. *J Cardiothorac Surg* 2007; **2**: 25.
52. Silvanus MT, Groeben H, Peters J. Corticosteroids and inhaled salbutamol in patients with reversible airway obstruction markedly decrease the incidence of bronchospasm after tracheal intubation. *Anesthesiology* 2004; **100**: 1052–7.
53. Su FW, Beckman DB, Yarnold PA, et al. Low incidence of complications in asthmatic patients treated with preoperative corticosteroids. *Allergy Asthma Proc* 2004; **25**: 327–33.
54. Hulzebos EH, Helders PJ, Favie NJ, et al. Preoperative intensive inspiratory muscle training to prevent postoperative pulmonary complications in high-risk patients undergoing CABG surgery: a randomized clinical trial. *JAMA* 2006; **296**: 1851–7.
55. Dronkers J, Veldman A, Hoberg E, et al. Prevention of pulmonary complications after upper abdominal surgery by preoperative intensive inspiratory muscle training: a randomized controlled pilot study. *Clin Rehabil* 2008; **22**: 134–42.
56. Sekine Y, Chiyo M, Iwata T, et al. Perioperative rehabilitation and physiotherapy for lung cancer patients with chronic obstructive pulmonary disease. *Jpn J Thorac Cardiovasc Surg* 2005; **53**: 237–43.
57. Inoue J, Ono R, Makiura D, et al. Prevention of postoperative pulmonary complications through intensive preoperative respiratory rehabilitation in patients with esophageal cancer. *Dis Esophagus* 2013; **26**: 68–74.
58. Bobbio A, Chetta A, Ampollini L, et al. Preoperative pulmonary rehabilitation in patients undergoing lung resection for non-small cell lung cancer. *Eur J Cardiothorac Surg* 2008; **33**: 95–8.

59. Stefanelli F, Meoli I, Cobuccio R, et al. High-intensity training and cardiopulmonary exercise testing in patients with chronic obstructive pulmonary disease and non-small-cell lung cancer undergoing lobectomy. *Eur J Cardiothorac Surg* 2013; **44**: e260–5.

60. Lucangelo U, Antonaglia V, Zin WA, et al. High-frequency percussive ventilation improves perioperatively clinical evolution in pulmonary resection. *Crit Care Med* **37**: 1663–9.

61. Mizuno Y, Iwata H, Shirahashi K, et al. The importance of intraoperative fluid balance for the prevention of postoperative acute exacerbation of idiopathic pulmonary fibrosis after pulmonary resection for primary lung cancer. *Eur J Cardiothorac Surg* 2012; **41**: e161–5.

62. Siemionow K, Cywinski J, Kusza K, et al. Intraoperative fluid therapy and pulmonary complications. *Orthopedics* 2012; **35**: e184–91.

63. Holte K, Klarskov B, Christensen DS, et al. Liberal versus restrictive fluid administration to improve recovery after laparoscopic cholecystectomy: a randomized, double-blind study. *Ann Surg* 2004; **240**: 892–9.

64. Ferraris VA, Davenport DL, Saha SP, et al. Surgical outcomes and transfusion of minimal amounts of blood in the operating room. *Arch Surg* 2012; **147**: 49–55.

65. Ortega R, Connor CW. Intraoperative management of patients with pulmonary hypertension. *Adv Pulm Hypertens* 2013; **12**: 18–23.

66. Overend TJ, Anderson CM, Lucy SD, et al. The effect of incentive spirometry on postoperative pulmonary complications: a systematic review. *Chest* 2001; **120**: 971–8.

67. Zarbock A, Mueller E, Netzer S, et al. Prophylactic nasal continuous positive airway pressure following cardiac surgery protects from postoperative pulmonary complications: a prospective, randomized, controlled trial in 500 patients. *Chest* 2009; **135**: 1252–9.

68. Perrin C, Jullien V, Venissac N, et al. Prophylactic use of noninvasive ventilation in patients undergoing lung resectional surgery. *Respir Med* 2007; **101**: 1572–8.

69. Lawrence VA, Cornell JE, Smetana GW. Strategies to reduce postoperative pulmonary complications after noncardiothoracic surgery: systematic review for the American College of Physicians. *Ann Intern Med* 2006; **144**: 596–608.

70. Jensen C, Tejirian T, Lewis C, et al. Postoperative CPAP and BiPAP use can be safely omitted after laparoscopic Roux-en-Y gatric bypass. *Surg Obes Relat Dis* 2008; **4**: 512–14.

71. Gould MK, Garcia DA, Wren SM, et al. Prevention of VTE in nonorthopedic surgical patients: antithrombotic therapy and prevention of thrombosis, 9th edn: American College of Chest Physicians Evidence-Based Clinical Practice Guidelines. *Chest* 2012; **141**: e227S–77S.

Anemia, blood transfusion, and coagulopathy

A. Cave

Anemia and blood transfusion are relatively common in high-risk surgical and critically ill patients. In recent years, blood transfusion in these patients has been questioned increasingly. In addition, the necessary collection, processing, testing, and storage infrastructure makes blood transfusion expensive and it should be our duty to use this scarce resource prudently.

Note: For hemoglobin (Hb), 1 g/dL = 10 g/L.

Anemia

Oxygen transport

Tissue oxygenation is a function of hemoglobin concentration, oxygenation of blood by the lungs, and cardiac output (CO) to deliver a supply of oxygenated blood to the tissues. The amount of blood delivered to the whole body (DO_2) is the product of CO and arterial blood content (CaO_2):

$$DO_2 = CO \times CaO_2$$

CaO_2 is determined primarily by the Hb concentration (Hb in g/dL) and the degree of Hb oxygen saturation (SaO_2) (HbO_2/Hb or SaO_2, as a fraction), so that:

$$CaO_2 = (Hb \times SaO_2 \times K) + (pO_2 \times 0.003)$$

where K is Huffner's constant (1.34) – the O_2-carrying capacity of 1g Hb, and pO_2 is arterial oxygen tension (i.e. partial pressure) in mmHg. The term ($pO_2 \times 0.003$) accounts for the amount of oxygen dissolved in blood.

It can be seen easily that a fall in Hb may have a profound effect on global DO_2 unless compensatory mechanisms occur. It is on this premise that red blood cells (RBCs) are often transfused, that is, to augment DO_2 at a time when the increased cellular oxygen demands of major surgery or critical illness put a strain on already stressed cardiorespiratory systems so that such demands may be met.

Physiological response to anemia

An acute reduction in Hb is sensed at the cellular level and several adaptive changes occur to optimize tissue oxygen delivery [1,2]:

Anesthesia and Perioperative Care of the High-Risk Patient, Third edition, ed. Ian McConachie. Published by Cambridge University Press.

Hemodynamic

An increase in CO is seen with normovolemic anemia. The most important mechanism is the effect of reduced blood viscosity. The decrease in plasma viscosity improves peripheral blood flow. There is also a disproportionate decrease in viscosity in the postcapillary venules compared to other vessels, which leads to a significant increase in venous return and left ventricular (LV) preload. By the Starling principle, an increase in stroke volume follows. This is nonsympathetically mediated. Ventricular afterload may also be reduced with decreased viscosity in the aorta, thereby increasing CO further. The second important mechanism is increased sympathetic stimulation of the cardiovascular effectors, which causes an increase in heart rate and contractility. This includes stimulation of aortic chemoreceptors and cardiac β-adrenergic receptors [3].

Microcirculatory

Increased capillary recruitment and density limits the diffusion distance to cells. In addition, as hemodilution with anemia increases, blood viscosity decreases disproportionately in capillary networks. This results in increased flow velocities of RBCs through capillary beds. This may increase the amount of oxygen supplied to the tissues.

Oxyhemoglobin dissociation curve (ODC)

A rightward shift in the ODC is seen, which increases the O_2 unloading by Hb for a given blood pO_2. This increases cellular O_2 extraction. The primary reason for this is the increased RBC 2,3-diphosphoglycerate (DPG) synthesis seen during anemia. Local temperature and pH cause a rightward shift in the curve, but their effect is thought to be less significant than that of 2,3-DPG.

Hypoxic cellular mechanisms

Activation of hypoxic cellular mechanisms such as neuronal nitric oxide synthase and hypoxia inducible factor helps to maintain oxygen homeostasis [4,5]. A fall in CaO_2, for example, due to a fall in Hb or decrease in oxygenation, results in an increase in erythropoietin production within minutes.

Note: these are the responses to anemia. When anemia is due to acute blood losses, the physiological responses to hypovolemia will also be triggered. In general, anemia is better tolerated than hypovolemia. A significant, acute fall in circulating blood volume, unless replaced or compensated for, is associated with progressive reductions in organ blood flow and function.

Anemia and the heart

The heart is particularly prone to adverse consequences in the face of anemia [1]. This is because normal myocardium has a high basal extraction, between 60% and 75%. As a result, DO_2 to the myocardium can increase only by increasing blood flow: it is "flow-restricted." In the presence of coronary artery disease (CAD), fixed coronary stenoses may prevent any increase in myocardial flow, thus limiting myocardial DO_2. Additionally, most of LV perfusion occurs during diastole and any shortening of the duration of diastole (e.g., tachycardia) limits coronary perfusion. Thus, during anemia, the increased mixed venous–oxygen blood brought about by the demands of an increased CO cannot be met, coronary blood flow is preferentially diverted to the subepicardial layers, and subendocardial ischemia or infarction ensues.

Effect of transfusion on oxygen transport

It is likely that transfusion improves oxygenation and outcome in severe, life-threatening anemia. However, it is unclear to what extent tissue oxygenation or outcome is improved in patients with moderate anemia (e.g., Hb: 7–10 g/dL) [6].

It has been assumed that an increase in global DO_2 (for example, by RBC transfusion) would result in an increase in oxygen consumption (VO_2) in critical illness.

- Creteur et al. [7] examined muscle tissue oxygenation, VO_2, and microvascular reactivity after RBC transfusion in medical-surgical intensive care patients. Patients were transfused if their Hb was <8 g/dL or between 8 g/dL and 9 g/dL in the presence of altered tissue perfusion (based on elevated lactate levels) or coronary artery syndromes. They found no improvement in muscle tissue oxygenation, VO_2, or microvascular reactivity after transfusion.
- In postcardiac surgery patients, the oxygen transport responses to transfusion vary. Orlov et al. [8] showed that in anemic patients transfused with RBCs in cardiac surgery, the oxygen extraction ratio (VO_2/DO_2) fell significantly following transfusion of RBCs only in patients whose pretransfusion oxygen extraction ratio was already increased. There was no change seen in those patients with a normal oxygen extraction ratio to start.

Thus, increasing DO_2 by RBC transfusion may not be of significant benefit in terms of increased oxygen uptake in the cells, but exposes the patient to the possible harmful effects of blood transfusion.

However, it must also be acknowledged that with significant, ongoing blood loss, at some point, blood transfusion *will* be required in addition to maintenance of blood volume and CO. Progressive anemia eventually will reduce DO_2 below its critical level (the point below which further falls in DO_2 cannot be compensated for by increased oxygen extraction by the tissues, with inevitable tissue hypoxia).

Role of anemia in morbidity and mortality

Anemia is independently associated with morbidity of multiple organ systems, including the heart, brain, and kidneys. Mortality is increased in patients with acute coronary syndromes, heart failure, and after non-cardiac and cardiac surgeries. Not surprisingly, anemia puts patients at risk for receiving blood transfusions, and the morbidity and mortality associated with that [9].

- In patients having acute coronary syndromes, the likelihood of death, myocardial infarction (MI), or recurrent ischemia increased as Hb fell below 11 g/dL [10].
- Saager et al. retrospectively assessed 30-day mortality in non-cardiac surgical patients using propensity matching for patients with and without preoperative anemia. They found an increased risk of mortality in the anemic group [9].
- Beattie et al. assessed 90-day mortality in non-cardiac surgical patients and found an increase in mortality in the anemic patients, regardless of whether they received transfusion [11].

- In a large retrospective cohort study, preoperative anemia was defined as a hematocrit of <36% in women and <39% in men, moderate anemia 29%–36% in women and 29%–39% in men, and moderate-severe anemia as ≤29% in both men and women. They found that preoperative anemia, even to a mild degree, is independently associated with an increased risk of 30-day mortality in patients undergoing major non-cardiac surgery. The study showed an association with increased risk of 30-day non-cardiac morbidity, including respiratory, urinary, wound, septic, and thromboembolic complications [12].

Blood transfusion

Indications for RBC transfusion

Despite extensive physiological and clinical studies, indications for RBC transfusion remain controversial. The term "transfusion trigger," coined to describe factors that motivate physicians to order blood, has become equated with a critical Hb value [13]. In truth, there is no optimal Hb level that can be applied to all patients, given their different physiologies and comorbid medical conditions.

Ideally, tests that indicate failing tissue oxygenation during acute blood loss or chronic anemia should guide the need for transfusion. Unfortunately no test has yet proven to be easy, reproducible, or sensitive to regional tissue hypoxia [13].

Clinical signs or symptoms of early tissue hypoxia are not reliable. Waiting for signs of end organ impairment, such as hypotension, oliguria, or impaired consciousness, before starting treatment is too late.

- Historically, Hb of 10 g/dL was accepted as the minimum level at which Hb should be maintained. In 1999, the Transfusion Requirements in Critical Care (TRICC) trial [14] was published. It remains the largest and most widely cited trial evaluating RBC transfusion thresholds. Patients (n=838) with Hb less than 9 g/dL were randomly allocated into two groups. The "liberal" transfusion group received RBC transfusions to maintain their Hb between 10 and 12 g/dL. The "restrictive" group received RBC transfusions to maintain Hb between 7 and 9g/dL [14]. Their primary outcome was 30-day mortality: 30-day mortality was 23.3% in the "liberal" group and 18.7% in the "restrictive" group (P=0.10). The "restrictive" group had a significantly lower rate of MI and congestive heart failure. In the "restrictive" group the average number of RBC units transfused was decreased by 54% and the exposure to any RBCs was decreased by 33%. The authors of this study recommend that a restrictive strategy of RBC transfusion be applied to critically ill patients. Of note, they suggest that the exception to this is patients with acute MI or unstable angina.
- This is in agreement with the study by Sabatine et al. mentioned earlier, who found that mortality and further ischemia increased in patients actively having acute coronary syndromes as their Hb fell below 11 g/dL [10].
- A Cochrane systematic review published in 2012 examined 19 trials involving 6264 patients that compared a restrictive versus liberal transfusion strategy. They concluded that existing evidence supports the use of the restrictive transfusion strategy with a transfusion threshold of 7–8 g/dL in patients, including those with pre-existing cardiac disease. They note that high-risk groups, such as those with acute

coronary syndromes, may need a higher transfusion threshold and that further studies are needed in this patient population [15].

- A similar study compared multiple organ dysfunction in children in the intensive care unit (ICU) [16]. The "restrictive" group was transfused at an Hb of <7 g/dL and the "liberal" group at an Hb of <9.5 g/dL. There was a 44% decrease in the number of RBC transfusions in the "restrictive" group. No significant difference was found in multiple organ dysfunction, mortality, or other adverse events between the two groups.

As a final word, recommendations by the American Society of Anesthesiologists (ASA) Task Force on Blood Component Therapy [17] and the Society of Cardiovascular Anesthesiologists [18] state that transfusion is:

- rarely required above an Hb of 10 g/dL
- reasonable and can be life-saving when Hb is <6 g/dL.

Harmful effects of blood transfusion

Acute hemolytic transfusion reaction

An estimated 1 in 250 000 transfusions result in an overt hemolytic reaction, most commonly secondary to minor RBC antigens.

ABO incompatibility

Catastrophic results can occur when the "wrong blood" in administered to the patient. The wrong ABO blood group is estimated to be administered in 1 in 38 000 units of RBCs [18]. Less than 10% of ABO-incompatible transfusions result in a fatal outcome [19]. Analysis of incident reports has revealed multiple errors of identification, often beginning when blood is collected from the blood bank [20]. The use of hospital protocols including systems for validation of patient identification by more than one person is vital.

RBC alloantibodies (non-ABO)

This results from patient immunization from a prior pregnancy or transfusion. Common alloantibodies include Rh, Kell, and Duffy. Patients may have antibody at levels below the detection capabilities of the antibody screening method or a clerical error may occur in the labeling of patient samples. Rarely is it caused by emergency uncross-matched blood given to an alloimmunized patient. The clinical reaction tends to be mild.

Old blood

The age of RBCs has been shown to increase transfusion-related complications in critically ill, postoperative, and trauma patients, although the evidence remains controversial. There are many preclinical studies showing that transfusion of stored blood impairs the microcirculation dynamics and the delivery of oxygen to tissues [21]. The clinical relevance at present is indeterminate [22].

- Stored blood has reduced levels of 2,3-DPG when stored for more than 24 hours, causing a leftward shift in the ODC and a reduced unloading of O_2 from Hb.
- The reduced membrane deformability of RBCs, brought about through their storage, is thought to impede their passage through the narrow confines of a capillary bed, with

potential implications for ischemic organs and tissues. The high hematocrit of packed RBCs will increase blood viscosity and further threaten perfusion of such areas.

- Transfusion of aged RBCs is associated with transfusion-related acute lung injury (TRALI) [23].

Transfusion-related acute lung injury

TRALI is the leading cause of transfusion-related death and is characterized by acute-onset lung injury within six hours of receiving an allogeneic blood product [24]. Recent evidence suggests the cause to be a "two-hit" hypothesis. The "first-hit" is patient derived and results in adherence of primed neutrophils to the pulmonary endothelium (e.g., in the setting of surgery or sepsis). The "second-hit" is caused by mediators in the blood transfusion that activate endothelial cells and pulmonary neutrophils, resulting in capillary leakage and subsequent pulmonary edema [25,26]. The resultant clinical picture is indistinguishable from acute respiratory distress syndrome (ARDS).

To reduce the incidence of TRALI, female donors of products with high plasma volume have been excluded. This has resulted in a roughly two-third decrease in the incidence of TRALI [26].

Transmission of infection by blood transfusion

Direct transmission of infection via contaminated blood is small but still possible.

Human immunodeficiency virus (HIV)

This risk is associated with the donation of blood during the immunologically silent "window period" of infection prior to the host antibody response. The current risk is estimated to be 1 in 7.8 million units of RBCs [27].

Hepatitis B

The current risk is estimated to be 1 in 153 000 unit transfusions [27]. The vast majority of cases resolve by developing immunity. In less than 5% of cases chronic infection occurs, usually followed by chronic liver disease [28].

Hepatitis C

The current risk is estimated to be 1 in 2.3 million unit transfusions [27]. Although an increasingly rare cause of hepatitis C infection, it has a high-associated morbidity.

West Nile virus

The current risk is estimated to be 1 in 1 million unit transfusions [29].

Parasites

Chagas disease is caused by the protozoan *Trypanosoma cruzi* and can lead to cardiac issues. The current risk is estimated to be 1 in 4 million unit transfusions, although this occurs mostly with platelet products rather than RBCs [30].

Prions

The potential for transmission by blood products of protein containing prion particles such as those responsible for human variant Creutzfeldt–Jacob disease (vCJD) represents an unknown risk. Four suspected cases have been reported in the U.K. [31]. In the absence of available blood diagnostic tests to identify preclinical prion infection, many countries have implemented precautionary measures to reduce the risk of transmission through blood and blood products. In the U.K. and France, previous recipients of blood components are deferred from blood donation to prevent potential transmission of the disease through transfusion [32]. In Canada and the U.S., blood deferral has been applied to persons who have spent significant periods of time in the U.K. or France [33].

Bacteria

The current risks of bacterial contamination, symptomatic septic reactions, and fatal bacterial sepsis are estimated to be 1 in 50 000, 1 in 250 000, and 1 in 500 000 unit RBC transfusions, respectively [34]. The incidence is much higher with platelets due to their storage at 20–24 °C.

Immunomodulatory effects of blood transfusion

Administration of blood products causes negative effects on the immune system, a condition termed transfusion-related immune modulation (TRIM) [35]. Mechanisms include suppression of cytotoxic cell and monocyte activity, release of immunosuppressive prostaglandins, inhibition of interleukin-2 production, and increase in suppressor T-cell activity [35].

Leukoreduction

White blood cells release many proinflammatory and prothrombotic mediators during storage. Leukoreduction is the removal of white blood cells from the blood component to be transfused. Removing them before storage helps to prevent the accumulation of cytokines such as interleukin-6, tumor necrosis factor-α, interleukin 1-β, and SD40 ligand that likely contribute to adverse transfusion reactions [36]. Leukoreduction has been shown to reduce febrile nonhemolytic transfusion reactions and cytomegalovirus (CMV) transmission [37]. There has been a widespread adoption of leukoreduction of blood in most countries.

Postoperative infection

The effects of blood transfusion-induced immunosuppression have been thought to increase the risk of postoperative infection including wound infections. The literature at present remains contradictory [13].

Cancer recurrence

Administration of perioperative blood transfusions in patients with colorectal cancer is associated with increased risk of cancer recurrence [38]. The best current evidence is provided by a meta-analysis by the Cochrane group published in 2006. They found that the pooled estimates of randomized control studies studying the effect of perioperative blood transfusions on recurrence of colorectal cancer yielded an odds ratio (OR) of 1.42 against transfused patients [39]. The evidence is less clear with other types of cancer [35].

Reducing the need for blood transfusion

The inherent risks, associated costs, and effect on blood inventory available have led to a greater reluctance to expose patients to the problems associated with allogeneic blood transfusion [40]. Thus, one should be able to justify the use of blood products at all times, and for each patient, question whether the benefits of transfusion are worth the risks.

Requirement for allogeneic blood transfusion can be reduced by:

- the detection and treatment of preoperative anemia
- accepting the appropriateness of a restrictive transfusion strategy for most patients
- preventing and reducing blood or RBC loss

Preoperative management

Anemia is the most important risk factor for transfusion [41], and 30% of surgical patients present preoperatively with anemia [12]. Preoperative assessment should include a thorough patient history, as well as relevant blood work depending on medical history, medications, type of surgery, and risk of major blood loss. Preadmission evaluation should take place as far in advance of elective surgery as possible (e.g., 30 days) to allow adequate time for evaluation and treatment of anemia [41].

- Erythropoiesis-stimulating agents (E-SA) can be considered in the preoperative setting for anemic patients. While originally recommended for patients undergoing orthopedic or cardiac surgery as a blood conservation strategy, their safety has been reassessed. A post-approval study showed that patients scheduled for elective spine surgery who received preoperative E-SAs had higher rates of thrombosis [42]. It should be noted that patients in this trial did not receive anticoagulation prophylaxis for thrombotic adverse events, in contrast to the clinical trials in joint replacement patients that resulted in the original approval of E-SAs in elective surgery [42,43]. Data from this study and others led the U.S. Food and Drug Administration (FDA) to restrict the use of E-SAs to nonvascular, non-cardiac patients undergoing major elective surgery. The European Union has restricted the use of E-SAs to elective orthopedic surgical patients. In clinical practice, the increased risks of death and thromboembolic events should be balanced against the benefits of treatment with E-SAs, considering each patient's clinical circumstances [43]. E-SAs remain a valuable treatment for patients such as Jehovah's witnesses or with significant antibodies for whom blood transfusion is not an option.
- Preoperative autologous blood donation is a potential strategy for patients undergoing elective surgery, particularly in patients with RBC alloantibodies. The increased costs associated with autologous donation, the reduced risk of infection associated with allogeneic transfusions, and advances in surgical techniques have made preoperative autologous donation poorly cost effective [40].

Prevention of blood loss

A detailed account of perioperative methods of reducing surgical blood loss lies outside the scope of this text, but these include:

- permissive hypotensive anesthetic techniques
- surgery under spinal or epidural anesthesia as opposed to general anesthesia
- appropriate attention to patient positioning, CO_2 tension, and venous drainage
- improved surgical technique, including minimally invasive surgery
- use of tourniquets and infiltration of vasoconstrictors

- use of antifibrinolytic and other drugs to reduce bleeding (see later)
- use of cell salvage and reinfusion
- acute normovolemic hemodilution (ANH) preventing the loss of RBCs

  Note: the benefit of ANH is the reduction of blood loss when whole blood is lost perioperatively at lower hematocrit values achieved with ANH. The blood collected by ANH is stored at room temperature and returned within eight hours of collection, thereby leaving the platelets and coagulation factors within the blood collected functionally intact. The current literature supports a role for ANH in patients undergoing open heart coronary artery bypass surgery and Jehovah's witnesses [40].

Management of surgical bleeding

First and foremost, bleeding from damaged blood vessels requires surgical control.

Occasionally with trauma patients, and less commonly with vascular surgery patients, conventional surgical techniques are ineffective and "damage control surgery" is recommended to prevent the lethal triad of coagulopathy, acidosis, and hypothermia and to prevent the development of irreversible shock. Damage control surgery [44] involves packing the abdomen, not closing the abdomen, ventilating the patient in ICU, and correcting coagulation defects, hypothermia, and acidosis. The patient undergoes definitive surgery when stable. This approach reduces the side effects of massive transfusion and saves the lives of trauma patients.

All other "nonsurgical" bleeding can be termed microvascular bleeding.

- Microvascular bleeding due to clotting factor deficiency is less common than surgical bleeding and hypothermia, and rarely occurs in surgery of under one hour and with transfusion of less than 10 units of blood. Prothrombin, factor V, and factor VII levels are critically reduced if losses exceed approximately twice the blood volume.
- Fresh frozen plasma for clotting factor replacement is recommended by the ASA [17] for:
  1. microvascular bleeding in the presence of a prothrombin time (PT) >1.5 times the middle of the reference range, an international normalized ratio (INR)≥ 1.6, or an activated partial prothromboplastin time (aPTT)$>1.5 \times$ normal
  2. emergency reversal of the effect of warfarin prior to surgery or during active bleeding episodes. As the hemostatic effect of plasma lasts for approximately eight hours, it should be given close to the start of any invasive surgical procedure and in conjunction with vitamin K administration
  3. plasma dose should be at least 10–15 mL/kg, including when being used for warfarin reversal
- Platelet replacement has also been recommended by ASA guidelines [17] for:
  1. microvascular bleeding with a platelet count of <50
  2. microvascular bleeding with $50<$platelet count<100 and a risk of more significant bleeding
  3. microvascular bleeding with a platelet count of <100 for surgery in a closed space (e.g., neurosurgery)
  4. microvascular bleeding with known platelet dysfunction (e.g., the presence of potent antiplatelet agents, cardiopulmonary bypass)

- Cryoprecipitate replacement for fibrinogen deficiency is recommended by the ASA [17] for:
    1. microvascular bleeding with fibrinogen concentration of <100–150 mg/dL
    2. in the setting of postpartum hemorrhage, fibrinogen levels may need to be >200 mg/dL for hemostasis

Massive transfusion

There are several definitions used for massive blood transfusion (MBT) in the literature. These include: ≥10 units RBCs in 24 hours; 1 blood volume in 24 hours; 0.5 blood volume within 3 hours; 6 units RBCs in 12 hours. The latest ASA guideline update on massive transfusion suggests a more practical and usable definition such as: a requirement for >4 RBC units in 1 hour with ongoing need for transfusion, or blood loss of >150 mL/min with hemodynamic instability and need for transfusion [17]. Full discussion of the management of MBT and prevention and treatment of coagulopathies is beyond the scope of this text, but the following is a summary of the principles recommended by the ASA Committee on Blood Management [17] and the European Society of Anaesthesiology (ESA) guidelines [45].

- Hospitals should have a Massive Transfusion Protocol in place to manage either surgical or medical emergencies effectively, where life-threatening hemorrhage is confronted [17,46]. This will involve contacting key personnel in the operating room and laboratories to ensure that blood products are made available quickly and transported to the patient.
- Surgical control of hemorrhage (including damage control surgery) and timely application of volume resuscitation with fluids and blood components to restore circulating volume and tissue oxygenation remain the cornerstone of treatment.
- Request suitable RBC products. O-negative blood is rarely essential, and most laboratories can supply group-specific blood very quickly (with ongoing cross-match checks while the blood is being delivered). Whole blood is ideal but not often available.
- Blood warmers and/or a rapid infusion device should be used. Rapid infusion devices are useful due to the speed at which blood may be pumped into the patient, but more crucially, they are able to warm blood adequately even at very high flow rates. This has been shown to limit the eventual total blood requirement by maintaining body temperature and preventing acidosis and coagulopathy [47].
- Employ cell-saver technology if available and if the wound is not heavily contaminated [45].
- Point-of-care (POC) coagulation testing (e.g., thromboelastography, thromboelastometry, Sonoclot) should be used to guide hemostatic therapy [45]. Standard coagulation tests such as PT, PTT, INR, platelet count, and fibrinogen usually require a minimum of 30–60 minutes and results may be clinically irrelevant if they are outdated by the time they are received [17].
- Request platelets (e.g., 1 unit/10 kg weight), fresh frozen plasma (FFP) (e.g,. 10–15 mL/kg), and cryoprecipitate (e.g., 6-unit pool) according to local guidelines. Evidence for the benefit of a 1:1:1 ratio-driven resuscitation is not supported by the current literature and increasingly it is being recommended that this be replaced by POC or other laboratory endpoints to direct therapy better [17,48].

- Fibrinogen replacement is indicated at levels of <1.5 g/L (150 mg/dL), or rotational thromboelastometry, or thromboelastography [46], showing signs of functional fibrinogen deficit. This can be achieved with fibrinogen concentrate doses of 3–4 g or cryoprecipitate of 50 mg/kg [17,45].
- Tranexamic acid (TXA) is recommended, particularly for trauma patients [45,48].
- Recombinant activated factor VII use is controversial. The risks of serious adverse effects advocate that its use be individualized based on a risk–benefit analysis [17].
- Base deficit and lactate levels should be monitored to assess adequacy of resuscitation in restoring oxygen deliveryVO_2 and tissue perfusion [17].
- Electrolyte abnormalities caused by dilution and transfusion should be corrected [17]:
  - hyperkalemia from large volume of banked RBCs
  - hypocalcemia from citrated anticoagulants
  - Na and Cl abnormalities from crystalloid infusion
- Suspect disseminated intravascular coagulation if clotting factor correction does not result in clinical improvement.

Coagulation and coagulopathy

POC testing

The literature supports a role for POC testing coupled with treatment algorithms in liver transplantation, cardiac, and trauma surgery [40]. A retrospective cohort study reviewed 3865 patients undergoing cardiac surgery before and after the implementation of POC testing coupled with a treatment algorithm. POC testing included activated clotting time, thromboelastometry, and whole-blood aggregometry. They found a significant decrease in blood and plasma transfusions, a significant increase in platelet, fibrinogen concentrate, and prothrombin complex concentrate administration, and a reduction by 50% of rates of reoperation for bleeding and for thrombotic complications [40,49].

Factor concentrates

Fibrinogen

Fibrinogen has a central role in the formation of the platelet plug [50]. Recommendations for minimum fibrinogen concentration is 1.5–2.0 g/L in surgical patients [51] and >2.0 g/L in postpartum bleeding [52].

- A recent systematic review shows that fibrinogen concentrates are more effective than plasma in the repletion of fibrinogen concentrations in patients with hemorrhage, with no adverse events reported [53].
- In a prospective randomized study in patients having aortic surgery on cardiopulmonary bypass with clinically relevant coagulopathy and bleeding after bypass, administration of fibrinogen guided by thromboelastometry decreased overall transfusion needs from 13 to 2 units of allogeneic blood products [54].

Prothrombin complex concentrates (PCC)

PCCs that contain all four (II, VII, IX, X) of the vitamin K-dependent clotting factors are approved for use internationally. Guidelines from several medical societies, including the 2012 American College of Chest Physicians (ACCP) practice guidelines, recommend that PCCs be given instead of plasma for acute reversal of warfarin coagulopathy [40,55].

- The safety of PCC in this setting remains controversial as several studies have shown increased risk of thrombotic events, although this has been contributed to cessation of anticoagulant therapy for underlying risk of thrombosis [43,56].
- PCCs are being used increasingly in the off-label setting of trauma and surgery associated with coagulopathy [51].
- A study of trauma patients used targeted treatment with PCCs and rotation thromboelastometry-based algorithms showed significant reductions in transfused blood components [57].
- At present, the role of PCCs in perioperative management of bleeding remains uncertain [40,58].

Recombinant activated factor VII (rFVIIa)

rFVIIa complexes bind directly with tissue factor released from the subendothelium at sites of vascular disruption. It also binds to activated platelets, which localizes factor X activation to sites of tissue injury.

- Current approved indications for rFVIIA include treatment of bleeding episodes in patients with congenital hemophilia A or B with inhibitors to Factors VIII or IX, patients with congenital Factor VII deficiency, and in patients with acquired hemophilia.
- In the European Union, it has also been approved for patients with inherited qualitative platelet defects [43].
- These approved indications have accounted for only 4.2% of the 73 747 cases reported to have used rFVIIa in the United States from 2000 to 2008 [59].
- A study in high-risk, bleeding cardiac surgery patients found that when rFVIIa was used postoperatively, there was a significant reduction in bleeding, transfusion requirements, and re-explorations [60].
- A systematic literature review found little evidence of efficacy for five off-label clinical settings: intracranial hemorrhage, cardiac surgery, trauma, liver transplantation, and prostatectomy. There was no reduction in mortality associated with the use of rFVIIa in any of these settings [61].
- In a systematic review analyzing 35 randomized clinical trials, a significantly increased risk of arterial (but not venous) thromboembolic events was found. This risk was especially high in patients 75 years of age or older [62].
- A Cochrane systematic review published in 2012 concluded that the effectiveness of rFVIIa as a hemostatic drug remains unproven, and that given the increased risk of arterial thromboembolic events, any use of rFVIIa outside of its current licensed indications should be restricted to clinical trials [63].
- Recent guidelines published by The Society of Thoracic Surgeons and the Society of Cardiovascular Anesthesiologist in 2011, as well as the ESA in 2013 for perioperative management of bleeding recommend rFVIIa only for use in intractable nonsurgical bleeding that is unresponsive to routine hemostatic therapy [18,64]. It is recommended that hypofibrinogenemia, thrombocytopenia, hypothermia, acidosis, and hyperfibrinolysis be treated prior to administration of rFVIIa [64].

Factor XIII (FXIII)

FXIII is activated by thrombin and crosslinks soluble fibrin monomers into insoluble fibrin strands. It also protects the developing clot from fibrinolysis [65].

- The blood conservation guidelines from the Society of Thoracic Surgeons and the Society of Cardiovascular Anesthesiologists have recommended that Factor XIII may be used as a hemostatic agent for clot stabilization in bleeding patients undergoing cardiac surgery with cardiopulmonary bypass when other treatments have not yielded satisfactory results [18].
- Current literature reveals mixed results and more studies are needed to support its routine use as a hemostatic agent.

Pharmacological adjuncts to coagulation

Many drugs have been used with varying success in an attempt to aid hemostasis without causing unwanted thrombosis or other side effects.

Antifibrinolytics

Antifibrinolytics inhibit the physiological fibrinolytic pathway that is responsible for dissolving clots [40].

- TXA is a lysine analog that acts by interfering with the activation of plasminogen to plasmin and its binding to fibrin clots [43]. In a clinical trial (CRASH 2) of 20 000 trauma patients with bleeding (or at risk of bleeding), early administration of 1 g of TXA before an eight-hour infusion of another 1 g resulted in a decrease in mortality and thrombotic complications when treatment was started within the first three hours after the trauma occurred [66].
- Aprotinin is a serine protease inhibitor that directly inhibits plasmin, thus reducing fibrinolysis [43]. Aprotinin was removed from the market in 2007 due to concerns of increased renal, cardiac, and cerebral complications. However, re-examination of the Blood Conservation Using Antifibrinolytics in a Randomized Trial (BART) study and other evidence have led to a reversal of this decision [43,67]. Aprotinin has been reintroduced in Canada and Europe for low-risk cardiac surgery.
- A Cochrane review concluded that antifibrinolytics provide worthwhile reductions in blood loss and allogeneic blood transfusions. Aprotinin seemed to be slightly more effective in this regard, but the lysine analogs appear to have no adverse events [67].
- Desmopressin or 1-deamino-8-D-arginine vasopressin is a synthetic analog of vasopressin. It contributes to hemostasis through increasing levels of von Willebrand factor and Factor VIII and improving platelet function. It is also thought to induce the production of nitric oxide and increase the level of tissue plasminogen activator [68]. It is indicated to maintain hemostasis in patients with hemophilia A or type-1 von Willebrand disease with Factor VIII activity of >5%. Desmopressin has also been used as a hemostatic agent in patients without pre-existing coagulation disorders undergoing high blood loss surgeries. A meta-analysis of 38 randomized, placebo-controlled trials reported that desmopressin had a statistically significant effect on reducing perioperative bleeding and transfusion of blood products. The effects were small, with blood loss reduced by 80 mL and transfusion reduced by 0.3 units. The risk of thromboembolic adverse events was not significantly increased [69]. Some studies suggest that in patients with platelet dysfunction (e.g., due to aspirin), there is increased benefit from desmopressin [70].

Topical hemostatics

Topical hemostatics act by activating/aggregating platelets, providing a physical scaffold for better clot formation, and compressing the bleeding vessels.

- Fibrin sealants are potent topical hemostatic products that contain both thrombin and fibrinogen. A meta-analysis evaluating 18 trials concluded that fibrin sealants reduced allogeneic RBC transfusions by 37% and reduced blood loss by an average of 161 mL per patient [71]. Previous concerns with inhibitory antibody formation have resulted in issuance of a black box warning on topical bovine thrombin. This risk appears to be eliminated when recombinant human protein is used [72].

Artificial oxygen carriers ("blood substitutes")

Artificial oxygen carriers are designed to improve tissue oxygenation by either supplying additional Hb molecules or by providing an inert medium capable of dissolving substantial amounts of oxygen [43]. The prospect of these products are very promising, as the infectious risks of blood transfusion may be avoided, there is no need for blood grouping and cross-matching, and an extended shelf life as well as possible storage at room temperature could make them universally available [73]. Unfortunately, the research into artificial oxygen carriers thus far finds that the risk far outweighs the benefits. None of these compounds has achieved market approval for Europe, the United States, or Canada.

- Perfluorocarbon (PFC) emulsion: PFC emulsions boost oxygen delivery by increasing the amount of dissolved oxygen. To maximize their effectiveness, they must be coupled with an increased FiO_2 to further increase the amount of dissolved oxygen [43]. One PFC that has reached clinical trials, Oxygent, has been shown in numerous studies to improve oxygen delivery and replace and reduce transfusions. However, there was an increase in stroke incidence in those patients receiving Oxygent compared to controls [74].
- Hemoglobin-based oxygen carriers (HBOCs): HBOCs increase oxygen delivery by increasing Hb levels. The Hb may be from human, animal, or recombinant sources. Studies have shown these products to be effective in reducing allogeneic transfusions, but all products studied to date have been associated with significantly higher risk of MI and death [75].

References

1. Hebert PC, Van der Linden P, Biro G, et al. Physiologic aspects of anemia. *Crit Care Clin* 2004; **20**: 187–212.

2. Hare GMT, Freedman J, Mazer CD. Review article: risks of anemia and related management strategies: can perioperative blood management improve patient safety? *Can J Anaesth* 2013; **60**: 168–75.

3. Shander A, Javidroozi M, Ozawa S, et al. What is really dangerous: anaemia or transfusion? *Br J Anaesth*; **107**: i41–59.

4. Tsui AK, Marsden PA, Mazer CD, et al. Priming of hypoxia-inducible factor by neuronal nitric oxide synthase is essential for adaptive responses to severe anemia. *Proc Natl Acad Sci U S A* 2011; **108**: 17544–9.

5. McLaren AT, Marsden PA, Mazer CD, et al. Increased expression of HIF-1 {alpha}, nNOS, and VEGF in the cerebral cortex of anemic rats. *Am J Physiol Regul Integr Comp Physiol* 2007; **292**: R403–14.

6. Roberson RS, Bennett-Guerrero E. Impact of red blood cell transfusion on global and regional measures of oxygenation. *Mt Sinai J Med* 2012; **79**: 66–74.

7. Creteur J, Neves AP, Vincent JL. Near infared spectroscopy technique to evaluate the effects of red blood cell transfusion on tissue oxygenation. *Crit Care* 2009; **13**: S11.

8. Orlov D, O'Farrell R, McCluskey SA, et al. The clinical utility of an index of global oxygenation for guiding red blood cell transfusion in cardiac surgery. *Transfusion* 2009; **49**: 682–8.

9. Saager L, Alparslan T, Reynolds LF, et al. The association between preoperative anemia and 30-day mortality and morbidity in noncardiac surgical patients. *Anesth Analg* 2013; **117**: 909–15.

10. Sabatine MS, Morrow DA, Giugliano SM, et al. Association of hemoglobin levels with clinical outcomes in acute coronary syndromes. *Circulation* 2005; **111**: 2042–9.

11. Beattie WS, Karkouti K, Wijeysundera DN, et al. Risk associated with preoperative anemia in noncardiac surgery. *Anesthesiology* 2009; **110**: 574–81.

12. Musallam KM, Tamim HM, Richards T, et al. Preoperative anaemia and postoperative outcomes in non-cardiac surgery: a retrospective cohort study. *Lancet* 2011; **378**: 1396–407.

13. Klein HG, Spahn DR, Carson JL. Red blood cell transfusion in clinical practice. *Lancet* 2007; **370**: 415–26.

14. Hebert PC, Wells G, Blajchman MA, et al. A multicenter, randomized, controlled clinical trial of transfusion requirements in critical care. *N Engl J Med* 1999; **340**: 409–17.

15. Carson JL, Carless PA, Hebert PC, et al. Transfusion thresholds and other strategies for guiding allogeneic red blood cell transfusion (Review). *Cochrane Database Syst Rev* 2012; **4**: CD002042.

16. Lacroix J, Hebert PC, Hutchinson JS, et al. Transfusion requirements for patients in paediatric intensive care units. *N Engl J Med* 2007; **365**: 1609–19.

17. American Society of Anesthesiologists Task Force on Perioperative Blood Transfusion and Adjuvent Therapies. Practice guidelines for perioperative blood transfusion and adjuvant therapies: an updated report. *Anesthesiology* 2006; **105**: 198–208.

18. Ferraris VA, Brown JR, Despotis GJ, et al. 2011 update to the Society of Thoracic Surgeons and the Society of Cardiovascular Anesthesiologists blood conservation clinical practice guidelines. *Ann Thorac Surg* 2011; **91**: 944–82.

19. Linden JV, Wagner K, Voytovich AE, et al. Transfusion errors in New York State: an analysis of 10 years' experience. *Transfusion* 2000; **40**: 1207–13.

20. Williamson LM, Lowe S, Love EM, et al. Serious hazards of transfusion (SHOT) initiative: analysis of the first two annual reports. *BMJ* 1999; **319**: 16–19.

21. Tinmouth A, Ferguson D, Yee IC, et al. Clinical consequences of red cell storage in the critically ill. *Transfusion* 2006; **46**: 2014–27.

22. Vamvakas EC. Meta-analysis of clinical studies of the purported deleterious effects of "old" (versus "fresh") red blood cells: are we at equipoise? *Transfusion* 2010; **50**: 600–10.

23. Sillimann CC, Boshkov LK, Mehdizadehkashi Z, et al. Transfusion related acute lung injury: epidemiology and a prospective analysis of etiologic factors. *Blood* 2003; **101**: 454–62.

24. Shander A, Javidroozi M. A reductionist approach to aged blood. *Anesthesiology* 2010; **113**: 1–3.

25. Vlaar APJ, Hofstra JJ, Levi M, et al. Supernatant of aged erythrocytes causes lung inflammation and coagulopathy in a "Two-hit" in vivo syngeneic transfusion model. *Anesthesiology* 2010; **113**: 92–103.

26. Vlaar APJ, Juffermans NP. Transfusion-related acute lung injury: a clinical review. *Lancet* 2013; **382**: 984–94.

27. O'Brien SF, Yi QL, Fan W, et al. Current incidence and estimated residual risk of transfusion-transmitted infections in donation made to Canadian Blood Services. *Transfusion* 2007; **47**: 316–25.

28. Callum JL, Lin Y, Pinkerton PH. Bloody easy 3: blood transfusions, blood alternatives and transfusion reactions, a

guide to transfusion medicine. 3rd edn. Canada: Ontario Regional Blood Coordinating Network, 2011.

29. Centers for Disease Control and Prevention. Transfusion associated transmission of West Nile virus–Arizona. *Morb Mortal Wkly Rep* 2004; **53**: 842–4.

30. Apagova M, Busch MP, Custer B. Cost-effectiveness of screening the US blood supply for *Trypanosoma cruzi*. *Transfusion* 2010; **50**: 2220–32.

31. Lescoutra-Etchegaray N, Sumian C, Culeux A, et al. Removal of exogenous prion infectivity in leukoreduced red blood cells unit by a specific filter designed for human transfusion. *Transfusion* 2013 [Epub ahead of print].

32. Cervia JS, Sowemimo-Coker SO, Ortolano GA, et al. An overview of prion biology and the role of blood filtration in reducing the risk of transfusion-transmitted variant Creutzfeldt–Jakob disease. *Transfus Med Rev* 2006; **20**: 190–206.

33. U.S. Department of Health and Human Services, Food and Drug Administration, Center for Biologics Evaluation and Research. Guidance for industry-revised preventative measures to reduce the possible risk of transmission of Creutzfeldt-Jakob disease (CJD) and variant Creutzfeldt-Jakob disease (vCJD) by blood and blood products. Available from: http://www.fda.gov/BiologicsBloodVaccines/GuidanceCompliance RegulatoryInformation/Guidances/default.htm.

34. Bracher ME, Hay SN. Bacterial contamination of blood components. *Clin Microbiol Rev* 2005; **18**: 195–204.

35. Cata JP, Wang H, Gottumukkala V, et al. Inflammatory response, immunosuppression, and cancer recurrence after perioperative blood transfusions. *Br J Anaesth* 2013; **110**: 690–701.

36. Lannan KL, Sahler J, Spinelli SL, et al. Transfusion immunomodulation–the case for leukoreduced and (perhaps) washed transfusions. *Blood Cells Mol Dis* 2013; **50**: 61–8.

37. Flohe S, Kobbe P, Nast-Kolb D. Immunological reactions secondary to blood transfusion *Injury* 2007; **38**: 1405–8.

38. Chung M, Steinmetz OK, Gordon PH. Perioperative blood transfusion and outcome after resection for colorectal carcinoma. *Br J Surg* 1993; **80**: 427–32.

39. Amato A, Pescatori M. Perioperative blood transfusions for the recurrence of colorectal cancer. *Cochrane Database Syst Rev*. 2006; **1**: CD005033.

40. Spahn DR, Goodnough LT. Alternatives to blood transfusion. *Lancet* 2013; **381**: 1855–65.

41. Goodnough LT, Maniatis A, Earnshaw P, et al. Detection, evaluation, and management of preoperative anaemia in the elective orthopaedic surgical patient: NATA guidelines. *Br J Anaesth* 2011; **106**: 13–22.

42. Stowell CP, Jones SC, Enny C, et al. An open-label, randomized, parallel-group study of perioperative epoeitin alfa versus standard of care for blood conservation in major elective spinal surgery: safety analysis. *Spine* 2009; **34**: 2479–85.

43. Goodnough LT, Shander A. Current status of pharmacologic therapies in patient blood management. *Anesth Analg* 2013; **116**: 15–34.

44. Germanos S, Gourgiotis S, Villias C, et al. Damage control surgery in the abdomen: an approach for the management of severe injured patients. *Int J Surg* 2008; **6**: 246–52.

45. Kozek-Langenecker SA, Afshari A, Albaladejo P, et al. Management of severe perioperative bleeding. Guidelines from the European Society of Anaesthesiology. *Eur J Anaesthesiol* 2013; **30**: 270–382.

46. Dente CJ, Shaz BH, Nicholas JM, et al. Improvements in early mortality and coagulopathy are sustained better in patients with blunt trauma after institution of a massive transfusion protocol in a civilian level I trauma center. *J Trauma* 2009; **66**: 1616–24.

47. Dunham CM, Belzberg H, Lyles R, et al. The rapid infusion system: a superior method for the resuscitation of

hypovolemic trauma patients. *Resuscitation* 1991; **21**: 207–27.

48. Dzik WH, Blajchman MA, Fergusson D, et al. Clinical review: Canadian National Advisory Committee on blood and blood products–massive transfusion consensus conference 2011: report of the panel. *Crit Care* 2011; **15**: R242.

49. Gorlinger K, Dirkmann D, Hanke AA, et al. First-line therapy with coagulation factor concentrates combined with point-of-care coagulation testing is associated with decreased allogeneic blood transfusion in cardiovascular surgery: a retrospective, single-center cohort study. *Anesthesiology* 2011; **115**: 1179–91.

50. Furie B, Furie BC. Mechanisms of thrombus formation. *N Engl J Med* 2008; **359**: 938–49.

51. Spahn DR, Bouillon B, Cerny V, et al. Management of bleeding and coagulopathy following major trauma: an updated European guideline. *Crit Care* 2013; **17**: R76.

52. Cortet M, Deneux-Tharaux C, Dupont C, et al. Association between fibrinogen level and severity of postpartum haemorrhage: secondary analysis of a prospective trial. *Br J Anaesth* 2012; **108**: 984–9.

53. Kozek-Langenecker S, Sorenson B, Hess JR, et al. Clinical effectiveness of fresh frozen plasma compared with fibrinogen concentrate: a systematic review. *Crit Care* 2011; **15**: R239.

54. Rahe-Meyer N, Solomon C, Hanke A, et al. Effects of fibrinogen concentrate as first-line therapy during major aortic replacement surgery: a randomized, placebo-controlled trial. *Anesthesiology* 2013; **118**: 40–50.

55. Guyatt GH, Akl EA, Crowther M, et al. Executive summary: antithrombotic therapy and prevention of thrombosis, 9th edn. American College of Chest Physicians evidence-based clinical practice guidelines. *Chest* 2012; **141**: 7–47.

56. Bobbitt L, Merriman E, Raynes J, et al. PROTHROMBINEX(®)-VF (PTX-VF) usage for reversal of coagulopathy: prospective evaluation of thrombogenic risk. *Thromb Res* 2011; **128**: 577–82.

57. Innerhofer P, Westermann I, Tauber H, et al. The exclusive use of coagulation factor concentrates enables reversal of coagulopathy and decreases transfusion rates in patients with major blunt trauma. *Injury* 2013; **44**: 209–16.

58. Sorenson B, Spahn DR, Innerhofer P, et al. Clinical review: prothrombin complex concentrates–evaluation of safety and thrombogenicity. *Crit Care* 2011; **15**: R201.

59. Logan AC, Yank V, Stafford RS. Off-label use of recombinant factor VIIa in U.S. hospitals: analysis of hospital records. *Ann Intern Med* 2011; **154**: 516–22.

60. Gill R, Herbertson M, Vuylsteke A, et al. Safety and efficacy of recombinant activated factor VII: a randomized placebo-controlled trial in the setting of bleeding after cardiac surgery. *Circulation* 2009; **120**: 21–7.

61. Yank V, Tuohy CV, Logan AC, et al. Systematic review benefits and harms of in-hospital use of recombinant factor VIIa for off-label indications. *Ann Intern Med* 2011; **154**: 529–40.

62. Levi M, Levy JH, Andersen HF, et al. Safety of recombinant activated factor VII in randomized clinical trials. *N Engl J Med* 2010; **363**: 1791–800.

63. Simpson E, Lin Y, Stanworth S, et al. Recombinant factor VIIa for the prevention and treatment of bleeding patients without haemophilia. *Cochrane Database Syst Rev* 2012; **3**: CD005011.

64. Levy JH, Greenberg C. Biology of Factor XIII and clinical manifestations of Factor XIII deficiency. *Transfusion* 2013; **53**: 1120–31.

65. Roberts I, Shakur H, Afolabi A, et al. The importance of early treatment with tranexamic acid in bleeding trauma patients: an exploratory analysis of the CRASH-2 randomized control trial. *Lancet* 2011; **377**: 1096–101.

66. Fergusson DA, Hebert PC, Mazer CD, et al. A comparison of aprotinin and lysine analogues in high-risk cardiac surgery. *N Engl J Med* 2008; **358**: 2319–31.

67. Henry DA, Carless PA, Moxey AJ, et al. Antifibrinolytic use for minimising perioperative allogeneic blood transfusion. *Cochrane Database Syst Rev* 2011; **3**: CD001886.

68. Kaufmann JE, Vischer UM. Cellular mechanisms of the hemostatic effects of desmopressin (DDAVP). *J Thromb Haemost* 2003; **1**: 682–9.

69. Crescenzi G, Landoni G, Biondi-Zoccai G, et al. Desmopressin reduces transfusion needs after surgery: a meta-analysis of randomized clinical trials. *Anesthesiology* 2008; **109**: 1063–76.

70. Ozier Y, Bellamy L. Pharmacologic agents: antifibrinolytics and desmopressin. *Best Pract Res Clin Anaesthesiol* 2010; **24**: 107–19.

71. Carless PA, Henry DA, Anthony DM. Fibrin sealant use for minimising peri-operative allogeneic blood transfusion. *Cochrane Database Syst Rev* 2009; **2**: CD004171.

72. Kessler CM, Ortel TL. Recent developments in topical thrombins. *Thromb Haemost* 2009; **102**: 15–24.

73. Shander A, Goodnough LT. Why an alternative to blood transfusion? *Crit Care Clin* 2009; **25**: 261–77.

74. Kocian R, Spahn DR. Haemoglobin, oxygen carriers and perioperative organ perfusion. *Best Pract Res Clin Anaesthesiol* 2008; **22**: 63–80.

75. Natanson C, Kern SJ, Lurie P, et al. Cell-free hemoglobin-based substitutes and risk of myocardial infarction and death: a meta-analysis. *JAMA* 2008; **299**: 2304–12.

Chapter 9

Diabetes

M. Banasch and I. McConachie

Diabetes can be defined as a disorder of glucose handling, characterized by elevated blood glucose and eventual organ dysfunction. Globally, diabetes is thought to affect 347 million people, with 3.4 million people dying in 2004 from hyperglycemia and related disease [1].

Diabetes broadly categorizes a spectrum of disease that includes, but is not limited to types 1, 2, and gestational diabetes.

- Type 1 diabetes refers to an inability of the pancreas to produce insulin, often being diagnosed in childhood or adolescence.
- Type 2 diabetes refers to the production of insulin being less than the body needs or ineffective use of that insulin (often associated with obesity or aging).
- Gestational diabetes occurs in pregnancy and will not be discussed here.

Current guidelines suggest a diagnosis of diabetes with either a fasting plasma glucose level of 7.0 mmol/L or greater, a random plasma glucose greater than 11.1 mmol/L, and symptoms of diabetes, or a two-hour plasma glucose after a 75-g oral glucose drink >11.1 mmol/L [2].

Diabetes has major implications for health and disease with population data suggesting the number of people affected continues to rise, with increases seen in fasting plasma glucose in nearly all countries surveyed [3]. The increase in the incidence of diabetes parallels the increase in obesity in the population.

General perioperative risks/considerations for the diabetic patient

Diabetes affects all body systems, leading to early development of atherosclerosis and numerous other end organ effects.

Airway manipulation

- In the early 1980s, it was found that patients with juvenile-onset diabetes had limited joint mobility.
- Stiff joint syndrome is found in type 1 diabetics, leading to impaired mobility of the atlanto-occipital joint.
- Elevated hemoglobin (Hb)A1C in morbidly obese patients is a known prognostic factor for difficult intubation. Increased HbA1C levels are correlated with more difficult laryngoscopy [4].

Anesthesia and Perioperative Care of the High-Risk Patient, Third edition, ed. Ian McConachie. Published by Cambridge University Press.

- The prayer sign (an inability to press the palms together without a gap remaining between the palms and fingers) [5] has been demonstrated to be useful for evaluating long-term type 2 diabetics.

Cardiovascular

The impact of diabetes on the cardiovascular system cannot be overstated. The perioperative risk of morbidity and mortality is thought to be doubled [6].

- Diabetics are at elevated risk for hypertension and stroke and lower limb amputations.
- American College of Cardiology (ACC) guidelines recommend heightened suspicion for coronary artery disease (CAD) in patients with diabetes.
- Insulin therapy has been identified as a significant risk factor for cardiac disease [7].
- In comparisons between diabetic and non-diabetic patients, atherosclerosis is found to develop earlier and be more widespread in diabetics.
- Silent myocardial infarctions (MIs) are more common in this patient group, possibly secondary to autonomic neuropathy and involvement of the sensory innervation of the heart, although a full understanding of the pathophysiology remains elusive [8].
- Diabetic autonomic neuropathy has multiple effects, causing significant morbidity and putting patients at risk for arrhythmias and sudden death. Commonly, patients have resting tachycardia, loss of heart rate variability, exercise intolerance, gastroparesis, and postural hypotension [8].
- Diabetics are at elevated risk for developing a cardiomyopathy specific to the disease and unrelated to CAD. Diastolic dysfunction predominates and may progress to heart failure, with preservation of the ejection fraction, and an eventual restrictive cardiomyopathy [9].

Nephropathy

- Diabetic nephropathy is increasingly common with aging with 40%–50% of patients expected to develop some degree of renal dysfunction. Diabetes is a leading cause of renal failure.
- There can be a profound effect on the renal clearance of drugs, placing the patients at risk for further nephrotoxicity.

Gastrointestinal (GI) effects

- Diabetic neuropathy affects the ganglion cells of the GI tract, which can delay gastric emptying and cause gastroparesis.
- This delayed emptying places patients at increased risk of aspiration and some clinicians administer metoclopramide to hasten transit, as well as prescribing medications to block acid production and neutralize stomach contents as pre-treatment.

Retinopathy

- A recent meta-analysis identified retinopathy as a possible screening tool for cerebral involvement of microvascular changes in diabetes [10].

- This study cited the embryological commonality of both the retina and the cerebral vasculature, suggesting this shared origin [10].

Surgery

- Diabetic patients, in general, have an increased risk of peri- and postoperative complications relating to the increased incidence of cardiac, microvascular, and renal disease. In addition, it is believed that there is an increased risk of wound and other infections and poor wound healing – especially where there is poor control of hyperglycemia.
- However, a recent, large retrospective study found no increase in complications in diabetic patients compared to non-diabetic patients after knee arthroplasty [11].
- A Cochrane review concluded "There is insufficient evidence to support strict glycemic control in the intra- and postoperative period among surgical patients for the prevention of surgical site infections." [12].

The surgical stress response

Surgery (and also trauma, sepsis, and burns) produces hormonal and metabolic changes referred to as the stress response. This results in increased secretion of hormones such as cortisol and growth hormone and activation of the sympathetic nervous system. The resultant changes produce a state of insulin resistance perioperatively, resulting in hyperglycemia after major surgery and impaired glucose control in diabetic patients.

Effect of anesthesia on blood glucose

Anesthetic agent effects

Many anesthetic agents and techniques affect glucose homeostasis in the perioperative period, especially if the surgical stress response is modified; however, the exact clinical significance of these changes is debatable. For example:

- A recent randomized control trial (RCT) demonstrated a significant decrease in blood glucose intraoperatively with preoperative premedication with ketamine [13].
- Propofol in the absence of a surgical stimulus has minimal effect on blood glucose [14], whereas propofol combined with a short-acting opiate infusion has been demonstrated to significantly decrease blood glucose intraoperatively when compared with inhalational anesthetic techniques, with minimal effect on blood glucose postoperatively [15,16].
- Since the 1980s, opiates have been known to modify the endocrine response to a surgical stimulus [17,18]. All of the different opiates available have been shown to have benefits in suppression of the hypothalamic-pituitary axis's response and blood glucose.
- Inhalational agents are a cornerstone of modern anesthesia; however, their effects on glucose homeostasis are being understood only more recently. There are significant increases in plasma glucose among patients anesthetized with sevoflurane when compared with propofol [14]. A number of authors have investigated this and determined that, as a group, inhalational agents cause a decoupling of the insulin response to hyperglycemia [14,16]. Sevoflurane and isoflurane anesthesia

impair glucose tolerance equally and independent of dosage up to 1.5 minimum alveolar concentration.

- The mechanism of impaired glucose regulation is thought to be secondary to the potassium adenosine triphosphate (ATP) channel present on β-cells of the pancreas, as recent rat models have demonstrated, in comparison between propofol and sevoflurane anesthetics [19,20].
- Whether there are further molecular mechanisms at work to account for the intergroup differences is undetermined as yet. However, these studies suggest significantly tighter glycemic control in patients anesthetized with propofol when compared with inhalational agents.

Antiemetic therapy

- Ondansetron and metoclopramide have little to no effect on blood glucose.
- Dexamethasone has been researched extensively and found to cause statistically significant increases in blood glucose; however, the clinical relevance of this effect is yet to be determined. Initial studies have demonstrated increased blood glucose after a single 10 mg bolus of dexamethasone, which appeared to have a peak effect at two hours, but a continued effect for ~24 hours postoperatively [21,22]. A more recent randomized controlled trial investigated the effects of dexamethasone in both non-diabetic and diabetic patients when compared with placebo. They observed a blood glucose increase of 1.6 mmol/L in the former, and no clinical increase in diabetic patients given dexamethasone when compared with placebo [23].
- The Society of Ambulatory Anesthesia has recommended that dexamethasone not be withheld from diabetic patients, recommending a dose of 4 mg, citing equal efficacy between this and higher doses for postoperative nausea prophylaxis [24].

Glycemic control: tight versus not

Tight control essentially means maintaining blood glucose within the normal laboratory range of 4.5–6.0 mmol/L. Less tight or moderate control may mean maintaining blood glucose at <10 or 11 mmol/L, depending on the study.

General population

- Since the early 1990s and the Diabetes Control and Complications Trial (DCCT), it has been known that tight glycemic control in the type 1 diabetic has significant benefits in reducing the risk of diabetic retinopathy, neuropathy, and nephropathy [25].
- In further follow-up, it was found that tight control of type 1 diabetics reduced cardiovascular disease by 42% and reduced the first occurrence of non-fatal stroke, (MIs), and death from cardiovascular disease by 57% [26].

The benefits observed with tight control of type 1 diabetics were then generalized to type 2 diabetics, with studies conducted to explore this possibility.

- The Action to Control Cardiovascular Risk in Diabetes study targeted middle-aged and elderly type 2 diabetics, with a HbA1C of >7.5% and cardiovascular disease risk factors, with an aim to decrease the HbA1C to <6.

- The study was terminated early due to increased mortality observed in the tight glycemic control group [27]. In long-term follow-up a decrease was found in non-fatal (MIs), but increased overall mortality was still observed.

Overall, it would appear that tight glycemic control in the type 1 diabetic is beneficial; however, the benefits are less clear in type 2 diabetics and may be harmful.

The critically ill patient

- Prior to 2001, most studies of intensive care unit (ICU) patients did not include normoglycemia among their aims.
- In a 2001 landmark study, Van den Berghe et al. demonstrated a 3.6% mortality reduction in patients placed on a tight glycemic control regimen [28]. However, this study contained a high proportion of cardiac surgery patients and may not be comparable to a more heterogenous ICU population. Indeed, later studies demonstrated less benefit from tight glucose control than seen in the original study.
- The possible harm of tight glycemic control was discovered more recently.
- In the NICE-SUGAR trial, a total of 6104 patients were randomized to receive either tight (4.5–6.0 mmol/L) or conventional (<10 mmol/L) glucose control. A statistically significant increase in mortality among the tight glycemic control group was observed [29].
- The Glucontrol trial, a multicenter RCT in Europe, observed significant hypoglycemia in their patients and was stopped prematurely secondary to this finding [30]. Hypoglycemia resulting from tight glucose control may be the causative agent for these increases in mortality. This hypothesis is supported further by retrospective data, which when corrected for organ failure, also demonstrate an increased mortality associated with hypoglycaemia [31].
- Interestingly, despite the known adverse effects of hyperglycemia on neurological outcome in neurologically impaired patients (such as patients with closed head injuries or cerebrovascular accidents), a systematic review and meta-analysis found similar results in neurocritical care patients [32]. That is, there were no benefits to tight glucose control with increases in hypoglycemia in those patients, poor control worsened outcome, and moderate control may be best.
- The lack of apparent benefit from tight glucose control has led to a number of different hypotheses, including that the degree of hyperglycemia may be a marker of the severity of disease. There has been interest in the potential beneficial effects insulin may have beyond simply decreasing glucose as long as hypoglycemia is avoided. These include a possible protein sparing effect and a lowering of serum cortisol levels – in one study seemingly related to insulin's beneficial effect [33]. In addition, a retrospective observational trial confirmed the general relationship between hyperglycemia in ICU and mortality but diabetic patients had no such association [34]. This suggests that hyperglycemia may have different biological and clinical implications in diabetic and non-diabetic patients.
- Overall, best outcomes may be seen if glycemic control targets in critically ill patients are closer to 7–11 mmol/L, that is, moderate control is best.

General surgical population

- Current evidence suggests an increased risk for complications secondary to poor glycemic control during the perioperative period. For example, an early case control trial in Europe found that preoperative hyperglycemia had an association with increased cardiovascular mortality in patients undergoing non-cardiac and nonvascular surgery [35].
- Further retrospective studies have identified additional complications related to hyperglycemia, with an increased risk of infection (odds ratio [OR] 2.0), reoperative intervention (OR 1.8), and death (OR 2.71) in both diabetic and non-diabetic cases with hyperglycemia [36]. Patients with hyperglycemia that were treated with insulin to a target blood glucose of <10 mmol/L had no significant increase in risk.
- Although there are limited prospective data, there may be benefit from avoiding poor control of hyperglycemia in the perioperative period in the non-cardiac patient, with vigilance to avoid hypoglycemia.

Cardiac surgery

- Traditional teaching suggested that tight glycemic control is beneficial in cardiac patients; however, the scrutiny given to the ICU literature has prompted further investigation.
- In 2007, an RCT comparing tight glycemic control with conventional treatment found an increased incidence of both stroke and death in the tight control group [37].
- Retrospective studies in both 2010 and 2011 demonstrated decreased mortality and complications in patients with moderate glycemic control when compared with tight control [38,39].
- These data suggest little benefit to tight versus moderate blood glucose control; however, recent data suggest there may be differences between diabetic and non-diabetic patients in their responses to hyperglycemia and its implications. Thus, there is increased hospital mortality in hyperglycemic post-coronary artery bypass grafting (CABG) non-diabetic patients while hyperglycemia in diabetic patients was not associated with increased mortality [40].
- Overall, recent trends would suggest there is benefit to moderate blood glucose control in the perioperative period, with fewer complications when compared with tight control and better outcomes than poor control.

Intraoperative management

- Currently, there is no evidence regarding the optimal management algorithm.
- The choice of method of glucose control is probably less important than the skill, organization, and coordination of the nurses and doctors involved.
- Current consensus statements from the Society of Ambulatory Anesthesia recommend a regime based on patient safety and avoidance of adverse outcomes, including the avoidance of hypo-/hyperglycemia [24]. They also recommend continuation of long-acting/basal insulin regimens (e.g., glargine) on the day of surgery, and holding intermediate-acting and oral medications.

- The decision to postpone surgery secondary to elevated blood glucose should be made only if there are significant complications (e.g., ketoacidosis) and there is time for optimization. Importantly, this decision should be made in consultation with the surgeon and taking all patient factors into account.
- Currently, there is little evidence as to the optimal intraoperative blood glucose level; however, experts recommend a target of <10.0 mmol/L [24].
- Newer insulins, such as basal glargine, with a peakless pharmacokinetic profile show promise. Glargine can provide better blood glucose control when compared with the glucose–insulin–potassium regimen commonly used in cardiac surgery [41].

Type 1 diabetic patients

- These patients differ from the type 2 group, in that glucose must be administered in order to prevent ketoacidosis.
- The recommended glucose administration is between 5 g/hr and 10 g/hr in the average 70-kg adult.
- This can be combined with insulin, and commonly, potassium for longer cases, with a glucose target of 10.0 mmol/L, as previously discussed.

Type 2 diabetic patients

- Current evidence suggests there can be more flexibility for the management of type 2 diabetic patients. It is recommended that hypoglycemia be avoided and to minimize the period of hyperglycemia.
- Caution must be taken in the management of patients with chronic poor control, as acute normalization of blood glucose can increase the risk of postoperative complications.

Hypoglycemia

- The management of hypoglycemia is comparatively simple.
- In the awake and cooperative patient, consumption of 10–25 g of glucose of clear sugary liquids (e.g., apple juice) will correct most hypoglycemic events. This will have negative implications in the fasted preoperative patient!
- In the anesthetised/unconscious/uncooperative patient, 20–50 mL of dextrose 50 can be administered, with careful monitoring for resolution of hypoglycemia in both cases.

References

1. Danaei G, Finucane MM, Lu Y, et al. National, regional, and global trends in fasting plasma glucose and diabetes prevalence since 1980: systematic analysis of health examination surveys and epidemiological studies with 370 country–years and 2.7 million participants. *Lancet* 2011; **378**: 31–40.
2. American Diabetes Association. Diagnosis and classification of diabetes mellitus. *Diabetes Care* 2013; **36**: S67–74.
3. Shaw J, Sicree R, Zimmet P. Global estimates of the prevalence of diabetes for 2010 and 2030. *Diabetes Res Clin Prat* 2009; **87**: 4–14.
4. Mashour GA, Kheterpal S, Vanaharam V, et al. The extended Mallampati score and a diagnosis of diabetes mellitus are predictors of difficult laryngoscopy in the morbidly obese. *Anesth Analg* 2008; **107**: 1919–23.
5. Kim RP, Edelman SV, DD. Musculoskeletal complications of diabetes mellitus. *Clin Diabetes* 2001; **19**: 132–5.

6. Kadoi Y. Anesthetic considerations in diabetic patients. Part I: preoperative considerations of patients with diabetes mellitus. *J Anesth* 2010; **24**: 739–47.

7. Fleisher LA, Beckman JA, Brown KA, et al. ACC/AHA 2007 guidelines on perioperative cardiovascular evaluation and care for noncardiac surgery: a report of the American College of Cardiology/American Heart Association Task Force on Practice Guidelines. *Circulation* 2007; **116**: e418–500.

8. Vinik AI, Erbas T, Casellini CM. Diabetic cardiac autonomic neuropathy, inflammation and cardiovascular disease. *J Diabetes Investig* 2013; **4**: 4–18.

9. Amour J, Kersten JR. Diabetic cardiomyopathy and anesthesia. *Anesthesiology* 2008; **108**: 524–30.

10. Patton N, Aslam T, MacGillivray T, et al. Retinal vascular image analysis as a potential screening tool for cerebrovascular disease: a rationale based on homology between cerebral and retinal microvasculatures. *J Anat* 2005; **206**: 319–48.

11. Adams AL, Paxton EW, Wang JQ, et al. Surgical outcomes of total knee replacement according to diabetes status and glycemic control, 2001 to 2009. *J Bone Joint Surg Am* 2013; **95**: 481–7.

12. Kao LS, Meeks D, Moyer VA, et al. Peri-operative glycaemic control regimens for preventing surgical site infections in adults. *Cochrane Database Syst Rev.* 2009; **3**: CD006806.

13. Du J, Huang Y, Yu X, et al. Effects of preoperative ketamine on the endocrine-metabolic and inflammatory response to laparoscopic surgery. *Chin Med J* 2011; **124**: 3721–5.

14. Zuurbier CJ, Keijzers PJM, Koeman A, et al. Anesthesia's effects on plasma glucose and insulin and cardiac hexokinase at similar hemodynamics and without major surgical stress in fed rats. *Anesth Analg* 2008; **106**: 135–42.

15. Schricker T, Carli F, Schreiber M, et al. Propofol/sufentanil anesthesia suppresses the metabolic and endocrine response during, not after, lower abdominal surgery. *Anesth Analg* 2000; **90**: 450–5.

16. Cok OY, Ozkose Z, Pasaoglu H, et al. Glucose response during craniotomy: propofol–remifentanil versus isoflurane–remifentanil. *Minerva Anestesiol* 2011; **77**: 1141–8.

17. Bovill JG, Sebel PS, Fiolet JW, et al. The influence of sufentanil on endocrine and metabolic responses to cardiac surgery. *Anesth Analg* 1983; **62**: 391–7.

18. Lacoumenta S, Yeo TH, Paterson JL, et al. Hormonal and metabolic responses to cardiac surgery with sufentanil–oxygen anaesthesia. *Acta Anaesthesiol Scand* 1987; **31**: 258–63.

19 Kitamura T, Ogawa M, Kawamura G, et al. The effects of sevoflurane and propofol on glucose metabolism under aerobic conditions in fed rats. *Anesth Analg* 2009; **109**: 1479–85.

20. Kitamura T, Sato K, Kawamura G, et al. The involvement of adenosine triphosphate-sensitive potassium channels in the different effects of sevoflurane and propofol on glucose metabolism in fed rats. *Anesth Analg* 2012; **114**: 110–16.

21. Hans P. Blood glucose concentration profile after 10 mg dexamethasone in non-diabetic and type 2 diabetic patients undergoing abdominal surgery. *Br J Anaesth* 2006; **97**: 164–70.

22. Pasternak JJ, McGregor DG, Lanier WL. Effect of single-dose dexamethasone on blood glucose concentration in patients undergoing craniotomy. *J Neurosurg Anesthesiol* 2004; **16**: 122–5.

23. Abdelmalak BB, Bonilla AM, Yang D, et al. The hyperglycemic response to major noncardiac surgery and the added effect of steroid administration in patients with and without diabetes. *Anesth Analg* 2013; **116**: 1116–22.

24. Joshi GP, Chung F, Vann MA, et al. Society for Ambulatory Anesthesia Consensus Statement on perioperative blood glucose management in diabetic patients undergoing ambulatory surgery. *Anesth Analg* 2010; **111**: 1378–87.

25. The Diabetes Control and Complications Trial Research Group. The effect of intensive treatment of diabetes on the development and progression of long-term complications in insulin-dependent diabetes mellitus. *N Engl J Med* 1993; **329**: 977–86.
26. Nathan DM, Cleary PA, Backlund JY, et al. Intensive diabetes treatment and cardiovascular disease in patients with type 1 diabetes. *N Engl J Med* 2005; **353**: 2643–53.
27. Action to Control Cardiovascular Risk in Diabetes Study Group. Effects of intensive glucose lowering in type 2 diabetes. *N Engl J Med* 2008; **358**: 2545–59.
28. Van Den Berghe G, Wouters P, Weekers F, et al. Intensive insulin therapy in critically ill patients. *N Engl J Med* 2001; **345**: 1359–67.
29. Finfer S, Chittock DR, Su SY-S, et al. Intensive versus conventional glucose control in critically ill patients. *N Engl J Med* 2009; **360**: 1283–97.
30. Preiser J-C, Devos P, Ruiz-Santana S, et al. A prospective randomised multi-centre controlled trial on tight glucose control by intensive insulin therapy in adult intensive care units: the Glucontrol study. *Intensive Care Med* 2009; **35**: 1738–48.
31. Hermanides J, Bosman RJ, Vriesendorp TM, et al. Hypoglycemia is associated with intensive care unit mortality. *Crit Care Med* 2010; **38**: 1430–4.
32. Kramer AH, Roberts DJ, Zygun DA. Optimal glycemic control in neurocritical care patients: a systematic review and meta-analysis. *Crit Care* 2012; **16**: R203.
33. Vanhorebeek I, Peeters RP, Vander Perre S, et al. Cortisol response to critical illness: effect of intensive insulin therapy. *J Clin Endocrinol Metab* 2006; **91**: 3803–13.
34. Egi M, Bellomo R, Stachowski E, et al. Blood glucose concentration and outcome of critical illness: the impact of diabetes. *Crit Care Med* 2008; **36**: 2249–55.
35. Noordzij PG, Boersma E, Schreiner F, et al. Increased preoperative glucose levels are associated with perioperative mortality in patients undergoing noncardiac, nonvascular surgery. *Eur J Endocrinol* 2007; **156**: 137–42.
36. Kwon S, Thompson R, Dellinger P, et al. Importance of perioperative glycemic control in general surgery: a report from the surgical care and outcomes assessment program. *Ann Surg* 2013; **257**: 8–14.
37. Gandhi GY, Nuttall GA, Abel MD, et al. Intensive intraoperative insulin therapy versus conventional glucose management during cardiac surgery: a randomized trial. *Ann Intern Med* 2007; **146**: 233–43.
38. Bhamidipati CM, LaPar DJ, Stukenborg GJ, et al. Superiority of moderate control of hyperglycemia to tight control in patients undergoing coronary artery bypass grafting. *J Thorac Cardiovasc Surg* 2011; **141**: 543–51.
39. Duncan AE, Abd-Elsayed A, Maheshwari A, et al. Role of intraoperative and postoperative blood glucose concentrations in predicting outcomes after cardiac surgery. *Anesthesiology* 2010; **112**: 860–71.
40. Székely A, Levin J, Miao Y, et al. Impact of hyperglycemia on perioperative mortality after coronary artery bypass graft surgery. *J Thorac Cardiovasc Surg* 2011; **142**: 430–7.
41. Kang H, Ahn KJ, Choi JY, et al. Efficacy of insulin glargine in perioperative glucose control in type 2 diabetic patients. *Eur J Anaesthesiol* 2009; **26**: 666–70.

Chapter 10

The obese or thin patient

P.M. Singh, N. Ludwig, I. McConachie, and A.C. Sinha

The obese patient

The subspecialty of medicine dealing with obese patients is called bariatric medicine. Bariatric patients are different! One unique aspect of anesthesia for an obese patient is that, unlike diabetes and hypertension, patients do not consider themselves to actually be ill, and a concept of an increased perioperative risk over the normal population does not, to them, seem to really be valid. These concerns become even more realistic when an ambulatory obese patient undergoes a bariatric surgery and suffers perioperative complications.

Obesity is a global problem with rising trends:

- Recent data suggests that in both Europe and the U.S., more than 50% of the adult population is overweight and 20%–25% are obese.
- By 2015, a total of 2.3 billion of the populations are likely to be overweight and 700 million will be obese.
- In the past three decades, the incidence of obesity in children has increased from 5% to 20% in the U.S.

When do we call a patient obese?

- The World Health Organization (WHO) defines the standard for obesity as body fat percentage of >25% and >35% in male and female adults, respectively [1].
- Body Mass Index (BMI) (Quetelet's index) is the most widely used convenient measure to diagnoses and quantify obesity. It is defined mathematically as:

weight (kg)/height^2 (m)

- BMI-based grading of obesity in the adult is shown in Table 10.1.
- This classification may be limited in subjects with large muscular mass (athletes etc.), who may falsely be falling into the overweight category.
- A waist to hip ratio of >0.9 and >1 in females and males, respectively, predisposes the individuals to higher rates of obesity-related complications.

Pathophysiological alterations and clinical relevance

The increased BMI indirectly affects multiple organ systems to alter physiological responses in the body, which predispose to higher risks for anesthesia.

Anesthesia and Perioperative Care of the High-Risk Patient, Third edition, ed. Ian McConachie. Published by Cambridge University Press.

Table 10.1. BMI grading of obesity in adults

WHO classification of obesity	
Weight class	BMI (kg/m^2)
Normal	18.5–24.9
Overweight	25–29.9
Obese	>30
Obesity grade 1	30–34.9
Obesity grade 2	35–39.9
Obesity grade 3 (morbidly obese)	40
Obesity grade 4 (Super obese)	>50
Obesity grade 5 (Super-super obese)	>60

Respiratory system

- Decrease in functional residual capacity, vital capacity, and total lung capacity, which may lead to early oxyhemoglobin desaturation.
- Increased closing volume, extension of West zone 4 (raised interstitial pressure), and basal atelectasis resulting in ventilation perfusion mismatch may occur. This also predisposes to desaturation, which may be unresponsive to raising FiO_2, responding only to recruitment maneuvers.
- Chronic hypoxemia can result in pulmonary hypertension and cor pulmonale. This also predisposes patients to poor tolerance to intraoperative hypoxemia and likely right heart failure, which is associated with very high mortality.
- Fat accumulation in the chest and abdominal wall decreases compliance of the respiratory system, necessitating higher ventilatory pressure to achieve optimal tidal volumes.

Expiratory reserve volume is the most sensitive indicator for obesity-associated changes on pulmonary function testing.

Cardiovascular system

- Those with a BMI of >25 kg/m^2 and >30 kg/m^2 (females and males) are around six and 16 times likely to have left ventricular (LV) hypertrophy, and even have increased perioperative diastolic failure.
- There is a strong association with hypertension (commonest) – every 10 kg increase in weight raises systolic and diastolic blood pressure by about 4 mmHg and 2 mmHg, respectively.
- With increased triglycerides and cholesterol, there is a higher possibility of atherosclerosis and thus coronary artery disease (CAD).
- If the cardiac conducting system shows fatty infiltration, there is a higher incidence of perioperative arrhythmias.
- An increase in cardiac output by 2–3 mL/100 gm of fat predisposes to an increased cardiac workload and hypertrophy.

Endocrine system

- Insulin resistance: with a BMI >30 kg/m^2, the person is 30 times more likely to develop diabetes when compared to a population of normal weight.
- Hypothyroidism: one-fourth of obese patients may have subclinical hypothyroidism predisposing to perioperative delayed awakening and prolonged/residual drug actions due to decreased metabolic rates.

Syndrome X

This is a metabolic syndrome with hypertension, diabetes, central obesity, hyperuricemia, and dyslipidemia (decreased HDL and increased LDL, triglycerides, and total cholesterol).

- The relative risk of associated postoperative complications increases approximately three-fold [2].
- Patients are at high-risk for cardiac morbidity, stroke, renal disease, and peripheral vascular disease.
- It is a proinflammatory state, increasing thrombotic complications (e.g., pulmonary embolism (PE), deep vein thrombosis (DVT), and wound infections) postoperatively.

Gastrointestinal system

- Increased stomach capacity, increased residual volume, and decreased gastric pH lead to a higher incidence of aspiration and regurgitation.
- Hiatal hernia and increased intragastric pressure is associated with reflux esophagitis and aspiration risk.
- Non-alcoholic steatohepatitis (NASH) is not directly related to the grade of obesity; however, it is related to chronicity of obesity. A small subgroup of patients has marginally elevated baseline serum transaminases.

Obstructive sleep apnea (OSA)

OSA is repetitive, partial (hypoapnea), or complete (apnea) obstruction of the upper airway, characterized by episodes of breathing cessation lasting 10 seconds or more during sleep. (See specific chapter on OSA and obesity hypoventilation syndrome.)

OSA and obesity

- Obesity causes fat deposition in the tongue and upper airway tissues, reducing luminal diameter and increasing the propensity to collapse.
- A 4 kg/m^2 increase is associated with about a four-fold increased risk of OSA.
- The most significant risk for OSA is obesity; 60%–90% of patients have a BMI of >29 kg/m^2.
- With a BMI of >40 kg/m^2, the incidence of OSA is up to 55% and 24% in males and females, respectively.
- Other risk factors associated with OSA (these should be accessed preoperatively) are: advanced age, male gender, postmenopausal females, first-degree relatives (odds ratio [OR] 1.5–2), smoking (OR 4.44), craniofacial anomalies, and hypertrophy of tonsils and adenoids.

Table 10.2. Comorbidities associated with OSA (adapted from Seet and Chung [3])

Comorbidities associated with OSA (in order of incidence)	
Organ system	**Condition**
Cardiac	Resistant hypertension Congestive cardiac failure Ischemic heart disease Dysrhythmias Atrial fibrillation
Respiratory	Pulmonary hypertension Asthma
Neurological	Stroke
Metabolic	Morbid obesity Metabolic syndrome (syndrome X) Hypothyroidism Type II diabetes
Miscellaneous	Head and neck cancer Gastroesophageal reflux disease Nocturia Open angle glaucoma

OSA and systemic comorbidities

The associated comorbidities with OSA are shown in Table 10.2 (in decreasing order of their incidence) [3].

- Long-standing OSA is associated with hypoxemia, hypercarbia, polycythemia, and cor pulmonale, which leads to systemic complications.
- An oxyhemoglobin saturation of <94% on breathing room air should alert to the possibility of long-term OSA and of systemic manifestations.

Diagnosing and grading of OSA (Table 10.3)

- OSA is diagnosed if the sum of the number of episodes of apnea and hypoapnea per hour of sleep is ≥5.
- The gold standard for classifying OSA is based on a sleep study; however, many surrogate sensitive questionnaires (STOP-Bang, Berlin) can be used while evaluating these patients [3].
- OSA must be distinguished from obesity hypoventilation syndrome (OHS), where the patient may have a resetting of basal CO_2 to a higher level along with permanent metabolic alkalosis (raised bicarbonate).
- Patients with a BMI ≥50 kg/m^2 or room air saturation ≤90% should be evaluated using room air arterial blood gas sampling to rule out OHS [4].

Perioperative continuous positive airway pressure (CPAP) and OSA – practical issues

- All patients may not need a sleep study for grading of OSA severity. Use of a screening questionnaire can help in assessment of severity. The Apnea–Hypopnea Index

Table 10.3. Preoperative grading of OSA

Preoperative grading of OSA			
Sleep study grading (apnea–hypopnea index)		**STOP-Bang (screening)**	
AHI	Grade	S	Snoring – audible across closed doors
0–5	None	T	Tiredness/fatigue during the day time
6–20	Mild OSA	O	Observed to have obstruction in sleep
21–40	Moderate OSA	P	Blood pressure – treatment for hypertension
>40	Severe OSA	B	BMI ≥35
		A	Age ≥50 years
		N	Neck circumference ≥40 cm
		G	Gender – male
		High-risk OSA if ≥3 positives Sensitivity 93% for AHI ≥15 Sensitivity almost 100% for AHI ≥30	

(AHI), especially in mild to moderate OSA, does not correlate well with perioperative complications.

- Suspected patients with severe OSA may undergo a sleep study preoperatively, if CPAP therapy is planned due to clinical symptoms. Improvement in AHI can guide titration of the level and duration of preoperative CPAP in such patients [5].
- If patients use CPAP preoperatively, they are likely to require it in the immediate postoperative period as well, and a low threshold should be maintained for its use in such patients.
- CPAP along with lung expansion therapy can be vital in preventing postoperative pulmonary complications in patients with symptoms of basal lung collapse (i.e., often unexplained dyspnea, desaturation, and hypercarbia) in the early postoperative period.
- Oronasal CPAP is more effective; however, nasal CPAP is tolerated better and can be used.
- Evidence exists in favor of prophylactic preoperative CPAP for reducing cardiac arrhythmias, stabilizing variable blood pressure, and decreasing myocardial oxygen consumption (VO_2) [6].
- Bowel anastomosis is no contraindication to low values of CPAP (5–10 cm of H_2O).

Difficult airway and obesity

- Many obese patients with abdominal distribution of fat may not have difficult airway.
- The reported incidence is around 14% – approximately three times higher than lean counterparts [7].
- Increasing BMI is associated with difficult mask ventilation; however, it correlates poorly with intubation difficulty.

- Predictors of possible difficult airway are restriction of neck extension (occipital pad of fat), high Mallampati score (≥3), increased neck circumference, associated OSA, increased age, and male gender. Recent reports suggest a neck circumference to thyromental distance ratio of >5 is one of the most sensitive predictors [7].
- Use of fiber-optic bronchoscopes or video laryngoscopes are valid rescue maneuvers in suspected difficult airway.
- Patients have a lower tolerance of apnea and desaturate rapidly despite adequate pre-oxygenation (due to low FRC, basal lung collapse on induction/paralysis, and higher basal VO_2). Use of slight (15°) head-up and positive end expiratory pressure (PEEP) (5–10 cm H_2O) on mask ventilation can increase this apneic duration.
- Use of an oral/nasal airway during mask ventilation and a ramped position during pre-oxygenation and intubation greatly assist in securing the airway.

Anesthetic drug pharmacology in the obese

General principles of drug dosage in obesity

- Volume of distribution of both lipid- and water-soluble drugs is increased (lipid-soluble more than water-soluble), thus loading doses needed after accounting for weight correction are higher.
- In obesity, lean body mass and adipose tissue increase disproportionately, thus altering drug kinetics.
- Oral bioavailability, metabolic drug clearance, and protein binding often remain unaltered.
- Most lipid-soluble drugs need dosing on the basis of either total or lean body weight. Nonlipid-soluble drugs need dosing on the ideal body weight (IBW) basis.
- Maintenance doses of lipid-soluble drugs need either dose or interval adjustments due to the possibility of accumulation in an increased fat mass.
- Lower solubility inhalation agents are preferred because of early, clear awakening and less accumulation in the fat compartment, leading to decreased residual effects.
- Order of preference is desflurane ≥ sevoflurane > isoflurane.
- Comparisons between desflurane and sevoflurane, however, have shown similar wakeup times and recovery profiles, thus choice must also be guided on the availability and economic basis [8,9].
- Limited data are available on the use of xenon, although it proved to have a significantly faster recovery time. However, the incidence of bradycardia, hypertension, and postoperative nausea and vomiting (PONV) is reported to be higher [10].
- Limited comparisons between desflurane and total intravenous anesthesia (TIVA) using propofol infusion in the morbidly obese patient are available. Results have shown shorter wakeup times and lesser oxyhemoglobin desaturation episodes in the desflurane group; however, the clinical benefit of this is questionable.
- TIVA using dexmedetomidine in OSA is promising, with a significant opioid sparing effect intra- and postoperatively [11].
- Opioids need careful titration in patients with OSA due to possible significant respiratory depressant effects. Shorter acting agents are preferred, with careful monitoring; supplement with multimodal analgesia.

Table 10.4. Dosage alterations for common anesthetic drugs

Dose protocols for intravenous drugs		
Drug	**Dose based on**	**Comments**
Thiopental	Induction: LBW	Induction dose action offset via redistribution
Propofol	Induction: LBW Maintenance: TBW	Propofol used for maintenance by infusion
Midazolam	Loading: TBW Maintenance: IBW	Significant increase in volume of distribution, T-half prolonged
Fentanyl Sufentanil	LBW LBW	High lipid solubility, increased volume of distribution and T-half
Remifentanil	LBW	Intraoperative drug of choice, minimal lipid accumulation
Morphine	IBW	Normal PCA dosage regimen
Succinylcholine	TBW	Increased metabolism due to increased pseudocholinesterase
Vecuronium Rocuronium Atracurium/cisatracurium	IBW IBW IBW	Unaltered pharmacokinetics when dosed on IBW

$IBW = A + 0.89 \times (\text{height in cm} = 152.4)$
For males $A = 49.9$
For females $A = 45.4$

$LBW = a \times TBW - b \times [TBW/\text{height (cm)}]^2$
For males $a = 1.10$, $b = 120$
For Females $a = 1.07$, $b = 148$
Roughly, LBW = IBW + 20%–30%

The dosing alterations needed for common anesthetic drugs used perioperatively are shown in Table 10.4 [12]. Doses for different drugs are based on IBW, lean body weight (LBW), or total body weight (TBW).

Choice of anesthetic technique (general or regional anesthesia)

- No randomized controlled trial (RCT) exists to prove superiority of one over the other. However, regional techniques should be used to supplement general anesthesia (GA) wherever possible.
- Regional anesthesia (RA) offers potential advantages in obese patients by having decreased opioid use, fewer pulmonary complications, improved postoperative pain control, decreased PONV, earlier ambulation, and decreased risk of thromboembolism [13].
- Technical problems exist due to the difficulty in identifying landmarks – the use of ultrasound (US)-guided blocks may be preferred. The failure rate of regional techniques is higher in morbidly obese patients.

- Epidural techniques may have a significant role in thoracoabdominal surgeries for intraoperative and postoperative analgesia. There is a significant opioid sparing effect.
- Lower epidural/intrathecal doses of LAs are required due to the decreased volume of epidural space and cerebrospinal fluid volume.

Preoperative evaluation

- Obese patients often have reduced physical activity, thus evaluating cardiorespiratory reserve has practical limitations. A high index of suspicion for cardiovascular ailments should be maintained as the obese patient may present with atypical symptoms.
- Pulmonary function testing often shows restrictive disease; however, unless severe limitation is present, this testing correlates poorly with clinical outcomes in obese patients. Thus, its routine use is not recommended [14].
- Consider anti-aspiration prophylaxis in view of the increased possibility of aspiration and regurgitation.

Preoxygenation and induction

The goal is to increase lung oxygen reserves while preventing lung collapse.

- For adequate pre-oxygenation at 100% oxygen use a tight-fitting mask for three to five minutes at tidal volume breathing. Additionally use CPAP of 5–10 cm.
- Alleviate increases in abdominal pressure by use of reverse Trendelenburg or beach chair position.
- Use ramped position of the patient for intubation – this aligns the oral, pharyngeal, and laryngeal axis better.
- Equipment for the management of unexpected difficult airway (American Society of Anesthesiologists [ASA] difficult airway algorithm) must be kept at hand.
- In very obese patients, the laryngeal mask airway should be used only as a rescue device if intubation fails and not as the primary airway device, due to the need for higher ventilatory pressures and possibility of aspiration.
- Use succinylcholine as a neuromuscular blocker (unless contraindicated), as early return of spontaneous breathing may prevent an airway catastrophe in the event of failed intubation.

Monitoring

All conventional monitoring suffers from limitations in the obese patient:

- Electrocardiograph (ECG) – this has low voltage due to increased chest wall fat insulation.
- Noninvasive blood pressure – inappropriate cuff size (often the arms have conical configuration) and applying the cuff has practical limitations. Additionally, noninvasive blood pressure may show falsely higher readings in obese patients.
- Central venous catheters overestimate pressure owing to raised intrathoracic pressure transmitted from the abdominal compartment and also because of associated diastolic dysfunction (LV hypertrophy) in the obese patient.
- Thus, maintain a low threshold for invasive arterial pressure monitoring.

- Recent evidence suggests dynamic fluid responsiveness variables (stroke volume variation, pulse pressure variation) can be used to access fluid requirements in the obese patient [15].
- Adequate neuromuscular blocking drug reversal with train-of-four monitoring prior to extubation prevents postoperative problems due to inadequate reversal or residual paralysis.

Patient positioning

- Special operating tables with extra width and supporting weight up to 455 kg (1000 lbs) may be needed for the ultra-obese patient.
- Use appropriate padding on pressure areas and "bean-bag" support devices wherever available.
- Rhabdomyolysis, pressure sores, and nerve injuries are positioning-related complications with a much higher incidence in the obese patient.
- Obese patients with OSA and raised hematocrit are at increased risk for intraoperative DVT. Consider perioperative thromboprophylaxis (mechanical calf compression devices and/or pharmacological intervention) in view of the increased incidence of DVT and PE, especially in patients with associated metabolic syndrome.

Ventilatory strategy

- Increased basal atelectasis and closing volume predispose to intraoperative decreases in oxygenation. This is more common in laparoscopic surgeries and surgeries requiring Trendelenberg positioning.
- Evidence suggests that a lung protective strategy using tidal volume of 6–8 ml/kg (IBW) with PEEP application, on a pressure control mode, improves oxygenation when compared to volume control modes [16].
- Use of recruitment maneuvers intraoperatively (CPAP of 30 cm H_2O for 30 seconds) significantly improves oxygenation in obese patients by decreasing basal atelectasis [17].

Postoperative analgesia

- Multimodal analgesia is vital in improving patient satisfaction, facilitating physical therapy and mobilization, and avoiding opioid-related side effects.
- RA techniques should be employed wherever feasible.
- Use non-opioids aggressively – high-efficacy non-steroidal anti-inflammatory drugs (NSAIDs) like ketorolac with acetaminophen (paracetamol) can provide satisfactory analgesia.
- Adjuvants like ketamine, clonidine, or dexmedetomidine have an opioid-sparing effect and may be beneficial.
- Methods like patient-controlled epidural analgesia (PCEA) and patient-controlled intravenous analgesia (PCA) are known to reduce opioid requirements significantly and decrease postoperative pulmonary complications [18].

Predicting postoperative complications

The majority of postoperative complications have shown only a direct correlation to obesity grade II or higher and associated metabolic syndrome. An interesting finding from various meta-analyses is the "obesity paradox," where complication rates were lower than normal in patients graded as overweight and grade I obesity [19].

- Visceral obesity (central distribution of fat) is a better predictor of risk than BMI [20]. Thus, evaluation of waist circumference has been shown to be a more reliable tool for risk assessment (e.g., waist circumference $\geq$102 cm = higher risk).
- The incidence of wound infections, cardiac complications, and mortality increases significantly with associated metabolic syndrome even with a mild to moderate increase in BMI.
- Preoperative poor lung condition, severe restricted pattern on pulmonary function tests, and limited effort tolerance are predictors of postoperative lung complications.
- Postoperative respiratory function may be improved by patient positioning in bed at a 45° angle, early mobilization, and aggressive use of physical therapy.
- Noninvasive ventilation may be useful in the postoperative period as there are suggestions that oxygenation may be bettered [21], and outcomes–including the incidence of respiratory failure, length of intensive care unit (ICU) and hospital stay, and overall hospital mortality–may also be improved [22].
- Wound infections, wound dehiscence, longer surgical time, and increased blood loss are complications showing a higher incidence even with small increments in BMI [23].

The underweight/thin patient

A BMI of less than 18.5 kg/m^2 classifies a patient as below normal weight and may have a variety of causes.

- Undernutrition, skeletal muscle depletion (sarcopenia), and cachexia related to end-stage organ dysfunction and malignancy represent overlapping etiological syndromes in the underweight and frail patient. Malignancy-related cachexia is outside the scope of this chapter.
- The combination of an acute illness, the catabolic stress of surgery, as well as perioperative immobilization in the underweight patient represents a high-risk for surgery.

Malnutrition (undernutrition)

Malnutrition refers to a general term that indicates a lack of some or all nutritional elements necessary for human health.

- Protein–energy malnutrition, also known as macronutrient deficiencies, signifies an imbalance between the supply of protein and energy and the body's demand for them to ensure optimal growth and function.
- Deficiencies in specific micronutrients (vitamins and minerals) represent a separate form of malnutrition.

A variety of malnutrition syndromes exist and contribute to increased perioperative risk.

Etiology and classification

Primary malnutrition is related to inadequate intake of nutrients:

- Poverty-related protein–energy malnutrition in children of the developing world represents one of the most significant unsolved world health issues.

- In the developed world, poverty as well as a lack of access to nutritious food in certain communities can lead to both macronutrient and micronutrient deficiencies.

Secondary malnutrition is the result of a variety of comorbid diseases:

- Psychiatric illness such as anorexia nervosa or bullimia nervosa can result in malnourishment.
- Various gastrointestinal (GI) disorders, malabsorption syndromes, and dysphagia can also lead to malnourishment.
- Endocrine disorders such as hyperthyroidism, medication side effects, as well as drug and alcohol abuse can contribute to malnutrition.

Assessment of malnutrition

All patients should be assessed for the presence and the risk of developing malnutrition in the perioperative period. A thorough history should be taken to assess for history of weight loss, periods of poor food intake, as well as periods of recent illness or immobilization.

Various criteria have been developed for the clinical assessment of the patient's nutritional status:

- The Malnutrition Universal Screening Tool (MUST) is a reliable and valid tool for determining the presence of malnutrition [24].
- Other available screening tools include the Subjective Global Assessment of Nutritional Status (SGA) and the Short Nutritional Assessment Questionnaire.

Laboratory investigations are often used in the assessment of malnutrition but are of limited utility:

- Serum proteins including albumin and pre-albumin may be used as a marker of protein status.
- Although pre-albumin may be more sensitive to acute changes in nutrition status due to its shorter half-life, its measured level is affected by hydration status, hepatic and renal dysfunction, as well as inflammation and drug interactions [25].

What are the clinical implications for the malnourished patient?

The underweight patient carries a significant perioperative risk. The lack of adipose tissue and lean body stores of energy combined with the catabolic state of surgery leads to a decreased functional reserve available for postoperative recovery.

- A large review of over 25 000 patients over the age of 65 years undergoing vascular surgery found the highest 30-day mortality among underweight patients with a BMI of <18.5. It was even greater than those with a BMI of >40 [26].
- Low BMI in the perioperative period has also been associated with the development of pressure ulcers [27] and delayed wound healing [28].
- Outcomes have been shown to be worse in patients with a low BMI undergoing cardiac surgery [29] and colonic surgery [30].
- In the ICU population, a low BMI has been shown to be independently associated with increased mortality [31,32].

Systems-based implications for the underweight patient

Respiratory system

- Starvation has the effect of decreasing lung elasticity, resulting in decreased pulmonary compliance.
- Respiratory rate may be low.
- In extreme eating disorders, self-induced vomiting can lead to aspiration pneumonia and spontaneous pneumothoraces.
- Malnourished patients have poor cough efforts, and hence are more prone to respiratory infections.

Cardiovascular system

- Malnourished patients have a low metabolic rate with resultant hypotension and bradycardia.
- Arrhythmias are common. ECG changes include atrioventricular (A-V) block, prolonged QT, ST depression, and T-wave inversion.
- Decreased myocardial and LV function has been demonstrated.

Others

- GI: esophageal strictures, gastric dilation, hyperamylasemia, and fatty liver
- renal: reduced glomerular filtration rare, proteinuria, raised blood urea nitrogen, and concentrated urine
- metabolic: electrolyte imbalances including hypomagnesemia, and hypocalcemia due to vitamin D deficiency
- hematological: anemia, leucopenia, and thrombocytopenia
- decrease in immune function
- neurological: alterations in autonomic nervous system, decreased pain sensitivity, neuropathies, and generalized weakness
- in ICU patients, impaired weaning off ventilator support

Pharmacokinetics

- Metabolic pathways are deranged with reductions in albumin and plasma cholinesterase.
- Fat-soluble drug redistribution and excretion is altered along with fluid and electrolyte imbalance, as is the neuromuscular junction activity and sensitivity to narcotics.
- Hypoalbuminemia results in increased nonprotein-bound active form of the drugs in plasma, and hence enhanced potency of many drugs.
- The low metabolic rate can delay drug breakdown and elimination. Consequently, the dose of most anesthetic drugs needs reduction on a weight-for-weight basis, and should be carefully titrated against response.

Treatment and prevention of malnutrition in the perioperative period

A great deal of research has gone into the use of enteral nutrition (EN) and parenteral nutrition in the perioperative period. EN is usually recommended over parenteral nutrition in all patients who can tolerate the feeds and in whom the GI system is working. A risk–benefit analysis regarding nutritional support must be made for each individual patient.

Preoperative nutritional support is generally reserved for patients that are judged to be moderately to severely malnourished. The indications for and timing of perioperative nutritional support are controversial:

- A seven to 10-day course of preoperative nutrition has been recommended in malnourished patients undergoing GI surgery when delaying surgery would not cause undue harm [33]. Consideration should be given to the potential morbidity associated with the increased hospitalization time required for this preoperative nutritional support.
- Early postoperative nutritional support in the form of total parenteral nutrition (TPN) is indicated in malnourished patients who are unable to take in adequate nutrition orally [34].
- Reported benefits to postoperative nutritional support include improved wound healing [35], improved quality of life [36], as well as maintenance of GI integrity [37].
- However, a meta-analysis of RCTs comparing enteral, parenteral, and no artificial nutrition in the perioperative period found no mortality difference between the groups [38].

Sarcopenia

Sarcopenia refers to loss of skeletal muscle mass that is often age related.

- It was previously defined as an absolute muscle mass less the two standard deviations below a young healthy adult mean [39].
- However, more recently there has been a movement to redefine sarcopenia as a geriatric syndrome producing functional impairments and disability.
- A recent European consensus on sarcopenia stressed the importance of both low muscle mass and low muscle function in the diagnosis of sarcopenia [40].
- Sarcopenia is not limited to patients with low BMI. The loss of lean body mass can occur even while masked by significant adipose tissue.

Prevalence and assessment tools

The prevalence of sarcopenia varies with the method of measurement but certainly increases with age.

- One commonly referenced study made use of duel-energy X-ray absorpitometry to estimate the muscle mass of the four limbs. Prevalence increased from 13% to 24% in persons under 70 years of age and to >50% in persons over 80 years old [39].
- Other body imaging techniques include magnetic resonance imaging (MRI) and computed tomography (CT) scans.
- Bioimpedence analysis has been used to estimate volume of fat and lean body mass [41].
- Anthropometric measures such as triceps skin fold thickness have been used, but the lack of validity has called their use into question [40].
- A common measurement of strength includes the hand grip strength.
- Other measurements of function include the Short Physical Performance Battery, Timed Get Up and Go Test, and the Usual Gait Speed.

Pathophysiology of sarcopenia

There are several mechanisms involved in the process of sarcopenia.

- The natural aging process includes a decrease in myofibrillar protein synthesis as well as loss of motor units via denervation, resulting in muscle atrophy. The conversion of type I muscle fibers to type II muscle fibers contributes to muscle wasting in the elderly [42].
- Inactivity and bed rest greatly accelerate this aging process.
- Increased catabolic catecholamines and corticosteroids, decreased anabolic factors such as testosterone and growth hormone, and increased insulin resistance represent contributing factors to muscle wasting.

Clinical implications of sarcopenia

Low muscle mass, rather than low BMI, may be a better indicator of a low functional reserve. The loss of muscle mass related to sarcopenia results in some elderly, frail patients functioning very near their maximal oxygen consumption ($VO_{2\ max}$) while completing even simple activities of daily living. The perioperative period exacerbates this situation as the stress response of surgery results in a catabolic state that accelerates muscle wasting. When combined with disuse atrophy-associated perioperative immobility, even previously active patients may lose the ability to perform basic tasks in a very short period of time. Maximal aerobic power may be exceeded simply with ventilation and attempts at mobility, leading to a rapid and sometimes irreversible decline that result in poor outcomes.

Indeed, several studies have specifically linked sarcopenia to poor outcomes:

- In a review of patients with (chronic obstructive pulmonary disease COPD), low muscle mass but not low BMI was associated with poor outcomes [43].
- Sarcopenia is also associated with increased mortality from cirrhosis and may be a better predictor than conventional indices of liver function [44].

In surgical patients:

- In one recent study, sarcopenia was associated with postoperative infection and delayed recovery from colorectal cancer resection surgery [45].
- Sarcopenia is also associated with increased mortality following breast cancer surgery [46] and pancreatic cancer surgery [47].
- Similarly, sarcopenia patients undergoing liver resection for metastasis had prolonged hospital stays and increased short-term postoperative morbidity associated with surgery [48].
- In a recent study of elderly trauma patients, sarcopenia was a better predictor of mortality, duration of ICU stay, and duration of ventilatory support than traditional measures of nutritional state [49].

Treatment and prevention of sarcopenia

The multifactorial nature of sarcopenia as well as the lack of standardized outcome measures represents challenges in the study of treatment of this syndrome. Although exercise and physical activity likely represent the most important intervention in both treatment and prevention of sarcopenia, few studies have attempted to study sarcopenic patients exclusively. In addition, it is not always feasible to implement exercise training in significantly deconditioned patients. Certainly, there is evidence that moderate activity and resistance training can improve function in elderly patients.

- A Cochrane review of 121 studies involving elderly patients undergoing progressive resistance training demonstrated improved performance in simple activities, improved strength testing, and reduced pain from osteoarthritis [50].
- It therefore seems prudent to promote even trivial amounts of activity in the perioperative period to slow or prevent further loss of muscle mass in surgical patients.

Anabolic drug interventions have yielded promising results in the treatment of sarcopenia:

- Testosterone supplementation can be used to increase muscle mass and has been shown to increase muscle contraction force in the elderly [51], but has not been studied specifically in the sarcopenia population.
- Similarly, growth hormone and dehydroepiandosterone supplementation can be used for its anabolic properties, but it has not been studied in the context of sarcopenia [52].

Nutritional status in the context of sarcopenia is a topic of much debate. Observational studies have linked inadequate intake of proteins, vitamin D, and antioxidant nutrients to the development of sarcopenia [53]. Studies involving nutritional supplementation of sarcopenic patients have yielded mixed results.

References

1. Romero-Corral A, Somers VK, Sierra-Johnson J, et al. Accuracy of body mass index to diagnose obesity in the US adult population. *Int J Obes (Lond)* 2008; **32**: 959–66.

2. Echahidi N, Pibarot P, Després J-P, et al. Metabolic syndrome increases operative mortality in patients undergoing coronary artery bypass grafting surgery. *J Am Coll Cardiol* 2007; **50**: 843–51.

3. Seet E, Chung F. Obstructive sleep apnea: preoperative assessment. *Anesthesiol Clin* 2010; **28**: 199–215.

4. Banerjee D, Yee BJ, Piper AJ, et al. Obesity hypoventilation syndrome: hypoxemia during continuous positive airway pressure. *Chest* 2007; **131**: 1678–84.

5. Epstein LJ, Kristo D, Strollo PJ Jr, et al. Clinical guideline for the evaluation, management and long-term care of obstructive sleep apnea in adults. *J Clin Sleep Med* 2009; **5**: 263–76.

6. Gula LJ, Krahn AD, Skanes AC, et al. Clinical relevance of arrhythmias during sleep: guidance for clinicians. *Heart* 2004; **90**: 347–52.

7. Kim WH, Ahn HJ, Lee CJ, et al. Neck circumference to thyromental distance ratio: a new predictor of difficult intubation in obese patients. *Br J Anaesth* 2011; **106**: 743–8.

8. Vallejo MC, Sah N, Phelps AL, et al. Desflurane versus sevoflurane for laparoscopic gastroplasty in morbidly obese patients. *J Clin Anesth* 2007; **19**: 3–8.

9. De Baerdemaeker LEC, Jacobs S, Den Blauwen NMM, et al. Postoperative results after desflurane or sevoflurane combined with remifentanil in morbidly obese patients. *Obes Surg* 2006; **16**: 728–33.

10. Abramo A, Di Salvo C, Foltran F, et al. Xenon anesthesia improves respiratory gas exchanges in morbidly obese patients. *J Obes* 2010; **2010**: 421593.

11. Hofer RE, Sprung J, Sarr MG, et al. Anesthesia for a patient with morbid obesity using dexmedetomidine without narcotics. *Can J Anaesth* 2005; **52**: 176–80.

12. Ingrande J, Lemmens HJM. Dose adjustment of anaesthetics in the morbidly obese. *Br J Anaesth* 2010; **105**: i16–23.

13. Brodsky JB, Mariano ER. Regional anaesthesia in the obese patient: lost landmarks and evolving ultrasound

guidance. *Best Pract Res Clin Anaesth* 2011; **25**: 61–72.

14. Ramaswamy A, Gonzalez R, Smith CD. Extensive preoperative testing is not necessary in morbidly obese patients undergoing gastric bypass. *J Gastrointest Surg* 2004; **8**: 159–64.
15. Jain AK, Dutta A. Stroke volume variation as a guide to fluid administration in morbidly obese patients undergoing laparoscopic bariatric surgery. *Obes Surg* 2010; **20**: 709–15.
16. Cadi P, Guenoun T, Journois D, et al. Pressure-controlled ventilation improves oxygenation during laparoscopic obesity surgery compared with volume-controlled ventilation. *Br J Anaesth* 2008; **100**: 709–16.
17. Reinius H, Jonsson L, Gustafsson S, et al. Prevention of atelectasis in morbidly obese patients during general anesthesia and paralysis: a computerized tomography study. *Anesthesiology* 2009; **111**: 979–87.
18. Charghi R, Backman S, Christou N, et al. Patient controlled i.v. analgesia is an acceptable pain management strategy in morbidly obese patients undergoing gastric bypass surgery. A retrospective comparison with epidural analgesia. *Can J Anaesth* 2003; **50**: 672–8.
19. Mullen JT, Moorman DW, Davenport DL. The obesity paradox: body mass index and outcomes in patients undergoing nonbariatric general surgery. *Ann Surg* 2009; **250**: 166–72.
20. Hu FB. Obesity and mortality: watch your waist, not just your weight. *Arch Intern Med* 2007; **167**: 875–6.
21. Zoremba M, Kalmus G, Begemann D, et al. Short term non-invasive ventilation post-surgery improves arterial blood-gases in obese subjects compared to supplemental oxygen delivery – a randomized controlled trial. *BMC Anesthesiol* 2011; **11**: 10.
22. El-Solh AA, Aquilina A, Pineda L, et al. Noninvasive ventilation for prevention of post-extubation respiratory failure in obese patients. *Eur Respir J* 2006; **28**: 588–95.
23. Doyle SL, Lysaght J, Reynolds JV. Obesity and post-operative complications in patients undergoing non-bariatric surgery. *Obes Rev* 2010; **11**: 875–86.
24. Malnutrition Advisory Group of the British Association for Parenteral & Enteral Nutrition (BAPEN). The MUST report. Nutritional screening for adults: a multidisciplinary responsibility. *BAPEN* 2003. http://www.bapen.org.uk/pdfs/must/must_exec_sum.pdf.
25. Robinson MK, Trujillo EB, Mogensen KM, et al. Improving nutritional screening of hospitalized patients: the role of prealbumin. *J Parenter Enteral Nutr* 2003; **27**: 389–95; quiz 439.
26. Nafiu OO, Kheterpal S, Moulding R, et al. The association of body mass index to postoperative outcomes in elderly vascular surgery patients: a reverse J-curve phenomenon. *Anesth Analg* 2011; **112**: 23–9.
27. Lindgren M, Unosson M, Krantz AM, et al. Pressure ulcer risk factors in patients undergoing surgery. *J Adv Nursing* 2005; **50**: 605–12.
28. Sullivan DH, Bopp MM, Roberson PK. Protein-energy undernutrition and life-threatening complications among the hospitalized elderly. *J Gen Intern Med* 2002; **17**: 923–32.
29. Perrotta S, Nilsson F, Brandrup-Wognsen G, et al. Body mass index and outcome after coronary artery bypass surgery. *J Cardiovasc Surg* 2007; **48**: 239–45.
30. Brown SC, Abraham JS, Walsh S, et al. Risk factors and operative mortality in surgery for colorectal cancer. *Ann R Coll Surg Engl* 1991; **73**: 269–72.
31. Tremblay A, Bandi V. Impact of body mass index on outcomes following critical care. *Chest* 2003; **123**: 1202–7.
32. Garrouste-Orgeas M, Troché G, Azoulay E, et al. Body mass index. An additional prognostic factor in ICU patients. *Intensive Care Med* 2004; **30**: 437–43.
33. Ward N. Nutrition support to patients undergoing gastrointestinal surgery. *Nutr J* 2003; **2**: 18.
34. Klein S, Kinney J, Jeejeebhoy K, et al. Nutrition support in clinical practice:

review of published data and recommendations for future research directions. Summary of a conference sponsored by the National Institutes of Health, American Society for Parenteral and Enteral Nutrition, and American Society for Clinical Nutrition. *Am J Clin Nutr* 1997; **66**: 683–706.

35. Schroeder D, Gillanders L, Mahr K, et al. Effects of immediate postoperative enteral nutrition on body composition, muscle function, and wound healing. *J Parenter Enteral Nutr* 1991; **15**: 376–83.

36. Beattie A, Prach, Baxter J, et al. A randomised controlled trial evaluating the use of enteral nutritional supplements postoperatively in malnourished surgical patients. *Gut* 2000; **46**: 813–18.

37. Fujita T, Daiko H, Nishimura M. Early enteral nutrition reduces the rate of life-threatening complications after thoracic esophagectomy in patients with esophageal cancer. *Eur Surg Res* 2012; **48**: 79–84.

38. Koretz RL, Avenell A, Lipman TO, et al. Does enteral nutrition affect clinical outcome? A systematic review of the randomized trials. *Am J Gastroenterol* 2007; **102**: 412–29.

39. Baumgartner RN, Koehler KM, Gallagher D, et al. Epidemiology of sarcopenia among the elderly in New Mexico. *Am J Epidemiol* 1998; **147**: 755–63.

40. Cruz-Jentoft AJ, Baeyens JP, Bauer JM, et al. Sarcopenia: European consensus on definition and diagnosis: Report of the European Working Group on Sarcopenia in Older People. *Age Ageing* 2010; **39**: 412–23.

41. Janssen I, Heymsfield SB, Baumgartner RN, et al. Estimation of skeletal muscle mass by bioelectrical impedance analysis. *J Appl Physiol* 2000; **89**: 465–71.

42. Jeejeebhoy KN. Malnutrition, fatigue, frailty, vulnerability, sarcopenia and cachexia: overlap of clinical features. *Curr Opin Clin Nutr Metab Care* 2012; **15**: 213–19.

43. Mador MJ. Muscle mass, not body weight, predicts outcome in patients with chronic obstructive pulmonary disease. *Am J Respir Crit Care Med* 2002; **166**: 787–9.

44. Montano-Loza AJ, Meza-Junco J, Prado CM, et al. Muscle wasting is associated with mortality in patients with cirrhosis. *Clin Gastroenterol Hepatol* 2012; **10**: 166–73.

45. Lieffers JR, Bathe OF, Fassbender K, et al. Sarcopenia is associated with postoperative infection and delayed recovery from colorectal cancer resection surgery. *Br J Cancer* 2012; **107**: 931–6.

46. Villaseñor A, Ballard-Barbash R, Baumgartner K, et al. Prevalence and prognostic effect of sarcopenia in breast cancer survivors: the HEAL Study. *J Cancer Surviv* 2012; **6**: 398–406.

47. Peng P, Hyder O, Firoozmand A, et al. Impact of sarcopenia on outcomes following resection of pancreatic adenocarcinoma. *J Gastrointest Surg* 2012; **16**: 1478–86.

48. Peng PD, van Vledder MG, Tsai S, et al. Sarcopenia negatively impacts short-term outcomes in patients undergoing hepatic resection for colorectal liver metastasis. *HPB (Oxford)* 2011; **13**: 439–46.

49. Moisey LL, Mourtzakis M, Cotton BA, et al. Skeletal muscle predicts ventilator-free days, ICU-free days, and mortality in elderly ICU patients. *Crit Care* 2013; **17**: R206.

50. Mangione KK, Miller AH, Naughton IV. Cochrane review: improving physical function and performance with progressive resistance strength training in older adults. *Phys Ther* 2010; **90**: 1711–15.

51. Ferrando AA, Sheffield-Moore M, Yeckel CW, et al. Testosterone administration to older men improves muscle function: molecular and physiological mechanisms. *Am J Physiol Endocrinol Metab* 2002; **282**: E601–7.

52. Malafarina V, Uriz-Otano F, Iniesta R, et al. Sarcopenia in the elderly: diagnosis, physiopathology and treatment. *Maturitas* 2012; **71**: 109–14.

53. Robinson S, Cooper C, Aihie Sayer A. Nutrition and sarcopenia: a review of the evidence and implications for preventive strategies. *J Aging Res* 2012; **2012**: 510801.

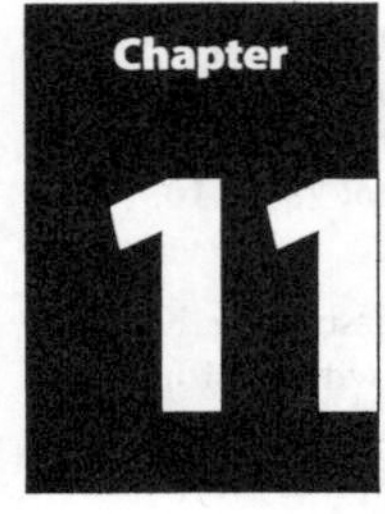

Obstructive sleep apnea and obesity hypoventilation syndrome

E.H.L. Chau, J. Wong, and F. Chung

Obstructive sleep apnea (OSA) is the most common type of sleep-disordered breathing.

- The prevalence of moderate OSA is 11.4% and 4.7% in men and women, respectively [1].
- Obesity hypoventilation syndrome (OHS) is characterized by a triad of obesity, daytime hypoventilation, and sleep-disordered breathing [2].
- OHS is a disease entity distinct from simple obesity and OSA.
- The prevalence of OHS is 10%–20% in patients with OSA and 0.15%–0.3% in the general population [3].
- OSA and OHS are often undiagnosed in patients presenting for elective surgery.

Diagnosis of OSA and OHS

The diagnosis of OSA is based on an overnight polysomnography, which measures the Apnea-Hypopnea Index (AHI). The AHI, defined as the average number of abnormal breathing events per hour of sleep, is used to determine the severity of OSA:

- mild OSA: AHI 5–15
- moderate OSA: AHI 15–30
- severe OSA: AHI >30

The diagnosis of OSA syndrome (OSAS) incorporates clinical signs and symptoms in addition to polysomnography findings [4]. These clinical findings include:

- excessive daytime sleepiness
- choking or gasping during sleep
- recurrent awakenings from sleep
- unrefreshing sleep
- daytime fatigue
- impaired concentration

The terms OSA and OSAS are often used interchangeably in the anesthesiology literature. The diagnosis of OHS requires the presence of [5]:

- obesity (Body Mass Index [BMI] $\geq$30 kg/m^2)
- daytime awake hypercapnia ($PaCO_2 \geq 45$ mmHg) and hypoxemia ($PaO_2 < 70$ mmHg)
- sleep disordered breathing (e.g., OSA)

Anesthesia and Perioperative Care of the High-Risk Patient, Third edition, ed. Ian McConachie. Published by Cambridge University Press.

- exclusion of other known causes of hypoventilation (e.g., severe obstructive or restrictive parenchymal lung disease, kyphoscoliosis, severe hypothyroidism, neuromuscular disease, and congenital central hypoventilation syndrome)

Pathophysiology of OSA and OHS

Pathophysiological mechanisms leading to OSA [6]:

Anatomical imbalance

- An excessive amount of soft tissue in the pharynx or small craniofacial size can result in narrowing of the pharyngeal airway space and obstruction of airflow.
- Body weight and neck circumference are important contributing factors.

Lung volume reduction during the perioperative period

- The reduction of functional residual capacity (FRC) causes cephalad displacement of the trachea, decreasing longitudinal tension of the pharyngeal airway wall and increasing pharyngeal collapsibility.

Pathophysiological mechanisms leading to OHS [2,7]

Increased mechanical load and impaired respiratory mechanics

- Obesity imposes a significant load on the respiratory system and could result in hypoventilation secondary to fatigue and weakness of the respiratory muscles.
- Mechanisms other than obesity may lead to hypoventilation as less than one third of the morbidly obese individuals develop hypercapnia.

Leptin resistance

- Leptin is a protein produced by adipose tissue that regulates appetite and energy expenditure.
- A higher level of leptin is found in individuals with simple obesity leading to an increase in ventilation to compensate for the increased CO_2 production associated with excess body mass.
- Patients with OHS exhibit an even higher serum leptin level than eucapnic individuals matched for BMI, suggesting ventilatory control in OHS patients may be resistant to leptin.

Impaired compensation of acute hypercapnia in sleep-disordered breathing

- Obstructive apneas and hypopneas during sleep lead to transient episodes of acute hypercapnia, which are compensated by hyperventilation during brief periods of arousal between the obstructive events.
- Compared to eucapnic subjects with OSA, OHS patients do not hyperventilate to the same extent between periods of apnea, resulting in acute hypercapnia that may cause renal bicarbonate (HCO_3^-) retention. A transition from acute to chronic hypercapnia in OHS may occur if these patients were not able to excrete the excess HCO_3^-.

Comorbidities associated with OSA and OHS

- OSA is associated with cardiovascular disease (coronary artery disease [CAD], heart failure, arrhythmias, hypertension), cerebrovascular disease, metabolic syndrome, gastroesophageal reflux disease, and obesity [1].
- Predisposing factors to OSA include altered upper airway anatomy (craniofacial abnormalities, macroglossia, retrognathia), endocrine diseases (Cushing disease, hypothyroidism), connective tissue diseases (Marfan syndrome), and lifestyle factors such as smoking and alcohol consumption.

OSA and obesity are prominent features in OHS. In addition, several clinical characteristics are present in OHS patients that may increase their perioperative risk for cardiac or pulmonary complications [3]:

Restrictive pulmonary physiology

- Simple obesity impairs respiratory mechanics through reduced lungs volumes, reduced chest wall compliance, increased respiratory resistance, and increased work of breathing. These parameters are further increased in OHS.
- Typical spirometry in OHS reveals a restrictive pattern (reduced forced expiratory volume (FEV_1) and forced vital capacity (FVC) but normal FEV_1/FVC). FRC, total lung capacity (TLC), and expiratory reserve volume (ERV) are reduced.

Blunted central respiratory drive

- OHS patients have a blunted central respiratory drive to both hypercapnia and hypoxia. Its etiology is currently unclear.

Pulmonary hypertension

- The incidence in OHS patients ranges from 30% to 88%.
- The etiology of pulmonary hypertension is likely secondary to chronic alveolar hypoxia and hypercapnia.

Postoperative complications and outcome in patients with OSA and OHS

- Long-standing untreated OSA is an independent risk factor for all-cause mortality [8].
- Postoperative complications occur more frequently in OSA than non-OSA patients due to their predisposition to upper airway obstruction and hypoxemia. A higher incidence of postoperative desaturation, respiratory failure, postoperative cardiac events (cardiac arrest, myocardial ischemia, and arrhythmias), and intensive care unit (ICU) transfers were observed in patients with OSA [9–12].
- Hospitalized patients with OHS experience higher morbidity and mortality than patients who are similarly obese and have OSA. They are more likely to develop heart failure, angina, cor pulmonale, and require invasive mechanical complications [13,14].
- OHS patients undergoing bariatric surgery suffer a higher mortality than non-OHS patients. The major causes of death include pulmonary embolus and intra-abdominal sepsis from anastomotic leaks [15].

Treatment modalities for OSA and OHS

Positive airway pressure (PAP)

- The mainstay of treatment for patients with OSA and OHS is the usd of PAP devices [4,16].
- Continuous PAP (CPAP) is the treatment of choice for OSA.
- CPAP significantly improves sleepiness, quality of life, and cognitive function in OSA patients.
- CPAP and bilevel PAP are both shown to be efficacious for OHS.
- Occasionally, CPAP may not improve upper airway obstruction or oxygenation in OHS completely. In these non-responders, bilevel PAP should be considered.
- In OHS, short-term ($\leq$3 wk) PAP therapy improves gas exchange (oxygenation and CO_2 elimination); long-term ($\geq$4 wk) PAP therapy improves lung volume and central respiratory drive to CO_2.

Bariatric surgery

- Bariatric surgery is the mainstay of treatment for morbidly obese patients in whom conservative measures have failed. It is the most effective method for sustained weight loss and should be considered in patients with OSA and OHS.
- Bariatric surgery significantly reduces upper airway obstruction in OSA. However, the effect is not complete as the AHI after surgery is still consistent with moderate OSA. These patients may still require PAP therapy [17].
- Additional benefits in OHS include an improvement in gas exchange and pulmonary function.

Supplemental oxygen

- Supplemental oxygen improves oxygen saturation (SaO_2) in patients with OSA. However, it does not reduce AHI and may cause a lengthening of apnea/hypopnea episodes when compared with patients breathing air [18].
- Approximately 40% of patients with OHS continue to desaturate during sleep while on adequate CPAP settings.
- The administration of supplemental oxygen prevents hypoxia but may worsen hypercapnia by reducing minute ventilation [19].
- The lowest concentration of oxygen should be applied to avoid worsening hypercapnia while maintaining adequate oxygenation.

Preoperative evaluation of patients with diagnosed OSA and OHS

Primary goals for preoperative evaluation of patients with diagnosed OSA and OHS are:

- Anticipate potential difficulties in airway management.
- Ensure adequate treatment for upper airway obstruction.
- Optimize significant cardiopulmonary comorbidities.

Anticipate potential difficulties in airway management

- A careful examination of patients should be performed to assess markers of difficult intubation and ventilation.

- OSA is a risk factor for both difficult mask ventilation and intubation [20].
- Obesity results in a three-fold increase in difficult mask ventilation [21].

Ensure adequate treatment for upper airway obstruction

- A review of patient's symptoms, polysomnography results, and compliance to PAP devices is key in evaluating relief of upper airway obstruction.
- Patients experiencing persistent or recurrent manifestations of upper airway obstruction (poor sleep quality interrupted by apneas/hypopneas, daytime tiredness, and snoring), significant weight gain, and hypoxemia (SaO_2 <94%) may require readjustment of PAP devices.

Optimize significant cardiopulmonary comorbidities

- The evaluation of cardiopulmonary comorbidities in OSA and OHS should include a focused assessment of arrhythmias, CAD, congestive heart failure, and pulmonary hypertension/right ventricular (RV) dysfunction.
- If these patients are undergoing major surgery, stress testing and transthoracic echocardiogram may be considered if this will improve perioperative management.

A clinical pathway was proposed for the preoperative evaluation of patients with diagnosed OSA [1]; this can also be applied to patients with diagnosed OHS (Figure 11.1):

- In patients with moderate-to-severe OSA, perioperative risk reduction strategies (see later) and PAP therapy should be emphasized. Patients who develop a significant

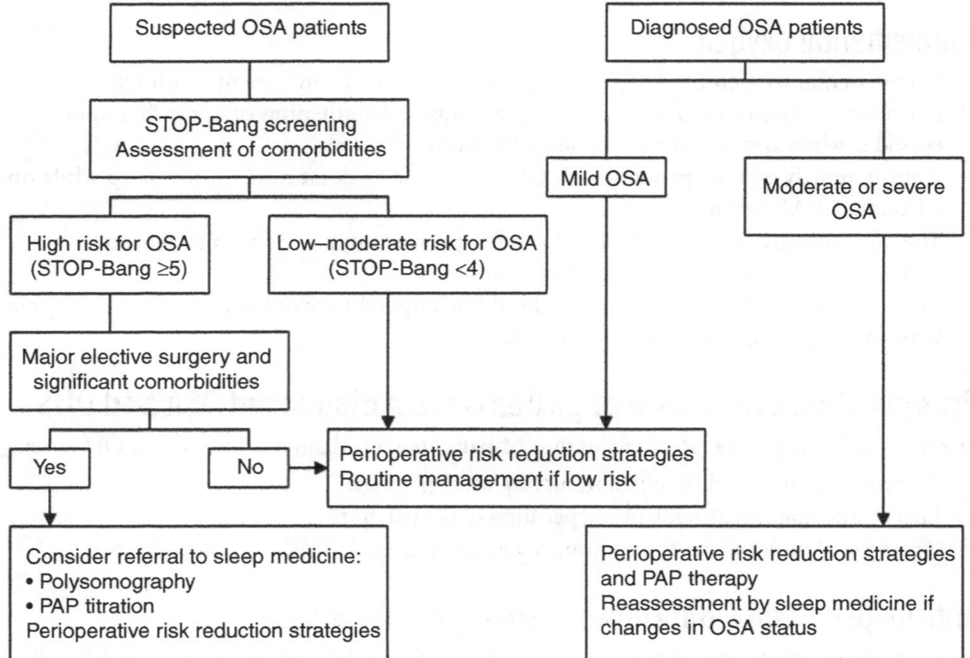

Figure 11.1. Preoperative evaluation of the patient with diagnosed or suspected OSA.

deterioration of OSA status warrant a reassessment by sleep medicine before major elective surgery.

- In patients with mild OSA, routine management is adequate.

Preoperative evaluation of patients with suspected OSA and OHS

- Patients with features of obesity and thick neck circumference should lead to a high index suspicion and screening for OSA should be performed.
- In patients with moderate to severe OSA or morbidly obese patients (BMI $\geq$40) with or without known OSA, we recommend screening for OHS [22,23].

Screening tools for OSA

- Questionnaire-based screening tools are practical and can be applied in the preoperative clinic.
- The STOP-Bang questionnaire is validated in surgical patients and is an easy-to-use scoring model based on yes/no answers to eight questions (Table 11.1) [24]. It facilitates risk stratification for OSA and triage for diagnostic evaluation. The higher the score, the more likely the patient has moderate to severe OSA [25].
- A STOP-Bang score of 0–2 indicates a low risk for OSA. A score of 3–4 indicates intermediate-risk and a score of 5–8 indicates a high-risk of OSA [25].

Screening tools for OHS

The screening for OHS involves evaluating for OSA and hypoventilation.

Screening for OSA can be accomplished using the STOP-Bang questionnaire, as mentioned earlier. Screening for hypoventilation consists of:

- Measurement of serum HCO_3^- as a surrogate for daytime hypercapnia. The higher the HCO_3^- ($\geq$27 mEq/L), the higher the likelihood of OHS [26].

Table 11.1. STOP-Bang questionnaire

S = snoring. Do you snore loudly (louder than talking or loud enough to be heard through closed doors)?
T = tiredness. Do you often feel tired, fatigued, or sleepy during daytime?
O = observed apnea. Has anyone observed you stop breathing during your sleep?
P = pressure. Do you have or are you being treated for high blood pressure?
B = BMI >35 kg/m^2
A = age >50 years
N = neck circumference >40 cm
G = male gender
Scoring and risk for OSA:
A positive answer to each item scores 1 point.
0–2 points: low-risk
3–4 points: intermediate-risk
5–8 points: high-risk for moderate to severe OSA

Adapted from Chung et al. [24] and Chung et al. [25].

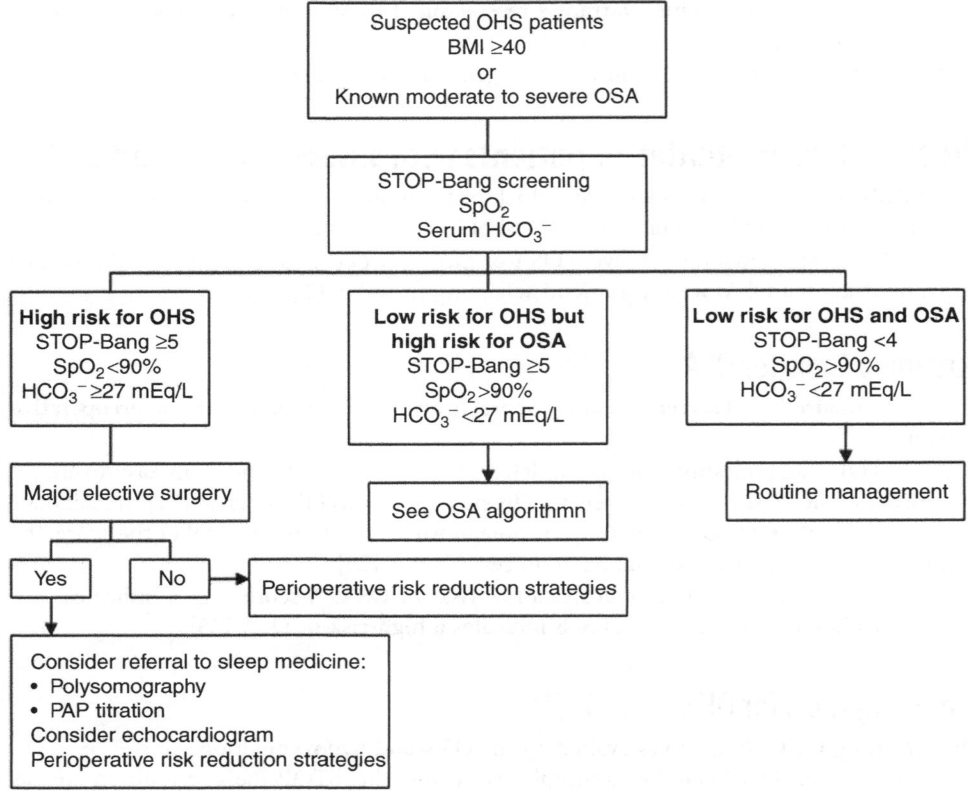

Figure 11.2. Preoperative evaluation of the patient with suspected OHS.

- Measurement of oxygen saturation via pulse oximetry (SpO_2) as a surrogate for daytime hypoxemia. A value of <90% with a PaO_2 of <70 mmHg should alarm physicians regarding the presence of OHS.
- If the serum HCO_3^- is elevated or SpO_2 is low, a measurement of arterial blood gases is recommended.

A clinical pathway was proposed for the preoperative evaluation of patients with suspected OSA (Figure 11.1) and OHS (Figure 11.2) [1,3]:

- In patients at high-risk of OSA or OHS with significant comorbidities and undergoing major elective surgery, a referral to sleep medicine should be considered for polysomnography and PAP titration study. Furthermore, in patients at high-risk for OHS, a transthoracic echocardiogram should be considered to assess RV dysfunction and pulmonary hypertension.
- In patients at high-risk of OSA or OHS but who are otherwise without significant comorbidities and not scheduled for major surgery, a preoperative referral to sleep medicine may not be necessary. However, perioperative risk reduction strategies should be undertaken (see later).
- Patients at low risk for OSA may be managed with routine perioperative care.

Perioperative risk reduction strategies

In the perioperative period, patients with OSA and OHS are at risk for the following:

- potential difficult airway
- residual post-anesthesia sedation
- opioid-induced ventilatory impairment
- post-extubation airway obstruction

Potential difficult airway

- A variety of airway adjuncts and skilled anesthesiology assistance should be available before the induction of anesthesia.
- Obese patients should be placed in the ramp position with elevation of the head and torso to improve the ease of ventilation and glottic view from the neutral position.
- Preoxygenation with 100% oxygen increases apnea tolerance time post-induction. The application of CPAP at 10 cmH_2O in a 25° head-up tilt position reduces atelectasis formation and improves oxygenation further [27,28].

Residual post-anesthesia sedation

- Patients with OSA and OHS are sensitive to the respiratory depressant effects of anesthetic agents.
- Rapid emergence from anesthesia using short-acting anesthetic agents such as insoluble volatile anesthetics (desflurane) or remifentanil minimize post-anesthesia sedation.
- If feasible, the use of the regional anesthetic (RA) technique with minimal sedation should be considered.

Opioid-induced ventilatory impairment

- The heightened sensitivity to opioids of patients with OSA and OHS predispose them to recurrent airway obstruction and hypoventilation in the post-anesthesia period.
- An opioid-sparing analgesic regimen, consisting of regional nerve blocks with local anesthetics (LAs) and non-opioid adjuncts (e.g., acetaminophen and nonsteroidal anti-inflammatory drugs [NSAIDs]), should be considered.
- Postoperative monitoring for opioid-induced ventilatory impairment is essential to ensure patient safety. Individuals at high-risk of postoperative complications may be identified in the post-anesthesia care unit (PACU) and warrant a higher level of monitoring after they are discharged from the PACU.

A clinical pathway to facilitate this decision making process is proposed for OSA patients [1,29] (Figure 11.3); this can also be applied to patients with OHS:

- Patients with known or suspected OSA/OHS should be observed in the PACU for a longer period. An extended PACU stay of at least 30–60 minutes after the patient has met criteria for discharge should be considered.
- In patients with suspected OSA, recurrent PACU respiratory events (apnea $\geq$10 s, bradypnea <8 breaths/min, desaturation to <90%, and pain-sedation mismatch defined by concurrent high pain and sedation score) suggest a higher risk for postoperative respiratory complications, and therefore continuous oximetry monitoring may be

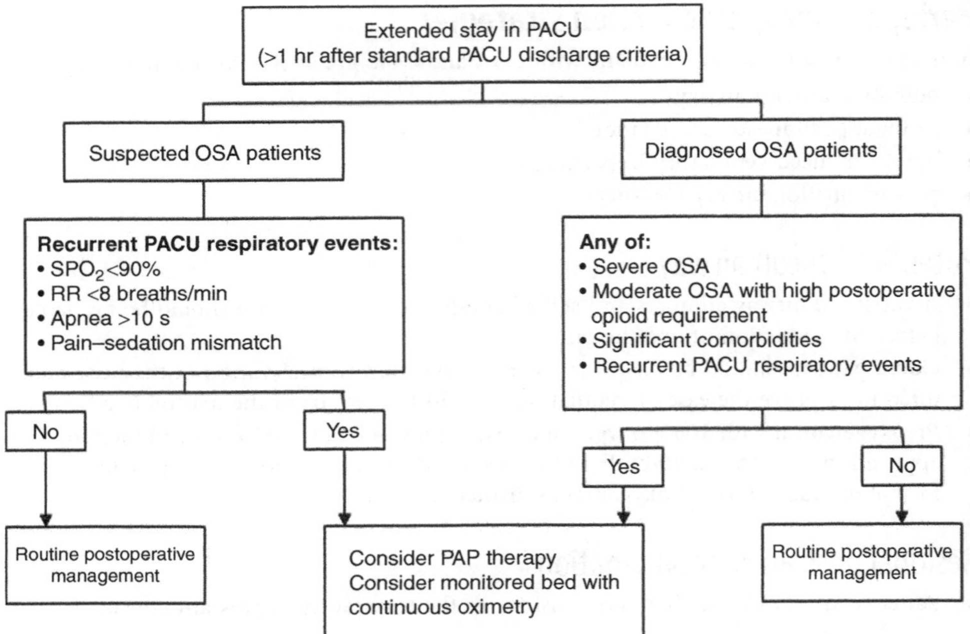

Figure 11.3. Postoperative management of the patient with diagnosed or suspected OSA.

required [30]. This can be achieved in a step-down unit, an inpatient ward near the nursing station, or by remote pulse oximetry with telemetry.

- In patients with diagnosed OSA, recurrent PACU respiratory events, severe OSA, significant comorbidities, and high postoperative opioid requirement are factors that indicate continuous oximetry monitoring.

Post-extubation airway obstruction

- Extubation should be carried out only after the OSA/OHS patient is fully conscious and cooperative. Neuromuscular blockade should be fully reversed.
- A semi-upright or lateral position is preferred for extubation and recovery.
- OSA/OHS patients who were prescribed PAP therapy at home should resume its use in the postoperative period.
- Empiric PAP therapy may be initiated in the PACU for patients with suspected but undiagnosed OSA/OHS who experience recurrent upper airway obstruction.

Postoperative rescue strategies for cardiopulmonary failure

- Outside the immediate post-extubation period, OSA and OHS patients remain at risk for cardiopulmonary failure due to multiple factors, such as sedation, sleep deprivation, and deconditioning. In particular, OHS patients are at high-risk secondary to increased respiratory load, blunted central drive, pulmonary hypertension, and impaired ventricular function.

- Postoperative cardiopulmonary failure in patients with OSA/OHS may assume various presentations [31]:
  - hypercapnic respiratory failure secondary to recurrent upper airway obstruction and hypoventilation
  - acute cardiogenic pulmonary edema secondary to myocardial ischemia and arrhythmias induced by intermittent hypoxemia
  - sudden death, an extreme manifestation, secondary to malignant arrhythmias or severe hypoxemia
- Early initiation of empiric PAP therapy could be used to treat cardiopulmonary failure without resorting to invasive mechanical ventilation [32].
- Other adjunctive interventions include judicious sedation/analgesia, optimization of volume status and cardiac output to prevent cardiogenic pulmonary edema, and minimal sleep disruption at night. A close follow-up with a sleep specialist is recommended.

Ambulatory surgery for OSA patients

Owing to the increasing number of procedures performed in the ambulatory settings, an increasing number of patients with OSA will present for outpatient surgical procedures. As OSA patients usually present with multiple comorbidities and a higher risk for postoperative complications, their suitability for ambulatory surgery is currently controversial.

- Multiple factors have to be considered to determine whether ambulatory surgery is appropriate for the OSA patient [33]. These include:
  - OSA status
  - status of comorbidities
  - age
  - nature of surgery
  - type of anesthesia
  - need for postoperative opioids
  - adequacy of post-discharge observation
  - capabilities of the outpatient facility
- The 2006 American Society of Anaesthesiologists (ASA) guidelines on the perioperative management of OSA patients suggested superficial/orthopedic surgery under LA/RA, and lithotripsy can be performed on an outpatient basis. However, OSA patients undergoing surgery to the upper airway and upper abdomen (laparoscopic) are not recommended to be discharged home on the same day.
- According to more recent studies, OSA patients who underwent ambulatory surgery experienced a higher incidence of transient hypoxemia requiring supplemental oxygen. However, there is no difference between the need for reintubation, ventilatory assistance, delayed discharge, unanticipated hospital admission, and death [34].

A recent consensus statement from the Society for Ambulatory Anesthesia made the following recommendations regarding the selection of OSA patients for ambulatory surgery [34]:

- The need for increased vigilance after discharge home should be emphasized to surgeons, patients, and their family (or caregivers).

- Patients receiving preoperative PAP therapy should be instructed to bring their device to the ambulatory care facility.
- In patients with suspected OSA, ambulatory surgery may be considered if their comorbidities are optimized and postoperative pain can be managed using non-opioid analgesia.
- In patients with diagnosed OSA, ambulatory surgery may be considered if their comorbidities are optimized and PAP therapy is complied with postoperatively. These patients are advised to use their PAP devices when sleeping, even in daytime, for several days postoperatively because potential risks can last for several days postoperatively.
- OSA patients with non-optimized comorbidities are not suitable for ambulatory surgery.
- Postoperatively, OSA patients who developed recurrent respiratory events (desaturation, bradypnea, apnea, and pain-sedation mismatch) in the PACU should be managed cautiously and admission for monitoring should be considered.

Summary

- OSA and OHS often remain undiagnosed in patients presenting for surgery.
- OSA is associated with multiple comorbidities including cardiovascular disease, cerebrovascular disease, metabolic syndrome, gastroesophageal reflux disease, and obesity.
- OHS is a disease entity distinct from OSA and simple obesity. It is characterized by severe upper airway obstruction, restrictive pulmonary physiology, blunted central respiratory drive, and pulmonary hypertension. These features place the OHS patient at high-risk for perioperative cardiopulmonary complications.
- Preoperative evaluation of patients with diagnosed OSA and OHS should focus on assessing potential difficulties in airway management, treatment for upper airway obstruction, and significant cardiopulmonary comorbidities.
- In patients with suspected OSA or OHS, screening tools, such as the STOP-Bang questionnaire, pulse oximetry, and serum HCO_3^- should be used to identify high-risk individuals.
- Preoperative sleep medicine consultation should be considered in the OSA/OHS patients undergoing major elective surgery.
- Perioperative risk reduction strategies for OSA and OHS include preparing for potential difficult airway, minimizing post-anesthesia sedation, monitoring for opioid induced ventilatory impairment, and preventing post-extubation airway obstruction.
- If OSA/OHS patients developed recurrent respiratory events (desaturation, bradypnea, apnea, and pain-sedation mismatch) in the PACU, they should be cared for post-PACU in a monitored bed with continuous oximetry.
- The PAP device is an important treatment modality for postoperative cardiopulmonary failure in patients with OSA/OHS.
- Ambulatory surgery may be considered in patients with OSA if they are optimized medically, comply with PAP therapy, and require minimal opioid for postoperative analgesia.

References

1. Seet E, Han T, Chung F. Perioperative clinical pathways to manage sleep-disordered breathing. *Sleep Med Clin* 2013; **8**: 105–20.
2. Mokhlesi B. Obesity hypoventilation syndrome: a state-of-the-art review. *Respir Care* 2010; **55**: 1347–62.
3. Chau E, Lam D, Wong J, et al. Obesity hypoventilation syndrome: a review of epidemiology, pathophysiology, and perioperative considerations. *Anesthesiology* 2012; **117**: 188–205.
4. Fleetham J, Ayas N, Bradley D, et al. Canadian Thoracic Society guidelines: diagnosis and treatment of sleep disordered breathing in adults. *Can Respir J* 2006; **13**: 387–92.
5. Olson A, Zwillich C. The obesity hypoventilation syndrome. *Am J Med* 2005; **118**: 948–56.
6. Isono S. Obstructive sleep apnea of obese adults: pathophysiology and perioperative airway management. *Anesthesiology* 2009; **110**: 908–21.
7. Piper AJ. Obesity hypoventilation syndrome–the big and the breathless. *Sleep Medicine Reviews* 2011; **15**: 79–89.
8. Marshall N, Wong K, Liu P, et al. Sleep apnea as an independent risk factor for all-cause mortality: the Busselton Health Study. *Sleep* 2008; **31**: 1079–85.
9. Kaw R, Chung F, Pasupuleti V, et al. Meta-analysis of the association between obstructive sleep apnoea and postoperative outcome. *Br J Anaesth* 2012; **109**: 897–906.
10. Gupta R, Parvizi J, Hanssen AD, et al. Postoperative complications in patients with obstructive sleep apnea syndrome undergoing hip or knee replacement: a case-control study. *Mayo Clin Proc* 2001; **76**: 897–905.
11. Kaw R, Pasupuleti V, Walker E, et al. Postoperative complications in patients with obstructive sleep apnea. *Chest* 2012; **141**: 436–41.
12. Liao P, Yegneswaran B, Vairavanathan S, et al. Postoperative complications in patients with obstructive sleep apnea: a retrospective matched cohort study. *Can J Anaesth* 2009; **56**: 819–28.
13. Berg G, Delaive K, Manfreda J, et al. The use of health-care resources in obesity-hypoventilation syndrome. *Chest* 2001; **120**: 377–83.
14. Nowbar S, Burkart KM, Gonzales R, et al. Obesity-associated hypoventilation in hospitalized patients: prevalence, effects, and outcome. *Am J Med* 2004; **116**: 1–7.
15. Fernandez AJ, Demaria EJ, Tichansky DS, et al. Multivariate analysis of risk factors for death following gastric bypass for treatment of morbid obesity. *Ann Surg* 2004; **239**: 698–702.
16. Fleetham J, Ayas N, Bradley D, et al. Canadian Thoracic Society 2011 guideline update: diagnosis and treatment of sleep disordered breathing. *Can Respir J* 2011; **18**: 25–47.
17. Greenburg D, Lettieri CJ, Eliasson AH. Effects of surgical weight loss on measures of obstructive sleep apnea: a meta-analysis. *Am J Med* 2009; **122**: 535–42.
18. Mehta V, Vasu T, Phillips B, et al. Obstructive sleep apnea and oxygen therapy: a systematic review of the literature and meta-analysis. *J Clin Sleep Med* 2013; **9**: 271–9.
19. Wijesinghe M, Williams M, Perrin K, et al. The effect of supplemental oxygen on hypercapnia in subjects with obesity-associated hypoventilation: a randomized, crossover, clinical study. *Chest* 2011; **139**: 1018–24.
20. Siyam M, Benhamou D. Difficult endotracheal intubation in patients with sleep apnea syndrome. *Anesth Analg* 2002; **95**: 1098–102.
21. Langeron O, Masso E, Huraux C, et al. Prediction of difficult mask ventilation. *Anesthesiology* 2000; **92**: 1229–36.
22. Kaw R, Hernandez AV, Walker E, et al. Determinants of hypercapnia in obese patients with obstructive sleep apnea: a systematic review and meta-analysis of cohort studies. *Chest* 2009; **136**: 787–96.
23. Mokhlesi B, Saager L, Kaw R. Q: Should we routinely screen for hypercapnia in sleep

apnea patients before elective noncardiac surgery? *Cleve Clin J Med* 2010; **77**: 60–1.

24. Chung F, Yegneswaran B, Liao P, et al. STOP questionnaire: a tool to screen patients for obstructive sleep apnea. *Anesthesiology* 2008; **108**: 812–21.

25. Chung F, Subramanyam R, Liao P, et al. High STOP-Bang score indicates a high probability of obstructive sleep apnoea. *Br J Anaesth* 2012; **108**: 768–75.

26. Mokhlesi B, Tulaimat A, Faibussowitsch I, et al. Obesity hypoventilation syndrome: prevalence and predictors in patients with obstructive sleep apnea. *Sleep Breath* 2007; **11**: 117–24.

27. Dixon B, Dixon JB, Carden JR, et al. Preoxygenation is more effective in the 25 degrees head-up position than in the supine position in severely obese patients: a randomized controlled study. *Anesthesiology* 2005; **102**: 1110–15.

28. Gander S, Frascarolo P, Suter M, et al. Positive end-expiratory pressure during induction of general anesthesia increases duration of nonhypoxic apnea in morbidly obese patients. *Anesth Analg* 2005; **100**: 580–4.

29. Swart P, Chung F, Fleetham J. An order-based approach to facilitate postoperative decision-making for patients with sleep apnea. *Can J Anaesth* 2013; **60**: 321–4.

30. Gali B, Whalen FX, Schroeder DR, et al. Identification of patients at risk for postoperative respiratory complications using a preoperative obstructive sleep apnea screening tool and postanesthesia care assessment. *Anesthesiology* 2009; **110**: 869–77.

31. Carr G, Mokhlesi B, Gehlbach B. Acute cardiopulmonary failure from sleep-disordered breathing. *Chest* 2012; **141**: 798–808.

32. Carrillo A, Ferrer M, Gonzalez-Diaz G, et al. Noninvasive ventilation in acute hypercapnic respiratory failure caused by obesity hypoventilation syndrome and chronic obstructive pulmonary disease. *Am J Respir Crit Care Med* 2012; **186**: 1279–85.

33. Gross J, Bachenberg K, Benumof J, et al. Practice guidelines for the perioperative management of patients with obstructive sleep apnea: a report by the American Society of Anesthesiologists Task Force on Perioperative Management of patients with obstructive sleep apnea. *Anesthesiology* 2006; **104**: 1081–93.

34. Joshi G, Ankichetty S, Gan T, et al. Society for Ambulatory Anesthesia consensus statement on preoperative selection of adult patients with obstructive sleep apnea scheduled for ambulatory surgery. *Anesth Analg* 2012; **115**: 1060–8.

Chapter 12

Smoking, alcohol, and recreational drug abuse

G. Evans

This chapter outlines anesthetic implications of several, unfortunately common, recreational habits (both legal and illegal), which are known to increase anesthetic and perioperative risk.

This chapter can provide only a brief overview of these topics and the reader is encouraged to review the suggestions for further reading.

Smoking

Oxygen delivery is impaired by carboxyhemoglobin and levels may exceed 10% in smokers. Carbon monoxide present in smoke reduces the amount of hemoglobin available to carry oxygen and also shifts the oxyhemoglobin dissociation curve to the left. These effects are important factors in exercise-induced angina and ventricular arrhythmias in smokers with coronary artery disease (CAD). Expired carbon monoxide concentration has been correlated with the frequency of significant ST depression during general anesthesia (GA) [1].

Quitting smoking for patients with CAD decreases risk for all-cause mortality by about one third; however, it is estimated that several months are required to realize the full benefit [2].

Current evidence supports the safety of nicotine replacement therapy (NRT) in patients with CAD [3]. In addition, NRT does not affect the patency of bypass grafts. Therefore, the benefit of NRT in patients with CAD outweighs the risks of continuing to smoke.

Respiratory function

- Chronic obstructive pulmonary disease (COPD) develops in almost 15% of smokers and up to another 50% have chronic bronchitis.
- Smokers produce greater amounts of mucus and clearance is impaired; in addition, immune function is decreased.
- Structural changes develop with chronic use, leading to smooth muscle proliferation and fibrosis.
- Mucociliary clearance shows some improvement with abstinence after one week.
- Smokers are at higher risk of perioperative pulmonary complications (PPC), including: respiratory failure, pneumonia, need for postoperative respiratory or aerosol therapy, airway events during induction (i.e., cough, laryngospasm), bronchospasm, and increased airway secretions. Children exposed to smoke at home are also at increased risk of PPCs.

Anesthesia and Perioperative Care of the High-Risk Patient, Third edition, ed. Ian McConachie. Published by Cambridge University Press.

- Retrospective analysis has determined that the frequency of PPCs in smokers who had coronary artery bypass grafting (CABG) and continued to smoke up until surgery was not different than those who quit within eight weeks of surgery (48% versus 56%). However, the rate of PPCs was significantly lower in those patients who quit more than eight weeks prior the surgery (17%) and similar to the rate of PPCs in non-smokers (11%) [4].
- Some studies have suggested an increase in rates of PPC in the first month of abstinence, possibly in relation to increased mucus production; however, a recent meta-analysis found that less than four weeks of smoking cessation did not increase or reduce the risk of postoperative respiratory complications [5].
- Long-term tobacco smoking increases the risk of postoperative admission to intensive care (in a dose-dependent fashion) with a trend toward increased mortality [6].
- Most perioperative problems due to smoking occur in the postoperative period but airway problems, and in particular, coughing during induction may vary with the anesthetic agent in use. For example, airway problems in smokers have been shown to be much more common with isoflurane compared to sevoflurane [7].
- Postoperative nausea and vomiting (PONV) are probably less in smokers compared with non-smokers [8], but this consideration does not outweigh the health benefits of encouraging smokers to quit before surgery.

Wound and bone healing

Bone healing may be impaired in smokers after orthopedic procedures [9]. Smoking cessation preoperatively dramatically decreases the rate of wound-related complications. The duration of cessation to realize this benefit is unknown but it appears to be at least four weeks [10].

Helping smokers quit

A primary recommendation from the U.S. Public Health Service Guideline on Tobacco Use and Dependence is to strongly urge all smokers who come in contact with the healthcare system to quit smoking and to aid them in doing so. This recommendation is based on the fact that physician advice to quit smoking increases abstinence rates even if the encounter is only brief, such as that in a preoperative clinic (i.e., <3 min duration of counseling). However, more intensive and multiple counseling formats will increase abstinence further. The use of medications will approximately double abstinence rates [11]. Perioperative interventions may be effective. For example:

- Varenicline, in a recent double-blind randomized controlled trial (RCT), has been shown to significantly increase smoking cessation in the perioperative period, with persisting increases in cessation at 12 months [12].
- A simple perioperative smoking cessation program (including counseling, brochures, and nicotine patches) performed in the pre-admission clinic has recently been shown to reduce the number of patients smoking by the date of surgery and for up to 30 days postoperatively [13].

Many smokers are reluctant to quit smoking preoperatively as cigarettes are used as a stress reliever. However, some recent data demonstrate that smokers do not report greater stress in the perioperative period than non-smokers, nor do they consistently develop withdrawal symptoms [14].

Alcohol

Ethanol is absorbed from the upper gastrointestinal (GI) track and reaches peak levels in the blood within 30 minutes. Hepatic alcohol dehydrogenase metabolizes ethanol to acetaldehyde, which then is converted to acetate. Acetate is metabolized to acetylcoenzyme A, then eventually to carbon dioxide and water. Thiamine is an essential cofactor in the final step of metabolism and deficiency contributes to build-up of metabolites.

Acetaldehyde directly impairs cardiac contractile function, disrupts cardiac excitation (contractile coupling), inhibits myocardial protein synthesis, interferes with phosphorylation, and inactivates coenzyme A. Alcohol dehydrogenase is saturated at relatively low blood levels, and this changes elimination from first-order to zero-order kinetics. Oxidative metabolism of ethanol indirectly results in lactate accumulation, ketone formation, and impaired gluconeogenesis, secondary to an overall decrease in redox potential.

Physical findings associated with long-term alcoholism are parotid enlargement, flushed faces, gynecomastia, cardiomyopathy, hepatomegaly, stigma of cirrhosis, testicular atrophy, palmar erythema, Dupyutren contractures, peripheral neuropathy, nutritional deficiencies, and recurrent infections. Table 12.1 summarizes the medical problems associated with alcoholism.

Toxicity

- Gross motor control and orientation may be significantly affected at 50 mg/dL (10.87 mmol/L).
- Classic signs of intoxication include ataxia, dysarthia, mydriasis, and nystagmus.
- Initially, ethanol causes central nervous system (CNS) stimulation via disinhibition, but then progresses to loss of protective reflexes, respiratory depression, and coma.
- Facial flushing associated with ethanol-induced vasodilation can lead to hypotension and tachycardia.
- In patients with cardiac disease, this may lead to decreased cardiac output, atrial fibrillation, nonsustained ventricular tachycardia and atrioventricular (A-V) block.
- Hypoglycemia is generally seen in children, binge drinkers with poor carbohydrate intake, and those who are malnourished.

Withdrawal and its management [15]

Ongoing stimulation of inhibitory γ-aminobutyric acid (GABA) receptor channel complex by ethanol leads to downregulation of this complex. Withdrawal is associated with a decrease in GABAergic activity and an increase in glutamatergic activity, which results in autonomic excitability and psychomotor agitation. Alcohol withdrawal may begin as early as six hours after cessation of drinking and is characterized as autonomic hyperactivity including tachycardia, tremor, hypertension, and psychomotor agitation.

Approximately 25% of patients with alcohol withdrawal syndrome (AWS) will develop hallucinations – as apposed to delirium tremens (DT), where the hallucinations are associated with a clear sensorium. AWS seizures occur in about 10% of patients – 40% of these will be isolated seizures and 3% will develop status epilepticus. Benzodiazepines are

Table 12.1. Summary of medical problems associated with alcoholism.

Central nervous system effects	• Psychiatric disorders (depression) • Nutritional disorders (Wernicke–Korsakoff) • Withdrawal syndrome • Cerebellar degeneration • Cerebral atrophy • Peripheral neuropathy
Cardiovascular effects	• Dilated cardiomyopathy • Cardiac dysrhythmias • Systemic hypertension • Autonomic insufficiency
Gastrointestinal and hepatobiliary effects	• Esophagitis • Gastritis • Pancreatitis • Hepatic cirrhosis (portal hypertension leading to varices and hemorrhoids)
Skin and musculoskeletal effects	• Spider angiomas • Myopathy • Osteoporosis
Endocrine and metabolic effects	• Decreased serum testosterone • Decreased gluconeogenesis (hypoglycemia) • Ketoacidosis • Hypoalbuminemia • Hypomagnesemia
Hematologic effects	• Thrombocytopenia • Leukopenia • Anemia

the first-line treatment for AWS seizures (note: there is no role for phenytoin in treatment or prevention of these seizures); for example, diazepam 5–10 mg IV every five minutes, titrated to achieve sedation and seizure control.

DT is the most serious complication of AWS and is usually seen between 48 and 96 hours after the last consumption of alcohol. It is associated with either a disturbance of consciousness or a change in cognition, or the development of a perceptual disturbance. DT can last for up to two weeks. Initial management of DT should include IV benzodiazepines for sedation, aiming to maintain spontaneous respiration with normal vital signs. Diazepam is generally the first-line drug due to its long half-life – unless the patient has advanced liver disease, in which case, lorazepam may be a better choice because of its lack of active metabolites.

If patients fail to respond to high doses of diazepam, then a second GABAergic drug should be used, such as phenobarbital or propofol – these patients will generally require airway management and intensive care unit (ICU) admission.

All patients should be assessed for dehydration and appropriate volume resuscitation instituted. Nutritional deficiencies are common in chronic alcohol users and all should receive thiamine to prevent the development of Wernicke encephalopathy. Ideally, this should be started before dextrose; however, it may be reasonable to co-administer dextrose with thiamine. Magnesium deficiency is common and should be corrected.

Although the mainstay of management of AWS remains the benzodiazepines, carbamazepine and valproic acid have been shown to increase the seizure threshold in alcohol withdrawal. These drugs may therefore be used as adjuncts to benzodiazepines [15]. In addition, the blunting of sympathetic activity by clonidine makes it an agent of potential value in AWS [16]. It is widely used for this purpose in Europe.

Anesthetic considerations for acute intoxication

- If possible, surgery and anesthesia should be delayed to allow the acute toxic effects to wear off and to allow rehydration and electrolyte corrections.
- If anesthesia is unavoidable, one should consider that there may be decreased minimum alveolar concentration (MAC), decreased level of consciousness, hypoventilation, full stomach, hypotension, hypothermia, impaired autonomic responses, and platelet dysfunction.
- Careful padding and positioning is essential as patients are at increased risk of peripheral nerve palsy.
- Consider Internal Medicine consultation for postoperative management of withdrawal.

Anesthesia for chronic alcohol abusers

- Chronic alcohol abusers may be on a downward spiral toward organ failure and death.
- Anesthesia requirements will vary. Initially, there is increased tolerance due to a degree of cross-sensitization and enzyme induction. As the patient's general health fails, s/he may become very sensitive to usual induction doses of anesthesia.
- Nutritional disorders, cardiomyopathy, liver disease, and frank cirrhosis may all develop.
- Cholinesterase levels may be reduced, but the clinical significance of this with regard to succinylcholine action is often small.
- The immune system will be impaired, leading to increased wound infections.
- Coagulation disturbances will also lead to increased problems with perioperative bleeding.
- In patients with advanced liver disease, acute liver failure may occur postoperatively.
- AWS with DT, resulting from abstinence during perioperative admission, is a significant factor in the increased morbidity seen in chronic alcohol abusers.
- However, as little as one month of preoperative abstinence can reduce postoperative morbidity in alcohol abusers [17]. This is likely due to improving organ function and a reduced surgical stress response.
- Complications appear to be directly related to the amount of alcohol consumed. The complication rate is 50% higher in those who consume three to four drinks per day and 200%–400% higher in those consuming five or more drinks per day [18].

Recreational drugs

Cocaine

Cocaine is an alkaloid benzoylmethylecgonine from the leaf of the *Erythroxylon coca* shrub. The hydrochloride salt forms a white crystalline compound, soluble in water, which may be absorbed through nasal mucosa. After being dissolved in ether and extracted via evaporation the "freebase" form is created, which can be inhaled. "Crack" cocaine is formed after dissolving the hydrochloride salt in water and adding sodium bicarbonate and then heating the substance to a hard rock-like substance.

Cocaine powder is absorbed from the nasal mucosa with a time to onset of one to three minutes, with peak effect in 20 minutes. Inhalation or injection results in faster onset of only seconds and peak effect in three to five minutes. The half-life of cocaine is 0.5–1.5 h; however, the half-life of active metabolites ranges from 3.5 to 8 h. The fatal dose is 1 g of pure cocaine orally or as little as 10 mg IV.

- Local anesthetic effects are via direct blockade of sodium channels and stabilization of the axonal membrane. Type IA and IC anti-arrhythmic effects on myocardial cells decrease the rate of depolarization and amplitude of action potentials [19].
- Cocaine causes an accumulation of catecholamines by interfering with the uptake of neurotransmitters by presynaptic sympathetic nerve terminals, with a secondary effect of release of norepinephrine. This results in increased concentrations of norepinephrine and epinephrine, causing vasoconstriction and tachycardia.
- Psychostimulant effects are secondary to inhibition of dopamine reuptake into presynaptic neurons, resulting in euphoria and alertness. Other central affects include mydriasis, headache, vomiting, and hallucinations.
- Between 1% and 5% of cocaine is excreted in the urine unaltered. Thus, cocaine or its metabolites can be identified by immunochemical assay of the urine for up to 24–48 hours after ingestion.
- Cocaine and ethanol together produce cocaethylene, which has direct cardiac depressant effects.

Cardiac toxicity

- The most frequent complications are coronary ischemia, myocardial infarction (MI), arrythmias, and cardiomyopathy. Cocaine use leads to premature atherosclerosis.
- Aspirin should be given to all cocaine users complaining of chest pain. Of those with cocaine-related chest pain, 6% will have enzymatic evidence of MI [20].
- Coronary vasoconstriction can produce vasospasm and decreases in vessel caliber by 10% [21].
- Acute toxicity can produce tachy- and bradydysrythmias, prolonged QRS, increased QTc, increased A-V conduction time, and refractory atrial periods.
- People abusing cocaine are at increased risk of ventricular fibrillation and sudden death because of increased sympathetic tone [22].
- Chronic cocaine use may result in myocarditis and left ventricular (LV) diastolic dysfunction.
- Cocaine abusers may develop cerebrovascular toxicity.
- Cocaine abuse is associated with generalized tonic-clonic or focal seizures.
- The increasing use of crack cocaine has led to increasing case reports of ischemic and hemorrhagic strokes [23].

Pulmonary toxicity

- As many as 25% of users experience pulmonary complications – most frequently associated with drug inhalation.

- Injury secondary to thermal injury generally involves the tracheobronchial tree.
- Damage to bronchial epithelium can stimulate vagal receptors and result in bronchospasm.
- Valsalva maneuver during inhalation or abrupt cough, resulting in increased intra-alveolar pressure, has been associated with pneumothorax, pneumomediastinum, and pneumopericardium [24].
- Cocaine can also act as a hapten or antigen when inhaled, inducing a hypersensitivity pneumonitis (the so-called Crack Lung) – this pneumonitis is characterized by diffuse alveolar and interstitial infiltrates [25].
- Massive hemoptysis occurs secondary to diffuse alveolar hemorrhage. The etiology is likely vasoconstriction-induced anoxia of epithelium and endothelium [24].
- Direct injury to the pulmonary capillary endothelial wall resulting in increased permeability can lead to non-cardiogenic pulmonary edema [24].
- Cardiogenic pulmonary edema is seen in the setting of LV dysfunction associated with chronic use, or acutely with increased sympathetic tone.

GI toxicity

- The most common serious GI complication is mucosal ischemia and perforation.
- The anticholinergic properties of cocaine decrease gastric motility, and increased acid exposure promotes ulcer formation [19].
- Infarction or hemorrhage of the spleen has been associated with cocaine abuse [26].

Renal toxicity

- Myocyte injury secondary to ischemia, seizures, and direct myocyte injury may manifest as rhabdomyolysis and acute renal failure.
- Thrombosis and renal artery spasm have been described as a mechanism for renal infarction [26].
- Renal scleroderma, Henoch–Schönlien purpura, and focal segmental glomerulosclerosis have all been associated with cocaine abuse [27].

Management

- Benzodiazepines appear to be the most effective in decreasing psychomotor agitation, seizures, and hyperthermia; high doses may be required (i.e., diazepam titrated up to 1 mg/kg or more, starting with 5–10 mg and repeated every 3–5 min).
- Pure β-blockers are contraindicated as they may precipitate unopposed α-adrenergic stimulation with catastrophic consequences (e.g., severe hypertension and vasospasm).
- Phentolamine, a pure α-adrenergic antagonist, is highly effective in reducing cocaine-induced vasoconstriction – dosage is 1–2.5 mg IV, repeated until symptoms resolve or hypotension develops.
- Nitrates such as nitroglycerin or nitroprusside are effective in the treatment of chest pain associated with cocaine use.
- Sodium bicarbonate appears to be effective in treating wide-complex tachycardias [20].
- Lidocaine continues to be a first-line agent in the management of tachyarrhythmias as per the American Heart Association (AHA), despite the concern over shared type IA profiles of both cocaine and lidocaine.

- Amiodarone has been suggested as a safer choice by some; however, validation in prospective studies is lacking, and others suggest that its β-blocking effects are of significant concern. Calcium channel blocking drugs have been shown in animal studies to enhance the occurrence of seizures [28].

Anesthesia considerations

- The potentiation of neuromuscular blockade has been demonstrated in patients receiving succinylcholine and cocaine [29]. This does not contraindicate its use in these patients, but caution should be used due to this possible interaction.
- Cocaine-intoxicated patients will require an increase in MAC and may experience severe hypertension with larnygoscopy.
- Increased risk of cardiac arrhythmias, such as ventricular tachycardia, frequent premature ventricular complexes, or *torsade de pointes* with use of potent volatile anesthetics (especially halothane, which should be avoided) [30].
- There may be concern over regional techniques if thrombocytopenia is present. One should consider requesting a platelet count in all patients prior to surgery.
- Treat intoxicated patients as full stomach.
- GA is considered by many to be safe [31] in non-toxic patients who present for elective surgery and have a positive screen for metabolites in their urine (i.e,. normal arterial pressure, normal heart rate, normothermic, a normal electrocardiograph (ECG) including a QTc interval <500 ms). Others would suggest that a one-week drug-free period is required before elective surgery [32].
- One should avoid using ketamine due to its sympathomimetic properties. Etomidate should be used with caution because of the risk of myoclonus, seizures, and hyperreflexia. Thus induction of GA with propofol or thiopental is considered most appropriate by the majority of authors.
- Patients may demonstrate hypotension unresponsive to ephedrine (in chronic users). Hypotension appears to respond well to low doses of phenylephrine.

Chronic abuse of opiates

Opium

Opium is derived from the seedpod of the poppy plant *Papaver somniferum*. Alkaloids derived directly from opium are referred to as opiates, such as morphine and codeine. Chemical alteration of these alkaloids is used to create semi-synthetic opioids such as heroin, naloxone, and oxycodone. Methadone and fentanyl are examples of synthetic opioids.

Heroin

Owing to its high lipid solubility, heroin is rapidly absorbed and crosses the blood–brain barrier within 20 seconds. This rapid absorption contributes to its euphoric effect. In the central nervous system, heroin is locally hydrolyzed to the active metabolites monoacetylmorphine and morphine within 30 minutes. Heroin is more appropriately known as diamorphine and is still widely used as a narcotic analgesic in the U.K.

Opiate toxicity

- Classic "toxidrome" consists of miosis, hypoventilation, lethargy, and ileus.
- Chemoreceptor sensitivity to hypercarbia and hypoxia is decreased, resulting in reduced ventilatory drive.
- Alveolar ventilation is decreased secondary to diminished respiratory rate and tidal volume.
- Heroin has been reported to cause non-cardiogenic pulmonary edema as far back as 1880 by Osler. Other similar reports have been described for virtually all opiates, although the etiology remains unclear.
- Heroin may stimulate status asthmaticus when inhaled. The likely mechanism is opiate-induced bronchial constriction compounded by histamine release; these attacks are often poorly or unresponsive to bronchodilators [33].
- Hypotension with opiates is secondary to arteriolar and venous dilation; this response is mediated by histamine release and increased vagal activity.
- Methadone can prolong the QT interval and predispose the patient to *torsades de pointes.*
- Meperidine (called pethidine in some countries), propoxyphene, and tramadol may all be associated with decreased seizure threshold.
- Meperidine is metabolized to normeperidine and accumulation, especially in patients with renal failure, can cause delirium, tremors, and seizures [34].

Naloxone

Naloxone acts as an antagonist at all opioid receptors, and its safety profile in opiate naïve patients has been well established. However, there is a small increase in the incidence of severe complications in opioid-dependent patients. These complications have been reported in approximately 2% of heroin users and include asystole, seizures, pulmonary edema, and acute withdrawal [35]. Therefore, the initial dose in intoxication should be small and titrated to effect, starting with 0.04–0.05 mg IV.

Anesthesia considerations in the opioid-abusing patient

- associated infections if the patient is an IV user (i.e., HIV, hepatitis, syphilis, endocarditis)
- potentially difficult IV access
- co-ingestion of other agents of abuse
- full stomach, decreased level of consciousness, respiratory depression
- potential for opiate "withdrawal"
- exaggerated postoperative pain
- need for larger doses of intraoperative and postoperative opiates. It is suggested that regular base opiate requirements should be continued both preoperatively and postoperatively [36].

Cannabinoids

The earliest recorded use of marijuana was in the fourth century in China, reaching Europe in AD 500. Marijuana is the most commonly used illicit drug in North America. In fact, at least 40% of the population over the age of 12 years has used the drug at least once.

Pharmacology and pathophysiology

Tetrahydrocannabinol (THC) binds to two specific cannabinoid-binding receptors, CB1 located throughout the brain and CB2 located in immune system tissues (splenic macrophages), peripheral nerve terminals, and the vas deferens. Binding at both receptors inhibits adenylyl cyclase and stimulates potassium channel conductance [37].

Between 10% and 35% of smoke containing THC is absorbed and peak plasma concentration occurs on average in eight minutes, with the onset of psychoactive effects within minutes. Ingestion of THC results in an unpredictable onset of psychoactive effects ranging from one to three hours.

THC is nearly completely metabolized in the liver by hepatic microsomal hydroxylation and oxidation via the P450 (CYP) system. Metabolites can be detected in the urine several days after use (THC-COOH average excretion half-life: 2–3 days, range: 0.9–9.8 days). Thus, in chronic users, detection may remain possible for up to several weeks.

Clinical effects

- Psychological effects are variable, but most commonly involve relaxation, giddiness or laughter, and increased appetite.
- Toxicity leads to decreased coordination, muscle strength, and hand steadiness, lethargy, sedation, postural hypotension, inability to concentrate, slurred speech, and slow reaction times.
- Users may also experience distrust, dysphoria, fear or panic, and transient psychotic episodes.
- Common cardiovascular changes are increases in heart rate (mean baseline increase from 66 to 89 beats/min) and decreased vascular resistance (these changes last for 2–3 h). Repeated ingestion may, however, result in decreased heart rate and blood pressure [38].
- Inhalation or ingestion produces decreased airway resistance and increased airway conductance in both normal patients and asthmatics.
- Ocular effects include conjunctival injection and decreased intraocular pressure.

Management and anesthesia considerations

- Agitation, anxiety, and transient psychotic episodes may be treated with benzodiazepines or antipsychotics.
- There are no specific antidotes.
- Co-ingestion or other illicit drug use should be identified so their effects can also be anticipated.
- It may be prudent to consider recent users as having a full stomach (decreased gastric emptying).
- If low or moderate doses of the drug have been consumed, an increase in sympathetic activity occurs, parasympathetic activity is reduced, and tachycardia with increased cardiac output is observed. Therefore, drugs that increase heart rate further should be avoided (e.g., ketamine, pancuronium, atropine, and epinephrine) [30].
- High doses result in inhibition of sympathetic activity but not of parasympathetic activity, and this leads to hypotension and bradycardia; this may cause profound myocardial depression with induction and initiation of potent inhalational agents.

- Increased incidence of life-threatening arrhythmias has not been reported; however, an increase in ectopic activity (supraventricular or ventricular) and ST-segment and T-wave changes can occur [39].
- Upper airway irritability may be increased and reports of oropharyngitis, acute upper airway edema, and obstruction have been reported in these patients undergoing GA [30].
- Cannabinoids are used in some countries as adjuncts for management of chronic pain.

Amphetamines

Amphetamine abuse was recognized as early as 1936, with "designer" amphetamines surfacing in the 1980s, the most well-known examples being MDMA (methylenedioxy-methamphetamine or "ecstasy") and MDEA (3,4-methylenedioxyethamphetamine).

Pharmacology

The primary mechanism of action of amphetamines is release of catecholamines from presynaptic terminals (particularly norepinephrine and dopamine). Binding affinity for select neurotransmitters largely determines pharmacological effects, that is, MDMA has high affinity for serotonin transporters, resulting in primarily serotonergic effects [40]. Higher levels of norepinephrine at the locus ceruleus in the brain results in increased alertness, and anorectic and locomotor stimulation. Increased levels of dopamine in the CNS mediates the stereotypical compulsive repetitive behaviors displayed by users. The effects of serotonin and dopamine on the mesolimbic system are responsible for altering perception and causing psychotic behavior.

As amphetamines are relatively lipophilic, they cross the blood–brain barrier readily. Elimination is via multiple pathways, including hepatic transformation and renal excretion.

Toxicity

- Clinical effects are similar to cocaine; however, duration of effects tends to be longer (up to 24 h).
- Amphetamines are, however, less likely to result in seizures, dysrhythmias, and myocardial ischemia than cocaine [41].
- Psychosis is more common.
- Patients who present to hospital are often anxious, volatile, aggressive, have visual and tactile hallucinations, and may progress to life-threatening agitation.
- Sympathetic findings include mydriasis, diaphoresis, hyperthermia, tachycardia, hypertension, vasospasm; severe complications include MI, aortic dissection, ischemic colitis, acute lung injury, and intracranial hemorrhage. Ecstasy use may present with hyperthermia as a predominant feature. Deaths from ecstasy may be idiosyncratic with fatal reactions claimed to occur on first use. Severe dehydration is also a feature in some reports.
- High levels of muscular activity and hyperthermia may result in metabolic acidosis, rhabdomyolysis, acute renal failure (acute tubular necrosis), and coagulopathy; multi-organ failure may then follow. Necrotizing vasculitis has also been associated with amphetamine use.
- Cardiomyopathy has been described as a complication of acute and chronic use.

- Death is most commonly secondary to hyperthermia, dysrhythmias, and intracerebral hemorrhage.
- Chronic use of MDMA in animals has been reported to produce irreversible destruction of neurons effected by dopamine and serotonin transporters (possibly by generation of toxic oxygen free radicals).
- Co-ingestion of other agents of abuse should also be considered.

Management and anesthesia considerations

- Hyperthermia requires interventions to achieve cooling. Dantrolene anecdotally has been used in ecstasy poisoning [42].
- Restraints may be required for agitated patients in order to protect from self-harm or harm to staff.
- Sedation with benzodiazepines or other medication should be instituted early to decrease heat generation and rhabdomyolysis with rapid titration until the patient is calm (antipsychotics such as haloperidol are recommended to treat delirium).
- One may consider intubation and muscle relaxation in severe cases.
- Blood and urine investigations for co-ingestion agents, glucose, blood urea nitrogen (BUN), creatinine (Cr), creatine phosphokinase (CPK), coagulation screen, blood gas, and electrolytes should be done.
- Patients may be significantly dehydrated and hyponatremia should be considered due to an increase in antidiuretic hormone (ADH) secretion [43].
- Urine output should be maintained at 1–2 mL/kg/h/.
- Patients with acute renal failure may require urgent hemodialysis secondary to hyperkalemia and acidosis.
- A full stomach must be considered if surgery is required.
- With GA, the risk of autonomic dysregulation is high – this may result in wide swings in blood pressure and tachycardia [30].
- Extreme caution should be used with administration of drugs such as ephedrine and ketamine, as these patients will exhibit exaggerated responses [30].
- In patients with a history of MDMA-induced hyperthermia, succinylcholine should not be used and avoidance of potent volatile agents should be considered [30].
- In MDMA users, drugs metabolized by the liver and eliminated by the kidneys will have a prolonged effect (possibly secondary to fatty infiltration of the liver and acute renal failure).
- Chronic methamphetamine users have decreased anesthetic requirements if not intoxicated (due to decreased levels of catecholamines in the CNS).

"Bath salts"

Synthetic cathinones have now become popular drugs of abuse in many regions. Cathinone is a naturally occurring β-ketone amphetamine analog found in the leaves of the *Catha edulis* plant; synthetic cathinones are derivatives of this compound. Commonly abused drugs include mephedrone, methedrone, and methylenedioxypyrovalerone (MDPV), but drug dealers will often turn to other cathinone derivatives, of which there are many, to avoid substance control laws. These drugs possess amphetamine-like properties, dopamine reuptake inhibition, and the ability to modulate serotonin [44]. They are often used along with alcohol and other drugs of abuse.

Animal studies have shown MDPV to be at least 10 times more potent than cocaine at producing locomotor activation, tachycardia, and hypertension [45].

Two components of bath salts, mephedrone and MDPV, produce opposite effects at human dopamine transporters that are comparable with methamphetamine and cocaine, respectively. In a recent study, mephedrone was shown to be nearly as potent as methamphetamine. MDPV was much more potent than cocaine and its effect was longer lasting [46].

Toxicity

- Agitation is very common, ranging from 28%–66%; other neurological side effects include dizziness, headache, memory loss, tremor, and seizures. Users may also complain of auditory and visual hallucinations, depression, dysphoria, euphoria, increased or decreased energy, increased and decreased concentration, panic, paranoia, perceptual distortions, and restlessness [41].
- Cardiovascular side effects include palpitations, shortness of breath, and chest pain.
- Gastrointestinal side effects include abdominal pain, anorexia, nausea, and vomiting.
- Other side effects include shortness of breath, nose bleeds, myoclonus, tinnitus, and blurry vision.
- Overdose may result in severe rhabdomyolysis with delayed development of acute compartment syndrome [47].
- Patients with fatal overdoses have often had symptoms similar to sympathomimetic toxicity, including metabolic acidosis, rhabdomyolysis, acute renal failure, and disseminated intravascular coagulation.

Management and anesthesia considerations

- Treatment of toxicity is largely supportive; benzodiazepines may be used to help treat agitation, tachycardia, hypertension, or seizures.
- Cooling should be instituted for hyperthermia.
- Antipsychotics have been used to treat agitation and psychosis, but there is reason to use some antipsychotics with caution due to their ability to lower seizure threshold (consider using haloperidol or risperidone; avoid using chlorpromazine and clozapine).
- Laboratory investigations: blood and urine for co-ingestions, electrolytes, BUN, Cr, CPK, glucose, blood gas, lactate, and coagulation screen.
- Patients may need significant rehydration and urine output should be maintained.
- Patients should likely be considered a full stomach if urgent surgery is required.
- Caution should be used with administration of drugs such as ephedrine and ketamine, as exaggerated responses may occur.
- Avoid tramadol, serotonin, and norepinephrine reuptake inhibitors.

References

1. Woehlck HJ, Connolly LA, Cinquegrani MP, et al. Acute smoking increases ST depression in humans during general anaesthesia. *Anesth Analg* 1999; **89**: 856–60.
2. Lightwood JM, Glantz SA. Short-term economic and health benefits of smoking cessation: myocardial infarction and stroke. *Circulation* 1997; **96**: 1086–97.
3. Benowitz NL, Gourlay SG. Cardiovascular toxicity of nicotine: implications for nicotine replacement therapy. *J Am Coll Cardiol* 1997; **29**: 1422–31.
4. Warner MA, Divertie MB, Tinker JH. Preoperative cessation of smoking and

pulmonary complications in coronary artery bypass patients. *Anesthesiology* 1984; **60**: 380–3.

5. Wong J, Lam DP, Abrishami A, et al. Short-term preoperative smoking cessation and postoperative complications: a systematic review and meta-analysis. *Can J Anesth* 2012; **59**: 268–79.
6. Møller AM, Pedersen T, Villebro N, et al. A study of the impact of long-term tobacco smoking on postoperative intensive care admission. *Anaesthesia* 2003; **58**: 55–9.
7. Wild MR, Gornall CB, Griffiths DE. Maintenance of anaesthesia with sevoflurane or isoflurane effects on adverse airway events in smokers. *Anaesthesia* 2004; **59**: 891–3.
8. Chimbira W, Sweeney BP. The effect of smoking on postoperative nausea and vomiting. *Anaesthesia* 2000; **55**: 540–4.
9. Kwiatkowski TC, Hanley EN Jr, Ramp WK. Cigarette smoking and its orthopedic consequences. *Am J Orthop* 1996; **25**: 590–7.
10. Sorensen LT, Karlsmark T, Gottrup F. Abstinence from smoking reduces incisional wound infection. A randomized controlled trial. *Ann Surgery* 2003; **238**: 1–5.
11. Warner DO. Helping surgical patients quit smoking: why, when and how. *Anesth Analg* 2005; **101**: 481–7.
12. Wong J, Abrishami A, Yang Y, et al. A perioperative smoking cessation intervention with varenicline: a double-blind, randomized, placebo-controlled trial. *Anesthesiology* 2012; **117**: 755–64.
13. Lee SM, Landry J, Jones PM, et al. The effectiveness of a perioperative smoking cessation program: a randomized clinical trial. *Anesth Analg* 2013; **117**: 605–13.
14. Warner DO, Patten CA, Ames SC, et al. Smoking behavior and perceived stress in cigarette smokers undergoing elective surgery. *Anesthesiology* 2004; **100**: 1125–7.
15. Mayo-Smith MF. Pharmacological management of alcohol withdrawal. A meta-analysis and evidence-based practice guideline. American Society of Addiction Medicine Working Group on Pharmacological Management of Alcohol Withdrawal. *JAMA* 1997; **278**: 144–51.
16. Dobrydnjov I, Axelsson K, Berggren L, et al. Intrathecal and oral clonidine as prophylaxis for postoperative alcohol withdrawal syndrome: a randomized double-blinded study. *Anesth Analg* 2004; **98**: 738–44.
17. Tønnesen H, Rosenberg J, Nielsen HJ, et al. Effect of preoperative abstinence on poor postoperative outcome in alcohol misusers: randomised controlled trial. *BMJ* 1999; **318**: 1311–16.
18. Tønnesen H, Nielsen PR, Lauritzen JB, et al. Smoking and alcohol intervention before surgery: evidence for best practice. *Br J Anaesth* 2009; **102**: 297–306.
19. Boghdadi MS, Henning RJ. Cocaine: pathophysiology and clinical toxicology. *Heart Lung* 1997; **26**: 466–83.
20. Lange RA, Hillis LD. Cardiovascular complications of cocaine use. *N Engl J Med* 2001; **345**: 351–8.
21. Karch SB. Cocaine cardiovascular toxicity. *South Med J* 2005; **98**: 794–9.
22. Frishman WH, Del Vecchio A, Sanal S, et al. Cardiovascular manifestations of substance abuse part 1: cocaine. *Heart Dis* 2003; **5**: 187–201.
23. Daras M. Neurologic complications of cocaine. *NIDA Res Monogr* 1996; **163**: 43–65.
24. Haim DY, Lippmann ML, Goldberg SK, et al. The pulmonary complications of crack cocaine. A comprehensive review. *Chest* 1995; **107**: 233–40.
25. Laposata EA, Mayo GL. A review of pulmonary pathology and mechanisms associated with inhalation of freebase cocaine ("crack"). *Am J Forensic Med Pathol* 1993; **14**: 1–9.
26. Shanti CM, Lucas CE. Cocaine and the critical care challenge. *Crit Care Med* 2003; **31**: 1851–9.
27. Crowe AV, Howse M, Bell GM, et al. Substance abuse and the kidney. *Quant J Med* 2000; **93**: 147–52.

28. Derlet RW, Albertson TE. Potentiation of cocaine toxicity with calcium channel blockers. *Am J Emerg Med* 1989; 7: 464–8.
29. Jatlow P, Barash PG, Van Dyke C, et al. Cocaine and succinylcholine sensitivity: a new caution. *Anesth Analg* 1979; **58**: 235–8.
30. Hernandez M, Birnbach DJ, Van Zundert AA. Anaesthetic management of the illicit-substance-using patient. *Curr Opin Anaesthesiol* 2005; **18**: 315–24.
31. Hill GE, Ogunnaike BO, Johnson ER. General anaesthesia for the cocaine abusing patient. Is it safe? *Br J Anaesth* 2006; **97**: 654–7.
32. Vagts DA, Boklage C, Galli C. Intraoperative ventricular fibrillation in a patient with chronic cocaine abuse – a case report. *Anaesthesiol Reanim* 2004; **29**: 19–24.
33. Cygan J, Trunsky M, Corbridge T. Inhaled heroin-induced status asthmaticus: five cases and review of the literature. *Chest* 2000; **117**: 272–5.
34. Stone PA, Macintyre PE, Jarvis DA. Norpethidine toxicity and patient controlled analgesia. *Br J Anaesth* 1993; **71**: 738–40.
35. Osterwalder JJ. Naloxone–for intoxications with intravenous heroin and heroin mixtures–harmless or hazardous? A prospective clinical study. *J Toxicol Clin Toxicol* 1996; **34**: 409–16.
36. Balasubramanian S, Hadi I. Perioperative pain management in patients with chronic pain. *CPD Anaesthesia* 2006; **8**: 109–13.
37. Onaivi ES, Leonard CM, Ishiguro H, et al. Endocannabinoids and cannabinoid receptor genetics. *Prog Neurobiol* 2002; **66**: 307–44.
38. Benowitz NL, Jones RT. Cardiovascular effects of prolonged delta-9-tetrahydrocannabinol ingestion. *Clin Pharmacol Ther* 1975; **18**: 278–97.
39. Kuckowski KM. Marijuana in pregnancy. *Ann Acad Med Singapore* 2004; **33**: 336–9.
40. Green AR, Mechan AO, Elliott JM, et al. The pharmacology and clinical pharmacology of 3,4-methylenedioxymethamphetamine (MDMA, "ecstasy"). *Pharmacol Rev* 2003; **55**: 463–508.
41. Zagnoni PG, Albano CZ. Psychostimulants and epilepsy. *Epilepsia* 2002; **43**: 28–31.
42. Watson JD, Ferguson C, Hinds CJ, et al. Exertional heat stroke induced by amphetamine analogues. Does dantrolene have a place? *Anaesthesia* 1993; **48**: 1057–60.
43. Wolff K, Tsapakis EM, Winstock AR, et al. Vasopressin and oxytocin secretion in response to the consumption of ecstasy in a clubbing population. *J Psychopharmacol* 2006; **20**: 400–10.
44. Prosser JM, Nelson LS. The toxicology of bath salts: a review of synthetic cathinones. *J Med Toxicol* 2012; **8**: 33–42.
45. Baumann MH, Partilla JS, Lehner KR, et al. Powerful cocaine-like actions of 3,4-methylenedioxypyrovalerone (MDPV), a principal constituent of psychoactive 'bath salts' products. *Neuropsychopharmacology* 2013; **38**: 552–62.
46. Cameron KN, Kolanos R, Solis E Jr, et al. Bath salts components mephedrone and methylenedioxypyrovalerone (MDPV) act synergistically at the human dopamine transporter. *Br J Pharmacol* 2013; **168**: 1750–7.
47. Levine M, Levitan R, Skolnik A. Compartment Syndrome after "bath salts" use: a case series. *Ann Emerg Med* 2013; **61**: 480–3.

Chapter 13

Intraoperative ventilatory management

R. Blank, L.R. Rochlen, and J.M. Blum

Rational and safe intraoperative ventilatory management depends on an understanding of the pathophysiology of the respiratory system subjected to general anesthesia (GA) and mechanical ventilation.

- Both normal and abnormal lungs will suffer alterations in gas exchange and mechanics under such artificial circumstances.
- In most cases, the anesthesia provider takes a patient without respiratory failure preoperatively, assumes total or partial control of ventilation intraoperatively, and aims to return the patient to comfortable spontaneous breathing postoperatively.
- There is, however, a subset of patients who enter the operating room (ORm) at heightened risk for serious postoperative pulmonary complications (PPCs) due to pre-existing or procedural risk factors.
- In recent years, clinical studies in the ORm have increasingly scrutinized the role of ventilator settings and strategies in the development and mitigation of postoperative lung injury in susceptible patients.

Respiratory pathophysiology – influences of general anesthesia and positive-pressure ventilation

The induction of GA and use of positive pressure invariably result in changes in pulmonary physiology, even in patients without co-existing pulmonary disease.

Atelectasis

- It is estimated that atelectasis in the most dependent portions of the lung occurs in approximately 90% of patients undergoing GA [1,2]. Atelectasis in itself can produce hypoxemia by means of increased intrapulmonary shunting, as well as lead to a decrease in lung compliance and inflammatory changes of the lung [3,4]. In addition, mechanical ventilation of a partially collapsed lung may redirect tidal volume to well-ventilated lung zones, causing regional hyperinflation and increased dead space that render overall ventilation less efficient.
- Atelectasis due to anesthesia is thought of primarily as collapse of alveoli at the acinar level, where respiratory gases are exchanged. Resting lung volume is reduced by 0.8–1.0 L when moving from upright to the supine position. An additional decrease

Anesthesia and Perioperative Care of the High-Risk Patient, Third edition, ed. Ian McConachie. Published by Cambridge University Press.

of 0.4–0.5 L is seen when anesthesia is induced [3]. These changes are present within five minutes after induction, as seen by computed tomography (CT) [2].

- Factors related to type of anesthetic used, type of surgery, and patient comorbidities modify the degree of atelectasis and the extent to which it can be prevented.
- Intraoperative atelectasis is present in patients undergoing GA both during spontaneous ventilation and following muscle paralysis accompanied by mechanical ventilation [3]. There is no difference in the amount of atelectasis between inhalational and intravenous anesthesia when muscle relaxation is used. However, if ketamine is used as the sole anesthetic without muscle relaxation, less atelectasis has been observed. Epidural analgesia as the sole anesthetic causes no or minimal atelectasis and no change in ventilation/perfusion matching [5].
- Positive fluid balance and transfusion of blood products will increase the degree of atelectasis formation.
- In the lateral decubitus position, atelectasis is seen more in the dependent lung compared to the non-dependent lung. Prone positioning may promote more even distribution of ventilation in anesthetized patients and overall less atelectasis.
- The type of surgery plays a role in frequency and degree of atelectasis. Atelectasis is more commonly seen in patients undergoing cardiac surgery with cardiopulmonary bypass, thoracic surgery with one-lung ventilation, vascular surgery, abdominal surgery, emergency surgery, and open procedures compared to laparoscopic procedures [2,6].
- Development of intraoperative atelectasis is independent of age and gender. Obesity and chronic restrictive pulmonary disease may predispose to atelectasis formation [2]. The amount of atelectasis that develops will also be more severe in the obese and chronic lung disease patient population.

Proposed mechanisms for the development of intraoperative atelectasis include:

Decreased functional residual capacity (FRC)

The decrease in FRC that occurs is multifactorial [2,4]. After induction of anesthesia, the relaxed diaphragm moves cephalad, resulting in increased pleural pressure, mainly in the dependent portions of the lungs. Muscle paralysis with the loss of intercostal muscle function and a decrease in transverse diameter of the thorax also contributes to decreased FRC. With this fall in FRC, lung compliance decreases and airway resistance increases, which promotes airway closure and further atelectasis [4].

- Decreases in FRC are evident within minutes of induction. Gas exchange continues to deteriorate progressively during abdominal and thoracic surgical procedures. FRC is not decreased further during peripheral surgery [7]. FRC is decreased 20%–25% in the supine position. Further decreases are seen when the patient is placed in the Trendelenburg position.
- Intraoperative lung collapse also occurs due to shift of central blood volume from the thorax to the abdomen, causing increased intra-abdominal pressure [2].
- Ventilatory dysfunction can extend into the postoperative period as a result of the combined effects of residual curarization, central respiratory depression, mechanical muscle injury from surgery/trauma, and pain [8].

Gas absorption

Oxygen absorption from alveoli into the circulation helps to explain intraoperative atelectasis [2]. When a high inspired oxygen concentration (FiO_2) is delivered, the alveolar partial pressure of oxygen is increased, promoting the uptake of oxygen from the alveoli to the capillaries at a rate that may exceed the inflow of fresh gas. Additionally, if gas uptake continues in the presence of airway closure, gas inflow is prevented and alveoli will collapse. These effects can be mitigated by combining oxygen with less soluble gases such as nitrogen and nitrous oxide.

Impairment of surfactant function

Pulmonary surfactant acts to reduce alveolar surface tension thereby stabilizing the alveoli and preventing collapse [2]. It is hypothesized that the stabilizing function of surfactant is diminished during anesthesia as a possible contributing cause of atelectasis.

The physiological changes incurred during GA may be unavoidable due to a combination of factors discussed here. However, there are mechanisms to prevent the severity of atelectasis that develops, thereby attempting to minimize complications.

- Prevention of atelectasis formation can begin prior to induction of GA. It is common practice to pre-oxygenate patients with 100% FiO_2. This may, however, contribute to absorption of oxygen and atelectasis formation as discussed earlier. Using a lower FiO_2, while reducing the margin of safety during the apneic period when securing the airway, may actually limit the amount of atelectasis formed [1]. Pre-oxygenation with less than 100% FiO_2 does not prevent the development of atelectasis completely; it will only delay the onset [4]. Use of continuous positive airway pressure (CPAP) before endotracheal intubation may provide sufficient positive pressure to the distal lung to avoid collapse. In healthy adults and children, ventilation with CPAP prior to intubation significantly reduces atelectasis formation compared to ventilation without CPAP [1]. In obese patients, higher levels of CPAP may be required. Regardless of induction strategy, strong consideration should be given to a recruitment maneuver (RM) followed by an appropriate positive end-expiratory pressure (PEEP) setting after the airway is secured (see later section on clinical strategies to improve respiratory outcomes).
- Similar arguments apply to emergence from anesthesia where use of less than 100% FiO_2 and CPAP may again have an important role [9]. Initiation of noninvasive positive pressure after extubation can be considered as a rescue therapy for hypoxemic patients [10], or as a pre-emptive strategy in patients at high-risk for PPCs such as obese patients or those after abdominal surgery [1]. Suctioning of the airways may promote atelectasis and should be minimized [4].

Postoperative pulmonary complications

Historically, studies of PPCs have focused on pneumonia and respiratory failure while variably including a variety of other conditions [11].

- For example, a recent large prospective study of PPCs defined seven possible complications – respiratory infection, respiratory failure, atelectasis, aspiration pneumonitis, bronchospasm, pleural effusion, and pneumothorax [12]. Using such broad definitions in a population-based surgical cohort, the authors identified at least one PPC in 5.0% of patients. Importantly, the presence of at least one PPC was associated with longer length of hospital stay and increased mortality. The strongest predictors of PPCs were intrathoracic surgery, preoperative oxygen saturation less than 90%, and operation duration of >3 hours.

- From this and other reports, additional identified patient risk factors include advanced age, American Society of Anesthesiologists (ASA) status, poor functional status, chronic obstructive pulmonary disease (COPD), congestive heart failure, recent respiratory infection, anemia, and hypoalbuminemia [11,12].
- Unfortunately, there are limited clinical data on effective strategies to reduce the burden of PPCs in general, with the strongest evidence supporting postoperative lung expansion modalities, selective nasogastric decompression, avoidance of long-acting neuromuscular blockers, and laparoscopic approaches when feasible [13].

Other recent studies have concentrated on the development of the less common but more severe entity of postoperative acute lung injury (ALI)/acute respiratory distress syndrome (ARDS) [14]. ALI/ARDS is a clinical syndrome of hypoxemic respiratory failure with multiple etiologies including sepsis, pneumonia, aspiration, trauma, multiple transfusions, and cardiopulmonary bypass – all of which are relevant in surgical patients. Despite advances in critical care and ventilator management, the mortality of ALI/ARDS remains high at approximately 30%–40%. Fortunately, the incidence of postoperative ALI/ARDS is low, measured at only 0.2% in a large retrospective study of more than 50 000 low-risk surgical procedures [15].

An appeal of ALI/ARDS as the outcome under scrutiny is ready identification of specific populations at heightened risk and as possible targets for intervention trials.

- By choosing a surgical cohort of 4366 patients undergoing major operations under GA for longer than three hours, the surgical lung injury prediction (SLIP) project documented an overall ALI/ARDS incidence of 2.6% with rates greater than 5% in complex thoracic and cardiac operations and as high as 22% after major aortic surgery [16].
- While type of surgery was by far the strongest predictor, other patient risk factors included alcohol abuse, COPD, gastroesophageal reflux disease, and diabetes mellitus.

Another advantage of a focus on ALI/ARDS is that there exists a knowledge base of pathophysiology and treatment/prevention strategies from the intensive care unit (ICU) environment. In particular, the phenomenon of ventilator-induced lung injury (VILI) has been a major topic of study [17].

- By the 1990s, increasing animal and human research implicated volutrauma (lung over-distention from high tidal volumes) and atelectrauma (cyclic opening and collapse of alveoli) as contributors to the development and perpetuation of lung injury in mechanically ventilated patients.
- The landmark ARMA (Acute Respiratory Distress Syndrome Management with Lower versus Higher Tidal Volume) trial showed a mortality benefit in patients with established ARDS, with the use of 6 mL/kg versus 12 mL/kg tidal volumes, based on predicted body weight (PBW) determined by gender and height [18].
- Subsequent ICU trials, both retrospective [19,20] and prospective [21], have identified high tidal volume as a risk factor for the development of ALI/ARDS in intubated patients without ALI/ARDS at the onset of mechanical ventilation.

- The optimal strategies for treating atelectasis and preventing atelectrauma in the ICU remain controversial, with multiple published methods for setting PEEP [22,23] with or without RMs [24].

Clinical strategies to improve respiratory outcomes

Ideal intraoperative ventilatory management should address the known phenomenon of atelectasis under GA and incorporate lung-protective strategies to decrease the incidence of PPCs including ALI/ARDS. Untreated atelectasis and associated atelectrauma may very well increase the risk of postoperative lung injury when other risk factors are present. Although these concerns are particularly relevant for high-risk patients and procedures, there is no reason not to apply sound ventilation principles to all patients under GA.

- One of the earliest and most influential reports of intraoperative atelectasis demonstrated resolution of both hypoxemia and low pulmonary compliance with periodic hyperinflations to airway pressures of 20 cm H_2O for 10 s, then 30 cm H_2O for 15 s, followed by 40 cm H_2O for 15 s [25]. These were meant to mimic the periodic deep breaths or sighs of normal breathing. Such hyperinflations, now known as RMs or vital capacity maneuvers, are readily achieved on anesthesia machines through manual bag ventilation with an adjustable pressure-limiting valve.
- Another strategy recommended by the same paper is the continuous use of large tidal volumes. Indeed, it is common practice among many anesthesia providers to apply supraphysiological tidal volumes (physiological tidal volumes are approximately 6 mL/kg PBW) and to omit PEEP entirely [26]. High tidal volumes indexed to PBW are particularly common in obese patients and women in whom there may be significant discrepancies between actual and predicted body weights.
- Such practices run against current intensive care standards, which emphasize limitation of tidal volumes (and plateau pressures) as well as judicious use of PEEP.
- The importance of the RM in reversing anesthesia-induced atelectasis has been verified in a series of radiographic and physiological studies. CT imaging of the lungs of healthy volunteers under GA showed that an airway pressure of 40 cm H_2O was required to eliminate visible atelectasis [27]. Even higher pressures may be necessary in patients with decreased chest wall compliance due to morbid obesity, ascites, pregnancy, abdominal compartment syndrome, or laparoscopic insufflation. Such atelectasis reversal is short-lived unless sufficient PEEP (e.g., at least 10 cm H_2O) is applied after the RM, especially in the presence of a high FiO_2 that promotes absorption atelectasis [28]. Recruitment has also been shown to minimize dead space and wasted ventilation, likely by reducing zones of regional over-distention that result during ventilation of partially collapsed pre-recruitment lung with conventional tidal volumes [1].
- More sophisticated alveolar recruitment strategies have been advocated that replace the static RM with a stepwise increase in airway pressures using pressure–control ventilation up to a PEEP of 20 cm H_2O and a peak inspiratory pressure (PIP) of 40 cm H_2O, followed by a decremental PEEP trail aiming to identify optimal oxygenation and compliance [1]. The advantages of such a method include more precise control of pressures and times, gradual conditioning of the patient's circulation to higher airway pressures, and early detection of hemodynamic compromise. Hypotension due to decreased venous return, most marked in hypovolemic patients, is a known complication of elevated intrathoracic pressure. There is also a risk of barotrauma with

all forms of RMs and they should be avoided in cases of known pneumothorax, bronchopleural fistula, or bullous disease. Elevated intracranial pressure (ICP) is also a relative contraindication to RMs and high levels of PEEP due to concerns that elevations in intrathoracic pressure may increase ICP further and decrease blood pressure, resulting in decreased cerebral perfusion.

While multiple studies have shown the benefit of alveolar recruitment on physiological parameters including oxygenation, ventilatory efficiency, and pulmonary compliance, it remains to be seen whether the routine use of intraoperative RMs will decrease PPCs.

- Interestingly, the strongest current evidence for PPC reduction is for postoperative lung expansion modalities such as incentive spirometry, deep breathing exercises, chest physical therapy, intermittent positive-pressure breathing, and CPAP, all of which likely work in part through minimization of atelectasis [13].
- Two recent randomized trials [29,30] of general surgery patients have compared a comprehensive protective ventilation strategy (moderate PEEP, prescribed RMs, and physiological tidal volumes) to conventional ventilation (no PEEP or RMs, slightly higher tidal volumes).
- The first, smaller trial included 56 open abdominal operations and found less radiographic atelectasis, improved oxygenation, better pulmonary function tests, and less suggestion of pulmonary infection postoperatively in the protective ventilation group, although length of hospital stay was not significantly reduced [29].
- The second, larger study of 400 major abdominal surgeries (mostly hepatobiliary and colorectal) found a significant decrease from 27.5% to 10.5% in the incidence of the primary outcome, a composite of pulmonary and extrapulmonary complications within seven days of surgery, in the protective ventilation group. Specifically, rates of atelectasis, pneumonia, need for postoperative mechanical ventilation, and sepsis were all higher in the non-protective group with a corresponding increased length of hospital stay [30].
- An additional large prospective multi-center randomized controlled trial (RCT) is ongoing with a comparison of protective ventilation (PEEP 12 cm H_2O and routine RMs) to conventional ventilation (PEEP 2 cm H_2O and no routine RMs), also in patients undergoing open abdominal surgery, with PPCs as the primary endpoint. [31].

The avoidance of excessive hyperinflation and volutrauma is the other side of lung-protective ventilation. While RMs intentionally create temporary hyperinflation in an effort to expand all collapsed lung fully, repetitive tidal hyperinflation is likely a major component of VILI.

- The best data that tidal volume limitation decreases risk of ALI/ARDS come from the ICU [19,20] and thoracic surgery procedures requiring one-lung ventilation [32,33].
- There have also been small positive trials involving esophagectomy patients [34], brain-dead lung donors [35], and cardiac surgery patients [36].
- However, retrospective cohort studies of postoperative ALI/ARDS have failed to identify intraoperative tidal volume as an independent risk factor [15,37,38]. Pressure-related parameters, specifically PIP [37] and drive pressure [15] (defined as PIP–PEEP), have emerged as modest predictors.
- A prospective multi-center observational study of intraoperative ventilatory management and PPCs has closed enrollment after recruiting over 10 000 patients,

and promises to shed more light on the relationship between intraoperative parameters and postoperative complications [39].

Conclusion

How should we ventilate patients in the ORm? General anesthesiology textbooks remain quiet on this fundamental and everyday question. Some important principles are:

- The common practice of using supraphysiological tidal volumes without PEEP will support oxygenation and not cause overt harm in the majority of patients, but carries the potential for volutrauma and atelectrauma in those at risk for postoperative lung injury due to other patient- and/or surgery-related risk factors.
- Atelectasis develops quickly and reliably after induction of anesthesia and can be minimized with RMs after induction and circuit disconnections, application of PEEP after RMs, minimization of FiO_2 when possible, and continuation of lung expansion modalities into the recovery room and postoperative ward.
- Although the data are not conclusive for surgical patients in general, use of physiological tidal volumes indexed to PBW with simultaneous avoidance of high airway pressures has proven beneficial for selected surgical populations. Moreover, there is no evidence that such lung-protective ventilator management confers clinical disadvantages to surgical patients.

References

1. Tusman G, Bohm SH. Prevention and reversal of lung collapse during the intra-operative period. *Best Pract Res Clin Anaesthesiol* 2010; **24**: 183–97.
2. Duggan M, Kavanagh BP. Pulmonary atelectasis: a pathogenic perioperative entity. *Anesthesiology* 2005; **102**: 838–54.
3. Hedenstierna G, Edmark L. The effects of anesthesia and muscle paralysis on the respiratory system. *Intensive Care Med* 2005; **31**: 1327–35.
4. Hedenstierna G. Oxygen and anesthesia: what lung do we deliver to the post-operative ward? *Acta Anaesthesiol Scand* 2012; **56**: 675–85.
5. Magnusson L, Spahn DR. New concepts of atelectasis during general anaesthesia. *Br J Anaesth* 2003; **91**: 61–72.
6. Tusman G, Bohm SH, Warner DO, et al. Atelectasis and perioperative pulmonary complications in high-risk patients. *Curr Opin Anaesthesiol* 2012; **25**: 1–10.
7. Wahba RW. Perioperative functional residual capacity. *Can J Anaesth* 1991; **38**: 384–400.
8. Sasaki N, Meyer MJ, Eikermann M. Postoperative respiratory muscle dysfunction: pathophysiology and preventive strategies. *Anesthesiology* 2013; **118**: 961–78.
9. Benoit Z, Wicky S, Fischer JF, et al. The effect of increased FIO(2) before tracheal extubation on postoperative atelectasis. *Anesth Analg* 2002; **95**: 1777–81.
10. Squadrone V, Coha M, Cerutti E, et al. Continuous positive airway pressure for treatment of postoperative hypoxemia: a randomized controlled trial. *JAMA* 2005; **293**: 589–95.
11. Smetana GW, Lawrence VA, Cornell JE. Preoperative pulmonary risk stratification for noncardiothoracic surgery: systematic review for the American College of Physicians. *Ann Intern Med* 2006; **144**: 581–95.
12. Canet J, Gallart L, Gomar C, et al. Prediction of postoperative pulmonary complications in a population-based surgical cohort. *Anesthesiology* 2010; **113**: 1338–50.
13. Lawrence VA, Cornell JE, Smetana GW. Strategies to reduce postoperative pulmonary complications after

noncardiothoracic surgery: systematic review for the American College of Physicians. *Ann Intern Med* 2006; **144**: 596–608.

14. Bernard GR, Artigas A, Brigham KL, et al. The American-European Consensus Conference on ARDS. Definitions, mechanisms, relevant outcomes, and clinical trial coordination. *Am J Respir Crit Care Med* 1994; **149**: 818–24.
15. Blum JM, Stentz MJ, Dechert R, et al. Preoperative and intraoperative predictors of postoperative acute respiratory distress syndrome in a general surgical population. *Anesthesiology* 2013; **118**: 19–29.
16. Kor DJ, Warner DO, Alsara A, et al. Derivation and diagnostic accuracy of the surgical lung injury prediction model. *Anesthesiology* 2011; **115**: 117–28.
17. Tremblay LN, Slutsky AS. Ventilator-induced lung injury: from the bench to the bedside. *Intensive Care Med* 2006; **32**: 24–33.
18. The Acute Respiratory Distress Syndrome Network. Ventilation with lower tidal volumes as compared with traditional tidal volumes for acute lung injury and the acute respiratory distress syndrome. *N Engl J Med* 2000; **342**: 1301–8.
19. Gajic O, Dara SI, Mendez JL, et al. Ventilator-associated lung injury in patients without acute lung injury at the onset of mechanical ventilation. *Crit Care Med* 2004; **32**: 1817–24.
20. Gajic O, Frutos-Vivar F, Esteban A, et al. Ventilator settings as a risk factor for acute respiratory distress syndrome in mechanically ventilated patients. *Intensive Care Med* 2005; **31**: 922–6.
21. Determann RM, Royakkers A, Wolthuis EK, et al. Ventilation with lower tidal volumes as compared with conventional tidal volumes for patients without acute lung injury: a preventive randomized controlled trial. *Crit Care* 2010; **14**: R1.
22. Talmor D, Sarge T, Malhotra A, et al. Mechanical ventilation guided by esophageal pressure in acute lung injury. *N Engl J Med* 2008; **359**: 2095–104.
23. Briel M, Meade M, Mercat A, et al. Higher vs lower positive end-expiratory pressure in patients with acute lung injury and acute respiratory distress syndrome: systematic review and meta-analysis. *JAMA* 2010; **303**: 865–73.
24. Fan E, Wilcox ME, Brower RG, et al. Recruitment maneuvers for acute lung injury: a systematic review. *Am J Resp Crit Care Med* 2008; **178**: 1156–63.
25. Bendixen HH, Hedley-Whyte J, Laver MB. Impaired oxygenation in surgical patients during general anesthesia with controlled ventilation. A concept of atelectasis. *N Engl J Med* 1963; **269**: 991–6.
26. Jaber S, Coisel Y, Chanques G, et al. A multicentre observational study of intra-operative ventilatory management during general anaesthesia: tidal volumes and relation to body weight. *Anaesthesia* 2012; **67**: 999–1008.
27. Rothen HU, Sporre B, Engberg G, et al. Re-expansion of atelectasis during general anaesthesia: a computed tomography study. *Br J Anaesth* 1993; **71**: 788–95.
28. Neumann P, Rothen HU, Berglund JE, et al. Positive end-expiratory pressure prevents atelectasis during general anaesthesia even in the presence of a high inspired oxygen concentration. *Acta Anaesthesiol Scand* 1999; **43**: 295–301.
29. Severgnini P, Selmo G, Lanza C, et al. Protective mechanical ventilation during general anesthesia for open abdominal surgery improves postoperative pulmonary function. *Anesthesiology* 2013; **118**: 1307–21.
30. Futier E, Constantin J-M, Paugam-Burtz C, et al. A trial of intraoperative low-tidal-volume ventilation in abdominal surgery. *N Engl J Med* 2013; **369**: 428–37.
31. Hemmes SN, Severgnini P, Jaber S, et al. Rationale and study design of PROVHILO – a worldwide multicenter randomized controlled trial on protective ventilation during general anesthesia for open abdominal surgery. *Trials* 2011; **12**: 111.
32. Licker M, Diaper J, Villiger Y, et al. Impact of intraoperative lung-protective

interventions in patients undergoing lung cancer surgery. *Crit Care* 2009; **13**: R41.

33. Yang M, Ahn HJ, Kim K, et al. Does a protective ventilation strategy reduce the risk of pulmonary complications after lung cancer surgery?: a randomized controlled trial. *Chest* 2011; **139**: 530–7.
34. Michelet P, D'Journo XB, Roch A, et al. Protective ventilation influences systemic inflammation after esophagectomy: a randomized controlled study. *Anesthesiology* 2006; **105**: 911–19.
35. Mascia L, Pasero D, Slutsky AS, et al. Effect of a lung protective strategy for organ donors on eligibility and availability of lungs for transplantation: a randomized controlled trial. *JAMA* 2010; **304**: 2620–7.
36. Sundar S, Novack V, Jervis K, et al. Influence of low tidal volume ventilation on time to extubation in cardiac surgical patients. *Anesthesiology* 2011; **114**: 1102–10.
37. Fernandez-Perez ER, Sprung J, Afessa B, et al. Intraoperative ventilator settings and acute lung injury after elective surgery: a nested case control study. *Thorax* 2009; **64**: 121–7.
38. Hughes CG, Weavind L, Banerjee A, et al. Intraoperative risk factors for acute respiratory distress syndrome in critically ill patients. *Anesth Analg* 2010; **111**: 464–7.
39. Hemmes SNT, de Abreu MG, Pelosi P, et al. ESA Clinical Trials Network 2012: Las Vegas – local assessment of ventilatory management during general anaesthesia for surgery and its effects on postoperative pulmonary complications: a prospective, observational, international, multicentre cohort study. *Eur J Anaesthesiol* 2013; **30**: 205–7.

Chapter 14

Analgesia for the high-risk patient

M. Pariser and C. Clarke

This chapter serves as a guide to evidence-based practices in the perioperative pain management of high-risk patients.

- The patient who is at high risk, either because of extensive surgery or poor physiological reserve, requires effective pain relief to avoid morbidity and even mortality.
- There are more potential limitations to certain drugs and regional techniques in the elderly and those with systemic illness.
- Multiple factors must be weighed by the Acute Pain Service (APS) in formulating an individual management plan.

The goals of this management should include, but are not limited to:

1. providing adequate postoperative pain control
2. reducing the incidence of side effects, including postoperative nausea and vomiting (PONV) and ileus
3. reducing the incidence of perioperative complications and morbidity
4. enabling early mobilization
5. minimizing emotional and physiological stress as a result of the procedure
6. reducing the evolution of acute pain to chronic pain
7. trying to achieve the above goals in a cost effective manner

The APS

A well-organized, multidisciplinary APS is essential to ensure optimal pain management is achieved in "high-risk" patients.

- A 2002 review of the literature concluded that an APS improves pain scores and patient satisfaction while significantly reducing cost, nausea, and patient morbidity [1].
- A 2010 cost-effectiveness analysis demonstrated that the increased cost of an APS service provides more effective pain management than conventional ward management [2].

The APS team, at most centers, now consists of at least one dedicated nurse and an anesthesia consultant. A pharmacist and/or a physical therapist may complement the team.

Anesthesia and Perioperative Care of the High-Risk Patient, Third edition, ed. Ian McConachie. Published by Cambridge University Press.

Pathophysiology of acute pain

The classic nociceptive system responsible for the transmission of pain sensations is well understood.

- Peripheral Aδ- and C-fibers sense the noxious stimuli of a pressure, cutting, thermal, or chemical nature and transmit them via an action potential in the axon to the dorsal horn of the spinal cord.
- At the dorsal horn, these signals are relayed to the ascending spinothalamic tract. The dorsal horn is more than a simple relay point; it acts as a signal modulator, enhancing or inhibiting signals from the periphery [3].
- From the thalamus, the signal is transferred to the somatosensory cortex, which is responsible for the localized perception of pain and activating either a withdrawal or non-movement response.

Clinical pain differs from the nociceptive model seen in the laboratory of the neurophysiologist. In order to appreciate the need for multimodal pain management in the perioperative period, one must understand the contributions of peripheral and central sensitization to the pain experience.

- Trauma releases inflammatory mediators from tissues, mast cells, macrophages, and lymphocytes.
- Vasodilation and increased capillary permeability augments the inflammatory response.
- The "sensitizing soup" of mediators promotes the depolarization of sympathetic and sensory nerve fibers. A stimulus that is normally perceived as non-painful, such as pressure, becomes painful. The excitation threshold of peripheral nociceptors is lowered causing stimuli to initiate a stronger pain response than occurs in the non-sensitized state [4].
- Central sensitization is the phenomenon of enhanced perception of peripheral stimuli via facilitated transmission at spinal cord synapses [5]. This amplified pain response after surgery appears to be mediated by up-regulation of prostaglandins and interleukins in the central nervous system [6]. The neurotransmitter, glutamate, plays a crucial role in sensitization at the dorsal horn by binding to the N-methyl-D-aspartate (NMDA) receptor and facilitating sodium conductance intracellularly [7].
- The involvement of NMDA receptors, prostaglandins, and calcium-permeable α-amino-3-hydroxy-5-methyl-4-isoxazolepropionic acid receptors in the development of central sensitization, explain why ketamine, non-steroidal anti-inflammatory drugs (NSAIDs) and gabapentin/pregabalin, are important pharmacological agents in treatment and prevention of post-surgical pain.
- Early identification and treatment of neuropathic pain, due to peripheral or central nervous system dysfunction, is important. Neuropathic pain is often described as "burning" or "shooting" and may be elicited by touch or pressure on the affected area. It is poorly responsive to opioids. Effective strategies for the prevention, management, and treatment of neuropathic pain remain largely unproven.

Pain assessment

Owing to cultural, social, and emotional influences, patients demonstrate broad variation in their reactions to pain, necessitating individualized assessment. This section focuses on effective tools for evaluating pain *intensity*.

- When assessing postoperative pain, it is important to differentiate between surgical incision pain and pre-existing pain from other causes.
- The preadmission consultation should identify high-risk patients and establish a pain management plan before the day of surgery, and determine whether inpatient or intensive care unit (ICU) admission will be required.
- The most practical tool for assessment of pain at the bedside is the Numerical Rating Scale (NRS). The patient is asked to rate their pain from 0–10; 0 represents no pain and 10 represents the worst imaginable pain. This scale consistently gives the most reproducible scores and is easy to apply [8].
- The Faces Pain Scale is a variation of the NRS containing a series of facial expressions ranging from happy to sad. Patients are asked to rate their pain by choosing the face they feel is most representative of their own pain. This will yield a score that depends on the number of faces the patient has to choose from. This scale has been shown to be effective in patients with cognitive impairment, particularly in the ICU setting [9].
- The Visual Analog Scale is a 10-cm line bordered by the phrase "no pain" and "worst imaginable pain." The patient is asked to place a mark on the line to demonstrate the intensity of her/his pain. This mark is measured, in mm, from 0, giving a pain score from 0–100. This pain scale has been demonstrated to give the most statistically robust data for research trials but can demonstrate user variability as great as 20%, with patients scoring different pain values without stating any difference in their perceived pain. This yields false results that may be determined as clinically significant [10].
- The key points in choosing a pain assessment tool are that it must be quick and easy to use, used regularly, repeated soon after any intervention, and applied both at rest and on movement.

From a clinical perspective, patients should comfortably be able to take a deep breath and cough. Changes in the *type* or *intensity* of the pain being experienced by the patient may indicate either failure of the analgesic technique, for example, an epidural catheter falling out or becoming disconnected, or possibly deterioration in the patient's condition, such as compartment syndrome.

Site of surgery/trauma

In assessing analgesia requirements for the high-risk patient, the site of surgery must be considered in conjunction with the patient's medical condition. Certain procedures have a higher incidence of severe acute pain, and potential for neuropathic postoperative pain. The list includes but is not limited to the following procedures: amputation, mastectomy, thoracotomy, coronary artery bypass grafting (CABG), cesarean section, and inguinal hernia repair [11]. Specific considerations for all procedures are beyond the scope of this chapter. Guidelines for specific procedures are available from many international anesthesia associations and can be readily accessed online (i.e., European PROSPECT Working Group [www.postoppain.org]).

Chest wall

Patients having chest surgery may experience severe postoperative pain that alters chest wall mechanics, making the patient vulnerable to atelectasis, ventilation/perfusion mismatching, hypoxemia, and infection [12].

Thoracic epidural analgesia (TEA) has long been the gold standard for pain control in this surgical population.

- A 2008 systematic review compared thoracic epidural, paravertebral, intrathecal, intercostal, and interpleural analgesic techniques to each other and to systemic opioid analgesia, in adult thoracotomy [13]. Continuous paravertebral block (PVB) was as effective as TEA with local anesthetic (LA) and had a reduced incidence of hypotension.

Choice of regional technique is dependent upon the clinical context, the competency of the anesthesia provider, and patient preference. Opioid adjuncts, including NSAIDs, gabapentin/pregabalin, and intravenous ketamine, may be useful.

Upper abdomen/lower abdomen

A significant proportion of patients in this category will present as emergency cases with the possibility of concomitant sepsis, dehydration, electrolyte imbalance, and other physiological deficits. Upper abdominal surgery adversely affects postoperative pulmonary function. A systematic review of the literature supports the ability of epidural analgesia to reduce perioperative pulmonary complications in the high-risk patient following abdominal surgery [14]. The majority of lower abdominal or pelvic surgery cases are elective (e.g., gynecologic) and tend to cope very well with patient-controlled analgesia (PCA) or traditional opioid dosing.

Peripheral sites

The main concern in those with peripheral limb surgery is impairment of mobility as this predisposes the patient to thromboembolic phenomenon as well as atelectasis [12]. The analgesic objectives should be to promote early mobilization. A multimodal analgesic regime, with consideration of regional anesthesia where appropriate, is optimal.

Pain in more than one location

This is a common problem following major trauma. Although epidural anesthesia (EA) may be indicated to treat pain from chest trauma or a laparotomy, it will not provide effective analgesia for concomitant limb fractures. One strategy is to use LA only in the epidural infusion and allow the patient to use a standard PCA to treat the pain not managed by the epidural. This strategy can also be used when epidural analgesia is inadequate due to a missed segment, or when low epidural placement misses the top end of a surgical wound.

Major considerations of pain management for coexisting disease

Coronary artery disease

- Uncontrolled pain initiates a sympathetic response increasing arterial pressure, heart rate, and myocardial contractility. In addition, this response may trigger hypercoagulability and vasospasm [15].
- All the factors can contribute to altering myocardial supply and demand ratios, resulting in ischemia or infarction [16].

The use of TEA has been well studied in cardiac disease. TEA seems to increase oxygen supply by increasing the diameter of coronary arteries while maintaining perfusion pressure [16]. This technique increases myocardial blood supply despite sympathetic stimulation [17].

There is little evidence that optimal pain control decreases the incidence of perioperative cardiac events. However, one clinical trial in patients undergoing revascularization demonstrated that superior pain control reduced the frequency and severity of ischemic events [18].

Ketamine decreases catecholamine reuptake, causing an increased sympathomimetic tone, increasing myocardial contractility at induction doses. No studies have examined the effect of ketamine on myocardial ischemia in the low doses used for pain management.

Patients with fixed cardiac output

In patients with severe aortic stenosis, severe mitral valve stenosis or hypertrophic obstructive cardiomyopathy, it may be necessary to obtain echocardiography before proceeding with neuraxial analgesia. Decreased afterload and venous return (preload) from the pharmacological sympathectomy may cause profound hypotension.

Respiratory system disease

Chronic obstructive pulmonary disease (COPD) and reactive airway disease are both prevalent in the surgical population.

- A large meta-analysis looked at various analgesic strategies to reduce postoperative respiratory complications. The studies reviewed looked at epidural opioid, epidural LA, epidural opioid with LA, thoracic versus lumbar insertion, intercostal nerve blocks, wound infiltration with LA and intrapleural LA. Outcomes assessed were clinically significant atelectasis, respiratory infection, and any pulmonary complication (e.g., hypoxia, need for ventilatory support).
- It was determined that patients undergoing abdominal and thoracic surgery had the greatest benefit from epidural analgesia with LA. Patients who received LA epidurals had higher PaO_2, and a lower incidence of atelectasis, pulmonary infections, and overall pulmonary complications [19].

This analgesic strategy should be considered when anesthetizing patients with COPD or asthma for thoracic procedures.

Despite studies demonstrating the efficacy of epidural analgesia in reducing perioperative pulmonary complications, there has been concern raised that it may actually be detrimental to the patient with obstructive pulmonary disease.

- Insertion of a high thoracic epidural block has been shown to initially reduce vital capacity and forced expiratory volume by 8%–10%, primarily as a result of the decreased function of the intercostal muscles [19].
- However, abdominal and thoracic surgery patients may have postoperative reductions in vital capacity and forced expiratory volume by as much as 60% due to diaphragmatic dysfunction.
- Later, protective effects compensate for small initial loss of lung volumes with epidural insertion [20].
- The theoretical concern of an increase in airway reactivity in sympathectomized patients does not appear to be borne out in reality as evidence shows that epidural analgesia

causes up to a 20% reduction in airway reactivity. This phenomenon appears to be explained mainly by the fact that intravenous LA blocks neutrally mediated airway constriction [21].

Ketamine is beneficial in the respiratory-compromised patient.

- It causes an increase in spontaneous respiratory rate.
- It has bronchodilatory effects.

These two qualities, in addition to its pain-relieving and opioid-sparing benefits, make it an excellent analgesic to consider in the patient with obstructive pulmonary disease.

The patient with reactive airway disease or nasal polyps may be more likely to manifest hypersensitivity to aspirin and other NSAIDs, even if s/he does not have a documented sensitivity.

Sleep apnea

Opioids contribute to obstruction in sleep apnea by preferential depression of upper airway muscle activity similar to the effect of sleep. It appears that both dose and route of administration are important for alteration of upper airway muscle function [22]. A 2007 study concluded that there is a dose-dependent relationship between opioids and obstructed/ataxic breathing [23]. Recent guidelines recommend a multimodal strategy to reduce the amount of opiate given, and limit the risk of respiratory depression [24].

Hepatic disease

Liver disease accounts for a significant proportion of hospitalized patients.

- The duration and effect of analgesics can be significantly affected secondary to alterations in pharmacodynamics and pharmacokinetics, depending on the degree of organ dysfunction.
- Patients with liver failure, particularly those with hepatic encephalopathy, are much more sensitive to the sedative effects of opioid analgesics.
- Finally, when planning the analgesic technique, one must be aware of the coagulation status of the patient leading to increased risk of an epidural hematoma.

The liver is the major site for biotransformation of essentially all opioids, with the exception of remifentanil, which is metabolized by ester hydrolysis in the plasma. In hepatic failure, remifentanil pharmacokinetics do not appear to change significantly [25]. If one chooses to administer opioids, it is important to titrate the dose specifically to the patient's level of pain and vital signs. Initial dosing should not occur on a standard scheduled regime until the duration of drug effect in that individual is determined.

Administration of codeine to patients with hepatic dysfunction is a poor choice. Codeine relies upon hepatic biotransformation into morphine. Thus, if metabolism of codeine is seriously impaired, the expected analgesic action will not occur.

The use of acetaminophen in patients with liver disease has been controversial in the past. However, a systematic review concluded that acetaminophen is safe to use in patients with chronic liver disease. Although the elimination of acetaminophen in hepatic dysfunction occurs more slowly than in patients without liver disease, repeated administration of the drug does not result in accumulation. Hepatotoxicity seems to be confined to those who misuse acetaminophen, intentionally or accidentally. The use of therapeutically recommended doses does not appear to increase hepatotoxicity in patients with chronic liver disease [26].

The literature carries conflicting reports as to whether or not NSAIDs contribute to acute hepatic toxicity or worsens chronic hepatic insufficiency. NSAIDs should be avoided in patients who are already taking potentially hepatotoxic drugs, or have autoimmune disease [27]. Patients with severe liver disease are also predisposed to gastrointestinal (GI) bleeds and hepatorenal syndrome, which could be exacerbated further by the use of NSAIDs. Treatment with NSAIDs in patients with liver disease should be undertaken only after a careful analysis of the risk–benefit ratio.

Renal disease

In selecting an analgesic regime for this patient population, it is important to consider which drugs possess active metabolites, that are renally excreted, or have a prolonged renal clearance.

- Alfentanil, sufentanil, remifentanil, fentanyl, ketamine, and acetaminophen may be safest for use in renal impairment, with no specific change in dosing required [28].
- In the presence of renal disease, one should not use NSAIDs as they have the potential to cause renal failure or worsen existing renal disease. This vulnerability is particularly enhanced during the use of angiotensin-converting enzyme (ACE) inhibitors, diuretics, and β-blockers [29].
- The active metabolite of meperidine, normeperidine, accumulates in renal insufficiency, causing central nervous system (CNS) excitatory symptoms of anxiety, agitation, hypereflexia, myoclonus, tremors, and seizures. Meperidine is clearly contraindicated in patients in renal failure.
- The active metabolite of morphine, morphine-6-glucuronide, is excreted renally. It is approximately ten times as potent as morphine. In renal insufficiency, it has the ability to accumulate and cause significant respiratory depression. Another opioid, hydromorphone or fentanyl, is preferable.

Other analgesics should have their doses adjusted according to the estimated renal clearance remaining.

Sepsis

Patients with sepsis are at risk of developing multi-organ dysfunction or failure. One must decrease the perception of pain while avoiding suppression, or deterioration, of the cardiovascular, respiratory, hepatic, or renal systems. Despite the proven benefits of neuraxial techniques in other classes of high-risk patients, this option is relatively contraindicated in sepsis due to the risk of CNS infection and the risk of coagulopathy. All systems must be assessed and considered carefully before implementing an analgesic strategy.

Obesity

Obese patients display a higher incidence of diabetes, renal failure, respiratory failure, hypertension, and coronary artery disease (CAD).

- Changes in tissue distribution produced by obesity can markedly affect the apparent volume of distribution of the anesthetic drugs. The loading dose of lipophilic opioids should be based on total body weight, but the maintenance doses should be reduced because of the higher sensitivity of the obese patient to the depressant effects of these agents [30].

- Other changes induced by obesity, which affect the pharmacokinetic profile of anesthetic drugs, include an absolute increase in total blood volume and cardiac output (CO), as well as alterations in plasma protein binding [31].
- Changes related to obesity can induce severe glomerular injury, leading to chronic renal disease [32]. In these cases, the estimation of creatinine clearance from standard formulae is inaccurate, and the dosing of renally excreted drugs must be adjusted according to the measured creatinine clearance [33].
- Although fatty infiltration of the liver is often seen in obese patients, hepatic metabolism of drugs may be preserved or even enhanced [32].

A multimodal approach, limiting the amount of opioid by using regional techniques and non-opioid adjuncts, is recommended.

Elderly patients

Pain in the elderly is often underdiagnosed and undertreated due to its myriad presentations. Inadequate pain management in the elderly can exacerbate emotional distress and depression, delirium, anxiety, and sleep disturbances, and delay mobilization. Compounding these concerns is the fact that they are subject to polypharmacy, and have a high prevalence of comorbidities.

The elderly patient demonstrates age-related reduction in organ function affecting pharmacokinetics and pharmacodynamics [34].

- Drugs display increased potency and prolonged duration of effect due to a reduced volume of distribution, decreased clearance, and reduction in protein binding [35].
- PCA appears to be the analgesic modality of choice in this patient population as it allows for individual tailoring of dosing to the patient. When compared with intramuscular narcotic administration, PCA has demonstrated superiority in that there is a lower incidence of confusion and pulmonary complications [36].

Multimodal analgesia is not contraindicated in elderly patients but should be implemented cautiously. Start low and go slow. More frequent pain assessment to monitor for treatment efficacy and side effects should be considered in this population [37].

Specific modalities

Multimodal analgesia

Multimodal analgesia is the use of two or more analgesic agents in combination to affect different targets in the pain pathway and minimize the use of opioids. One can optimize pain relief while minimizing potential side effects of any one specific treatment.

- A multimodal approach has been shown to produce better pain relief, to reduce the total amount of analgesics required, and to lower side effects.
- In addition to opioids, many other compounds have been added to the multimodal regimen including LA, acetaminophen, NSAIDs, ketamine, anticonvulsants, and atypical antipsychotics.

- Although there exist small studies to support the use of the individual adjuncts, the most significant results have been demonstrated with neuraxial and regional techniques, as well as ketamine and NSAIDs.

Intravenous PCA

The patient self-titrates an opioid, most commonly morphine, in small doses, generally 1–2 mg, using a patient request button. Each time a dose is administered, the system "locks out" for a set period during which time the request button is ineffective, a feature integral to patient safety. Subsequent requests, after each lockout will result in further doses.

- This method is excellent for maintaining analgesia once achieved.
- Pre-loading of the patient via the intravenous (IV) or intramuscular (IM) routes is mandatory to the success of the technique, as using the button alone can take hours to achieve a steady serum level of analgesic drug.
- The patient must have the mental and physical capabilities to understand the concept and to press the button.
- A recent Cochrane review demonstrated that PCA yields greater patient satisfaction and lower pain scores while showing a higher rate of opioid consumption and pruritis when compared to traditional staff-administered dosing. The PCA group had a similar incidence of other adverse events [38].

Individuals vary widely in their metabolism of opioids and serum levels required for analgesia. This technique offers the potential to address inter-individual variability. PCA also provides for increased analgesia during periods where pain intensity is increased due to therapeutic interventions such as physical therapy, dressing changes, etc.

EA and patient-controlled epidural analgesia (PCEA)

The pros and cons of EA are much debated.

- When comparing EA of all types with PCA, superior postoperative analgesia is demonstrated with the epidural technique [39].
- A 2006 meta-analysis concluded that adding EA to a conventional anesthetic for thoracic and abdominal surgery results in a number of benefits including reduced time to extubation, need for re-intubation, ICU stay, pain scores, and opioid consumption [40].
- A 2012 Cochrane review further demonstrates the benefits of EA, stating that after abdominal aortic surgery, epidural LA decreases overall cardiac complications, myocardial infarctions (MIs), and gastric and renal complications when compared to systemic opioid analgesia [41].
- With the exception of this small high-risk subset of the surgical population, EA has failed to demonstrate a significant reduction in postoperative morbidity and mortality [42].
- EA has not been associated with improved outcomes in patients undergoing minimally invasive thoracic or abdominal procedures.

Alternatives to EA may provide analgesia with lower side-effect profiles; these will be discussed below. The role of regional anesthesia in preventing cancer recurrence is discussed in its own chapter.

Epidural opioids are effective when used in conjunction with LA.

- This synergism reduces the required dose and side-effects associated with either the LA or opioid alone [43].
- Infusion regimes vary, but usually incorporate mixtures of bupivacaine at a concentration of 0.0625%–0.15% combined with a lipid soluble opioid. These mixtures are infused at rates of up to 14 mL/h, depending upon the site of insertion.
- Insertion of the EA at an appropriate segmental level is important as spread of drugs within the epidural space is limited.
- In practice, hypotension due to autonomic blockade by the LA is a far bigger problem than respiratory depression. Lowering the dose of the opioid may be wise if respiratory depression is a significant patient risk factor.

The addition of non-opioid epidural adjuncts, including clonidine, ketamine, and magnesium, is beyond the scope of this chapter.

PCEA is a modification of EA. Similar opioid/local anesthetic mixtures tend to be used but with a lower background infusion rate.

- The main difference is that the patient is able to self-administer extra doses of the mixture to supplement analgesia if required. PCEA allows greater flexibility of dose and better patient response to increases in pain intensity such as during physical therapy.

A typical setting for PCEA would be 6 mL background infusion of bupivacaine 0.125% with hydromorphone: 10–20 ug/mL with 5 mL bolus permitted every 15 min.

There are always situations where EA is impossible or should be used with care. These include:

- patient refusal (absolute contraindication)
- infection at the site of insertion (absolute contraindication)
- anticoagulation (consider reversal if for elective surgery)
- fixed cardiac output states (e.g., aortic stenosis, hypertrophic obstructive cardiomyopathy)
- epidural blockade may precipitate profound cardiovascular collapse in these patients (use with care including full hemodynamic monitoring and ICU monitoring)

Paravertebral block

Continuous PVB involves placing a catheter percutaneously, or with surgical assistance close to intervertebral foramen, where nerves exit the spinal cord, causing nerve conduction blockade. Many methods have been described in the literature.

- Recent studies have demonstrated that it provides analgesia non-inferior to EA, with fewer side effects, including decreased rates of hypotension and decreased respiratory suppression [44].

Absence of protocols, non-standardization of catheter placement, and provider inexperience, may partially explain the slow adoption of this technique, which may be optimal in patients with significant cardiac and respiratory comorbidities.

Regional blocks are discussed further in a separate chapter.

Continuous peripheral nerve blocks

Continuous peripheral nerve blocks by infusion of LA through an indwelling catheter have been demonstrated to yield reduced pain scores and lower side effects compared to PCA or IM opioid regimes [45].

- A 2012 systematic review and meta-analysis demonstrated that continuous peripheral nerve blocks were superior to single shot nerve blocks, especially for aggressive early rehabilitation [46].
- Some single-shot blocks of the brachial plexus have a prolonged action, often extending into the first or even second postoperative day, and should be considered in patients where avoidance of opioids is desirable, but the resources for continuous blocks are not available.

It is worthwhile to note that a 2007 meta-analysis failed to demonstrate any reduction in morbidity and mortality with the use of peripheral nerve analgesia, compared to traditional analgesic techniques [47].

Wound catheters

Placing a catheter directly in the wound, for continuous or bolus administration of local anesthetic (with or without adjuncts), is a simple technique.

- A 2006 systematic review found that continuous wound catheters improve analgesia, reduce opioid use and side effects, and increase patient satisfaction [48].
- In contrast, a 2011 meta-analysis demonstrated that injection of LA through wound catheters did not reduce pain intensity, except at 48 hours in a subgroup of patients undergoing obstetric and gynecological surgery. The authors conceded that their findings should be interpreted with caution due to the heterogeneity of procedures among other factors [49].

Ongoing research into the concentration and volume of LA drugs, the risk of toxicity, the potential role of adjuncts, and procedure specific considerations, is required.

Wound infiltration

Wound infiltration involves the injection of long-acting LA (ropivicaine or bupivacaine), with or without adjuvant (ketorolac, an opioid like morphine, and epinephrine), into the surgical site at the time of surgery.

- A 1998 qualitative systematic review demonstrated that infiltration of the surgical incision provided clinically relevant pain relief, limited by the short duration of action of LA available [50].
- A 2012 review of wound infiltration analgesia in orthopedic patients undergoing total hip and knee arthroplasty found it provided analgesia superior to standard care [51]. A similar technique has been adopted as part of a multimodal approach to theses procedures at our center.

Drug delivery systems, using liposomal and microcapsule technology, may yield longer-acting LA formulations with significantly longer duration of analgesia at the surgical site [52].

Specific medications

Opioids

It is well known that all opioids may produce the same general side effects including respiratory depression, urinary retention, cough suppression, nausea, rigidity, pruritis, and sedation-related hypotension. This section will highlight distinct points to consider regarding specific opioids in the management of high-risk patients.

Morphine

Morphine has the potential for histamine release. In human studies, 10% of patients receiving morphine had increased levels of plasma histamine; these levels have been directly correlated with hypotension. One should avoid large bolus doses of morphine in the hemodynamically unstable patient. As mentioned previously, morphine should not be administered in renal failure, due to accumulation of the morphine-6 glucuronide metabolite.

Hydromorphone

Hydromorphone has a lower incidence of histamine release compared to morphine. It is a fast-acting opioid with five to eight times the potency of morphine. The most beneficial quality of hydromorphone is that, at usual postoperative dosing, its metabolites rarely cause concern.

Oxycodone

Oxycodone (6-deoxy-7,8-dihydro-14-hydroxy-3-O-methyl-6-oxomorphine) is a semi-synthetic opioid analgesic first synthesized and prescribed for clinical use in Germany in the early twentieth century. Its North American consumption increased following the release of immediate, controlled-release, and acetaminophen combinations in the mid-1990s. Controlled studies demonstrating its efficacy have been performed in postoperative pain, cancer pain, osteoarthritis-related pain, post-herpetic neuralgia, and diabetic neuropathy. Oxycodone has 60%–80% bioavailability, and less than 10% is excreted unchanged in urine. Oxycodone's pharmacokinetics are dependent on age, and hepatic and renal function [53]. Caution should be used prescribing to affected patient populations.

Codeine

Patients in hepatic failure may be unable to convert codeine to morphine, resulting in diminished analgesia from codeine. Administration of morphine, or a different opioid not dependent upon hepatic metabolism, is recommended in this population.

Meperidine

The most important consideration with meperidine is the possibility of the accumulation of the excitatory metabolite, normeperidine. Normeperidine has a long half-life of up to 40 hours. Thus, patients with renal impairment or those that have been receiving the drug over several days are at increased risk of seizures or agitation.

Fentanyl

Fentanyl and its analogs, sufentanil and alfentanil, have minimally active metabolites. They do not cause histamine release or direct myocardial depression. Fentanyl, in particular, has been demonstrated to be safe for use in PCA. Studies have demonstrated that fentanyl and morphine PCA have the same safety, side effect, and patient satisfaction profile [54].

Development of the patient-controlled fentanyl hydrochloride iontophoretic transdermal system (fentanyl ITS) uses an electric current to administer patient-controlled, pre-programed doses of fentanyl transdermally.

- A 2005 study demonstrated comparable pharmacokinetics with IV fentanyl [55].
- A 2007 comparison of fentanyl ITS with intravenous morphine PCA, using data from three active controlled trials (including 1941 patients), demonstrated that fentanyl ITS was non-inferior and had a similar adverse event and side effect profile [56].

Given the transdermal route, one should monitor for signs of redness, skin irritation, or breakdown at the site of administration.

Methadone

Methadone is a synthetic, long-acting opioid, developed in Germany in 1937, that is now commonly used for the treatment of chronic pain and opioid dependence. It has opioid agonist and NMDA receptor antagonist activity.

- A 2011 study demonstrated that a one-time administration of methadone (0.2 mg/kg), administered before skin incision for complex spine surgery, reduced pain scores and opiate consumption with comparable adverse effects [57].

Use of methadone may be limited in high-risk patients due to its long duration of action, variable pharmacokinetics, and hepatic metabolism.

Tramadol

Tramadol is an atypical opioid as it is only a weak μ-opioid agonist and exerts its primary action as a serotonin and noradrenaline reuptake inhibitor. Its analgesic activity is dependent on metabolism by cytochrome P-450 2D6 to its active form, o-demethyltramadol. Consequently, 5%–10% of patients that are slow-metabolizers receive less effect.

- Tramadol, at equianalgesic doses, appears to have a lower side effect profile than the other opioids. This includes a smaller effect on bowel motility, and less respiratory depression [58,59].

It has been available in several European countries since the 1970s where it has been used intravenously in trauma, labor, myocardial emergencies, intraoperatively, and postoperatively.

Tapentadol

Tapentadol (3-[(1R,2R)-3-(dimethylamino)-1-ethyl-2-methylpropyl]phenol hydrochloride) acts centrally, on ascending pain pathways, as a norepinephrine reuptake inhibitor and μ-opioid agonist [60]. It is indicated for the treatment of acute moderate-to-severe pain. Unlike tramadol (which requires metabolic activation by the cytochrome P-450), tapentadol is a non-racemic molecule, which does not require metabolism to its active form, and has no active metabolites.

- A 2009 study of patients undergoing bunionectomy demonstrated similar analgesic efficacy, but increased GI tolerance, of tapentadol compared to oxycodone [61].

Tapentadol should not be prescribed to individuals suspected of having conditions that may increase intracranial pressure or individuals with severe liver impairment.

Acetaminophen/paracetamol

Acetaminophen has been shown to be a useful adjunct to opioids in the management of postoperative pain. The analgesic effect occurs centrally by activating descending serotonergic pathways [62]. Paracetamol also acts peripherally to block pain impulse generation but its mechanism of action is not fully understood.

- A 2005 meta-analysis demonstrated an opioid-sparing effect of 20%, but no change in the incidence of opioid-related side effects [63].

Intravenous paracetamol has been available in European countries for over 20 years.

NSAIDs

NSAIDs posses opioid-sparing capabilities. Whether this contributes to a significant clinical difference in patient outcome remains open for debate.

- NSAIDs produce analgesia by inhibiting cyclooxygenase (COX), an enzyme that converts arachidonic acid into thromboxane and prostaglandins, important messengers in the inflammatory pathway.
- Non-selective NSAIDs inhibit both COX-1 and COX-2 enzymes and selective NSAIDs inhibit only COX-2.
- The anti-inflammatory properties are derived from COX-2 inhibition whereas the adverse GI and renal events are derived from COX-1 inhibition. The major side effects of non-selective NSAIDs include platelet inhibition, inhibition of renal function, and erosion of gastric mucosa.
- The chance of worsening renal failure appears significant for patients with renal disease, or on ACE inhibitors, as well as those patients that are volume depleted [29].
- The selective COX-2 inhibitors, although they do not have as high an incidence of GI complications or platelet inhibition, do have their own side effects including adverse renal and cardiac events. Prolonged use may predispose patients to an increased risk of thrombotic cardiovascular events [64]. Several COX-2 inhibitors have been withdrawn from the market due to concerns over cardiovascular side effects.

Combination paracetamol and NSAIDs

Previous recommendations advocated for the use of paracetamol and an NSAID together, as part of multimodal analgesia, were based on the absence of strong evidence.

- A 2010 systematic review, however, demonstrated that combining paracetamol with NSAIDs provides superior analgesia when compared to either drug used independently with no increase in side effects [65].

Ketamine

Ketamine is a non-competitive antagonist of the NMDA receptor that induces significant sedation and analgesia. Intraoperative subanesthetic doses have been demonstrated to possess opioid-sparing properties in addition to the ability to prevent central and peripheral sensitization from surgical interventions [66].

- A 2006 Cochrane review found that the addition of subanesthetic doses of ketamine reduced PCA opioid consumption in the first 24 hours, reduced the incidence of PONV, and showed minimal occurrence of adverse events (hallucinations, bad dreams) [67].
- A 2011 systematic review of intravenous ketamine administration, which included 70 studies involving 4701 patients, further demonstrated benefit for patients undergoing upper abdominal, thoracic, and major orthopedic surgery [68].
- A 2010 review of morphine/ketamine PCA concluded that the addition of ketamine to morphine in a 1:1 ratio was beneficial for patients undergoing thoracic surgery but was of limited benefit in patients undergoing abdominal and orthopedic procedures. Ketamine/morphine PCA was not compared to perioperative ketamine infusion [69].

Ketamine should not be used in patients with the potential to develop increased intracranial pressure.

Gabapentin and pregabalin

Both act via modulation of the α_2-δ subunit of voltage-gated calcium channels. Binding to the α_2-δ subunit results in attenuation of calcium flux into the neuron, which in turn inhibits the release of various pain-inducing neurotransmitters. Although they function at the same receptor, pregabalin achieves its efficacy at lower doses than gabapentin, and thus seems to have a lower side effect profile.

- Gabapentin and pregabalin have both been shown to be effective adjuncts to perioperative analgesia providing reductions in pain scores, opioid consumption, and opioid-related side effects [70].
- A 2011 systematic review demonstrated that perioperative administration of gabapentin and pregabalin may prevent chronic post-surgical pain; however, more trials are needed to confirm these findings [71].

Lidocaine

Intraoperative intravenous lidocaine infusions for the reduction of postoperative pain and opioid sparing have been mentioned in the literature since the 1960s. However, until recently, intravenous lidocaine had been primarily utilized for the treatment of chronic pain [72].

- The perioperative use of lidocaine has been featured in the literature demonstrating opioid sparing, decreased pain scores, and shortened hospital stays [73].
- The mechanism of action is postulated to be a combination of anti-inflammatory effects and antagonism of the NMDA receptor [74].
- A 2011 meta-analysis of perioperative lidocaine infusion use during thoracic, abdominal, and orthopedic surgeries, including 29 studies, demonstrated decreased time to first flatus, decreased time to first bowel movement, decreased nausea and vomiting, and decreased time to discharge when compared to the control groups for patients undergoing abdominal procedures [75].

Magnesium

The use of intravenous magnesium, administered as a bolus or continuously, has been reported to reduce opioid requirements and improve postoperative pain. The exact mechanism of action is unknown. It is postulated that it acts as an NMDA receptor antagonist and reduces the influx of sodium and calcium into neurons following noxious stimuli.

- A 2013 quantitative systemic review found that perioperative magnesium may decrease opioid consumption and pain scores [76].

Standardization of protocols to determine the optimal dose and regimen, bolus versus infusion, for magnesium use as part of a multimodal strategy is still required. Caution should be used in hypotensive patients.

Capsaicin

Capsaicin, 8-methyl-N-vanillyl-6-nonenamide, is an alkaloid derived from the seeds and stems of chilli peppers. It can be used in topical and injectable forms. It acts peripherally on the TRPV-1 (transient receptor potential cation channel subfamily V, member 1), a non-selective cation channel, found on unmyelinated C-fibers [77]. Activation of TRPV-1 receptors is thought to induce high intensity impulses and the release of proinflammatory peptides due to calcium influx into the neuron. Prolonged application of capsaicin, and activation of the receptor, decreases TRPV1 activity and C-fiber activation through desensitization.

- Topical capsaicin cream, usually combined with topical NSAIDs and opioid analgesics, has been used to treat acute injuries, as well as lower back pain, arthritic pain, and post-herpetic neuralgia [78].
- Opioid-sparing effects have been demonstrated in randomized controlled trials (RCTs), when the injectable form has been used for the treatment of postoperative pain following hernia repair, bunionectomy, and joint replacement [79].

Following its initial administration, capsaicin can produce an undesired burning sensation in its area of application. Injection should occur following general or regional anesthesia.

Cannabinoids

Cannabinoids produce analgesia by acting on the endogenous cannabinoid system at peripheral, spinal, and supraspinal sites. Specific description of these mechanisms is beyond the scope of this chapter. Cannabinoids have been used with modest benefit in patients suffering from various chronic pain conditions.

- A 2006 dose escalation study demonstrated that cannabinoids may have an opioid-sparing effect when administered as part of a multimodal strategy [80].
- In contrast, a 2006 Canadian study demonstrated no benefit from nabilone 2 mg, and increased pain scores in the nabilone group [81].

Despite animal models, their use remains controversial due to numerous political, cultural, and social considerations.

Selective serotonin and norepinephrine reuptake inhibitors

These medications are thought to affect the descending inhibitory pain pathways of the brain and spinal cord by increasing the amount of serotonin and norepinephrine available at the synapses. Their specific mechanism of action to modulate pain has not been elucidated. There are numerous studies detailing their effectiveness for the treatment of chronic pain. Recent studies of venlafaxine and duloxetine have demonstrated a potential role for these medications as part of a multimodal strategy to treat acute pain and prevent chronic pain.

- A 2010 study of patients undergoing total knee arthroplasty, demonstrated an opioid-sparing effect following the perioperative administration of two doses of duloxetine [82].
- A 2010 study of patients undergoing mastectomy, found venlafaxine to be non-inferior to gabapentin in the treatment of acute postoperative pain, and decreased the incidence of post-mastectomy pain, relative to gabapentin, at six months [83].

Further study is required to determine the role of these medications as part of multimodal strategies for acute pain management and chronic pain prevention.

Dexamethasone

Glucocorticoids are routinely utilized in the perioperative period to decrease inflammation and prevent PONV. Recent meta-analyses have concluded that steroids, as part of a multimodal strategy, may also have opioid-sparing effects in addition to known antiemetic properties.

- A 2013 systematic review and meta-analysis concluded that a single dose of dexamethasone improved pain scores, opioid requirement, and time in the post-anesthesia care unit (PACU), with no increase in adverse events (wound infection and wound healing) [84].

Caution should be exercised in administering glucocorticoids to patients at risk of adverse events including, but not limited to, hyperglycemia, steroid psychosis, systemic infection, and peptic ulcer disease.

α_2-adrenergic agonists

Clonidine and dexmedetomidine are centrally acting α_2-adrenergic agonists.

Clonidine has been used for many indications including hypertension, attention deficit hyperactivity disorder (ADHD), opiate withdrawal, and pain. Dexmedetomidine is commonly used as an infusion for procedural sedation in the operating room or in ICU. Oral clonidine has been associated with hypotension and bradycardia. The use of clonidine as an adjunct in neuraxial analgesia is beyond the scope of this chapter.

- A 2012 systematic review and meta-analysis found decreased opioid consumption, pain intensity, and incidence of PONV, with an increased incidence of postoperative bradycardia. Hypotension was limited to the group that was given clonidine [85].

Of note, a 2013 retrospective study comparing patients undergoing coronary artery bypass surgery, with and without valve replacement, who received dexmedetomidine infusion, showed a decrease in postoperative mortality up to one year, as well as a decreased incidence of postoperative complications and delirium [86].

Peripheral opioid μ-receptor antagonists

Prolonged-release naloxone, alvimopan, and naltrexone are opioid μ-receptor antagonists. They do not significantly reduce opiate-induced analgesia or cause withdrawal symptoms when administered orally or subcutaneously. These medications have been found to decrease opioid-induced bowel dysfunction and postoperative ileus [87].

- A 2012 meta-analysis of three double-blinded, randomized, controlled trials (including 1388 patients who underwent abdominal surgery), showed that alvimopan accelerated GI recovery and decreased patient discomfort [88].

Research into the efficacy and safety of these drugs is ongoing. The potential for incorporating these medications into a multimodal strategy to minimize perioperative bowel dysfunction, a side effect of opioid analgesia that delays hospital discharge, is a promising strategy.

Non-pharmacological interventions

Transcutaneous electrical nerve stimulation (TENS)

TENS involves the placement of electrodes over peripheral nerves close to the site of pain and applying electrical impulses to stimulate these nerves. It is thought to stimulate γ-aminobutyric acid (GABA) and opioid receptors at the spinal level and inhibit transmission of the pain signal.

- A 2008 trial of 60 open-heart surgery patients, demonstrated decreased pain and analgesic intake in the group randomized to TENS and medications, when compared to the sham TENS with medications, and medications only groups over the first postoperative 24 hours [89].
- A 2009 review concluded that TENS, as part of a multimodal treatment strategy, decreases pain intensity and opioid consumption while improving respiratory function and physical therapy tolerance, when used for treatment of post-thoracotomy pain [90].

Given the low incidence of side effects, incorporation of TENS into a multimodal strategy may be of benefit for those patients in whom drug interactions limit pharmacological options. Broader use may be limited by the cost of the unit itself and training of allied health professionals unfamiliar with the equipment.

Acupuncture

Acupuncture, a group of procedures that involve the placement of needles in the skin at precise pressure points, and using manual or electrical stimulation has been used for thousands of years in the practice of traditional Chinese medicine.

- A 2008 systematic review concluded that this technique may be beneficial for relieving postoperative pain and reducing opioid-associated side effects [91].

Integrating acupuncture into perioperative treatment may pose significant challenges.

Analgesia for the high-risk patient

Optimal pain management in the high-risk patient to reduce the stress response to surgery remains challenging. Studies are ongoing into multimodal combinations to reduce postoperative opioid consumption. In deciding upon a perioperative plan, one must account for patient-specific risk factors, procedure-specific risk factors, and perioperative pathophysiology. Development of evidence-based, procedure-specific recommendations is an ongoing process. Changes to individual clinical practice tend to occur more slowly than the rate of evidence. Minimally invasive surgical techniques, new medications, new medication delivery systems, and advances in regional anesthesia are promising new methods for achieving this goal. The adoption of multimodal analgesia should continue as part of a strategy to decrease time to mobilization and discharge from hospital. Long-term studies on persistent postoperative pain and quality of life are lacking. Appropriate perioperative care must extend beyond the immediate perioperative period. It should account for the long-term impact of treatment decisions for each patient undergoing surgery.

References

1. Werner M, Soholm L, Rotboll-Nielsen P, et al. Does an Acute Pain Service improve postoperative outcome? *Anesth Analg* 2002; **95**: 1361–72.
2. Lee A, Chan SK, Ping Chen P, et al. The costs and benefits of extending the role of the Acute Pain Service on clinical outcomes after major elective surgery. *Anesth Analg* 2010; **111**: 1042–50.
3. Willis WD, Westlund KN. Neuroanatomy of the pain system and of the pathways that modulate pain. *J Clin Neurophysiol* 1997; **14**: 2–31.
4. Woolf CJ, Ma Q. Nociceptors–noxious stimulus detectors. *Neuron* 2007; **55**: 353–64.
5. Woolf CJ, Salter MW. Neuronal plasticity: increasing the gain in pain. *Science* 2000; **288**: 1765–8.
6. Buvanendran A, Kroin JS, Berger RA, et al. Upregulation of prostaglandin E2 and interleukins in the central nervous system and peripheral tissue during and after surgery in humans. *Anesthesiology* 2006; **104**: 403–10.
7. Neugebauer V, Lucke T, Schailble HG. N-methyl-D-aspartate (NMDA) and non-NMDA antagoniststs block the hyperexcitability of dorsal horn neurons during development of acute arthritis in rat's knee joints. *J Neurophysiol* 1993; **70**: 1365–77.
8. Williamson A, Hoggart B. Pain: a review of three commonly used pain rating scales. *J Clin Nurs* 2005; **14**: 798–804.
9. Terai T, Yukioka H, Asada A. Pain evaluation in the intensive care unit: observer-reported faces scale compared with self-reported visual analog scale. *Reg Anesth Pain Med* 1998; **23**: 147–51.
10. Richardson J, Sabanathan S, Shah R. Post-thoracotomy spirometric lung function: the effect of analgesia. *J Cardiovasc Surg* 1999; **40**: 445–56.
11. Borsook D, Kussman BD, George E, et al. Surgically induced neuropathic pain: understanding the perioperative process. *Ann Surg* 2013; **257**: 403–12.
12. Liu SS, Wu CL. Effect of post-operative analgesia on major post-operative complications: a systematic update of the evidence. *Anesth Analg* 2007; **104**: 689–702.
13. Joshi GP, Bonnet F, Shah R, et al. A systematic review of randomized trials evaluating regional techniques for postthoracotomy analgesia. *Anesth Analg* 2008; **107**: 1026–40.
14. Lewis KS, Whipple JK, Michael KA, et al. Effect of analgesic treatment on the physiologic consequences of pain. *Am J Hosp Pharm* 1994; **15**: 1539–54.
15. Devereaux PJ, Goldman L, Cook DJ, et al. Perioperative cardiac events in patients undergoing non-cardiac surgery: a review of the magnitude of the problem, the pathophysiology of events and methods to estimate and communicate risk. *Can Med Assoc J* 2005; **173**: 727–34.
16. Warltier DC, Pagel PS, Kersten JR. Approaches to the prevention of perioperative myocardial ischemia. *Anesthesiology* 2000; **92**: 253–9.
17. Meissner A, Rolf N, Van Aken H. Thoracic epidurals and the patient with heart disease: benefits, risks and controversies. *Anesth Analg* 1997; **85**: 517–28.
18. Nygard E, Kofoed KF, Freiberg J, et al. Effects of high thoracic epidural analgesia on myocardial blood flow in patients with ischemic heart disease. *Circulation* 2005; **111**: 2165–70.

19. Ballantyne JC, Carr DB, deFerranti S, et al. The comparative effects of postoperative analgesic therapies on pulmonary outcome: cumulative meta-analyses of randomized controlled trials. *Anesth Analg* 1998; **86**: 598–612.

20. Groeben H, Schwalen A, Irsfeld S, et. al. High thoracic epidural anesthesia does not alter airway resistance and attenuates the response to an inhalational provocation test in patients with bronchial hyperreactivity. *Anesthesiology* 1994; **81**: 868–74.

21. Groeben H. Epidural anesthesia and pulmonary function. *J Anesth* 2006; **20**: 290–9.

22. Catley DM, Thornton C, Jordan C, et al. Pronounced, episodic oxygen desaturation in the postoperative period: its association with ventilatory pattern and analgesic regimen. *Anesthesiology* 1985; **63**: 20–8.

23. Walker JM, Farney RJ, Rhondeau SM, et al. Chronic opioid use is a risk factor for the development of central sleep apnea and ataxic breathing. *J Clin Sleep Med* 2007; **3**: 455–61.

24. Joshi GP, Ankichetty SP, Gan TJ, et al. Society for Ambulatory Anesthesia Consensus Statement on preoperative selection of adult patients with obstructive sleep apnea scheduled for ambulatory surgery. *Anesth Analg* 2012; **115**: 1060–8.

25. Dershwitz M, Hoke JF, Rosow CE, et al. Pharmacokinetics and pharmacodynamics of remifentanil in volunteer subjects with severe liver disease. *Anesthesiology* 1996; **84**: 812–20.

26. Benson GD, Koff RS, Tolman KG. The therapeutic use of acetaminophen in patients with liver disease. *Am J Ther* 2005; **12**: 133–41.

27. O'Connor N, Dargan PI, Jones AL. Hepatocellular damage from non-steroidal anti-inflammatory drugs. *QJM* 2003; **96**: 787–91.

28. Murphy EJ. Acute pain management pharmacology for the patient with concurrent renal or hepatic disease. *Anaesth Intensive Care* 2005; **33**: 311–22.

29. Whelton A. Nephrotoxicity of nonsteroidal anti-inflammatory drugs: physiologic foundations and implications. *Am J Med* 1999; **106**: 13S–24S.

30. Casati A, Putzu M. Anesthesia in the obese patient: pharmacokinetic considerations. *J Clin Anesth* 2005; **17**: 134–45.

31. Adams JP, Murphy PG. Obesity in anaesthesia and intensive care. *Br J Anaesthesiol* 2000; **85**: 91–108.

32. Henegar JR, Bigler SA, Henegar LK, et al. Functional and structural changes in the kidney in the early stages of obesity. *J Am Soc Nephrol* 2001; **12**: 1211–17.

33. Snider RD, Kruse JA, Bander JJ, et al. Accuracy of estimated creatinine clearance in obese patients with stable renal function in the intensive care unit. *Pharmacotherapy* 1995; **15**: 747–53.

34. Feely J, Coakley D. Altered pharmacodynamics in the elderly. *Clin Geriatr Med* 1990; **6**: 269–83.

35. Owen JA, Sitar DS, Berger L, et al. Age-related morphine kinetics. *Clin Pharmacol Ther* 1983; **34**: 364–8.

36. Egbert AM, Parks LH, Short LM, et al. Randomized trial of postoperative patient-controlled analgesia vs intramuscular narcotics in frail elderly men. *Arch Int Med* 1990; **150**: 1897–903.

37. Aubrun F. Postoperative analgesia in elderly patients. *Drugs Aging* 2013; **30**: 81–90.

38. Hudcova J, McNicol ED, Quah CS, et al. Patient controlled opioid analgesia versus conventional opioid analgesia for postoperative pain. *Cochrane Database Syst Rev* 2006; **4**: CD003348.

39. Wu C, Cohen S, Richman J, et al. Efficacy of postoperative patient-controlled and continuous infusion epidural analgesia versus intravenous patient-controlled analgesia with opioids: a meta-analysis. *Anesthesiology* 2005; **103**: 1079–88.

40. Guay J. The benefits of adding epidural analgesia to general anesthesia: a metaanalysis. *J Anesth* 2006; **20**: 335–40.

41. Nishimori M, Low JHS, Zheng H, et al. Epidural pain relief versus systemic opioid-based pain relief for abdominal aortic

surgery. *Cochrane Database Syst Rev* 2012; 7: CD005059.

42. Manion SC, Brennan TJ. Thoracic epidural analgesia and acute pain management. *Anesthesiology* 2011; **115**: 181–8.

43. Block BM, Liu SS, Rowlingson AJ, et al. Efficacy of postoperative epidural analgesia: a meta-analysis. *JAMA* 2003; **290**: 2455–63.

44. Wenk M, Shug SA. Perioperative pain management after thoracotomy. *Curr Opin Anaesthesiol* 2011; **24**: 8–12.

45. Richman JM, Liu SS, Courpas G, et al. Does continuous peripheral nerve block provide superior pain control to opioids? *Anesth Analg* 2006; **102**: 248–57.

46. Bingham AE, Fu R, Horn JL, et al. Continuous peripheral nerve block compared with single-injection peripheral nerve block: a systematic review and meta-analysis of randomized controlled trials. *Reg Anesth Pain Med* 2012; **37**: 583–94.

47. Bonnet F, Marret E. Postoperative pain management and outcome after surgery. *Best Pract Res Clin Anaesthesiol* 2007; **21**: 99–107.

48. Liu SS, Richman JM, Thirlby RC, et al. Efficacy of continuous wound catheters delivering local anesthetic for postoperative analgesia: a quantitative and qualitative systematic review of randomized controlled trials. *J Am Coll Surg* 2006; **203**: 914–32.

49. Gupta A, Favaios S, Perniola A, et al. A meta-analysis of the efficacy of wound catheters for post-operative pain management. *Acta Anaesthesiol Scand* 2011; **55**: 785–96.

50. Moiniche S, Mikkelsen S, Wetterslev J, et al. A qualitative systematic review of incisional local anaesthesia for postoperative pain relief after abdominal operations. *Br J Anaesth* 1998; **81**: 377–83.

51. McCarthy D, Iohom G. Local infiltration analgesia for postoperative pain control following total hip arthroplasty: a systematic review. *Anesthesiol Res Pract* 2012 [Epub ahead of print]

52. Whiteman A, Bajaj S, Hasan M. Novel techniques of local anaesthetic infiltration. Continuing Education in Anaesthesia. *Crit Care Pain* 2011: **11**: 167–71.

53. Liukas A, Kuusniemi K, Aantaa R, et al. Plasma concentrations of oral oxycodone are greatly increased in the elderly. *Clin Pharmacol Ther* 2008; **84**: 462–67.

54. Woodhouse A, Hobbes AF, Mather LE, et al. A comparison of morphine, pethidine and fentanyl in the postsurgical patient-controlled analgesia environment. *Pain* 1996; **64**: 115–21.

55. Sathyan G, Jaskowiak J, Evashenk M, et al. Characterisation of the pharmacokinetics of fentanyl HCl patient-controlled transdermal system (PCTS): effect of current magnitude and multiple-day dosing, and comparison with IV fentanyl administration. *Clin Pharmacokinet* 2005; **44**: 7–15.

56. Viscusi ER, Siccardi M, Damaraju CV, et al. The safety and efficacy of fentanyl iontophoretic transdermal system compared with morphine intravenous patient-controlled analgesia for postoperative pain management: an analysis of pooled data from three randomized, active-controlled clinical studies. *Anesth Analg* 2007; **105**: 1428–36.

57. Gottschalk A, Durieux ME, Nemergut EC. Intraoperative methadone improves postoperative pain control in patients undergoing complex spine surgery. *Anesth Analg* 2011; **112**: 218–23.

58. Wilder-Smith CH, Bettiga A. The analgesic tramadol has minimal effect on gastrointestinal motor function. *Br J Clin Pharmacol* 1997; **43**: 71–5.

59. Tarrkila P, Tuominen M, Lindgren L, et al. Comparison of respiratory effects of tramadol and pethidine. *Eur J Anaesthesiol* 1998; **15**: P64–8.

60. Tzschentke TM, Christoph T, Kögel B, et al. (-)-(1R,2R)-3-(3-dimethylamino-1-ethyl-2-methyl-propyl)-phenol hydrochloride (tapentadol HCl): a novel mu-opioid receptor agonist/norepinephrine reuptake inhibitor with broad-spectrum analgesic properties. *J Pharmacol Exp Ther* 2007; **323**: 265–76.

61. Stegmann JU, Weber H, Steup A, et al. The efficacy and tolerability of multiple-dose tapentadol immediate release for the relief of acute pain following orthopedic (bunionectomy) surgery. *Curr Med Res Opin* 2008; **24**: 3185–96.

62. Graham GG, Scott KF. Mechanism of action of paracetamol. *Am J Ther* 2005; **12**: 46–55.

63. Remy C, Marret E, Bonnet F. Effects of acetaminophen on morphine side-effects and consumption after major surgery: meta-analysis of randomized controlled trials. *Br J Anesth* 2005; **94**: 505–13.

64. Iezzi A, Ferri C, Mezzetti A, et al. COX-2 friend or foe? *Curr Pharmacol Design* 2007; **13**: 1715–21.

65. Ong CK, Seymour RA, Lirk P, et al. Combining paracetamol (acetaminophen) with nonsteroidal antiinflammatory drugs: a qualitative systematic review of analgesic efficacy for acute postoperative pain. *Anesth Analg* 2010; **110**: 1170–9.

66. DeKock MF, Lavand'homme PM. The clinical role of NMDA receptor antagonists for the treatment of postoperative pain. *Best Pract Res Clin Anaesthesiol* 2007; **21**: 85–98.

67. Bell RF, Dahl JB, Moore RA, et al. Perioperative ketamine for acute postoperative pain. *Cochrane Database Syst Rev* 2006; **1**: CD004603.

68. Laskowski K, Stirling A, McKay WP, et al. A systematic review of intravenous ketamine for postoperative analgesia. *Can J Anaesth* 2011; **58**: 911–23.

69. Carstensen M, Moller AM. Adding ketamine to morphine for intravenous patient-controlled analgesia for acute postoperative pain: a qualitative review of randomized trials. *Br J Anaesthesiol* 2010; **104**: 401–6.

70. Tiippana EM, Hamunen K, Kontinen VK. Do surgical patients benefit from perioperative gabapentin/pregabalin? A systematic review of efficacy and safety. *Anesth Analg* 2007; **104**: 1545–56.

71. Clarke H, Bonin RP, Orser BA, et al. The prevention of chronic postsurgical pain using gabapentin and pregabalin: a combined systematic review and meta-analysis. *Anesth Analg* 2012; **115**: 428–42.

72. Omote K. Intravenous lidocaine to treat postoperative pain management: novel strategy with a long-established drug. *Anesthesiology* 2007; **106**: 5–6.

73. Hollmann MW, Durieux ME. Local anaesthetics and the inflammatory response: a new therapeutic indication? *Anesthesiology* 2000; **93**: 858–75.

74. Sugimoto M, Uchida I, Mashimo T. Local anaesthetics have different mechanisms and sites of action at the recombinant N-methyl-D-aspartate (NMDA) receptors. *Br J Pharmacol* 2003; **138**: 876–82.

75. Vigneault L, Turgeon AF, Cote D, et al. Perioperative intravenous lidocaine infusion for postoperative pain control: a meta-analysis of randomized controlled trials. *Can J Anaesth* 2011; **58**: 22–37.

76. Albrecht E, Kirkham KR, Liu SS, et al. Peri-operative intravenous administration of magnesium sulphate and postoperative pain: a meta-analysis. *Anaesthesia* 2013; **68**: 79–90.

77. Kissin I. Vanilloid-induced conduction analgesia: selective, dose-dependant, long-lasting, with a low level of potential neurotoxicity. *Anesth Analg* 2008; **107**: 271–81.

78. Mason L, Moore RA, Derry S, et al. Systematic review of topical capsaicin for the treatment of chronic pain. *BMJ* 2004; **328**: 991–8.

79. Hartrick CT, Pestano C, Carlson N, et al. Capsaicin instillation for postoperative pain following total knee arthroplasty: a preliminary report of a randomized, double-blind, parallel-group, placebo-controlled, multicentre trial. *Clin Drug Invest* 2011; **31**: 877–82.

80. Holdcroft A, Maze M, Doré C, et al. A multicenter dose-escalation study of the analgesic and adverse effects of an oral cannabis extract (cannador) for postoperative pain management. *Anesthesiology* 2006; **104**: 1040–6.

81. Beaulieu P. Effects of nabilone, a synthetic cannabinoid, on postoperative pain. *Can J Anaesth* 2006; **53**: 769–75.

82. Ho KY, Tay W, Yeo MC, et al. Duloxetine reduces morphine requirements after knee replacement surgery. *Br J Anaesth* 2010; **105**: 371–6.

83. Amr YM, Yousef AA. Evaluation of efficacy of the perioperative administration of venlafaxine or gabapentin on acute and chronic postmastectomy pain. *Clin J Pain* 2010; **26**: 381–5.

84. Waldron NH, Jones CA, Gan TJ, et al. Impact of perioperative dexamethasone on postoperative analgesia and side-effects: systematic review and meta-analysis. *Br J Anaesth* 2013; **110**: 191–200.

85. Blaudszun G, Lysakowski, Elia N, et al. Effect of perioperative systemic α2 agonists on postoperative morphine consumption and pain intensity: systematic review and meta-analysis of randomized controlled trials. *Anesthesiology* 2012; **116**: 1312–22.

86. Ji F, Li Z, Nguyen H, et al. Perioperative dexmedetomidine improves outcomes of cardiac surgery. *Circulation* 2013; **127**: 1576–84.

87. Holzer P. Opioid antagonists for prevention and treatment of opioid-induced gastrointestinal effects. *Curr Opin Anaesthesiol* 2010; **23**: 616–22.

88. Vaughan-Shaw PG, Fecher IC, Harris S, et al. A meta-analysis of the effectiveness of the opioid receptor antagonist alvimopan in reducing hospital length of stay and time to gi recovery in patients enrolled in a standardized accelerated recovery program after abdominal surgery. *Dis Colon Rectum* 2012; **55**: 611–20.

89. Emmiler M, Solak O, Kocogullari C, et al. Control of acute postoperative pain by transcutaneous electrical nerve stimulation after open cardiac operations: a randomized placebo-controlled prospective study. *Heart Surg Forum* 2008; **11**: E300–3.

90. Freynet A, Falcoz PE. Is transcutaneous electrical nerve stimulation effective in relieving postoperative pain after thoracotomy? *Interact Cardiovasc Thorac Surg* 2010; **10**: 283–8.

91. Sun Y, Gan TJ, Dubose JW, et al. Acupuncture and related techniques for postoperative pain: a systematic review of randomized controlled trials. *Br J Anaesthesiol* 2008; **101**: 151–60.

Chapter 15

Regional anesthesia for the high-risk patient

J. Brookes and S. Dhir

Regional anesthesia and analgesia (RA) has many benefits for this population of patients, including provision of high quality analgesia, reduced requirements for opioids and non-steroidal anti-inflammatory drugs (NSAIDs), avoidance of general anesthesia (GA), and reduced autonomic system activation. However, these advantages must be balanced against potentially significant drawbacks such as hemodynamic instability, difficulty in assessing the extent of nerve block, and risks associated with motor block including patient falls.

Regional techniques may be used to either supplement or entirely replace GA, but even when used in combination with GA, advantages may be gained in terms of reduced postoperative pain, quicker recovery, and reduced incidence of nausea and vomiting.

The objective of this chapter is to describe the indications, limitations, and practical aspects of regional techniques in high-risk patients, based on current evidence. Complete descriptions of the relevant anatomy and doses and concentrations of local anesthetic (LA) drugs are beyond the scope of this chapter. Pediatric RA is not discussed.

Central neuraxial blocks

Potential physiological advantages of neuraxial analgesia include:

- Cardiovascular system – abolition of pain afferent signals lead to a reduction in the stress response, with a subsequent reduction in cardiac work and cardiac oxygen demand.
- Respiratory system – effective analgesia can improve respiratory dynamics, which may lead to increased functional residual capacity and arterial oxygenation.
- Gastrointestinal (GI) system – there may be a reduction in nausea and vomiting rates.
- Postoperative mobilization – effective analgesia can improve compliance with physical therapy.
- Cardiac output may be improved in patients with regurgitant cardiac valvular lesions due to a reduction in systemic vascular resistance.

There are also potential disadvantages:

- Sympatholysis can reduce blood pressure due to vasodilation and reduced cardiac output secondary to sympathetic blockade. This may reduce organ perfusion in pressure dependent regions.

Anesthesia and Perioperative Care of the High-Risk Patient, Third edition, ed. Ian McConachie. Published by Cambridge University Press.

- Decrease in systemic vascular resistance due to sympathetic block may be particularly problematic in patients with fixed cardiac output states such as mitral and aortic stenosis.
- Too dense a block may result in undesirable motor blockade, which can impair the ability to mobilize, and increase the risk of falls.

Neuraxial analgesia has been shown to be superior when compared to opioid-based techniques, including those based on patient controlled analgesia [1]. Techniques that allow its use on frail patients therefore are desirable:

- Unpredictable block height and resultant hemodynamic instability secondary to single shot blocks can be minimized by using continuous catheter-based techniques, which allow careful titration of the extent of block.
- Extended spinal anesthesia using a microcatheter as a primary method of anesthesia for colorectal surgery in high-risk patients in whom GA would have been associated with higher morbidity and mortality has also been used with success [2].
- RA alone (spinal or epidural) has been shown to be a feasible and safe option for abdominal surgery in selected high-risk patients with severe pulmonary impairment [3].

Intensive care unit (ICU) patients can also benefit from regional analgesia. Epidural analgesia (EA) is the technique most often used in this setting. Mortality reduction has not been shown, but the technique eases management and improves patient comfort in the ICU in patients with chest trauma, thoracic and abdominal surgeries, major orthopedic surgery, acute pancreatitis, paralytic ileus, cardiac surgery, and intractable angina pain [4]. Particular points to consider in this setting are:

- altered conscious level will affect the ability of the patient to consent
- safety of epidural insertion in the sedated patient, which is controversial [5]
- likely difficult in optimal positioning of the patient if EA is sited preoperatively
- difficulty in neurological assessment of the sedated patient, and potential for delayed recognition of vertebral canal hematoma or abscess
- challenges to aseptic technique and increased infection risk when siting catheters in a non-operative environment
- increased risk of hematoma in patients receiving prophylactic anticoagulation or suffering from a coagulopathy
- block-related hemodynamic changes in a patient with reduced physiological reserve

Truncal blocks

Thoracic paravertebral block (PVB)

PVB has been shown to be effective for both abdominal [6] and thoracic [7,8] surgery with reduced rates of hypotension, urinary retention, pulmonary complications, and failure compared to epidural block.

- PVB also has the advantages of avoiding needling the neuraxis, particularly relevant in the presence of coagulopathy or spinal abnormalities.
- Use of ultrasound (US) brings the advantages of identifying the location and depth of the epidural space, rather than relying on blind needle advancement and loss of resistance alone [9].

Transversus abdominis plane block (TAPB)

Originally described as a single-shot injection in the triangle of Petit, TAPB is now commonly performed under US guidance, and has been shown to provide effective analgesia following cesarean section [10] and several abdominal procedures [11]. It has also been shown to be feasible to place catheters in the subcostal region [12], bringing the promise of effective analgesia for upper abdominal surgery.

Multiple catheter techniques carry the potential to provide an alternative to EA but no published studies have demonstrated this to date.

Peripheral nerve blocks for upper limb surgery

Advances in US technology have led to a resurgence in the use of peripheral nerve blocks, with improvements in block efficacy, onset times, and success rate.

Brachial plexus nerve blocks and individual terminal nerve blocks are capable of providing stand-alone anesthesia as well as high-quality analgesia for shoulder and upper limb surgery in high-risk patients.

- Benefits are primarily avoidance of GA and reduced opioid and NSAID requirement in the postoperative period.
- These advantages may be particularly desirable in patients with renal failure, a high-risk of delirium, or sleep apnea.
- Nausea and vomiting are also reduced.

Interscalene block

- Owing to the close proximity of the phrenic nerve to the trunks of the brachial plexus, phrenic nerve blockade has been described in up to 100% of patients. Although the use of US has permitted large reductions in the required volume and dose of LA, avoidance of phrenic nerve palsy cannot be guaranteed. Predicted inability to tolerate hemidiaphragmatic paresis therefore should be viewed as an absolute contraindication. Combined suprascapular and axillary nerve block may be a satisfactory alternative in this situation [13].
- The proximity of an interscalene catheter to a tracheostomy should be considered due to the risk of catheter site contamination.
- Cervical spine injury or reduced neck movement may lead to challenging access to the insertion site.

Supraclavicular blocks

- US guidance has led to a surge in the popularity of this block as the pleura can usually be visualized and avoided, but pneumothorax risk is still a factor to be considered.

Infraclavicular block

- This block also carries a risk of pneumothorax, especially in the patient with increased chest wall tissue.
- A particular advantage is that catheter placement is ideal in this location, with a low likelihood of dislodgement due to relatively immobile tissues.

Axillary block

- This block has the advantage of a low incidence of serious complications, which are unlikely to be tolerated by the high-risk patient – in particular, pneumothorax, phrenic nerve palsy, and major vessel puncture.
- Catheter techniques are unreliable due to the existence of tissue septae, which may prevent the easy spread of LA from a single catheter tip.
- It does not provide full anesthesia reliably for mid-arm/elbow surgery.

Peripheral nerve blocks for lower limb surgery

The lower limb does not lend itself well to regional blocks as a primary technique for all surgical operations.

- Anesthesia to the knee and above requires blockade of multiple nerves.
- Anesthesia for hip surgery is extremely challenging, with peripheral nerve blockade alone requiring blockade of the femoral, obturator, sciatic, and lumbar segmental nerves.
- Anesthesia for surgery below the knee is much more straightforward, requiring only a femoral or saphenous block, in combination with a sciatic nerve block.

A further problem with lower limb techniques is motor block. To some extent this is inevitable, and the increased risk of falls is a significant concern. In addition, the potential for delayed mobilization must be considered.

Specific considerations for individual lower limb blocks are as follows:

Lumbar plexus block

- This block is an effective method of achieving anesthesia of the obturator, femoral, and lateral femoral cutaneous nerves.
- It is a deep block, and may lead to an unrecognized hemodynamically significant hemorrhage, especially in the coagulopathic patient.
- Epidural and/or spinal spread has been reported, as has renal injury and peritoneal puncture.
- The need for lateral positioning of the patient may require IV analgesics in the trauma patient.
- It is a challenging block to learn.
- The depth of the lumbar plexus means structures often cannot be seen clearly with US.

Femoral nerve block

- This block provides good analgesia for knee surgery, but is associated with significant quadriceps weakness. Mobility can be impaired and the risk of falls must be considered.

Sciatic nerve block

- The sciatic nerve can be blocked with a number of approaches.
- The anterior approach permits blockade in the supine position but is significantly more challenging to achieve, and this approach may increase the risk of neurovascular injury in the thigh.
- Patient positioning may be difficult, requiring other approaches in trauma patients.

Additives to LAs [14]

Epinephrine

- Vasoconstriction of perineural vessels leads to decreased block site LA uptake, and prolonged LA duration. Reduced blood levels of drug also result, lowering the risk of systemic LA toxicity.
- Is useful as a marker of intravascular injection in the non-parturient.
- Epinephrine may accentuate injury in nerves with disrupted neural blood flow.

Clonidine

- Clonidine may increase the duration of LA in single-shot blocks.
- There is no apparent benefit in continuous peripheral nerve blocks.
- It significantly prolongs spinal anesthesia.
- Side effects include hypotension, bradycardia, and sedation.

Ketamine

- Ketamine blocks sodium and potassium currents in peripheral nerves.
- It causes central antinociception through NMDA (N-methyl-D-aspartate) receptors.

Opioids

- There are uncertain clinical effects in peripheral nerve blocks.
- Pruritus, urinary retention, and sedation may occur when used in central neuraxial blocks.
- Opioids increase hypotension when given intrathecally.

NSAIDs

- Effects of NSAIDs may depend on the presence of inflammation at the site.
- They may attenuate the hyperalgesic state caused by prostaglandin-induced afferent nerve sensitization.
- They may improve postoperative analgesia and prolong tourniquet tolerance in intravenous (IV) RA.

Verapamil

- Verapamil has no significant advantage over epinephrine if expected duration of surgery is <3.5 h.

Hyaluronidase

- Hyaluronidase does not hasten block onset, reduce incidence of failed block, or affect LA blood concentration.
- May shorten block duration.

Dexmedetomidine

- No change in block onset time occurs.
- There is considerable prolongation of block duration.
- Potential adverse events are hypotension, bradycardia, and sedation.
- It has not been approved for perineural use in some countries, yet.

IV RA

- IV RA is simple, reliable, easy to administer and cost-effective.
- Block duration is very short following tourniquet deflation.
- Due to more favorable toxicity profiles, prilocaine and lidocaine are commonly used agents.
- A successful block requires exsanguination of the limb, which may not be tolerated in trauma patients.
- Unplanned cuff deflation can result in LA toxicity and a purpose-designed cuff must be used.
- IV RA is not a suitable technique for prolonged and repeated procedures.

Indications for the use of RA in high-risk patients

Cardiac surgery

- Thoracic EA may be very beneficial in a selected population of cardiac surgery patients. The risks like those related to anticoagulation may be acceptable if strict protocols are followed with appropriate neurological monitoring.
- Unstable angina – increased coronary perfusion has been shown in multiple studies.
- Careful patient selection and procedure is crucial, including screening of preoperative drug use and an initial normal coagulation profile. Attempts at placement should be limited.
- Much of the debate on the value of EA following cardiac surgery through a median sternotomy centers around whether the risks of hematoma formation are worth the benefits of improved analgesia [15]. On critical review of the literature, enhanced postoperative analgesia appears to be the only clear benefit, as neuraxial techniques have no other clinically important effect on outcome [16].

Carotid surgery

- RA may be a suitable technique when carotid endarterectomy is performed in high-risk patients. This is further discussed in the chapter on anesthesia for vascular surgery.

The elderly patient

- Continuous regional techniques have been used to provide effective analgesia with lower pain scores and better physical therapy for the perioperative management of high-risk elderly patients undergoing major abdominal, vascular, or orthopedic surgery [17].
- Isolated orthopedic injuries in high-risk geriatric patients managed by RA have a lower risk of thromboembolism. With the use of minimal sedation, mental status and respiratory function is preserved.

Obesity

Delayed recovery from GA and postoperative hypoxemia can be avoided if a regional technique is adopted for ambulatory surgery in obese patients. However, these patients are more likely to have a failed block [18].

Additional effects of regional techniques

Stress response and regional techniques

- RA blocks efferent autonomic neuronal pathways to adrenal medulla, liver, etc., and blocks afferent input from the operative site to the central nervous system and the hypothalamic–pituitary axis.
- RA better preserves immune function.
- RA leads to reduced IL-6 and other cytokine responses.
- RA leads to smaller increases in cortisol, catecholamines, and other stress hormonal changes.
- Reduction of stress and the catabolic response with regional techniques provides enhanced recovery and dynamic pain control [19].
- However, it should be kept in mind that the attenuated inflammatory response in the immunocompromised patient may diminish the clinical signs and symptoms associated with infection [20].

Mortality and morbidity

- A global reduction in postoperative complications such as deep vein thrombosis (DVT), pulmonary embolism (PE), pneumonia, and cardiac events has been shown in meta-analyses including older trials [21].
- There is also a clear reduction in mortality in older studies, but no statistical difference has been seen in recent studies [22]. This may be explained partially by the widespread modern use of thromboprophylaxis that was absent in older studies. Lower odds ratio [OR] of death at seven and 30 days, but no difference in overall major morbidity [23] have been observed.

Coagulation and DVT

There is a hypercoagulable state after surgery due to:

- potentiation of the stress response
- endothelial damage with tissue factor activation
- synergy with inflammatory responses

This may result in vaso-occlusive and thrombotic events, e.g. DVT, PE, graft failure.

- The use of RA in high-DVT-risk surgery is thought to reduce this risk in comparison with GA.
- The sympathetic block leads to vasodilation of the limbs and increased blood flow, resulting in less stasis both intra- and postoperatively, with reduced blood cell adhesion to damaged vessel walls. RA also reduces platelet aggregation, lowers mean arterial pressure, and alters coagulation and fibrinolytic responses to prevent clotting further (whereas GA is thought to inhibit fibrinolytic function completely) [24].

Vascular graft function

- GA results in reduced blood flow in the deep veins with increased risk for graft occlusion.
- Sympatholysis due to RA improves regional blood flow and microcirculation.
- RA promotes fibrinolytic activity:
  - reduced postoperative rise in plasminogen activator inhibitor-1
  - reduced postoperative rise in platelet aggregation
  - rapid return of antithrombin III levels to normal
- Systemic LA absorption impairs platelet aggregation.
- Benefits may be seen only if RA is continued postoperatively.

In addition to the aforementioned benefits, patients undergoing major vascular procedures may have a lower cardiac morbidity with EA; however, there is little effect on mortality/morbidity in peripheral vascular surgery [25]. Postoperative thoracic EA has been shown to reduce postoperative myocardial infarction (MI) by as much as 40% [26].

GI

Effects of RA on the GI tract are due to:

- blockade of afferent and efferent limbs of the nociceptive arc (parasympathetic innervation by the vagus is intact)
- systemic absorption of LA – improves bowel motility (direct excitatory effect in GI smooth muscle)
- reduction of opioid use
- blockade of inhibitory spinal reflex arc
- pharmacological sympathectomy – increases GI blood flow, resulting in improved colonic motility

There is good evidence that RA techniques with the avoidance of GA (particularly opioid-based analgesia) are associated with reduced incidence of postoperative GI dysfunction. It has also been demonstrated that ileus during intra-abdominal surgery is shorter if EA is used with LA without the addition of epidural opioids [27].

Excessive fluid loading in an attempt to correct epidural-induced hypotension may have a potential adverse effect on anastomotic integrity by compromising microcirculation. Vasoparesis rather than absolute hypovolemia is usually the cause of hypotension, and therefore it is illogical to treat it with fluids alone, especially in high-risk patients where GI tract perfusion may be critical [28].

Pulmonary

- Postoperative EA with LA and/or opioids is known to reduce pulmonary morbidity and decrease atelectasis [29].
- The use of RA techniques in high-risk patients undergoing non-cardiac surgery has been shown to decrease the incidence of postoperative pulmonary complications [30].
- The protective effect of EA against pneumonia has persisted over the last 35 years, although the relative benefit has fallen due to a reduction in the baseline pneumonia risk [31].

Blood loss

- It has been shown that there is a significant positive correlation between morphine consumption and blood loss in providing good-quality pain relief.
- Sympathectomy can lead to vasodilation, pooling, and decrease of preload.
- This collectively reduces blood loss and has been demonstrated in cesarean section, hysterectomy, prostatectomy, and hip arthroplasty.

Joint mobility

Early mobilization after major orthopedic surgery plays a vital role in successful functional rehabilitation, as postoperative pain often reduces or even prevents effective physical therapy. There is enough evidence that improved joint mobility, most likely resulting from potent analgesia provided by the nerve block [32,33], helps in early functional recovery and achieves therapy goals with lower narcotic consumption.

Other morbidity

- Postoperative sleep disturbance – the anesthesia-related causes are thought to be pain, volatile agents, stress responses, and use of opioids. RA is known to reduce postoperative sleep disturbances by influencing all of these factors.
- Cognitive changes are discussed in the chapter on the elderly patient.
- Fatigue – this depends on surgical stress, and the causes are thought to be opioid use, postoperative sleep disturbances, and the inflammatory/endocrine response. RA improves fatigue, facilitating early mobilization and return to normal activities.

Costs

Increased direct costs:

- equipment, pumps for continuous blocks, and time to perform blocks
- some institutions staff-specific "block room" with associated costs

Reduced indirect costs (although often difficult to identify) due to potential:

- reduction in length of stay and superior pain control
- reduction in mortality, pulmonary/cardiac/other morbidity, graft failure
- early achievement of discharge criteria
- facilitation of early ambulation and enteral nutrition

Role of the acute pain service

Authors have recommended that patients with continuous EA should be seen at least on a daily basis [34], and this minimum requirement should also be met for patients receiving continuous peripheral nerve blockade.

Continuous EA requires close monitoring of block parameters:

- Adequate analgesia and sympatholysis mandates coverage of surgical site dermatomes.
- Blockade of unnecessary segmental levels will lead to hypotension, reducing organ perfusion and risking increased fluid requirements. This will increase interstitial edema, jeopardizing bowel anastomoses and impairing pulmonary and renal function.

- Lower limb motor block due to EA will, particularly in combination with reduced sensation over bony prominences, increase the risk of pressure sores and increase the falls risk.
- Fluid balance must be closely monitored. Hypotension may be incorrectly ascribed to sympathetic blockade by clinicians unpracticed in assessing epidural block height, and the epidural infusion inappropriately reduced. Conversely, a proportion of patients may experience resistant hypotension despite a block height that is required to provide analgesia. In this situation, a decision must be made to alter the patient position, resite the EA at a different level, switch to an opioid-only epidural solution, utilize another form of analgesia, or use vasoactive medications.
- Regular assessment of the catheter entry site is essential to detect early signs of infection and catheter displacement.
- Regular assessment looking for signs of spinal canal infection or hematoma is also mandatory in view of the narrow window for intervention should one of these potentially devastating complications occur.

Peripheral nerve blocks also require regular assessment.

- As with neuraxial anesthesia, motor block can lead to the risk of limb injury, pressure sores, and falls.
- Apparently innocuous degrees of motor block can predispose to falls; for example, foot drop can cause a disproportionate tendency to catch the foot while mobilizing.
- Lower limb blocks of more than one nerve territory require appropriate knowledge when troubleshooting inadequate or overly effective blocks. Consequences from incorrect management due to inadequate monitoring and supervision may outweigh benefits bestowed by the block.

Anticoagulation and RA

Pharmacological prophylaxis against DVT is now well established for moderate and high-risk surgery. This has major implications with regard to both central and peripheral RA: the operator must consider routinely whether the benefits to be gained from a regional technique outweigh the risks of bleeding complications. Of note, the 2010 American Society of Regional Anesthesia (ASRA) recommendations make no distinction between neuraxial and even superficial nerve blocks [35]. A more recent guideline from the a working party from the Association of Anaesthetists of Great Britain and Ireland (AAGBI) emphasized that risk falls on a spectrum, and operator judgment plays an important role in balancing risks and benefit [36].

When assessing risk, blocks may be divided into those where adjacent blood vessels can and cannot be compressed easily.

- Neuraxial techniques carry the potential risk of devastating neurological complications resulting from a relatively small volume of blood in the confined spinal canal.
- The largest study to provide information on the prevalence of spinal hematoma after neuraxial blocks included 1 260 000 spinal blocks and 450 000 epidural blocks [37]. Thirty-three cases of spinal hematoma were found. The incidence was found to differ markedly between patient groups – as high as 1 in 3600 for elderly females receiving knee arthroplasty to 1 in 200 000 for obstetric epidurals. Risk factors can be patient, surgical, or anesthetic in nature.

With respect to the particular prophylaxis drug in question, factors to be considered include timing, duration of action, duration of administration, and co-administration of other antithrombotic agents. Suggested intervals to respect prior to RA may be referenced easily in both the 2010 ASRA [35] and 2013 U.K. guidelines [36].

New thromboprophylactic drugs are reaching the market on a frequent basis. These may provide great challenges for the anesthetist as safety data, with specific regard to RA, may not yet exist. A cautious approach with emphasis on patient safety is recommended.

Table 15.1 provides a brief summary and comparison between the 2010 ASRA guidelines [35] and those from the British working party [36].

Meta-analyses and outcomes

Numerous studies have compared RA techniques to systemic analgesia, and RA to GA. There have also been multiple meta-analyses and systematic reviews. Many focused on the quality of analgesia and short-term transient side effects (nausea and vomiting, pruritus, etc.), while others have examined major morbidity and mortality.

- In 2000, Rodgers et al. [21] carried out a large systematic review of nearly 10 000 patients in trials between 1971 and 1997, who were randomized to intraoperative neuraxial blockade with or without GA. The authors found statistically significant and very large (approximately 30%–60%) reductions in mortality and morbidity (which included thromboembolic disease, transfusion requirements, pneumonia, and respiratory depression).
- A large multicenter Australasian randomized controlled trial (the "MASTER" trial) in 2002 [22], comparing high-risk patients undergoing major surgery under GA with and without intra- and postoperative EA, found substantially better analgesia in the epidural group but no significant differences in mortality or morbidity. Likely reasons for this are that the earlier meta-analysis included a very disparate group of patients (receiving intrathecal or EA, with and without GA), from a wide period over which perioperative techniques have changed markedly: a good example is widespread modern use of thromboprophylaxis.
- Block et al., in 2003 [38], carried out a large meta-analysis including 100 trials comparing EA to parenteral opioids, and also found significantly improved analgesia in the epidural group. They had inadequate data to compare major morbidity, however. Of interest, the thoracic analgesia group had higher nausea and vomiting rates compared to the parenteral opioid group, consistent with other authors' analyses.
- With regard to cognitive complications, a systematic review and meta-analysis by Mason et al. showed a non-significant tendency among patients receiving general rather than regional techniques to suffer increased levels of postoperative cognitive decline, but not postoperative delirium [39].
- In 2008, a large retrospective matched-pairs cohort study [40] examined the effect of EA on 30-day mortality for patients undergoing intermediate- to high-risk non-cardiac surgery, including a wide selection of vascular, abdominal, or orthopedic procedures. Cases were identified from physician billings for commencement of EA, so this was clearly an effectiveness rather than efficacy study as it was not possible to identify which EA s provided successful analgesia. Mortality was slightly lower (1.74% versus 1.95%) in the epidural group. This was statistically significant due to the large numbers but the number needed to treat (NNT) was high at 477.

Table 15.1. Summary of anticoagulation guidelines for regional anesthesia (Adapted from [35,36].)

	Time between last dose and block		Time between last dose and catheter removal		Time between block/catheter removal and subsequent dose	
	AAGBI	ASRA	AAGBI	ASRA	AAGBI	ASRA
Unfractionated subcutaneous prophylactic dose	4 h or normal APTTR	No period specified for bid regime with <10 000 U/24 h. Place epidural before next dose	4 h or normal APTTR	No specified period, but TID dosing not advised when catheter in place	1 h	Ideally remove catheter 1 h before next dose with BID dosing
Unfractionated intravenous treatment dose	4 h or normal APTTR	No recommendation	4 h or normal APTTR	2–4 h Recommends neurological testing for 12 h following procedure	4 h	Delay for 1 h after block. Mention made that in studies looking at intraoperative anticoagulation, 1 h interval left between block and heparinization (24 h for cardiac), and high-risk patients excluded
LMWH subcutaneous prophylactic dose	12 h[1]	10–12 h. 24 h if bid dosing. Administer half of usual dose 24 h before if LMWH is for bridging therapy following discontinuation of warfarin	12 h[1]	With single daily dosing, 10–12 h. Catheter techniques not advised if BID dosing	4 h.[1] Consider only one dose in 1st 24 h after block	After block, 6–8 h postop. if once daily dosing, 24 h if twice daily AND adequate hemostasis. 24 h if traumatic block. Do not use with catheter *in situ* if BID dosing. 2 h minimum after catheter removal

Table 15.1. *(cont.)*

	Time between last dose and block		Time between last dose and catheter removal		Time between block/catheter removal and subsequent dose	
	AAGBI	**ASRA**	**AAGBI**	**ASRA**	**AAGBI**	**ASRA**
LMWH subcutaneous treatment dose	24 h	24 h	Not recommended while catheter is *in situ*	Minimum of 10–12 h if once daily	4 h minimum after neuraxial catheter removal. May increase to 24 h if block is traumatic	
NSAIDs	No additional precautions	No concerns alone; does not recommend in presence of anticoagulants, including LMWH. Advises consideration of COX-2 inhibitors	No additional precautions	No concerns alone; does not recommend in presence of anticoagulants, including LMWH. Advises consideration of COX-2 inhibitors		
Aspirin	No additional precautions	As per NSAIDs	No additional precautions	As per NSAIDs		
Clopidogrel	7 d	At least 7 d. If between 5 and 7 d, normalization of platelet function should be demonstrated	Not recommended while catheter is *in situ*	Not recommended while catheter is *in situ*	6 h	Not stated

Warfarin	INR <1.4	INR <1.5 on initiation with warfarin. Long-term warfarin stopped 4–5 d previously and INR normalized	Warfarinization not recommended with catheter *in situ*	No specified interval, but recommended that INR be <1.5 and duration of therapy be <48 h	Immediately	
Dabigatran (prophylaxis or treatment)						
(CrCl >80 mL/min)	48 h	States only cautious approach	Not recommended while catheter is *in situ*	States only cautious approach	6 h	States only cautious approach
(CrCl 50–80 mL/min)	72 h	States only cautious approach	Not recommended while catheter is *in situ*	States only cautious approach	6 h	States only cautious approach
(CrCl 30–50 mL/min)	96 h	States only cautious approach	Not recommended while catheter is *in situ*	States only cautious approach	6 h	States only cautious approach
Thrombolytics	10 d	Suggest avoid due to insufficient data	Drug not recommended if catheter in place	Suggests fibrinogen level if thrombolytics given	10 d	10 d

[1] U.K. prophylactic dosing is typically at 24 h intervals.

- More recently in 2013, a post-hoc analysis [41] was reported to ascertain the effects of RA on the outcomes of the Perioperative Ischemic Events (POISE) Trial (cardiovascular death, non-fatal MI, and non-fatal cardiac arrest). Outcomes of 7925 from the original 8351 patients were analyzed, and outcomes were either worse or non-significantly different in the neuraxial groups. Hypotension, reduced organ perfusion, and resultant increased fluid administration were proposed as possible causative factors. Confounders were certainly possible, but the results undoubtedly contrasted with previous studies, which have suggested either no difference or benefits from neuraxial anesthesia.
- Published in 2013 as well, a very large database review of 382 236 U.S. patients undergoing primary hip or knee arthroplasty [42] in around 400 different hospitals showed large reductions in 30-day mortality and major morbidity in the group receiving neuraxial rather than GA or a combined technique. Length of stay was also lower. An analysis of a subgroup of these patients [43] with a diagnosis of obstructive sleep apnea also showed significantly lower rates of major morbidity in the neuraxial group.

While the potential confounders inherent in these studies cannot be ignored, retrospective reviews are likely to be the only practical way to compare rates of very rare outcomes [44].

Looking at peripheral nerve blockade rather than neuraxial anesthesia, almost all studies comparing these blocks to systemic analgesia have shown reductions in pain scores and minor side effects (e.g., nausea and vomiting, pruritus) but not at all time-points. The meta-analysis by Richman et al. in 2006 [45] confirmed these benefits at all time-points assessed. Data concerning effects on major morbidity by peripheral nerve blocks is lacking, due to the numbers required for rare outcomes.

References

1. Wu CL, Cohen SR, Richman JM, et al. Efficacy of postoperative patient-controlled and continuous infusion epidural analgesia versus intravenous patient-controlled analgesia with opioids: a meta-analysis. *Anesthesiology* 2005; **103**: 1079–88.
2. Kumar CM, Corbett WA, Wilson RG. Spinal anaesthesia with a micro-catheter in high-risk patients undergoing colorectal cancer and other major abdominal surgery. *Surg Oncol* 2008; **17**: 73–9.
3. Savas JF, Litwack R, Davis K, Miller TA et al. Regional anesthesia as an alternative to general anesthesia for abdominal surgery in patients with severe pulmonary impairment. *Am J Surg* 2004; **188**: 603–5.
4. Schulz-Stübner S, Boezaart A, Hata JS. Regional analgesia in the critically ill. *Crit Care Med* 2005; **33**: 1400–7.
5. Krane EJ, Dalens BJ, Murat I, et al. The safety of epidurals placed during general anesthesia. *Reg Anesth Pain Med* 1998; **23**: 433–8.
6. Serpetinis I, Bassiakou E, Xanthos T, et al. Paravertebral block for open cholecystectomy in patients with cardiopulmonary pathology. *Acta Anaesthesiol Scand* 2008; **52**: 872–3.
7. Davies RG, Myles PS, Graham JM. A comparison of the analgesic efficacy and side-effects of paravertebral vs epidural blockade for thoracotomy–a systematic review and meta-analysis of randomized trials. *Br J Anaesth* 2006; **96**: 418–26.
8. Joshi GP, Bonnet F, Shah R, et al. A systematic review of randomized trials evaluating regional techniques for postthoracotomy analgesia. *Anesth Analg* 2008; **107**: 1026–40.
9. Pusch F, Wildling E, Klimscha W, et al. Sonographic measurement of needle insertion depth in paravertebral blocks in women. *Br J Anaesth* 2000; **85**: 841–3.
10. Belavy D, Cowlishaw PJ, Howes M, et al. Ultrasound-guided transversus abdominis plane block for analgesia after Caesarean delivery. *Br J Anaesth* 2009; **103**: 726–30.

11. McDonnell JG, O'Donnell B, Curley G, et al. The analgesic efficacy of transversus abdominis plane block after abdominal surgery: a prospective randomized controlled trial. *Anesth Analg* 2007; **104**: 193–7.

12. Hebbard PD, Barrington MJ, Vasey C. Ultrasound-guided continuous oblique subcostal transversus abdominis plane blockade: description of anatomy and clinical technique. *Reg Anesth Pain Med* 2010; **35**: 436–41.

13. Price DJ. The shoulder block: a new alternative to interscalene brachial plexus blockade for the control of postoperative shoulder pain. *Anaesth Intensive Care* 2007; **35**: 575–81.

14. Marri SR. Adjuvant agents in regional anaesthesia. *Anaesth Intensive Care Med* 2012; **13**: 559–62.

15. Castellano JM, Durbin CG Jr. Epidural analgesia and cardiac surgery: worth the risk? *Chest* 2000; **117**: 305–7.

16. Chaney MA. Intrathecal and epidural anesthesia and analgesia for cardiac surgery. *Anesth Analg* 2006; **102**: 45–64.

17. Michaloudis D, Petrou A, Bakos P, et al. Continuous spinal anaesthesia/analgesia for the perioperative management of high-risk patients. *Eur J Anaesthesiol* 2000; **17**: 239–47.

18. Servin F. Ambulatory anesthesia for the obese patient. *Curr Opin Anaesthesiol* 2006; **19**: 597–9.

19. Kehlet H, Dahl JB. Anaesthesia, surgery, and challenges in postoperative recovery. *Lancet* 2003; **362**: 1921–8.

20. Horlocker TT, Wedel DJ. Regional anesthesia in the immunocompromised patient. *Reg Anesth Pain Med* 2006; **31**: 334–45.

21. Rodgers A, Walker N, Schug S, et al. Reduction of postoperative mortality and morbidity with epidural or spinal anaesthesia: results from overview of randomised trials. *BMJ* 2000; **321**: 1493.

22. Rigg JRA, Jamrozik K, Myles PS, et al. Epidural anaesthesia and analgesia and outcome of major surgery: a randomised trial. *Lancet* 2002; **359**: 1276–82.

23. Wu CL, Hurley RW, Anderson GF, et al. Effect of postoperative epidural analgesia on morbidity and mortality following surgery in medicare patients. *Reg Anesth Pain Med* 2004; **29**: 525–33.

24. Edmonds MJR, Crichton TJH, Runciman WB, et al. Evidence-based risk factors for postoperative deep vein thrombosis. *ANZ J Surg* 2004; **74**: 1082–97.

25. Bode RH Jr, Lewis KP, Zarich SW, et al. Cardiac outcome after peripheral vascular surgery. Comparison of general and regional anesthesia. *Anesthesiology* 1996; **84**: 3–13.

26. Beattie WS, Badner NH, Choi P. Epidural analgesia reduces postoperative myocardial infarction: a meta-analysis. *Anesth Analg* 2001; **93**: 853–8.

27. Marret E, Remy C, Bonnet F, et al. Meta-analysis of epidural analgesia versus parenteral opioid analgesia after colorectal surgery. *Br J Surg* 2007; **94**: 665–73.

28. Low J, Johnston N, Morris C. Epidural analgesia: first do no harm. *Anaesthesia* 2008; **63**: 1–3.

29. Ballantyne JC, Carr DB, deFerranti S, et al. The comparative effects of postoperative analgesic therapies on pulmonary outcome: cumulative meta-analyses of randomized, controlled trials. *Anesth Analg* 1998; **86**: 598–612.

30. Stevens RD, Fleisher LA. Strategies in the high-risk cardiac patient undergoing non-cardiac surgery. *Best Pract Res Clin Anaesthesiol* 2004; **18**: 549–63.

31. Pöpping DM, Elia N, Marret E, et al. Protective effects of epidural analgesia on pulmonary complications after abdominal and thoracic surgery: a meta-analysis. *Arch Surg* 2008; **143**: 990–9.

32. Capdevila X, Barthelet Y, Biboulet P, et al. Effects of perioperative analgesic technique on the surgical outcome and duration of rehabilitation after major knee surgery. *Anesthesiology* 1999; **91**: 8–15.

33. Ilfeld BM, Wright TW, Enneking FK, et al. Joint range of motion after total shoulder

arthroplasty with and without a continuous interscalene nerve block: a retrospective, case-control study. *Reg Anesth Pain Med* 2005; **30**: 429–33.

34. Ready LB, Oden R, Chadwick HS, et al. Development of an anesthesiology-based postoperative pain management service. *Anesthesiology* 1988; **68**: 100–6.

35. Horlocker TT, Wedel DJ, Rowlingson JC, et al. Regional anesthesia in the patient receiving antithrombotic or thrombolytic therapy: American Society of Regional Anesthesia and Pain Medicine Evidence-Based Guidelines, 3rd edn. *Reg Anesth Pain Med* 2010; **35**: 64–101.

36. Harrop-Griffiths W, Cook T, Gill H, et al. Regional anaesthesia and patients with abnormalities of coagulation: the Association of Anaesthetists of Great Britain & Ireland The Obstetric Anaesthetists' Association Regional Anaesthesia UK. *Anaesthesia* 2013; **68**: 966–72.

37. Moen V, Dahlgren N, Irestedt L. Severe neurological complications after central neuraxial blockades in Sweden 1990–1999. *Anesthesiology* 2004; **101**: 950–9.

38. Block BM, Liu SS, Rowlingson AJ, et al. Efficacy of postoperative epidural analgesia: a meta-analysis. *JAMA* 2003; **290**: 2455–63.

39. Mason SE, Noel-Storr A, Ritchie CW. The impact of general and regional anesthesia on the incidence of post-operative cognitive dysfunction and post-operative delirium: a systematic review with meta-analysis. *J Alzheimers Dis* 2010; **22**: 67–79.

40. Wijeysundera DN, Beattie WS, Austin PC, et al. Epidural anaesthesia and survival after intermediate-to-high risk non-cardiac surgery: a population-based cohort study. *Lancet* 2008; **372**: 562–9.

41. Leslie K, Myles P, Devereaux P, et al. Neuraxial block, death and serious cardiovascular morbidity in the POISE trial. *Br J Anaesth* 2013; **111**: 382–90.

42. Memtsoudis SG, Sun X, Chiu Y-L, et al. Perioperative comparative effectiveness of anesthetic technique in orthopedic patients. *Anesthesiology* 2013; **118**: 1046–58.

43. Memtsoudis SG, Stundner O, Rasul R, et al. Sleep apnea and total joint arthroplasty under various types of anesthesia: a population-based study of perioperative outcomes. *Reg Anesth Pain Med* 2013; **38**: 274–81.

44. Neuman MD, Brummett CM. Trust, but verify: examining the role of observational data in perioperative decision-making. *Anesthesiology* 2013; **118**: 1008–10.

45. Richman JM, Liu SS, Courpas G, et al. Does continuous peripheral nerve block provide superior pain control to opioids? A meta-analysis. *Anesth Analg* 2006; **102**: 248–57.

Chapter 16

Postoperative deterioration

J. Vergel de Dios and I. McConachie

Today's hospitals face a high throughput of surgical cases of increasing complexity and in patients with multiple comorbidities. In addition, many institutions may face problems with:

- inadequate funding
- staff recruitment problems
- less senior, experienced staff (both medical and nursing) on the floor
- less continuity of medical care due to the introduction of shift systems
- inability of junior medical staff to recognize and manage a deteriorating patient and/or seek senior help

Inadequate care

There is a consistent body of evidence which shows that patients who become, or who are at risk of becoming, acutely unwell on general hospital wards receive inadequate care [1–3].

- In the U.K., the National Confidential Enquiry into Patient Outcome and Death (NCEPOD) identified the prime causes of this as being both delayed recognition and the institution of inappropriate therapy that subsequently culminated in a late referral to critical care [3]. Admission to an intensive care unit (ICU) was thought to have been avoidable in 21% of cases, and suboptimal care contributed to about a third of the deaths that occurred.
- Delays in ICU referral and admission and length of stay in hospital prior to ICU admission have been shown to be factors in poor outcome [4]. This implies that early diagnosis, referral, and intervention may improve outcome.
- In July 2007, the U.K. National Institute for Health and Clinical Excellence (NICE) published a document entitled *Acutely Ill Patients in Hospital – Recognition of and Response to Acute Illness in Adults in Hospital* [5]. They concluded that patients who are or become acutely unwell in hospital may receive suboptimal care. This may be because their deterioration is not recognized, is not appreciated, or is not acted upon sufficiently rapidly.

The importance of abnormal physiology

It is well established that abnormal physiology is associated with adverse clinical outcomes.

- A multicenter, prospective, observational study found that the majority (60%) of primary events (deaths, cardiac arrests, and unplanned ICU admissions) were preceded

Anesthesia and Perioperative Care of the High-Risk Patient, Third edition, ed. Ian McConachie. Published by Cambridge University Press.

by documented abnormal physiology, the most common being hypotension and a fall in the Glasgow Coma Score [6].
- In the U.K. NICE report of 2007, the majority (66%) of inpatients who had been in hospital for more than 24 hours before ICU admission exhibited physiological instability for more than 12 hours [5].
- Mortality has been shown to increase with the number of abnormal physiological parameters ($P<0.001$), being 0.7% with no abnormalities, 4.4% with one, 9.2% with two, and 21.3% with three or more [4].

A careful consideration of the progress of each patient and a review of their vital signs should reveal those patients who are failing to progress. However, those of us involved in caring for patients after admission to ICU realize that, only too often, deteriorating vital signs have been diligently charted without either recognition of their significance or appropriate intervention. While there remains a place for clinical acumen, there is an essential need for more comprehensive observations and objective assessments.

Possible solutions

- increased funding and more staff
- more high-care beds in the hospital
- education of staff
- shared care, staff rotations, and skill sharing
- early recognition and intervention in deteriorating patients
- Medical Emergency Teams (METs) and/or Critical Care Outreach Teams (CCOTs)

This chapter will address the last two possible solutions.

Identification of deterioration

Clinical deterioration can occur at any stage of a patient's illness. However, there are certain periods when patients are at their most vulnerable:

- the onset of their illness
- during surgical intervention
- discharge from critical care

The postoperative period is when close observation and monitoring are crucial in order to detect deterioration. Physiological systems are subjected to significant challenges:

- oxygen supply and demand imbalances
- cardiorespiratory stresses
- fluid and electrolyte shifts
- pain and anxiety
- gastrointestinal ileus
- catabolism
- energy supply and demand imbalance
- infection and sepsis

The role of the anesthesiologist

Prior to surgery, the opportunity exists to recognize the at-risk patient. Preoperative assessment and early recognition of those patients who are likely to deteriorate through their own comorbidities or through the complexity of the surgical procedure is vital. This enables appropriate investigations and risk stratification to be carried out and improves awareness of those caring for the sick patient.

Anesthesiologists are acutely aware of patients who deteriorate on the operating table during surgical procedures. Such information should be conveyed to receiving ward staff, either in critical care units or general wards, as intraoperative events can have a significant impact on a patient's postoperative course. Unanticipated events, such as more complex surgery of longer duration, prolonged aortic cross-clamp times, uncontrolled bleeding, emergency splenectomy, fat emboli, damage to surrounding structures, etc., can all influence outcome. They need to be recognized, communicated, and their implications monitored in the postoperative period.

Are hospitals safe?

We admit patients to hospital after surgery (rather than send them home) so they can be looked after in a place of safety and because we offer them better care than they could get at home. However, medical errors and other iatrogenic problems are responsible for significant morbidity and mortality in every health system studied. There are numerous causes of failures within hospital systems (beyond the scope of this chapter). Patient monitoring often can be one of those failures.

- Traditional monitoring of surgical (and other) patients involves measurement of vital signs and other clinical indicators. However, it can be argued that the act of merely assessing a patient and recording the findings is observation and not monitoring.
- Monitoring should require the presence of an alarming system and/or the detection of an abnormality should result in specific staff actions.
- Even after vital signs are measured, junior medical and nursing staff often are unable to recognize and initiate treatment of the deteriorating or critically ill patient. Standard textbooks on clinical examination often are poorly equipped to help students understand the principles of assessing the critically ill patient [7].
- In order to fill this gap, many have developed multidisciplinary courses aimed at addressing the suboptimal ward care often seen prior to admission to critical care units.

Prediction of postoperative deterioration

Numerous studies have demonstrated that certain patient comorbidities are associated with increased risk of serious adverse outcomes in the postoperative period. These include increased age, high American Society of Anesthesiologists (ASA) scores and congestive heart failure [8]. Patients from nursing homes and those presenting as emergencies are also at increased risk of adverse outcomes [8].

Patient factors during surgery can also suggest postoperative complications; for example:

- increasing oxygen requirements
- increasing ventilator pressures
- failure to respond to fluids

- vasopressor support
- difficult temperature control with subsequent hypothermia
- acidemia and/or increasing lactate levels
- poor intraoperative urine output
- poor glycemic control
- worsening tachycardia
- ST-segment or T-wave changes on the electrocardiograph (ECG)
- the use of blood products in the intraoperative period

Deterioration of respiratory status postoperatively has been well studied:

- A study of a large database of patients undergoing major general and vascular surgery found that the rate of intubation postoperatively due to deterioration was 2.6% [9]. Emergency surgeries, loss of functional independence preoperatively, and the presence of renal failure or significant COPD preoperatively were predictive factors. The majority of the reintubations occurred in patients admitted to ICU with sepsis.
- Another study of unplanned intubation found it occurred in approximately 2% of patients undergoing major surgery [10]. Perhaps not surprisingly, the factors most associated with postoperative intubation included age of >80 years, high ASA score, preoperative sepsis, and total operative time of >6 hours.
- Similar risk factors as found in these two studies are also predictive of the development of postoperative respiratory failure [11].
- Acute respiratory distress syndrome (ARDS) is uncommon after surgery (0.2% of surgical patients) and rare in ASA 1 or 2 patients. Postoperative ARDS is more common in emergency patients and those with COPD, with renal failure, and undergoing multiple surgeries. Additional intraoperative risk factors are increasing airway pressures and inspired oxygen concentration, excessive fluid administration, and blood transfusion [12].

The importance of early recognition

Focusing on improvement of response to patient crises may have limited success in terms of patient outcomes. We have seen how adverse events are preceded by a significant period of physiological deterioration. Therefore, it makes sense that lack of early recognition of physiological decline plays a major role in poor hospital outcomes.

As long ago as 1992, hospital deaths after surgical adverse events and postoperative complications were described as "failure-to-rescue" [13]. Rescuing failure-to-rescue patients requires:

1. early recognition of adverse events, complications, and physiological deterioration
2. systems to rapidly respond to such crises

Together, this approach involves the creation of rapid response systems (RRS) and appropriate hospital teams.

Rapid response systems

There are three components to rapid response systems [14]:

1. Afferent limb: notification of a deteriorating patient and activation of the RRS – the afferent limb is typically composed of individuals who are working on the ward

(physicians, nurses). Examples include activation criteria as set out by physiological track-and-trigger systems. More recently, the tracking of physiological variables has become automated in some centers.
2. Efferent limb: members of the RRS who respond to the afferent limb – the efferent limb is typically composed of individuals who work in the ICU. Examples include METs, patient-at-risk team (PART), rapid response teams (RRTs), and CCOTs. They differ slightly in team composition and whether patient follow-up is incorporated. In many centers, these teams also have a role in reviewing patients after discharge from ICU to improve their management, support the ward staff, and prevent readmission to ICU.
3. Administrative/quality improvement: the team that collects data to improve the system over time – important, but not discussed further here.

Afferent limb

There have been two main approaches to the afferent limb of rapid response systems:

1. physiological track-and-trigger systems
2. continuous monitoring systems

Physiological track and trigger systems

Physiological track-and-trigger systems rely on periodic observation of selected basic physiological signs ("tracking"), with predetermined calling or response criteria ("trigger") for requesting the attendance of staff who have specific expertise in the management of acute illness and/or critical care. These systems allow a large number of patients to be monitored and effectively screened for deterioration without a large increase in workload. A number of systems have been developed internationally:

Aggregate scoring systems

Aggregate scoring systems have been developed predominantly in the U.K. The original basic Early Warning Score (EWS) was developed at the James Paget Hospital in Norfolk [15], and other hospitals have taken the template idea and modified it for local use. The Modified Early Warning System (MEWS) [16] is probably the most widely studied variant in the U.K. [16]. The MEWS score is calculated by assessing five variables – respiratory rate, heart rate, blood pressure, central nervous system (CNS) by the AVPU method (alert, voice, pain, unresponsive), and temperature. A score from 0–3 is assigned to each, according to the degree of physiological derangement, and the combination of scores provides the MEWS. Other early versions also included urine output.

More recently, in 2012, the U.K. Royal College of Physicians recommended the nationwide adoption of a similar, standardized EWS – the National Early Warning System (NEWS) [17]. This is similar to the MEWS score but oxyhemoglobin saturation and administration of supplemental oxygen are added to give seven variables in total.

Aggregated weighted scoring systems score every parameter of a set of bedside observations and add the scores to give a final figure. The more abnormal a single parameter, the higher the weighting, and therefore the higher the aggregate score. If the score reaches a predetermined value, nursing staff trigger the appropriate response. The assistance requested is proportional to the severity of the score; low scores require a junior doctor response, higher scores require a more senior review or referral to critical care outreach services.

Continuous monitoring systems

EWS systems are limited by the intermittent nature of vital sign checks performed by nursing staff.

- What if nobody checks the vital signs?
- What if nobody recognizes the pattern or significance of deteriorating vital signs?

Continuous monitoring systems represent a more proactive approach to identifying patient deterioration, based on the premise that physiological changes can indicate and perhaps predict deterioration episodes. Multiple technologies are in use for both the measuring of physiological data and their analysis.

- Continuous ECG monitoring has long been used for cardiac patients, but studies have shown limited usefulness for ECG monitoring of low-risk patients and that an ECG is unreliable in predicting cardiac arrest. In addition, physicians overestimate the usefulness of ECG monitoring.
- Widespread use of pulse oximetry in postoperative patients has been shown to reduce the need for attendance of the hospital response team and need for transfer to ICU [18]. This was a study of true surveillance with pulse oximetry data wirelessly transmitted to a central computer server and nurses were notified directly by pager when values were outside set limits.
- Continuous, integrated monitoring of multiple variables is the logical extension of these concepts. The Biosign system continuously monitors blood pressure, respiratory rate, heart rate, skin temperature, and pulse oximetry and combines them into a single patient score. Studies have established proof of concept [19] but have not been shown to reduce mortality or the incidence of adverse events [20].
- In a trauma "step down" unit, early detection of instability patterns using continuous electronic monitoring led to a reduced incidence of critical instability events [21].
- Thus far, "The promise of electronic physiologic monitoring for continuous detection and prediction of deterioration has not been fully realized." [22].

It seems that the high technology solution (continuous monitoring systems) is favored in the U.S. over simpler (and cheaper) track-and-trigger systems. In addition to the resource implications, concerns may be raised over the potential impersonal nature of such systems and problems related to alarm fatigue and motion artifacts. Continuous monitoring systems should not replace other means of monitoring, such as nurses at the bedside, or lull institutions into a false sense of security.

The efferent limb

Various team concepts and structures have been established in hospitals worldwide. The original described system was the MET.

- The concept of the MET was introduced in Australia by Lee et al. in 1995 [23]. The aim of the team was to provide assistance in the peri-arrest situation. The team could be triggered by a patient meeting one or more of a set criteria or simply a patient causing concern. The team would consist of nursing and medical staff with appropriate resuscitation skills. This is a simple system but does not allow a patient's progress to be tracked or a graded response.

- The PART concept was similar with the aim of recognizing deteriorating patients at an earlier stage and preventing or expediting admission to critical care areas. The PART concept also allowed for direct referral from senior residents on the ward [24].
- The calling criteria for both METs and PARTs have typically used single parameter systems – the presence of one or more criteria triggering a response rather than the graded response associated with the EWS.
- In the U.S., RRTs are a key component of the Institute for Healthcare Improvement 100 000 Lives Campaign (most recently updated as the Five-Million Lives Campaign) [25]. After this report, RRTs were rapidly introduced across the U.S., followed by several enthusiastic (but often poorly designed or controlled) studies.
- While much of the original evidence has come from the U.K. and Australia, teams are now commonplace in North America and many other countries.
- Outreach is a similar (and overlapping concept) where the teams, typically composed of senior ICU nurses and/or physicians, provide support of patients identified as being appropriate for the efferent limb of an RRS and also follow up reviews and support of recently discharged ICU patients. This has been referred to as "ICU without walls."

Evaluation of rapid response and outreach systems

- The available track-and-trigger scores were not designed to predict outcome but to alert staff to potential problems in individual patients.
- In those studies that purport to show improved outcome with some variant of an outreach system, it is difficult to try and distinguish (and may be inappropriate to do so) between the role of the scoring trigger system used and any triggered interventions and resultant changes in outcomes.
- Single parameter systems, as used by MET systems, have low sensitivity, low positive predictive values, but high specificity. Multiple parameter systems, like EWS and continuous electronic monitoring systems, require the presence of one or more abnormal physiological variables. These systems have comparatively high sensitivity but relatively low specificity when one abnormal observation is present (that is, at low scores). Sensitivity decreases and specificity increases as the number of abnormal variables increase.
- Few studies are randomized and adequately powered. Rigorous evaluation of the published studies in this field, like Cochrane reviews, criticize the majority of studies published as being of poor methodological value [26]. They did not believe that meta-analysis was possible. However, it can be questioned whether randomized controlled trials (RCTs) are the appropriate gold standard in assessing the role of METs and RRTs.

Accuracy of predictions

Predictions of cardiac arrest, ICU admission, and mortality have been examined:

- In one case control study, the ability of a track-and-trigger system to predict in-hospital cardiac arrest based on 10 MET parameters was assessed. An receiver operating characteristic (ROC) analysis determined that a score of 4 has 89% sensitivity and 77% specificity for cardiac arrest; a score of 8 has 52% sensitivity and 99% specificity. Only 1% of patients who do not have a cardiac arrest score 8 or more and all patients scoring greater than 10 suffered a cardiac arrest [27].

- The ability of a PART to predict admission to ICU in hospital ward patients (patients triggered the system if they had three out of six abnormal physiological variables or reduced consciousness with increased heart or respiratory rate) had a sensitivity and specificity for patients with three abnormal observations of 27% and 57%, respectively. For patients with one abnormal observation, the sensitivity was 97% and specificity 18%. The presence of two abnormal observations had a sensitivity of 80% and specificity of 41% [28].
- In a third study, also based on the PART calling criteria, stepwise multiple regression identified five significant predictors of 30-day mortality (consciousness, heart rate, age, blood pressure, and respiratory rate) – sensitivity and specificity were 7.7% and 99.8%, respectively [6].
- With regard to aggregate scoring systems and MEWS in particular, a trigger score was associated with an increased risk of death (odds ratio [OR] 5.4, 95% confidence interval [CI_{95}] 2.8–10.7) and ICU admission (OR 10.9, CI_{95} 2.2–55.6) [29].
- The use of the EWS to predict mortality in a sample of 110 patients admitted with acute pancreatitis had sensitivities on days 1, 2, and 3 following admission of 85.7%, 71.4%, and 100%. Specificities were 28.3%, 67.4%, and 77.4%, respectively [30].
- A study from the Worthing Physiological Scoring System showed that the use of rigorous statistical methods in identifying both physiological parameters and abnormal physiological values enables the sensitivities and specificities of the system to be increased. At an intervention score of 2, its sensitivity and specificities are 78% and 57%, respectively [31].
- In 2012, the U.K. NCEPOD's prospective review on in-hospital cardiopulmonary resuscitation (CPR) after cardiac arrest found that, of the cases in which CPR was performed, 21% appeared to not have a track-and-trigger system in place [32]. Additionally, warning signs of patient deterioration were apparent 75% of the time, but reviewers of the cases felt that these signs were not recognized 36% of the time.

Improvements in outcome with rapid response and outreach systems

Improvements in outcome could arise from reductions in cardiac arrest and better survival from cardiac arrests, avoidance of ICU admission, and/or improved overall mortality. Full assessment of the effect of outreach systems on outcome is difficult due to different systems studied (EWS, METs, outreach teams, etc.), different hospitals, countries, and patient population types, and often lack of randomization or controlling for other changes in practice. Further potential problems are that many of the published studies are underpowered or investigate too short a period. Additionally, many of the studies of cardiac arrests recorded cardiac arrest calls rather than specific cardiac arrests. The Hawthorne effect in control groups is another possible confounding factor.

- Reductions in the incidence of cardiac arrest may be due to better education of ward staff in caring for patients and new "do not attempt resuscitation" (DNAR) orders being made on sick patients, as well as to improvements in care of pre-arrest patients. All are arguably of benefit.
- However, Bellomo et al. [33], also in Australia, showed that the introduction of a MET system reduced the number of cardiac arrests and also the deaths from cardiac arrest

when comparing the period before the introduction of the system and the time after its introduction. This was not found to be due to increased DNAR orders. Bellomo et al. also demonstrated reduced overall inpatient mortality even after adjusting for other factors contributing to long-term surgical mortality.

- Buist et al. found in a six-year audit that the introduction of a MET system, after adjustment for case mix, was associated with a 50% reduction in the incidence of cardiac arrest [34].
- Jones et al. assessed the effect of a MET service on patient mortality in the four years since its introduction into a teaching hospital [35]. They found fluctuating and variable effects on surgical mortality with apparent increases in mortality in medical patients, perhaps reflecting differences in the degree of disease complexity and reversibility between medical and surgical patients.
- One of only two RCTs in this field was the MERIT (Medical Early Response Intervention and Therapy) study from Australia [36]. This multicenter trial randomized 23 hospitals without a MET system to introduce such a system or maintain current practices. Results were disappointing for METs enthusiasts. The number of emergency calls for sick patients increased greatly over the course of the study period in the MET hospitals. However, both groups of hospitals showed a reduction in overall mortality over the study period with no statistically significant difference in outcome seen in the MET hospitals. Using their call-out criteria, many patients were not identified until less than 15 minutes before either cardiac arrest or ICU admission. It appears that the study may have been underpowered.
- The other published RCT from the U.K. randomized the wards in a single, large hospital. Priestley et al. [37] found that the interventions associated with an outreach team reduced hospital mortality (OR 0.52) and length of stay. They also found a possible increased length of stay associated with outreach which, after further analysis, may not have been statistically significant.
- Ball et al. [38] found that the introduction of a CCOT improved survival to discharge from hospital, after discharge from critical care, by 6.8%. Readmission to critical care decreased by 6.4%.
- Pittard [39] showed that, in his hospital, following the introduction of an outreach service, the emergency admission rate to ICU fell from 58% to 43%, with a shorter length of stay (4.8 days versus 7.4 days) and a lower mortality (28.6% versus 23.5%, P=0.05). The readmission rate also fell from 5.1% to 3.3% (P=0.05).
- The type of institution may be important. Shah et al. [40] found that introduction of RRTs to their academic center did not alter cardiac arrest rates or hospital mortality significantly. The presence of in-house physicians and house staff may lessen the benefit of such teams compared to hospitals without in-house medical staff.
- Over a period of seven years, a prospective non-randomized comparison before and after the introduction of a MET in Sweden found a 26% reduction in cardiac arrests (1.12/1000 admissions/yr versus 0.83, P=0.035). Hospital mortality reductions of 10% in the total population, 12% for medical patients, and 28% in unoperated surgical patients were also found [41].
- Outside of North America, the introduction of intensivist-led RRTs into an academic center in Saudi Arabia has recently been shown to result in improvements in all hoped-for areas – reduced cardiac arrests, decreased mortality of ward patients, improved

outcomes of patients requiring ICU admission, and reduced readmissions and mortality of patients recently discharged from the ICU [42].

- However, Karpman and colleagues offer a cautionary note. Their large retrospective study found that the introduction of RRTs increased admissions to ICU – often of lower illness severity, compared to previous admission data. In addition, they were unable to demonstrate an improved outcome in patients transferred from the ward, after adjusting for severity of disease [43].
- As Santamaria et al. pointed out, these large-scale changes in hospital systems will require time and patience to see any changes in cardiac arrest rates and hospital mortality [44].

Specific surgical and postoperative studies

- In a surgical ward population in the U.K., 17% of patients triggered a MEWS response. The MEWS in surgical patients was found to be 75% sensitive and 83% specific for admission to a high-care area, with an aggregate score threshold of 4 or more [45].
- The introduction of a nurse-based outreach system in a large Australian hospital led to a reduction in the incidence of serious adverse events and myocardial infarction in the first three days after surgery [46].
- Additionally in Australia, the introduction of an ICU-based MET into a university hospital seemed of benefit to patients having major surgery [47]. Although not a randomized trial, the results are of interest. The introduction of the MET team was associated with reductions in several adverse events:

Adverse event	Relative risk reduction
Overall adverse events	57.8%
Respiratory failure	79.1%
Renal failure	88.5%
Emergency ICU admissions	44.4%
Postoperative deaths	36.6%

The average length of stay after major surgery was also reduced.

- A combined CCOT and anesthesia-based acute pain team [48] reviewed high-risk patients on the wards during the first three days after surgery. They were also able to demonstrate a reduction in the incidence of adverse events and 30-day mortality (from 9% to 3%).
- Introduction of a MET service in a teaching hospital in Australia was associated with increased long-term survival in surgical patients (65.8% in the control period and 71.6% during the MET period (P=0.001), even after adjusting for other factors that contribute to long-term surgical mortality [49].
- All Medicare patients in the U.S. undergoing six major surgical procedures from 2005 to 2006 were studied [50]. Hospitals were ranked according to risk-adjusted mortality to identify the “best” hospitals. The best hospitals obviously had the lowest overall mortality for these procedures but all hospitals had similar incidences of major

complications and adverse events! Thus, a failure-to-rescue rate could be calculated for all hospitals. The failure-to-rescue rate varied from 6.8% in the best hospitals to 16.7% in the worst hospitals. This implies that significant improvements in outcome are possible if failure-to-rescue is addressed in individual hospitals (e.g., with RRS).

- This important finding was confirmed from Medicare data for three common high-risk cancer surgeries [51].
- It is worth emphasizing that the two aforementioned studies challenged two common surgical perceptions – the first [50] that complication rates are an important factor in adverse outcome, and the second [51] that hospital volume is an important factor in good outcomes. It is not so much that these are unimportant but that failure-to-rescue issues may overshadow them.
- Two hundred and eighty emergency surgery patients had their EWS measured preoperatively and changes were followed postoperatively. An "improving" EWS was associated with significantly improved survival compared with a "deteriorating or failing-to-improve" EWS [52]. The EWS predicted both mortality and the need for postoperative critical care.
- Incidence rates of unplanned intubation did not change significantly after MET deployment, suggesting that other strategies are needed to prevent this rare but highly morbid and mortal event [9].
- In a recent study, 0.2% of patients discharged from the post-anesthesia care unit (PACU) after surgery required the attention of an RRTs – 62% within 12 hours of discharge. These were matched with other patients as controls. Neurological comorbidity (cerebrovascular disease, seizures, dementia), preoperative opioid use, intraoperative phenylephrine infusion, and intraoperative fluid boluses increased the risk of RRTs activation [53].

Recent systematic review and meta-analysis

- RRTs have been associated with reduced cardiac arrest events but without an overall change in adult hospital mortality, according to a recent systematic review of a meta-analysis of 18 studies and 26 low-quality before-and-after studies [14].
- A different review [54] additionally focusing on EWS systems added that aggregate scoring systems seemed more effective than single parameter-based MET systems, and that the efferent limb of a system is more effective when led by clinicians with ICU skills.

References

1. McQuillian P, Pilkington S, Allan A, et al. Confidential enquiry into quality of care before admission to intensive care. *BMJ* 1998; **316**: 1853–8.
2. McGloin H, Adam SK, Singer M. Unexpected deaths and referrals to intensive care of patients on general wards. Are some cases potentially avoidable? *J R Coll Physicians Lond* 1999; **33**: 255–9.
3. NCEPOD. An acute problem? A report of the National Confidential Enquiry into Patient Outcome and Death (NCEPOD). London: NCEPOD, 2005.
4. Goldhill DR, McNarry AF. Physiological abnormalities in early warning scores are related to mortality in adult inpatients. *Brit J Anesth* 2004; **92**: 882–4.
5. Centre for Clinical Practice at NICE, UK. *Acutely ill patients in hospital: Recognition of and Response to Acute Illness in Adults in Hospital.* London: National Institute for Health and Clinical Excellence, 2007.
6. Kause J, Smith G, Prytherch D, et al. A comparison of antecedents to cardiac

arrests, deaths and emergency intensive care admissions in Australia and New Zealand, and the United Kingdom – the ACADEMIA study. *Resuscitation* 2004; **62**: 275–82.

7. Cook CJ, Smith GB. Do textbooks of clinical examination contain information regarding the assessment of critically ill patients? *Resuscitation* 2004; **60**: 129–36.
8. Leung JM, Dzankic S. Relative importance of preoperative health status versus intraoperative factors in predicting postoperative adverse outcomes in geriatric surgical patients. *J Am Geriatr Soc* 2001; **49**: 1080–5.
9. Snyder CW, Patel RD, Roberson EP, et al. Unplanned intubation after surgery: risk factors, prognosis, and medical emergency team effects. *Am Surg* 2009; **75**: 834–8.
10. Hua M, Brady JE, Li G. A scoring system to predict unplanned intubation in patients having undergone major surgical procedures. *Anesth Analg* 2012; **115**: 88–94.
11. Gupta H, Gupta PK, Fang X, et al. Development and validation of a risk calculator predicting postoperative respiratory failure. *Chest* 2011; **140**: 1207–15.
12. Blum JM, Stentz MJ, Dechert R, et al. Preoperative and intraoperative predictors of postoperative acute respiratory distress syndrome in a general surgical population. *Anesthesiology* 2013; **118**: 19–29.
13. Silber JH, Williams SV, Krakauer H, et al. Hospital and patient characteristics associated with death after surgery. A study of adverse occurrence and failure to rescue. *Med Care* 1992; **30**: 615–29.
14. Winters BD, Weaver SJ, Pfoh ER, et al. Rapid-response systems as a patient safety strategy: a systematic review. *Ann Int Med* 2013; **158**: 417–25.
15. Morgan RJM, Williams F, Wright MM. An early warning scoring system for detecting developing critical illness. *Clin Intensive Care* 1997; **8**: 100.
16. Subbe CP, Kruger M, Rutherford P, et al. Validation of a modified early warning score in medical admissions. *QJM* 2001; **94**: 521–6.
17. McGinley A, Pearse RM. A national early warning score for acutely ill patients. *BMJ* 2012; **345**: e5310.
18. Taenzer AH, Pyke JB, McGrath SP, et al. Impact of pulse oximetry surveillance on rescue events and intensive care unit transfers: a before-and-after concurrence study. *Anesthesiology* 2010; **112**: 282–7.
19. Hravnak M, Edwards L, Clontz A, et al. Defining the incidence of cardiorespiratory instability in patients in step-down units using an electronic integrated monitoring system. *Arch Intern Med* 2008; **168**: 1300–8.
20. Watkinson PJ, Barber VS, Price JD, et al. A randomised controlled trial of the effect of continuous electronic physiological monitoring on the adverse event rate in high risk medical and surgical patients. *Anaesthesia* 2006; **61**: 1031–9.
21. Hravnak M, Devita MA, Clontz A, et al. Cardiorespiratory instability before and after implementing an integrated monitoring system. *Crit Care Med* 2011; **39**: 65–72.
22. Taenzer AH, Pyke JB, McGrath SP. A review of current and emerging approaches to address failure-to-rescue. *Anesthesiology* 2011; **115**: 421–31.
23. Lee A, Bishop G, Hilman KM. The Medical Emergency Team. *Anaesth Intensive Care* 1995; **23**: 183–6.
24. Goldhill DR, Worthington L, Mulcahy A, et al. The patient-at-risk team: identifying and managing seriously ill ward patients. *Anaesthesia* 1999; **54**: 853–60.
25. Berwick DM, Calkins DR, McCannon CJ, et al. The 100,000 Lives Campaign. *JAMA* 2006; **295**: 324–7.
26. McGaughey J, Alderdice F, Fowler R, et al. Outreach and Early Warning Systems (EWS) for the prevention of intensive care admission and death of critically ill adult patients on general hospital wards. *Cochrane Database Syst Rev* 2007; **3**: CD005529.
27. Hodgetts TJ, Kenward G, Vlachonikolis IG, et al. The identification of risk factors for cardiac arrest and formulation of activation criteria to alert a medical emergency team. *Resuscitation* 2002; **54**: 125–31.

28. Goldhill DR, McNarry AF, Mandersloot G, et al. A physiologically based early warning score for ward patients: the association between score and outcome. *Anaesthesia* 2005; **60**: 547–53.
29. Subbe CP, Davies RG, Williams E, et al. Effect of introducing the Modified Early Warning score on clinical outcomes, cardio-pulmonary arrests and intensive care utilisation in acute medical admissions. *Anaesthesia* 2003; **58**: 797–802.
30. Garcea G, Jackson B, Pattenden CJ, et al. Early warning scores predict outcome in acute pancreatitis. *J Gastrointest Surg* 2006; **10**: 1008–15.
31. Duckitt RW, Buxton-Thomas R, Walker J, et al. Worthing physiological scoring system: derivation and validation of a physiological early-warning system for medical admissions. An observational, population-based single centre study. *Br J Anaesth* 2007; **98**: 769–74.
32. Perkins GD, Temple RM, George R. Time to intervene: lessons from the NCEPOD report. *Resuscitation* 2012; **83**: 1305–6.
33. Bellomo R, Goldsmith D, Uchino S, et al. A prospective before-and-after trial of a medical emergency team. *Med J Aust* 2003; **179**: 283–287.
34. Buist M, Harrison J, Abaloz E, et al. Six year audit of cardiac arrests and medical emergency team calls in an Australian outer metropolitan teaching hospital. *BMJ* 2007; **335**: 1210–12.
35. Jones D, Opdam H, Egi M, et al. Long-term effect of a Medical Emergency Team on mortality in a teaching hospital. *Resuscitation* 2007; **74**: 235–41.
36. Hillman K, Chen J, Cretikos M, et al. Introduction of the medical emergency team (MET) system: a cluster-randomised controlled trial. *Lancet* 2005; **365**: 2091–7.
37. Priestley G, Watson W, Rashidian A, et al. Introducing Critical Care Outreach: a ward-randomised trial of phased introduction in a general hospital. *Intensive Care Med* 2004; **30**: 1398–404.
38. Ball C, Kirkby M, Williams S. Effect of the critical care outreach team on patient survival to discharge from hospital and readmission to critical care: non-randomised population based study. *BMJ* 2003; **327**: 1014–7.
39. Pittard AJ. Out of our reach? Assessing the impact of introducing a critical care outreach service. *Anaesthesia* 2003; **58**: 882–5.
40. Shah SK, Cardenas VJ Jr, Kuo YF, et al. Rapid response team in an academic institution: does it make a difference ? *Chest* 2011; **139**: 1361–7.
41. Konrad D, Jäderling G, Bell M, et al. Reducing in-hospital cardiac arrests and hospital mortality by introducing a medical emergency team. *Int Care Med* 2010; **36**: 100–6.
42. Karpman C, Keegan MT, Jensen JB, et al. The impact of rapid response team on outcome of patients transferred from the ward to the ICU: a single-center study. *Crit Care Med* 2013; **41**: 2284–91.
43. Al-Qahtani S, Al-Dorzi HM, Tamim HM, et al. Impact of an intensivist-led multidisciplinary extended rapid response team on hospital-wide cardiopulmonary arrests and mortality. *Crit Care Med* 2013; **41**: 506–17.
44. Santamaria J, Tobin A, Holmes J. Changing cardiac arrest and mortality rates through a medical emergency team takes time and constant review. *Crit Care Med* 2010; **38**: 445–50.
45. Gardner-Thorpe J, Love N, Wrightson J, et al. The value of Modified Early Warning Score (MEWS) in surgical in-patients: a prospective observational study. *Ann R Coll Surg Engl* 2006; **88**: 571–5.
46. Story DA, Shelton AC, Poustie SJ, et al. The effect of critical care outreach on postoperative serious adverse events. *Anaesthesia*. 2004; **59**: 762–6.
47. Bellomo R, Goldsmith D, Uchino S, et al. Prospective controlled trial of effect of medical emergency team on postoperative morbidity and mortality rates. *Crit Care Med* 2004; **32**: 916–21.
48. Story DA, Shelton AC, Poustie SJ, et al. Effect of an anaesthesia department led critical care outreach and acute pain service

on postoperative serious adverse events. *Anaesthesia* 2006; **61**: 24–8.

49. Jones D, Egi M, Bellomo R, et al. Effect of the medical emergency team on long-term mortality following major surgery. *Crit Care* 2007; **11**: R12.

50. Ghaferi AA, Birkmeyer JD, Dimick JB. Complications, failure to rescue, and mortality with major inpatient surgery in medicare patients. *Ann Surg* 2009; **250**: 1029–34.

51. Ghaferi AA, Birkmeyer JD, Dimick JB. Hospital volume and failure to rescue with high-risk surgery. *Med Care* 2011; **49**: 1076–81.

52. Garcea G, Ganga R, Neal CP, et al. Preoperative early warning scores can predict in-hospital mortality and critical care admission following emergency surgery. *J Surg Res* 2010; **159**: 729–34.

53. Weingarten TN, Venus SJ, Whalen FX, et al. Postoperative emergency response team activation at a large tertiary medical center. *Mayo Clin Proc* 2012; **87**; 41–9.

54. McNeill G, Bryden D. Do either early warning systems or emergency response teams improve hospital patient survival? A systematic review. *Resuscitation* 2013; **84**: 1652–67.

Chapter 17

Acute kidney injury in surgical patients

R. Kishen

It is important to understand what causes compromise in renal function and acute kidney injury (AKI) in surgical patients. Perioperative AKI has serious consequences as it increases length of intensive care unit (ICU) and hospital stay as well as mortality. A significant number of these patients will progress to end-stage renal disease (ESRD) should they survive the original insult. The importance of recognizing the patients at risk, factors that cause or worsen AKI, and steps to prevent or at least lessen the impact of renal insults in vulnerable patients cannot be overemphasized.

Introduction

The main functions of the kidneys are maintenance of fluid and electrolyte homeostasis, excretion of waste products of metabolism, control of vascular tone and blood pressure, and regulation of hematopoiesis and bone metabolism. Kidneys are robust organs and will function under many adverse physiological conditions; however, AKI is not uncommon in surgical patients. Perioperative AKI increases morbidity, length of ICU and hospital stay as well as mortality, not to mention increased healthcare costs, both immediately and in the long term. These patients are critically ill and should be managed in ICU where various organ support facilities are immediately available. In hospital patients, the diagnosis of AKI is frequently delayed and subsequent management is often inadequate [1]. It is thus imperative for anesthetists, surgeons, intensivists, and all those caring for surgical patients to understand the pathophysiology of and risk factors for development of AKI as well as its prevention and management [2].

Basic applied physiology

In order to appreciate the various mechanisms and processes involved in renal dysfunction and AKI, it is important to revise some basic physiological principles [3]:

- Kidneys receive 20%–25% of cardiac output (CO) – the highest blood supply per unit weight of any organ system (after carotid body). Oxygen delivery to the kidney is about 80 mL/min/100 g of tissue, making kidneys one of the best perfused organs.
- Distribution of this blood flow in the kidney is not uniform; the cortex receives about 90% of the total blood flow – necessary to produce large volumes of glomerular filtrate. The renal medulla, metabolically very active, receives only about 10% of blood flow; low

Anesthesia and Perioperative Care of the High-Risk Patient, Third edition, ed. Ian McConachie. Published by Cambridge University Press.

blood flow in the medulla is to maintain the high osmolality in the medullary interstitium.

- Kidneys have complex blood supply patterns. The renal artery divides into segmental arteries, which are end arteries in that there is no collateral circulation between them. These segmental arteries divide into interlobular arteries, which in turn give rise to afferent arterioles (each arteriole has a sphincter) that supply blood to the glomerular tuft of capillaries. Glomerular capillaries drain into efferent arterioles (each also has a sphincter), which then divide to become peritubular capillaries (for cortical nephrons) or vasa recta (for juxtamedullary nephrons). Afferent and efferent arteriolar sphincters regulate blood flow to glomerular capillaries in response to various stimuli, especially tubuloglomerular feedback (TGF).
- Under normal physiological conditions, there is little change in renal blood flow (RBF) despite variations in mean arterial pressure (MAP). However, this may not be so under pathological conditions.
- The nephron is the metabolically active unit of the kidney. Most of the excreted sodium in glomerular filtrate is reabsorbed in the proximal convoluted tubule and medullary thick ascending part of the loop of Henlé (mTAL). Sodium reabsorption (against medullary interstitial osmotic gradient) is an energy consuming process, involves an Na/K-ATPase carrier, and accounts for about 80%–90% of the kidney's oxygen consumption. Most of the filtered water is reabsorbed in the loop of Henlé and collecting ducts.
- Although the kidney has high oxygen delivery, its overall oxygen extraction is low, there being regional differences in oxygen extraction within the kidney. The renal cortex extracts only about 18% of oxygen delivered to it whereas the medulla extracts about 80%. Thus medullary structures, like mTAL, because of low medullary blood flow and high oxygen extraction, work virtually at the verge of hypoxia; these metabolically active medullary structures are highly vulnerable to hypoperfusion and tissue hypoxia.
- Various regulatory mechanisms exist in the kidneys for preserving local blood flow and oxygen delivery. These include:
  - elaboration of nitric oxide, various dilating prostaglandins (e.g., prostaglandin E_1, prostacyclin), dopamine, and urodilatin (urinary analog of atrial natriuretic factor)
  - formation of vasoconstrictors like endothelins and angiotensin II
  - TGF: a mechanism that can feed back to the afferent (and the efferent) arterioles to regulate glomerular filtrate (decrease or increase it) depending on hydration, perfusion, and other factors. At times of low perfusion, TGF causes afferent arteriolar sphincter constriction, reduced filtration pressure in the glomerulus, and less filtrate is presented to the tubule; this reduces tubular function as less sodium needs to be reabsorbed, reducing tubular oxygen consumption and preserving tubular cell integrity at times of hypoperfusion
  - Medullary tubular growth factors like insulin-like growth factor I and epidermal growth factor are also elaborated; however, their role in pathogenesis or renal recovery in humans has not been studied fully

It should be appreciated that a large proportion of CO received by the kidneys is designed to produce large quantities of glomerular filtrate (necessary to excrete adequate quantities of toxins and metabolic waste) that is subsequently modified in the renal tubules and collecting ducts to form urine – most (99%) of the glomerular filtrate being reabsorbed.

In hypovolemic conditions (regardless of whether hypotension is present), dehydration and reduced CO, TGF, and other mechanisms come into play to preserve body fluid, which clinically manifests as oliguria. *Thus, oliguria is not always a sign of renal dysfunction* [4].

Acute renal failure is now called AKI

Defining AKI in the critically ill patient has suffered from inconsistency and wide variation. This has confounded the clinicians as it is difficult to make sense of published literature and make informed decisions [5]. Clinicians also need to appreciate that small and even transient increases in serum creatinine are associated with increased risk of death.

- Acute cessation of urine formation and rise in uremic toxins (urea and creatinine) in the blood is indicative of "renal failure" [6]. However, clinicians should be aware that sudden, absolute and total anuria is a blocked urinary catheter unless proven otherwise.
- More than 30 definitions of AKI have appeared in the literature in the past, making it difficult to analyze the literature meaningfully and to compare treatment strategies [7,8].
- Acute renal failure describes a process rather than a single stage of disease – the traditional "all or nothing" phenomenon [2]. The term AKI is an important step forward because it includes even those patients in whom complete failure of kidney function has not, as yet, set in. It allows clinicians to recognize renal dysfunction earlier when early appropriate actions may interrupt a process of decline into total failure of kidney function.
- Definitions based on glomerular filtration rate (GFR) and creatinine clearance (CC) are not practical in the critically ill patient as results of these tests are not available immediately.
- Work to assess the feasibility and diagnostic utility of biomarkers of renal injury is ongoing. Thus cystatin C, neutrophil gelatinase-associated lipocalin, interleukin 18, and kidney injury molecule 1 (KIM1) are being studied extensively [3,9,10]. Any or all of these markers may become available as easy bedside tests in the future; at present, they are not recommended for routine use in the clinical setting [10].
- Measurement of serum creatinine (SCr) and urine output (UO) has its own problems. Creatinine is influenced by age, gender, diet, muscle mass, etc., and UO is affected by the state of the patient's hydration, MAP, CO, and use of diuretics. In patients with pre-existing renal dysfunction, SCr rises disproportionately to kidney injury, and although indicative of emerging AKI, does not reflect its severity accurately.
- However, SCr and UO are easily measurable bedside parameters. Hence, any definition incorporating these two parameters is easy to employ in clinical practice.
- Emerging data have shown that even small or modest rises in SCr are associated with an adverse outcome in hospitalized patients [11,12]. Studies in patients having had cardiac surgery and with other cardiac conditions have also shown a similar pattern [13]. Hence, new definitions based on relatively small changes in SCr and UO have been proposed.
- Acute Dialysis Quality Initiative (ADQI) [14] has proposed RIFLE (risk, injury, failure, loss, and ESRD) criteria for AKI. The RIFLE criteria define AKI severity grades based on GFR/SCr, UO, and clinical outcome (Table 17.1) [15]. This definition inevitably will

Table 17.1. RIFLE criteria for AKI

	GFR criteria	UO criteria	
Risk	↑ in serum creatinine × 1.5 or ↓ in GFR >25%	UO <0.5 ml/kg/h over 6 h	High sensitivity
Injury	↑ in serum creatinine × 2 or ↓ in GFR >50%	UO <0.5 ml/kg/h over 12 h	
Failure	↑ in serum creatinine × 3 or ↓ in GFR >75% or serum creatinine > μmol/L or an acute rise of 48 μmol/L	UO <0.3 ml/kg/h over 24 h or anuria for 12 h (oliguria)	
Loss	Persistent AKI – complete loss of renal function >4 wk		High specificity
ESRD	End-stage renal disease (>3 mo)		

Table 17.2. Staging criteria for AKI

Stage	Creatinine	UO
1	≥26 μmol/L or 1.5- to 2-fold increase	<0.5 mL/kg/h >6 h
2	Increase by 2-fold to 3-fold	<0.5 mL/kg/h >12 h
3	Increase by >3-fold	< 0.3 mL/kg/h or anuria >12 h

increase the prevalence of AKI in that more patients who hitherto would not have been classified as suffering from "acute renal failure" will be identified as having AKI. The majority of the studies suggest that the use of RIFLE criteria convey significant prognostic information, at least in the ICU setting.

- More recently, the Acute Kidney Injury Network (AKIN) [16] has suggested a simplified definition, which depends on a smaller rise of creatinine (>25 μmol/L or a >50% rise from base line) or the development of oliguria (as defined by a UO of <0.5 mL/kg/hr for 6 hr or more) (Table 17.2) within 48 hours. These have simply been called "AKIN Staging Criteria." AKIN criteria also increase the prevalence of AKI, like ADQI RIFLE criteria.
- RIFLE and AKIN criteria are being extensively validated in terms of universal applicability and studies have shown that these definitions are clinically useful. Neither RIFLE nor AKIN criteria clearly define the points at which renal replacement therapy (RRTh) should be commenced or stopped.
- The author has used a simple working definition (similar to RIFLE and AKIN criteria, but predating them) based on SCr and UO for clinical decision making [17]. Thus, an adequately fluid-loaded patient with a precipitating etiological factor and/or risk factors (see later), with a normal or near normal MAP and CO (whether measured or clinically judged) and who exhibits:
  - a urine output of <0.25 mL/kg/hr for 6 hr (<500 mL/d in a 80 kg adult)
  - a rise of 50% in SCr in 12–24 hr
  - metabolic acidosis – not explained by clinical condition (e.g., sepsis, hyperchloraemia, etc.)

  fulfills a clinical definition indicating that renal function has failed (criterion F of RIFLE and stage III in AKIN criteria). This is also helpful in making the clinical decision for starting RRTh. It must be emphasized that the definition is only applied when all causes of the so-called pre-renal azotemia or failure have been eliminated (see later) and the irreversibility of AKI is established.

It cannot be overemphasized that RIFLE and AKIN criteria allow us to be aware of deteriorating renal function early so that adequate appropriate steps can be taken to prevent further decline into anuric AKI. This is an important advance in our day-to-day management of all critically ill patients.

Classification, pathophysiology, diagnostic tests, and incidence of AKI

Types of renal failure

Traditionally, textbooks have taught generations of doctors that renal failure is of three types: pre-renal, renal, and post-renal. It is still the popular teaching.

- Pre-renal failure describes renal failure due to factors before blood reaches the kidneys for purification (e.g., hypovolemia, hypotension, low CO, hemorrhage, etc.).
- Renal failure is due to intrinsic pathology of renal parenchyma caused by a variety of conditions, such as various nephropathies (vasculitides, pigment-induced renal damage, contrast-induced nephropathy, interstitial nephritides, etc.), and drug- and antibiotic-induced AKI. Traditionally, collectively these conditions are referred to as acute tubular necrosis (ATN). However, the term ATN does not convey the true pathophysiology of AKI in the critically ill patient.
- Post-renal failure is due to obstruction to the collecting system within the kidney (e.g., renal pelvis) or outside (e.g., ureteric obstruction).
- Pre-renal failure implies etiological factors outside the kidney affecting kidney function (but not including obstruction to urinary excretory pathways). It is not too difficult to imagine why this simplistic view gained popularity, has withstood the passage of time, and has been a popular paradigm for the last half a century [18]. The term is "neat" and helps organize some causes of oliguria as a separate and distinct entity. It is also easy to suggest that this pre-renal state, if not treated, progresses to the next phase – the intrinsic renal phase or so-called ATN, as it is assumed that the untreated pre-renal situation progresses to renal damage by ischemia (a natural consequence of prolonged hypovolemia, hypotension, or low CO!).
- However, there are problems with this concept. Consider, for example, a patient with severe diarrhea and oliguria (due to dehydration, and who may even exhibit raised SCr), classified as having pre-renal failure! In this case, pre-renal failure is not actually failure of kidney function; the kidneys are working normally in preserving the body's fluids and it is simply physiological oliguria [18]. In this situation, fluid therapy will restore kidney function (e.g., normal UO) – therefore, the kidneys have not actually failed. Hence, we need to rethink the utility of this term in the clinical context and abandon this traditional classification of emerging AKI, the pathology of which we do not yet understand fully [19]. It is also difficult to define the point at which pre-renal failure progress to intrinsic renal failure.
- These classical subdivisions of AKI neither explain nor represent the true clinical situations (except in post-renal or obstructive AKI). Simply put, pre-renal AKI is unrecognized resuscitation failure and should prompt immediate evaluation of the fluid and hemodynamic status of the patient. Post-renal AKI should prompt evaluation of the renal outflow tract, as the management of obstructive AKI is dramatically different. As the following section on pathophysiology will show, these three forms of AKI can be present at the same time in these patients.

Traditional classification of AKI into pre-renal, renal, and post-renal types seriously needs rethinking as evidence is emerging that pre-renal cannot be distinguished from renal or persistent AKI by biochemical or clinical markers, and does little for our understanding of its pathophysiology [20]. There is also evidence that even the so-called pre-renal stage shows a rise in some biomarkers of AKI, suggesting that renal injury is present, albeit in a milder form [21].

Pathophysiology

There is a paucity of data about the pathophysiology and morphology of AKI. Traditionally, postoperative AKI is thought to be mostly pre-renal, that is, due to hypovolemia. Established renal failure is thought to be ATN due to ischemia/reperfusion. Animal models have enhanced our understanding of renal physiology but have done little to advance our knowledge of AKI in the critically ill patient [22].

- Experimentally, AKI has been studied in small animal models where, under anesthesia, renal artery clamps are applied for a variable time and the animal's temperature is kept normal. In this situation, there is no blood flow nor are the kidneys carrying out any of their functions – a scenario far removed from clinical situation [19,22].
- Although RBF perturbations in AKI in critical illness are not known with certainty and RBF may be low, it is never zero; thus compromised kidneys are functioning, albeit under a low perfusion state. A few blood flow studies undertaken in humans and large animals have shown that, in the critically ill patient (especially with sepsis), RBF is CO dependent and is usually either normal or increased [23,24].
- Biopsy specimens from critically ill patients are lacking; thus, the true nature of renal parenchymal injury is not known [19,22]. The belief that the ultimate pathophysiological picture is that of necrosis or ATN has also been challenged with newer insights into AKI. The few biopsy specimens that are available to us do not show widespread necrosis; on the contrary (in patients with previously normal kidneys), the renal architecture looks remarkably normal [25] despite severely compromised kidney function.
- Abnormalities in renal parenchyma do occur; however, glomerular and tubular cell destruction and necrosis are rare or non-existent and the histology of such kidneys shows an absence of glomerulopathy (for instance, vasculitic renal disorders) [25,26].
- These abnormalities include a reversal of polarity in the tubular cells (the Na/K-ATPase carrier pump relocates to the luminal side of the cell from its basolateral site), cell swelling, and disruption of tight junctions, causing back-leak of tubular luminal fluid into medullary and cortical parenchyma [26]. Tubular cells may come off the basement membrane, and together with cell swelling, this causes tubular obstruction. Tubular obstruction along with disruption of tight junctions and back-leak of tubular fluid manifests as oliguria.
- Disrupted tubular cells may undergo apoptosis, which may be accelerated by cytokines and other by-products of inflammation. Apoptosis is an oxygen-consuming process (necrosis that results from total anoxia due to ischemia) [26].
- Thus the true pathophysiological picture of AKI in the critically ill patient is that of a non-functioning but structurally relatively normal kidney [19]. It is also clear that ATN is a misnomer and its use in describing AKI in the critically ill should be abandoned [27].

AKI in the critically ill surgical patient differs from renal failure seen on nephrology wards or in ESRD [17], having a multifactorial etiology and often being part of the multiple organ dysfunction syndrome. Thus, clinical management of this condition is also different from that of ESRD. AKI may be superimposed on pre-existing renal dysfunction in many patients. In patients with pre-existing renal dysfunction, even slight insults (that would not affect normal kidneys) can cause AKI. Clinicians should appreciate that coexisting hypovolemia, shock, hypotension, possible cardiac dysfunction (one or more may be present perioperatively), and morphological changes in the kidney (cell swelling, back-leak, etc.) may cause tubular cell dysfunction and obstruction – pre-renal, intrinsic, and post-renal situations co-exist in AKI at the same time.

Renal function tests

Classical tests of renal function such as measurement of GFR and CC are established and time-honoured tests in patients with renal failure.

- These tests are useful in patients who are stable and in whom SCr or renal function does not change quickly over short periods of time.
- Critically ill patients are not metabolically stable; biochemical markers for AKI (urea and SCr) change rapidly and there is ever-changing fluid balance, at least in the initial period of critical illness.
- CC requires urine collection over 24 hours, making the test tedious in the postoperative and critical care setting. Although collections over shorter periods (2 or 6 hr) have been shown to be equally valid in some studies [28], others have challenged their accuracy and validity in the critically ill [29].
- Various tests like urine microscopy, fractional excretion of sodium, and urine/plasma ratios are equally not applicable in these patients.
- That kidney dysfunction is present and can be defined (according to RIFLE or AKIN criteria) is enough to make clinical decisions in these patients. These newer definitions also allow early recognition and early appropriate steps to be taken to prevent possible decline to anuric AKI.
- Classical renal function tests performed preoperatively to evaluate renal function are useful in assessing patients and establishing base-line renal function, and may also have a place in special circumstances. However, they will not be discussed further here. Estimated GFR (eGFR), as reported by most laboratories, is a useful indicator of renal function that should be looked for in any preoperative blood tests.

Traditional renal function tests (blood and urine) have limited applicability in the critically ill patient with AKI, and contrary to classical thinking and teaching, certainly do not help to distinguish the so-called pre-renal from other forms of AKI [30].

Incidence

- Until recently, the true incidence of AKI in critically ill surgical patients has been difficult to estimate because of varying definitions of acute renal failure. AKI in the perioperative period has variously been estimated at 0.7%–35%, depending on the definition used.
- In cardiac surgery, the incidence of AKI is estimated at 1%–15% [5]. In patients undergoing cardiopulmonary bypass, other studies have estimated AKI to occur in

7%–8% of cases, with 1%–2% requiring RRTh [31,32]. However, with RIFLE and AKIN criteria, it should now be possible to estimate the true incidence of AKI, which may well be higher.

- In the U.K., data from the Intensive Care National Audit and Research Centre show that the incidence of acute renal failure in patients admitted to critical care areas after major surgery is 0.5%, with ICU mortality of 25% and hospital mortality of 38% [33]. This certainly is an underestimate as patients who develop mild AKI on the surgical wards postoperatively (e.g., AKIN stage I or even II), and which may not be recognized as AKI, are not counted in these numbers. Defining kidney injury based on RIFLE criteria (creatinine rise by 50%) with a minimum SCr of ≥180 μmol/L on admission from theater, AKI increased to 10.5%, with ICU mortality of 32.7% and hospital mortality of 46.3% in the same patient population [33].

Etiology of AKI in surgical patients

AKI in surgical patients is multifactorial in origin. The incidence is higher in patients undergoing complex surgery and prolonged operations, and certain situations are more prone to result in AKI.

Effect of anesthesia on renal function

- Anesthesia per se has little effect on renal function [3]. Most anesthetic agents are vasodilators and depress CO, which may affect renal perfusion; this is of little consequence in patients with normal renal function. However, such hemodynamic alterations may affect renal function in patients at risk and those with pre-existing renal dysfunction [3]. Positive pressure ventilation can reduce CO and renal perfusion, especially in dehydrated and hypovolemic patients [3].
- Certain fluorinated anesthetic agents have been known to cause renal dysfunction due to the liberation of the fluoride ion. Methoxyflurane, which caused high-output renal failure with elevation of SCr and urea, is no longer in clinical use. This nephrotoxicity, thought to be related to the production of fluoride by its metabolism, was seen at fluoride levels of 50–80 mM/L. However, other fluorinated volatile anesthetic agents like enflurane, isoflurane, and sevoflurane are not clinically nephrotoxic, despite fluoride levels of >50 mM/L obtained during their use [34]. Unlike methoxyflurane, which is metabolized to a significant degree in the kidneys, these later agents are relatively insoluble in body tissue and undergo biotransformation in the liver. The site of biotransformation/metabolism may be crucial for the occurrence of nephrotoxicity [34,35].
- Renal toxicity is also caused by haloalkenes produced by inhalation anesthetic agents, which react with CO_2 absorbents. Halothane, enflurane, isoflurane, and sevoflurane are all known to react with CO_2 absorbents. Halothane nephrotoxicity with haloalkenes occurred in rats but was never demonstrated clinically [34]. Sevoflurane reacts with CO_2 absorbents to form a haloalkene, compound A, especially when used in high concentrations, with low fresh gas flows, with baralyme (instead of soda lime), at higher CO_2 absorbent temperatures, and at higher CO_2 production. Despite this, sevoflurane anesthesia with low flows has been found to be safe and renal toxicity has not been convincingly demonstrated in humans [34,35].

- Suxamethonium (succinylcholine) has been known to cause rhabdomyolysis and may contribute to AKI in exceptional circumstances, such as suxamethonium-induced hyperpyrexia [36].
- Epidural anesthesia has been found to be as safe as general anesthesia for renal transplant surgery [37].
- Most other anesthetic agents and other drugs used in anesthesia do not demonstrate any significant nephrotoxicity, although drug and drug metabolite excretion may be affected when renal dysfunction occurs perioperatively.

Effect of surgery on renal function

- Major surgery is associated with an increased incidence of renal dysfunction and AKI is more common after emergency surgical procedures, and cardiac vascular surgery.
- AKI is more common after cardiac than any other surgery; up to 15% of patients may experience elevation of SCr at some point in the postoperative period. AKI following cardiac surgery increases morbidity, length of hospital stay, and mortality (about 60%) [31,32]. AKI in cardiac surgery is associated particularly with reduced CO, increased cardiopulmonary bypass (CPB) time, diabetes requiring therapy, pre-existing renal dysfunction, and age >70 years. Cytokine release, oxidant stress due to neutrophil activation by CPB, and possible pigment nephropathy (due to release of hemoglobin during CPB) are additional factors responsible for AKI [38]. The incidence of AKI is reduced in off-pump compared to on-pump heart operations [39].
- Major vascular and hepatic surgery are also associated with increased risk of AKI. Aortic surgery is a bigger risk factor than operations on peripheral vessels [40]; risks for AKI are increased by advanced age, raised preoperative SCr, large volume blood transfusion, duration of aortic cross-clamping, and requirement of inotropes in the postoperative period. Suprarenal cross-clamping is more of a risk than infrarenal cross-clamping; however, AKI is still related to the total duration of cross-clamping, whatever the site [40]. There is an increased incidence of AKI in emergency aortic surgery than in planned operations [41].
- Any major or prolonged surgery, large intraoperative blood loss, and emergency operations are also important factors for the development of AKI, especially in at-risk patients.

Other etiological factors responsible for AKI in the perioperative period

- Sepsis and/or septic shock are the major causes of AKI in the critically ill. Surgical patients may be septic before surgery or may acquire sepsis in postoperative period. Despite timely and the best treatment, AKI develops in a significant number of septic patients. Mortality of AKI associated with sepsis is unacceptably high despite advances in antibiotics and organ support technologies.
- Concomitant medication used before, during, or after surgery may adversely affect renal function. Thus, nephrotoxic antibiotics, non-steroidal anti-inflammatory drugs (NSAIDs), a combination of nephrotoxic antibiotics, and diuretics will all increase the risk of AKI [42]. With an aging population and multiple prescription drug usage, especially in the elderly, mention must also be made of angiotensin-converting enzyme

inhibitors and angiotensin receptor blockers; their preoperative use has been shown to increase the incidence of AKI; stopping them before surgery may reduce this risk [43].

- Radiological contrast media can cause severe renal impairment, especially if followed by major surgery shortly afterward. Mechanisms of contrast-induced nephropathy (CIN) are not fully understood; local renal vasoconstriction, direct tubular toxic effects, and contrast osmolality have all been implicated [44].
- Multiple trauma, especially requiring large-volume blood transfusion, and rhabdomyolysis (due to crush injuries) are all associated with the increased incidence of AKI. Mechanisms of tubular injury by myoglobin are still being debated. The most commonly accepted mechanism–tubular obstruction by precipitated myoglobin casts in acidic urine [45]–is being challenged and alternative explanations offered. One such explanation is that in acidic urine (pH <5.6), myoglobin dissociates into ferrihemate and globulin; ferrihemate causes impairment of renal tubular transport mechanisms, cell death, and deterioration of renal function [46].
- Abdominal compartment syndrome is an additional factor for AKI in postoperative patients or in victims of multiple trauma. Increased intra-abdominal pressure (IAP) may be caused by ileus, large intra-abdominal hematomata, abdominal organ edema, and intra-abdominal packs. Increased IAP directly compresses the renal parenchyma, reduces renal perfusion, and increases the release of antidiuretic hormone (ADH) and aldosterone (by stimulation of abdominal wall stretch receptors), thus reducing GFR and causing AKI.

Risk factors predisposing patients to AKI during the perioperative period

Recognizing patients who are at increased risk of AKI allows steps to be taken to minimize their exposure to renal insults as well as optimize their pre- and perioperative fluid status [2,47,48]. There are a variety of factors that increase risk of AKI in the perioperative period.

- Elderly patients are at increased risk of AKI. This probably reflects their reduced GFR, reduced nitric oxide production, and associated comorbidities like hypertension, diabetes, and other degenerative vascular disorders [47].
- Chronic kidney disease is a major risk factor. These patients exhibit a more pronounced rise in SCr than those with normal kidneys for the same degree of renal impairment. They are also affected more by trivial renal insults.
- Diabetes (requiring oral hypoglycemics or insulin), cirrhosis, acute or chronic liver dysfunction, pregnancy, pre-eclampsia or eclampsia all increase risk of AKI. Low CO states, cardiogenic shock, use of the balloon pump, and the need for inotropes after cardiac surgery are additional risk factors.
- Preoperative NSAIDs use, inadvertent NSAIDs, COX-1 and COX-2 inhibitor prescription postoperatively especially in patients with risk factors (e.g., diabetes), sodium-depleted patients, those receiving concomitant diuretics and other nephrotoxic drugs, and intravascular volume depletion increase the risk of AKI.
- Sepsis is a major risk, because of hypovolemia, hemodynamic instability, and the effects of endotoxin and various cytokines on renal tubules.
- Multiple myeloma, acid base disturbance, and hypoalbuminemia may increase risk as well.

- Retrospective (n=1166 non-cardiac postoperative patients) [49] as well as prospective studies (n=152 244 surgical procedures) [50] in surgical patients have identified a number of risk factors for AKI. They include: age ≥56 years, male gender, congestive cardiac failure, presence of ascites, hypertension, or diabetes, high-risk (e.g., vascular) surgery, emergency surgery, preoperative SCr >106 μmol/L, duration of surgery, requirement of blood transfusion, American Society of Anesthesiologists physical status score of IV or V, and revised cardiac risk index score of >2 (for detailed discussion, see references 2,49,50).

How can renal function be preserved in surgical patients?

The most important strategies in preserving renal function are: recognition that renal function is deteriorating, awareness of patients at risk, and the steps taken to minimize renal insult. Clinicians should understand that even small increases in SCr (and not its absolute value) are indicative of developing AKI and mechanisms should be in place to review, communicate, and act upon these changes in their patients [2]. Most instances of renal dysfunction in the perioperative period are due to lack of adequate fluid loading, suboptimal perfusion pressure, or low CO – the so-called pre-renal failure. Less than adequate hydration can creep up on the patients insidiously and must be addressed as the first priority. The same is true of inadequate perfusion (blood) pressure and CO. The following section addresses these issues briefly.

- There are no definitely proven strategies that prevent the development of AKI in the perioperative period or in the critically ill patient [51].
- Adequate fluids should be infused so that a urine flow of at least 0.5 mL/kg/hr (without diuretic use) is maintained during and after surgery. Although not scientifically proven, it seems logical and ensures that patients are well hydrated. Fluid resuscitation expands intravascular volume, increases CO, raises blood (hence perfusion) pressure, and improves oxygen delivery; all designed to improve renal perfusion, RBF, and glomerular filtration.
- Specific evidence about the benefits of adequate hydration in preventing AKI is lacking; however, adequate hydration is the first step in ameliorating oliguria. Functioning kidneys, under normal (and even under abnormal) physiological conditions will preserve fluid in conditions of dehydration and hypovolemia – this almost always manifests as oliguria and is not necessarily AKI.
- Benefits of fluid resuscitation are seen daily in our clinical practice. However, the most definitive evidence is seen in studies involving radiocontrast media-induced AKI. One of the most important conclusions drawn from these studies is that pre-contrast hydration reduces the incidence of CIN. Volume expansion, avoiding operations immediately after angiography, and using low-osmolality contrast media are suggested interventions that reduce CIN [44,52].
- Although it has its limitations, central venous pressure monitoring may be adequate in routine surgery to monitor fluid therapy. In complex patients and/or surgery, more sophisticated monitoring may be required. Many devices that monitor heart chamber functions and their filling are available now and being used to good effect.
- Avoiding nephrotoxins in perioperative periods in patients at risk cannot be overemphasized. Clinicians should be aware that nephrotoxin use in the perioperative period can creep up on their patients by well-intentioned desire to

provide pain relief (e.g., use of NSAIDs for pain relief in a patient who has just had an angiographic procedure).

- Choice of fluid for resuscitation is important. Excess chloride-containing fluids (e.g., 0.9% saline) have been shown to be detrimental to renal circulation. There are data indicating that saline-based fluids in both man and experimental animals may adversely affect renal function [53,54]. Studies in dogs have shown that raised serum chloride can reduce renal blood flow, GFR, and urine formation [55].
- An excellent randomized trial of 0.9% saline versus Plasma-Lyte®(a balanced electrolyte solution) in healthy human volunteers has demonstrated reduced RBF velocity as well as reduced renal cortical perfusion with 0.9% saline [56]. A recent observational study in critically ill patients has shown deleterious renal effects of a chloride-liberal fluid strategy; these harmful effects were reduced with a chloride-restricted fluid prescription [57].
- Balanced electrolyte solutions have been recommended as the fluid of choice in surgical patients by a consensus body in the U.K. [58].
- For some inexplicable reason, colloids are preferred by the clinical community in surgical patients in the U.K. Although some studies do show their beneficial effects on circulation, recent studies have cast doubts on their safety. They have also been found to have deleterious effects on renal function, as they increase AKI incidence and the need for RRTh, especially in sepsis [59–62].

Do pharmacological agents prevent AKI?

The prevailing view is that most cases of AKI are due to renal ischemia. This view is perpetuated by inappropriate animal models [19,22] and has led to many preventive therapies that cause renal vasodilation. Smaller trials favor various strategies; however, convincing evidence that one strategy is superior to other, or indeed any strategy works at all, is lacking. There has been a crusade to find a simple, single pharmacological "magic bullet" for prevention of AKI; unfortunately, this "penicillin of AKI" has eluded us thus far.

Dopamine

- Low-dose dopamine stimulates DA_1 and DA_2 receptors, causing renal arteriolar vasodilation and an increase in RBF, as demonstrated in well-hydrated animals (mice) and healthy humans. Dopamine also inhibits proximal tubular sodium reabsorption, thus causing natriuresis [63,64]. On the basis of these effects, it is suggested that low-dose dopamine affords protection in patients at risk of AKI [65].
- More than 200 articles, 60 studies, 17 randomized controlled trials (RCTs), many meta-analyses, reviews, and a Cochrane systematic review have been published since 1966. None of them show any benefit of a low or renal dose of dopamine in either prevention or amelioration of AKI [51,66]. Two large multicenter RCTs in patients with early signs of renal dysfunction have also failed to show any beneficial effect on prevention or outcomes in AKI [67,68].
- Due to its diuretic and natriuretic effects, low-dose dopamine may worsen hypovolemia as well as increase the metabolic load on the mTAL segment. Thus, dopamine may worsen kidney injury. In addition, low-dose dopamine has a direct adverse effect on renal vascular resistance (RVR). Whereas low-dose dopamine reduces RVR in the

normal kidney, it has the opposite effect in a dysfunctioning kidney – worsening hemodynamics in the very situation where it is thought to be useful [69,70].

- Besides, dopamine increases the risk of arrhythmias, has some undesirable neuroendocrine effects, and preferentially increases renal cortical blood flow without enhancing renal medullary blood flow [70].

Furosemide

Furosemide is the most commonly used drug to increase UO, convert oliguria into polyuria, and prevent AKI.

- Furosemide reduces sodium reabsorption by mTAL, thus reducing tubular oxygen consumption and increasing UO. Increased UO may dislodge the tubular obstruction and augment RBF. It also induces cyclooxygenases (COXs) and thereby increases the release of vasodilatory prostaglandins [71]. Furosemide may also cause COX-2 inhibition, which in turn inhibits TNF-induced apoptosis in tubular cells, especially in renal mesangial cells [72].
- Many studies have failed to show any benefit in terms of prevention of AKI, need for reduced RRTh, or reduced mortality. Studies in patients with AKI after cardiac surgery, radiological contrast media, and other forms of AKI have been equally disappointing [73].
- Recent meta-analyses and reviews have also failed to show any benefits other than increased UO in AKI with furosemide, with one study showing a tendency to increased mortality with higher doses of furosemide, probably due to immunosupression [74,75].

Mannitol

- Mannitol, an osmotic diuretic, increases UO, is a free radical scavenger, and in animal studies induces dilatory prostaglandin synthesis (and may thus improve RBF).
- Along with $NaHCO_3$, mannitol is recommended for prevention of AKI in rhabdomyolysis by promoting diuresis and flushing out myoglobin and preventing its precipitation in renal tubules [76]. It has also been recommended for prophylaxis in obstructive jaundice and major vascular surgery.
- However, studies have shown no benefit with mannitol in AKI induced by rhabdomyolysis [77], obstructive jaundice [78], or major vascular surgery [79,80].
- Mannitol can cause endothelial and epithelial cell apoptosis and hypernatremia. Tubular cells also take up mannitol molecules by pinocytosis, which causes cell swelling and cellular damage as well as induces renal vasoconstriction. If the diuretic response is minimal, mannitol induces volume expansion and hyponatremia [81].

Other pharmacological agents

- Fenaldopam, another DA-1 agonist, causes natruresis, and increases in RBF and UO. The RBF increase is dose dependent and equally distributed to the cortex and medulla. It can be safely infused peripherally but causes hypotension and reflex tachycardia. In various studies with small numbers of patients, fenaldopam has been shown to be reno-protective in CIN [82,83] and after CPB [84] and major vascular surgery [85].
- A recent meta-analysis of RCTs suggested that fenaldopam affords renal protection in AKI [86]. However, the studies included in the meta-analysis were of substandard quality, randomization was not obvious in many, and most were underpowered.

- $NaHCO_3$ has been recommended for prevention of CIN as well as AKI in cardiac surgery [87]. A recent meta-analysis has shown a small but statistically insignificant benefit with $NaHCO_3$ in CIN [88], and a recent study showed no benefit but increased mortality with $NaHCO_3$ in cardiac surgery [89].
- Atrial natriuretic peptide, calcium channel blockers, growth factors, N-acetylcysteine, adenosine antagonists, endothelin inhibitors, modulators of the complement system and NO, antioxidants, dobutamine, and dopexamine have all been tried; however, none have proven to be useful [51,81].

Managing AKI in at-risk surgical patients

- The first and most important step is to identify patients at risk. Pre-existing renal dysfunction is the single most important predictor of AKI and identification of such patients cannot be overemphasized. Particularly at risk are diabetic patients scheduled for cardiac or major vascular surgery. Patients with established AKI need monitoring and management in a critical care setting.
- In the U.K., pathology laboratories routinely report eGFR [90]. Although it does not accurately predict GFR in all patients, it is an indicator of existing renal dysfunction.
- SCr and UO should be reviewed regularly. Even small changes in SCr (as little as 25 μmol/L) should be taken seriously and senior and/or expert help sought.
- As AKI results from multiple factors, it is imperative to take note of factors causing AKI and avoid them, especially in patients at risk.
- Thus, as an example, close proximity of angiographic studies and surgery should be avoided. If surgery cannot be delayed, patients should be well hydrated preoperatively.
- Nephrotoxins should be avoided during surgery. Examples are: nephrotoxic antibiotics, diuretics, combination of nephrotoxic antibiotics and diuretics, NSAIDs (even if used by patients preoperatively), hyperosmolar contrast media, etc.
- Along with hydration, blood pressure and CO are determinants of RBF and glomerular filtration. Efforts must be made to keep these parameters as near normal as possible, with appropriate use of inotropes and/or vasoactive drugs if required. MAP should be adequate for the patient; hypertensive patients will require higher MAP to maintain adequate renal perfusion.
- Fluid loading is of utmost importance. There is no consensus on the type of fluid that is better at preventing AKI. However, excess use of 0.9% saline should be avoided as its harmful effects on renal function are now well documented.
- Guidelines for fluid therapy in surgical patients recommend a balanced salt solution like Hartmann's, Ringer's lactate, or similar solutions [58].
- Steps should be taken to establish the reversibility of AKI. This may include but is not limited to careful fluid challenges, optimization of cardiovascular status and MAP, stopping of all nephrotoxic drugs if possible, and re-evaluation of the patient's clinical condition.
- Sepsis must be treated (if necessary by surgical drainage), appropriate antibiotics started, and fractures fixed and stabilized.
- In established AKI, RRTh should be started without avoidable delay; if necessary and depending on the institutional protocols, advice from nephrologists used to dealing with critically ill cases should be sought.

- Detailed description of RRTh specific to critically ill patients is outside the scope of this chapter. Continuous forms of RRTh (CRRT) are preferred as they have various clinical advantages for the critically ill. CRRT should be delivered by healthcare workers familiar with the techniques and equipment management. Detailed standards for delivering CRRT and which contain up-to-date information have recently been described in the critically ill [91].

Conclusions

Although individual anesthetic agents have little direct effect on the kidneys, surgery and anesthesia do affect renal function, especially in patients at risk. There are no definitely proven strategies or pharmacological agents that prevent AKI in the perioperative period except adequate fluid loading. Awareness of factors that increase the risk of AKI, avoiding nephrotoxins, and good hemodynamic management along with adequate hydration are the key to preventing AKI. Such patients should be monitored in critical care areas. In established AKI, RRTh may be required, which should be provided in a critical care setting without undue delay. Most importantly, awareness of AKI, appropriate preventative steps, and obtaining senior and expert (intensivist or nephrologist) advice and help cannot be overemphasized.

Note

Guidelines for the prevention, detection, and management of AKI in hospitalized patients have been prepared by the National Institute of Health and Clinical Excellence (NICE), and were published in August 2013. (Available from: http://guidance.nice.org.uk/CG169.)

References

1. Stewart J, Findlay G, Smith N, et al. Adding insult to injury. A review of patients who died in hospital with primary diagnosis of acute kidney injury. NCEPOD, 2009. Available from: www.ncepod.org.uk/2009aki.htm (Accessed May 11, 2013.)
2. Brothwick E, Ferguson A. Perioperative acute kidney injury: risk factors, recognition, management and outcomes. *BMJ* 2010; **341**: 85–91.
3. Wagener G, Berntjens TE. Renal disease: the anesthesiologist's perspective. *Anesthesiol Clin* 2006; **24**: 523–47.
4. Thurau K, Boylan JW. Acute renal success. The unexpected logic of oliguria in acute renal failure. *Am J Med* 1976; **61**: 308–15.
5. Sadovnikoff N. Perioperative acute renal failure. *Int Anesthesiol Clin* 2001; **39**: 95–109.
6. Nolan C, Anderson R. Hospital-acquired acute renal failure. *J Am Soc Nephrol* 1998; **9**: 710–18.
7. Mehta RL, Chertow GM. Acute renal failure definitions and classification: time for change? *J Am Soc Nephrol* 2003; **14**: 2178–87.
8. Farley SJ. Acute kidney injury/acute renal failure: standardizing nomenclature, definitions and staging. *Nat Clin Pract Nephrol* 2007; **3**: 405.
9. Mori K, Nako K. Neutrophil gelatinase-associated lipocalin as the real-time indicator of active kidney damage. *Kidney Int* 2007; **71**: 967–70.
10. Devarajan P. Emerging biomarkers of acute kidney injury. *Contrib Nephrol* 2007; **156**: 203–12.
11. Chertow GM, Burdick E, Honour M, et al. Acute kidney injury, mortality, length of stay and costs in hospitalized patients. *J Am Soc Nephrol* 2005; **16**: 3365–70.
12. Himmelfarb J, Ikizler TA. Acute kidney injury: changing lexicography, definitions and epidemiology. *Kidney Int* 2007; **71**: 971–6.

13. Lassnigg A, Schmidlin D, Mouhieddine M, et al. Minimal changes of serum creatinine predict prognosis in patients after cardiac surgery: a prospective cohort study. *J Am Soc Nephrol* 2004; **15**: 1597–605.
14. Acute Dialysis Quality Initiative Group. Available from: www.adqi.net (Accessed November 15, 2007.)
15. Bellomo R, Ronco C, Kellum JA, et al. Acute renal failure – definitions, outcome measures, animal models, fluid therapy and information technology needs: the Second International Consensus Conference of the Acute Dialysis Quality Initiative (ADQI) Group. *Crit Care* 2004; **8**: R204–10.
16. Ronco C, Levin A, Warnock DG, et al. Improving outcomes from acute kidney injury (AKI): report on an initiative. *Int J Artif Org* 2007; **30**: 373–76.
17. Kishen R. Acute renal failure. In: McConachie I, ed. *Handbook of ICU Therapy*. London: Greenwich Media, 1999; 161–72.
18. Bellomo R, Bagshaw S, Langenberg C, et al. Pre-renal azotemia: a flawed paradigm in critically ill septic patients? *Contrib Nephrol* 2007; **156**: 1–9.
19. Kellum JA, Ronco C. Controversies in acute kidney injury: the 2011 Brussels Roundtable. *Crit Care* 2011; **15**: 155.
20. Schnider AG, Bellomo R. Urinalysis and pre-renal–kidney injury: time to move on. *Crit Care* 2013; **17**: 141.
21. Nejat M, Pickering JW, Devarajan P, et al. Some biomarkers of acute kidney injury are increased in pre-renal acute injury. *Kidney Int* 2012; **81**: 1254–62.
22. Heyman SN, Rosenberger C, Rosen S. Experimental ischaemia-reperfusion: biases and myths–the proximal vs. distal hypoxic tubular injury debate revisited. *Kidney Int* 2010; **77**: 9–16.
23. Di Giantomasso D, Morimatsu H, May CN, et al. Intra-renal blood flow distribution in hyperdynamic septic shock: effect of norepinephrine. *Crit Care Med* 2003; **31**: 2509–13.
24. Langenberg C, Bellomo R, May C. Renal blood flow in sepsis. *Crit Care* 2005; **9**: R363–74.
25. Solez K, Racusen C. Role of the renal biopsy in acute renal failure. *Contrib Nephrol* 2001; **132**: 68–75.
26. Sheridan AM, Bonventre JV. Pathophysiology of ischaemic acute renal failure. *Contrib Nephrol* 2001; **132**: 7–21.
27. Bock HA. Pathogenesis of acute renal failure: new aspects. *Nephron* 1997; **76**: 130–42.
28. Sladen RN, Endo E, Harrison T. Two hour versus 22-hour creatinine clearance in critically ill patients. *Anesthesiology* 1987; **67**: 1013–16.
29. Cherry RA, Eachempati SR, Hydo L, et al. Accuracy of short-duration creatinine clearance determinations in predicting 24-hour creatinine clearance in critically ill and injured patients. *J Trauma* 2002; **53**: 267–71.
30. Pons B, Lautrette A, Oziel J, et al. Diagnostic accuracy of early urine index changes in differentiating transient from persistent acute kidney injury in critically ill patients: multicentre cohort study. *Crit Care* 2013; **17**: R56.
31. Mangano CM, Diamonstone LS, Ramsay JG, et al. Renal dysfunction after myocardial revascularisation: risk factors, adverse outcomes and hospital utilisation. *Ann Intern Med* 1998; **128**: 194–203.
32. Conlon PJ, Stafford-Smith M, White WD, et al. Acute renal failure following cardiac surgery. *Nephrol Dial Transplant* 1999; **14**: 1158–62.
33. Intensive Care National Audit and Research Centre–ICNARC–Case Mix Patients Database; November 2007 (1996–2006).
34. Mazze RI. Fluorinated anaesthetic nephrotoxicity: an update. *Can J Anaesthesia* 1984; **31**: S16–22.
35. Reichle F, Conzen PF, Peter C. Nephrotoxicity of halogenated inhalation anaesthetics: fictions and facts. *Eur Surg Res* 2002; **34**: 188–95.

36. Coco TJ, Klasner AE. Drug-induced rhabdomyolysis. *Curr Opin Paediatr* 2004; **16**: 206–10.

37. Akpek EA, Kayhan Z, Dönmez A, et al. Early postoperative renal function following renal transplant surgery: effect of anaesthetic technique. *J Anesth* 2002; **16**: 114–18.

38. Haase M, Haase-Fielitz A, Bagshaw SM, et al. Cardio-pulmonary bypass-associated acute kidney injury: a pigment nephropathy? *Contrib Nephrol* 2007; **156**: 340–53.

39. Massoudy P, Wagner S, Thielmann M, et al. Coronary artery bypass surgery and acute kidney injury–impact of the off-pump technique. *Nephrol Dial Transplant* 2008; **23**: 2853–60.

40. Tallgren M, Niemi T, Pöyhiä R, et al. Acute renal injury and dysfunction following elective abdominal aortic surgery. *Eur J Vasc Endovasc Surg* 2007; **33**: 550–5.

41. Braams R, Vossen V, Lisman BA, et al. Outcome in patients requiring renal replacement therapy after surgery for ruptured and non-ruptured aneurysm of the abdominal aorta. *Eur J Endovasc Surg* 1999; **18**: 323–7.

42. Kishen R. Drug-induced nephropathy and acute renal injury in the critically ill. In: Nayyar V, Peter JV, Kishen R, et al., eds. *Critical Care Update 2006*. New Delhi: Jaypee Brothers, 2006; 68–75.

43. Arora P, Rajagopalam S, Ranjan R, et al. Preoperative use of angiotensin converting enzyme inhibitors/angiotensin receptor blockers is associated with increased risk for acute kidney injury after cardiovascular surgery. *Clin J Am Soc Nephrol* 2008; **3**: 1266–73.

44. Thomsen HS, Morcos SK. Contrast media and the kidney: European Society of Urogenital Radiology (ESUR) guidelines. *Br J Radiol* 2003; **76**: 513–18.

45. Prendergast BD, George CF. Drug-induced rhabdomyolysis: mechanisms and management. *Postgrad Med J* 1993; **69**: 333–6.

46. Thompson PD, Clarkson P, Karas R. Statin-associated myopathy. *JAMA* 2003; **289**: 1681–90.

47. Novis BK, Roizen MF, Aronson S, et al. Association of preoperative risk factors with postoperative renal failure. *Anesth Analg* 1994; **78**: 143–9.

48. Chertow GM, Lazarus JM, Christiansen CL, et al. Perioperative renal risk stratification. *Circulation* 1997; **95**: 878–84.

49. Abelha FJ, Botelho M, Fernandes V, et al. Determinants of postoperative acute kidney injury. *Crit Care* 2009; **13**: R79.

50. Kheterpal S, Tremper K, Heung M, et al. Development and validation of an acute injury risk index for patients undergoing general surgery: results from a national data set. *Anesthesiology* 2009; **110**: 505–15.

51. Zacharias M, Gilmore ICS, Herbison GP, et al. Interventions for protecting renal function in the perioperative period. *Cochrane Database Syst Rev* 2005; **3**: CD003590.

52. Solomon R, Deray G. How to prevent contrast-induced nephropathy and manage risk patients: practical recommendations. *Kidney Int* 2006; **69**: S51–3.

53. Wilkes NJ, Woolf R, Mutch M, et al. The effects of balanced versus saline-based hetastarch and crystalloid solutions on acid–base and electrolyte status and gastric mucosal perfusion in elderly surgical patients. *Anesth Analg* 2001; **93**: 811–16.

54. Wilcox CS. Regulation of renal blood flow by plasma chloride. *J Clin Invest* 1983; **71**: 726–35.

55. Heidemann HT, Jackson EK, Gerkens JF, et al. Intrarenal hypertonic saline infusions in dogs with thoracic caval constriction. *Kidney Int* 1987; **32**: 488–92.

56. Chowdhury AH, Cox EF, Francis ST, et al. A randomized, controlled, double-blind crossover study on the effects of 2-L infusions of 0.9% saline and on renal blood flow velocity and renal cortical tissue perfusion in healthy volunteers. *Ann Surg* 2012; **256**: 18–24.

57. Yunos NM, Bellomo R, Hegarty C, et al. Association between a chloride-liberal vs

chloride-restrictive intravenous fluid administration strategy and kidney injury in critically ill adults. *JAMA* 2012; **308**: 1566–72.

58. Powell-Tuck J, Gosling P, Lobo DN, et al. British consensus guidelines on intravenous fluid therapy for adult surgical patients. 2011. Available from: http://www.bapen.org.uk/pdfs/bapen_pubs/giftasup.pdf (Accessed May 28, 2013.)

59. Hodgson E, Teboul JL, Kishen R. Current views on fluid therapy in the critically ill. *Fluids* 2013; **2**: 7–13.

60. Bunkhorst FM, Engel C, Bloos F, et al. Intensive insulin therapy and pentastarch resuscitation in severe sepsis. *N Eng J Med* 2008; **358**: 125–39.

61. Penner A, Hasse N, Guttormsen AB, et al. Hydroxyethyl starch versus Ringer's acetate in sepsis. *N Eng J Med* 2012; **367**: 124–34.

62. Myburgh JA, Finfer S, Bellomo R, et al. Hydroxyethyl starch or saline for fluid resuscitation in intensive care. *N Eng J Med* 2012; **367**: 1901–11.

63. McDonald R, Goldberg I, McNay J, et al. Effects of dopamine in man: augmentation of sodium excretion, glomerular filtration rate and renal plasma flow. *J Clin Invest* 1964; **43**: 1116–24.

64. Hollenberg MK, Adams DF, Mendall P, et al. Renal vascular responses to dopamine: haemodynamic and angiographic observations in normal man. *Clin Sci* 1973; **45**: 733–42.

65. Cuthbertson BH, Noble DW. Dopamine in oliguria. *BMJ* 1997; **314**: 690–1.

66. Kellum JA. Use of dopamine in acute renal failure: a meta-analysis. *Crit Care Med* 2001; **29**: 1526–31.

67. Chertow GM, Sayegh MH, Allgern RL, et al. Is the administration of dopamine associated with adverse or favourable outcome in acute renal failure? Auriculin Anaritide Acute Renal Failure Study Group. *Am J Med* 1996; **101**: 49–53.

68. Bellomo R, Chapman M, Finer S, et al. Low dose dopamine in patients with early renal dysfunction: a placebo-controlled randomised trial. Australian and New Zealand Intensive Care Society (ANZICS) Clinical Trials Group. *Lancet* 2000; **356**: 2139–43.

69. Lauschke A, Teichgräber MA, Frei U, et al. 'Low-dose' dopamine worsens renal perfusion in patients with acute renal failure. *Kidney Int* 2006; **69**: 1669–74.

70. Tang IY. Prevention of perioperative acute renal failure: what works? *Best Pract Res Clin Anaesthsiol* 2004; **18**: 91–111.

71. Liguori A, Casini A, Di Loreto M, et al. Loop diuretics enhance the secretion of prostacyclin in vitro, in healthy persons, and in patients with chronic heart failure. *Eur J Clin Pharmacol* 1999; **55**: 117–24.

72. Ishaque A, Dunn MJ, Sorokin A. Cyclooxigenase -2 inhibits tumour necrosis alpha-mediated apoptosis in renal glomerular mesangial cells. *J Biol Chem* 2003; **278**: 10629–40.

73. Schetz M. Should we use diuretics in acute renal failure? *Best Pract Res Clin Anaesthesiol* 2004; **18**: 75–89.

74. Ho KM, Sheridan DJ. Meta-analysis of frusemide to prevent or treat acute renal failure. *BMJ* 2006; **333**: 420.

75. Sampath S, Moran JL, Graham PL, et al. The efficacy of loop diuretics in acute renal failure: assessment using Bayesian evidence synthesis techniques. *Crit Care Med* 2007: **35**: 2516–24.

76. Better OS, Rubinstein I. Management of shock and acute renal failure in casualties suffering from the crush syndrome. *Renal Failure* 1997; **19**: 647–53.

77. Homsi E, Barreiro MF, Orlando JM, et al. Prophylaxis of acute renal failure in patients with rhabdomyolysis. *Renal Failure* 1997; **19**: 283–8.

78. Gubern JM, Sancho JJ, Simo J, et al. A randomized trial on the effect of mannitol on postoperative renal function in patients with obstructive jaundice. *Surgery* 1988; **103**: 39–44.

79. Pass LJ, Eberhart RC, Brown JC, et al. The effect of mannitol and dopamine on the renal response to thoracic aortic cross-clamping. *J Thor Cardiovasc Surg* 1988; **95**: 608–12.

80. Baker AB, Lloyd G, Fraser TA, et al Retrospective review of 100 cases of endoluminal aortic stent-graft surgery from an anaesthetic perspective. *Anaesth Intensive Care* 1997; **25**: 378–84.

81. Jarnberg P-O. Renal protection strategies in the perioperative period. *Best Pract Res Clin Anaesthesiol* 2004; **18**: 645–60.

82. Tumlin JA, Wang A, Murray PT, et al. Fenaldopam mesylate blocks reduction in renal plasma flow after radiocontrast dye infusion: a pilot trial in the prevention of contrast nephropathy. *Am Heart J* 2002; **143**: 894–903.

83. Kini AS, Mitre CE, Kamran M, et al. Changing trends in incidence and predictors of radiographic contrast nephropathy after percutaneous coronary intervention with use of fenaldopam. *Am J Cardiol* 2002; **89**: 999–1002.

84. Halpenny M, Lakshmi S, O'Donnell A, et al. Fenaldopam: renal and splanchnic effects in patients undergoing coronary artery bypass grafting. *Anaesthesia* 2001; **56**: 953–60.

85. Halpenny M, Rushe C, Breen P, et al. The effect of fenaldopam on renal function in patients undergoing elective aortic surgery. *Eur J Anaesthesiol* 2002; **19**: 32–9.

86. Landoni G, Biondi-Zoccai GG, Tumlin JA, et al. Beneficial effects of fenaldopam in critically ill patients with or at risk for acute renal failure: a meta-analysis of randomised clinical trials. *Am J Kidney Dis* 2007; **49**: 56–68.

87. Hasse M, Hasse-Fielitz A, Bellomo R, et al. Sodium bicarbonate to prevent increase in serum creatinine after cardiac surgery: a pilot double blind, randomised controlled trial. *Crit Care Med* 2009; **37**: 39–47.

88. Hoste EAJ, De Waele JJ, Gevaert SA, et al. Sodium bicarbonate for prevention of contrast-induced acute kidney injury: a systematic review and meta-analysis. *Nephrol Dial Transplant* 2010; **25**: 747–58.

89. Haase M, Haase-Fielitz A, Plass M, et al. Prophylactic preoperative sodium bicarbonate to prevent acute kidney injury following open heart surgery: a multicenter double-blinded randomised controlled trial. *PLOS Med* 2013; **10**: e1001426. Available from: www.plosmedine.org (Accessed May 23, 2013.)

90. Levey A, Greene T, Kusek J, et al. A simplified equation to predict glomerular filtration rate from serum creatinine. *J Am Soc Nephrol* 2000; **11**: A0828.

91. Kishen R, Blakeley S, Bray K. *Intensive Care Society–Standards for Renal Replacement Therapy*. 2009. Available from: http://www.ics.ac.uk/icmprof/standards.asp?menuid=7 (Accessed May 16, 2013.)

Chapter 18

The role of simulation in managing the high-risk patient

M. Chin and A. Antoniou

Caring for the high-risk surgical patient with multiple comorbidities is frequently challenging, not least because the resulting physiological instabilities and perioperative complications are seen relatively infrequently by many anesthesiologists, especially if working in community hospitals. Training residents to deal with these problems once they have qualified often faces similar problems. Simulation training represents one promising approach to these concerns.

Background

Historically, medical education has often relied upon the apprenticeship model, and in fact, the mainstay of technical skills training in anesthesia remains supervised initial practice on patients.

- By completing a certain number of years of this apprenticeship model training, the hope is that the learner will encounter a sufficient number of situations to acquire an expert level of knowledge and skill.
- In recent years, there have been a number of concerns regarding this model of education, especially with the increasing complexity of patients and decreasing tolerance of medical error [1].

In 2000, the U.S. Institute of Medicine released a landmark publication entitled *To Err is Human: Building a Safer Health System* [2]. In this document, the Committee on Quality of Health Care in America revealed the startling statistic that as many as 98 000 patients die as a result of medical error every year, surpassing the mortality rates of motor vehicle accidents, breast cancer, or AIDS [2]. The committee proposed a number of recommendations for improving the rates of medical error; among them the use of simulation-based training.

In its broadest sense, simulation refers to the imitation or representation of one act or system by another. In healthcare, it is used in a variety of different settings from technical skills training to team and crisis resource management training. The need to provide students with the ability to learn through simulation has been apparent for many years. It is only in the last decade that this need is being met through the development of new technologies and teaching methods and the continued "buy-in" of the utility of simulation.

The evolution of simulation techniques and equipment has provided unlimited opportunities for education and research into how students learn, which learning methods are

Anesthesia and Perioperative Care of the High-Risk Patient, Third edition, ed. Ian McConachie. Published by Cambridge University Press.

better suited for certain aspects of patient care, and how healthcare professionals can function better as a team in any situation including the management of a high-risk patient in an acute crisis.

Changing landscape of medical education

Decreasing acceptance of the "learning curve"

The term "learning curve" has often been used to explain higher complication rates and mortalities associated with inexperienced practitioners and teams. With the increasing availability of technology to teach technical skills, there has been a paradigm shift within medical education, questioning the ethical nature of learning on patients. For example:

- A review in *BMJ* deplored that "training in technical procedures is often unsystematic and unstructured" [3].
- An editorial in the *New England Journal of Medicine* stated that "It is no longer acceptable, or appropriate, for students at any level of training to practice new skills on patients, even if they have a patient's explicit consent" [4].
- More recently, in *Chest*: "It is time to put see one, do one, teach one behind us. Procedure training should involve a combination of didactics and simulation, with objective evidence of technical competency before exposing patients to the risk of procedures performed by novice operators" [5].

Decreasing availability and increasing complexity of patients

Increasing numbers of medical learners combined with work hour reductions have resulted in a more limited exposure to patients with potentially life-threatening conditions. As a result, medical learners may not gain the necessary experience in order to be confident and competent in early recognition and management of these low-frequency, high-acuity situations – also known as critical incidents.

Critical incidents are defined as occurrences that, if not discovered or corrected in time, can lead to undesirable outcomes ranging from increased length of hospital stay to death. This includes medical error. Patients and the surgeries that are offered to them, particularly at academic centers, are becoming increasingly complex, escalating the risk of medical error and decreasing the number of appropriate encounters for medical learners [6].

The rates published by the Institute of Medicine represent an overall statistic; thus, it is not surprising that high-risk patients are at an even greater risk for experiencing critical incidents [7]. Simulation has an important role to play in providing trainees with the opportunities to acquire and refine the skills needed to provide competent care for their patients while protecting them from preventable error. These changes in the culture of medical education combined with the theoretical advantages of simulation have stimulated the interest in developing a more efficient and effective way of producing skilled, competent physicians.

Simulation in history

There has been a dramatic increase in the utilization of simulation in the twenty-first century. However, simulation as a teaching and learning platform has been around for decades. Many in the healthcare field identify the origins of high-fidelity simulation from the airline industry and their flight simulators. The history of flight simulation has led to a better understanding of the learning process of both an individual and a team when they are involved in critical situations [8]. This has paved the way for the credibility and acceptance of simulation as a training tool in healthcare.

1960s

- At the encouragement of anesthesiologist, Asmund Laerdal, a Norwegian plastic toy manufacturer developed Resusci-Anne, designed to teach cardiopulmonary resuscitation [9].
- SimOne, the first computer-controlled mannequin patient simulator was designed. It was created at the University of Southern California based on work by Dr. Judson Denson, a physician, and Dr. Stephen Abrahamson, an engineer. Unfortunately, it did not gain much acceptance in the medical field, and as a result, only one model was ever made [10].

1980s

Two teams at Stanford University and the University of Florida developed the next generation of mannequin patient simulators [11]:

- Gainesville Anesthesia Simulator, developed in Florida, began as a method to diagnose faults in anesthesia machines. It was developed eventually into a complete mannequin with software that automatically recognized injected drugs and enabled both predefined physiological changes as well as responses that depend on the actions of the learner.
- Dr. David Gaba, an anesthesiologist, and his colleagues created the Stanford Comprehensive Anaesthesia Simulation Environment (CASE) system. CASE was used to develop the Anesthesia Crisis Resource Management (ACRM) training curriculum, based on the Crew Resource Management aviation model.

1990s

- Higher-fidelity mannequins such as SimMan were developed [10].

Crisis resource management

Traditional medical training has focused on individuals learning to care for individual patients, yet as highlighted by the Institute of Medicine's *To Err is Human...*, most medical errors result from problems in the systems of care, rather than individual mistakes. High-reliability organizations (HROs) are institutions where individuals, working together in high-acuity situations facing great potential for error and disastrous consequences, consistently deliver care and positive results with minimal errors. While great strides have taken place in recent years to improve patient safety, healthcare today, unfortunately, still does not qualify as an HRO [11].

In the 1980s, Gaba and colleagues looked into the postgraduate training model in anesthesia and found gaps in several critical aspects of decision making and crisis management. While there was some existing literature on decision making in medicine, they found that the principles outlined did not apply to the highly dynamic decisions being made by anesthesiologists in the operating room [12]. The unique environment of the operating room, where crises and events change on a minute-to-minute basis, was found to be comparable with what is described by Orasanu and Connolly as a "complex dynamic world" [13]. In this environment:

- Problems are ill-defined.
- Environment is dynamic, and full of uncertainty.
- There is intense time pressure.
- Goals are ill-defined, shift, and compete with each other.
- Action/feedback loops are tightly coupled.
- Stakes are high.
- There are multiple "players."
- Personnel operate under strong organizational and cultural norms [13].

Another complex dynamic world to which anesthesia has often been compared is that of commercial aviation. In the 1980s, it was shown that the vast majority of errors in aviation were in large part due to failure of crew to manage their resources effectively despite possessing the appropriate technical skills [14]. Crew Resource Management was developed to address this disconnect. Using commercial aviation as a model, Gaba and colleagues developed a simulation-based course entitled Crisis Resource Management, reflecting terminology more familiar to anesthesiologists [12].

Crisis resource management is a training course based on the concept of a shared mental model. Mental models are knowledge and mechanisms that can be leveraged to describe, explain, and predict events. Effective teams use a shared mental model to achieve a mutually agreed upon goal in the safest possible manner [12]. To do this, team members must have proper knowledge, skills, and attitudes. Five core components of team effectiveness that have been identified are:

- team leadership
- mutual performance monitoring
- backup behavior
- adaptability
- team orientation [15]

Some of the key principles of crisis resource management described by Murray et al. are:

- establishing leadership and support for the leader
- recognizing specific functions of a leader
- importance of communication
- the need for continuous reassessment
- the use of all available resources
- avoidance of fixation of ideas and goals
- consideration of personality traits for optimal group performance [16]

Leadership

- It is strongly recommended that the leader should stand back and not get physically involved in doing any task. This frees the leader to observe from a distance, constantly assimilating information from team members, and allows him/her to assess the "big picture" situation more accurately.

Members

- Members should be careful not to overstep the role of the leader, but direct all communication through him/her to maximize team situational awareness.

Communication

- The Joint Commission on the Accreditation of Health Organizations analysis of sentinel events and root causes lists lack of effective communication as the number three reason for the occurrence of sentinel events from 2004 to 2012 [17].
- Leonard proposed the SBAR method for ensuring standardization in communication in aviation, which has now been utilized in crisis resource management training [18]:

  Situation – what is going on with the patient?
  Background – what is the clinical background or context?
  Assessment – what do I think the problem is?
  Recommendation – what would I do to correct it?

Global assessment

- The leader should reassess the situation continuously, without getting fixated on individual acts. The default assumption should be that the correct management plan should result in a positive response. If this is not occurring, the role of each member is to question the assumptions and conditions on which the management plan was made.

Resources and support

- In crisis situations, it is important to assess and utilize all resources to their maximal capacity. A leader in this situation should be prepared to request fresh ideas and resources as needed.

Advantages of simulation training

Simulation offers a number of unique benefits in medical education that have been well described previously [6,19,20]:

- Consistent and easy access to learning opportunities – because any clinical situation can be imitated at will, simulation training offers the opportunity to schedule many excellent teaching cases that are rare or difficult to obtain in real life. Simulation offers the ability to gain experience in a controlled fashion, and cases that can be reflected on at leisure.
- Safe environment in which to make mistakes without having to be rescued by a supervisor for patient safety – by removing the danger of causing harm to their patients, learners are able to follow their decisions through to their logical conclusions. This allows them to gain invaluable insight into the consequences of right or wrong actions.
- Customizable learning experiences from novice to expert levels – simulation scenarios can be tailored to a wide range of learners, from focusing on technical skills for beginners, to handling crisis situations that require an expert level of knowledge, technique, and clinical judgment.

- Detailed feedback and evaluation – the hectic pace of actual patient care often does not allow for ideal time to discuss with learners how to improve their performance or why certain events or actions took place. In contrast, simulation allows the debriefing of a scenario immediately after it has been played out. This allows detailed review of the events, promoting reflective practice among learners.

Much of this is especially important for the high-risk patient.

Evidence for simulation training

In describing educational research, it has been stated that: "Defining true effectiveness, separating out the part played by the various components of an educational intervention, and clarifying the real cost:benefit ratio are as difficult in educational research as they are in the evaluation of a complex treatment performed on a sample group of people who each have different needs, circumstances, and personalities" [21]. Research in simulation is no different. It presents an interesting challenge to the evidence-minded clinician, as there are many factors that complicate the assessment of its effectiveness. These include[12]:

- High inter-individual and inter-crew variability – even when scenarios presented are exactly the same, different personalities and interactions result in different outcomes. In order to examine patient outcomes of simulation, a large number of subjects would be required to conduct an adequately powered study.
- Simulation bias – to measure clinician performance in simulation, one of the few tools we have is simulation. Bias can arise when testing the usefulness of simulation-training by using a simulator as a test.
- Time frame of learning – learning and altering complex behaviors occurs over time, and evaluating the effectiveness of simulation would require longitudinal assessment over an extended period of time.
- Potential dilution of effect – it is possible that team training programs have not yet been able to involve all personnel in a given patient care environment, thus diluting the impact of individual simulator-trained members. While simulator training may indeed improve crisis resource management skills, unless these behaviors are reinforced by the healthcare organization in real clinical settings, the impact of simulator training could potentially be negated entirely.

The Kirkpatrick model of grading quality of evidence in educational research proposes four levels or stages of evaluation [21]:

- Level 1 is the evaluation of reaction, measuring the attributes of the learner such as satisfaction or happiness.
- Level 2 is the evaluation of learning, measuring the acquisition of knowledge and skills.
- Level 3 is the evaluation of behavior, attempting to measure the transfer of learning to the workplace.
- Level 4 is the highest level of evaluation, aimed at measuring the transfer of learning to patient outcome, such as morbidity and mortality.

Level 4 evidence for simulation is extremely difficult to achieve, and is still lacking, although these studies are beginning to increase in number. The vast majority of studies on simulation are at levels 1 to 3, and taken together, they suggest a trend toward benefit from simulator-based training.

Acquisition of knowledge and skills

A number of studies have shown improvement in skills in subsequent simulated scenarios.

- Looking at retention of skills, Morgan et al. showed that practicing anesthesiologists who had been trained with mannequin-based simulation with debriefing improved in their clinical management of simulated critical events even up to nine months after a single training session [22].
- A small study of anesthesia residents by Yee et al. showed improvement in nontechnical skills after a single ACRM-type simulator session, which involved participating in three simulated scenarios using a high-fidelity patient simulator followed by instructor-facilitated debriefing [23].
- Schwid et al. showed that even screen-based training for anesthesia residents resulted in better management of mannequin-based anesthetic emergencies than those who studied the same material from a handout [24].
- Kuduvalli et al. showed that anesthesiologists who had simulator training demonstrated a more structured approach and less misuse of equipment during simulated difficult airway scenarios [25].
- Chopra et al. showed that anesthesiologists who had received mannequin-based training for the management of malignant hyperthermia subsequently were able to respond more quickly, and deviate less from management guidelines for following simulated malignant hyperthermia scenarios [26].

Transfer of learning to the workplace

- Wayne et al. showed that residents who had simulation training adhered more closely to the ACLS guidelines during real cardiac events than their traditionally trained counterparts [27].
- A prospective single-blinded randomized controlled trial showed that anesthesia residents who participated in simulator training on weaning from cardiopulmonary bypass had superior performance in the real clinical setting [28].
- One study comparing the use of traditional teaching on patients versus simulation-based training for residents in the placement of central lines in a medical intensive care unit demonstrated that simulator-trained residents required fewer needle passes, showed lines placed resulted in fewer infections, and gained increased resident self-confidence in their procedural skills [29].

Despite these promising results, there are, however, studies that have failed to show any improvements following simulator-based sessions:

- Olympio et al. reported in their study that there was no improvement in resident management of esophageal intubation after simulation-based training [30].
- Borges et al. did not observe any significant change in consultant management of a "cannot intubate, cannot ventilate" simulated scenario following simulation training [31].
- Wenk et al. showed that problem-based learning was equally effective as a simulation session in teaching residents the proper technique of a rapid sequence induction. The difference between groups was that those who had participated in the simulation session were more confident in their skills than the control [32].

Key elements of simulator-based training

It is clear from the literature that while simulation has the potential to enhance learning, it does not consistently do so. Some simulation sessions appear to be more effective than others. Perhaps it is not simulation, in the broad sense, that is important, but key aspects included within simulation sessions that may be invaluable in enhancing learning.

Fidelity

Simulation exists in many shapes and forms, from the practice of interosseus needle insertion using frozen chickens to the replication of an operating theater in a simulation center using the same equipment found in the hospital and a high-fidelity simulated patient capable of countless tasks and responses. There are four main categories of simulators used for healthcare purposes, including anesthesia:

- Part task trainers simulate only part of the patient or task that is of interest. Examples include: Resusci-Anne, medical phantoms for intravenous or central line insertion, and torsos for airway management [10].
- Whole task trainers can reproduce all relevant aspects of a task including visual and auditory feedback. This term is often used to describe a mannequin patient simulator. Those that exist today can simulate an incredible range of physiological, pharmacological, and clinical parameters.
- Screen-based simulators, an example of which is the Virtual Anesthesia Machine created at the University of Florida.
- Virtual reality simulators, an example being the laparoscopic surgery box trainer.

These different types of simulators are sometimes referred to as high- or low-fidelity models, based on the degree of realistic imitation provided by the model. High-fidelity simulators are associated with significant cost, resulting in one of the barriers to the widespread use of this form of simulation. Research has thus been focused on determining what the relationship is between the level of fidelity and the degree of effectiveness of simulation sessions.

- High-fidelity and low-fidelity simulators can have equally positive impacts on learning for novice students [33].
- Nyssen et al. found that there were no significant differences between a low-fidelity computer-based simulator compared to a mannequin-based simulator for training novice and experienced anesthesia residents in the management of simulated anaphylactic shock [34].

The consensus now is that the degree of fidelity could and should increase with the level of training of the learner, as part of a progressive training program [35].

Debriefing

Debriefing is a process involving the active participation of learners in a "facilitated or guided reflection in the cycle of experiential learning" [36]. In simulation, it refers to the feedback process that follows a scenario and encourages the learner to reflect on his/her performance.

Researchers at Harvard University and the Massachusetts Institute of Technology have found the "reflective practitioners," those who learn to scrutinize their assumptions and mental routines, have a greater ability to self-correct and improve their professional skills compared to those without this reflective practice.

- The central idea behind reflective practice is that people make sense of, or process, their external stimuli through internal cognitive "frames" or mental models. These frames influence the course of action that someone takes.
- This is important because, by this token, many mistakes can be understood as the result of a logical course of thinking based on how a person is framing any given situation at that moment.
- Rudolph et al. give an excellent example of a trainee who has only learned to resuscitate a patient with a bag-valve mask. In a situation where s/he is required to treat a hypoxic patient without it, treatment might be delayed in search of this equipment. S/he has framed the situation such that a bag-valve mask is essential to resuscitation, whereas a trainee who has more experience might consider that passive oxygenation or mechanically optimizing the airway opening are other options.
- The role of the instructor in debriefing is to help trainees elicit these frames and develop new, correct frames where they have made errors [36].

Debriefing usually involves expert facilitation, and requires the instructors to create an environment in which participants feel simultaneously challenged and psychologically safe. A rash statement from the instructor during a debriefing can have serious ramifications for a participant: humiliation, dampened motivation, and a reluctance to raise questions [36]. Interestingly, while the structure and content of each debriefing session appear to have a significant effect on learning [37], the format (either video, multimedia, or self-debrief) does not [38]. Regardless of format, it has been shown that providing feedback is likely the most critical element in learning from simulation sessions [39].

Summary

- Simulation is becoming widespread in medical education for a number of reasons:
  - reduced training hours
  - reduced access to patients
  - decreasing tolerance for the "learning curve"
  - increasing public concern for patient safety
  - reduced opportunity for high-acuity, low-frequency scenarios
- Simulation has a role in training the competent anesthesiologist to manage high-risk patients as they are at increased risk for critical incidents. This will only increase in relevance in the future.
- There is no clear proof to date that simulation training results in overall improvements in patient outcomes but there is a definite trend toward benefit from a number of different studies.
- Key elements that may contribute to the usefulness of simulation include:
  - different levels of fidelity
  - debriefing
- While there is much yet to be learned and studied in the area of simulation, it has been said that "we should not wait to broadly adopt this tool in our teaching and in our assessment of competency...we have reached the tipping point (where simulation is fully integrated and accepted into medical education) [5].

References

1. Leblanc VR. Simulation in anesthesia: state of the science and looking forward. *Can J Anaesth* 2012; **59**: 193–202.

2. Kohn LT, Corrigan JM, Donaldson M, eds. *To Err is Human: Building a Safer Health System*. Washington, DC: National Academies Press, 2000.

3. Grantcharov TP, Reznick RK. Teaching procedural skills. *BMJ* 2008; **336**: 1129–31.

4. Aggarwal R, Darzi A. Technical-skills training in the 21st century. *N Engl J Med* 2006; **355**: 2695–6.

5. Murin S, Stollenwerk N. Simulation in procedural training. *Chest* 2010; **137**: 1009–11.

6. Castanelli DJ. The rise of simulation in technical skills teaching and the implications for training novices in anaesthesia. *Anaesth Intensive Care* 2009; **37**: 903–10.

7. Maaløe R, la Cour M, Hansen A, et al. Scrutinizing incident reporting in anaesthesia: why is an incident perceived as critical? *Acta Anaesthesiolog Scand* 2006; **50**: 1005–13.

8. Page R. Lessons from aviation simulation. In: Riley RH, ed. *Manual of Simulation in Healthcare*. Oxford: Oxford University Press, 2008; 37–50.

9. Cooper JB, Taqueti VR. A brief history of the development of mannequin simulators for clinical education and training. *Qual Saf Health Care* 2004; **13**: i11–18.

10. Lampotang S. Medium and high integration mannequin patient simulators. In: Riley RH, ed. *Manual of Simulation in Healthcare*. Oxford: Oxford University Press, 2008; 51–64.

11. Sundar E, Sundar S, Pawlowski J, et al. Crew resource management and team training. *Anesthesiol Clin* 2007; **25**: 283–300.

12. Gaba DM, Howard SK, Fish KJ, et al. Simulation-based training in anesthesia crisis resource management (ACRM): a decade of experience. *Simul Gaming* 2001; **32**: 175–93.

13. Orasanu J, Connolly T. The reinvention of decision making. In: Klein G, Orasanu J, Calderwood R, eds. *Decision Making in Action: Models and Methods*. Norwood, NJ: Ablex, 1993; 3–20.

14. Billings CE, Reynard WD. Human factors in aircraft incident: results of a 7-year study. *Aviat Space Environ Med* 1984; **55**: 960–5.

15. Salas E. Is there a "big five" in teamwork? *Small Group Res* 2005; **36**: 555–99.

16. Murray WB, Foster PA. Crisis resource management among strangers: principles of organizing a multidisciplinary group for crisis resource management. *J Clin Anesth* 2000; **12**: 633–8.

17. Joint Commission on the Accreditation of Health Organizations. *Sentinel event dataroot causes by event type 2004–2012*. 2013.

18. Leonard M. The human factor: the critical importance of effective teamwork and communication in providing safe care. *Qual Saf Health Care* 2004; **13**: i85–90.

19. Fanning RM, Gaba DM. The role of debriefing in simulation-based learning. *Simul Healthc* 2007; **2**: 115–25.

20. Society for Simulation in Healthcare–About Simulation [Internet]. Available from: http://ssih.org/about-simulation (Accessed June 22, 2013.)

21. Hutchinson L. Evaluating and researching the effectiveness of educational interventions. *BMJ* 1999; **318**: 1267–9.

22. Morgan PJ, Tarshis J, LeBlanc V, et al. Efficacy of high-fidelity simulation debriefing on the performance of practicing anaesthetists in simulated scenarios. *Br J Anaesth* 2009; **103**: 531–7.

23. Yee B, Naik VN, Joo HS, et al. Nontechnical skills in anesthesia crisis management with repeated exposure to simulation-based education. *Anesthesiology* 2005; **103**: 241–8.

24. Schwid HA, Rooke GA, Michalowski P, et al. Screen-based anesthesia simulation with debriefing improves performance in a

mannequin-based anesthesia simulator. *Teach Learn Med* 2001; **13**: 92–6.

25. Kuduvalli PM, Jervis A, Tighe SQM, et al. Unanticipated difficult airway management in anaesthetised patients: a prospective study of the effect of mannequin training on management strategies and skill retention. *Anaesthesia* 2008; **63**: 364–9.
26. Chopra V, Gesink BJ, de Jong J, et al. Does training on an anaesthesia simulator lead to improvement in performance? *Br J Anaesth* 1994; **73**: 293–7.
27. Wayne DB, Didwania A, Feinglass J, et al. Simulation-based education improves quality of care during cardiac arrest team responses at an academic teaching hospital: a case-control study. *Chest* 2008; **133**: 56–61.
28. Bruppacher HR, Alam SK, LeBlanc VR, et al. Simulation-based training improves physicians' performance in patient care in high-stakes clinical setting of cardiac surgery. *Anesthesiology* 2010; **112**: 985–92.
29. Barsuk JH, McGaghie WC, Cohen ER, et al. Use of simulation-based mastery learning to improve the quality of central venous catheter placement in a medical intensive care unit. *J Hosp Med* 2009; **4**: 397–403.
30. Olympio MA, Whelan R, Ford RPA, et al. Failure of simulation training to change residents' management of oesophageal intubation. *Br J Anaesth* 2003; **91**: 312–18.
31. Borges BCR, Boet S, Siu LW, et al. Incomplete adherence to the ASA difficult airway algorithm is unchanged after a high-fidelity simulation session. *Can J Anaesth* 2010; **57**: 644–9.
32. Wenk M, Waurick R, Schotes D, et al. Simulation-based medical education is no better than problem-based discussions and induces misjudgment in self-assessment. *Adv Health Sc Educ Theory Pract* 2009; **14**: 159–71.
33. Friedman Z, You-Ten KE, Bould MD, et al. Teaching lifesaving procedures: the impact of model fidelity on acquisition and transfer of cricothyrotomy skills to performance on cadavers. *Anesth Analg* 2008; **107**: 1663–9.
34. Nyssen A-S, Larbuisson R, Janssens M, et al. A comparison of the training value of two types of anesthesia simulators: computer screen-based and mannequin-based simulators. *Anesth Analg* 2002; **94**: 1560–5.
35. Aggarwal R, Mytton OT, Derbrew M, et al. Training and simulation for patient safety. *Qual Saf Health Care* 2010; **19**: i34–43.
36. Rudolph JW, Simon R, Dufresne RL, et al. There's no such thing as "nonjudgmental" debriefing: a theory and method for debriefing with good judgment. *Spring* 2006; **1**: 49–55.
37. Park CS, Rochlen LR, Yaghmour E, et al. Acquisition of critical intraoperative event management skills in novice anesthesiology residents by using high-fidelity simulation-based training. *Anesthesiology* 2010; **112**: 202–11.
38. Boet S, Bould MD, Bruppacher HR, et al. Looking in the mirror: self-debriefing versus instructor debriefing for simulated crises. *Crit Care Med* 2011; **39**: 1377–81.
39. Issenberg SB, McGaghie WC, Petrusa ER, et al. Features and uses of high-fidelity medical simulations that lead to effective learning: a BEME systematic review. *Med Teach* 2005; **27**: 10–28.

Chapter 19

Anesthesia, surgery, and palliative care

V. Schulz, C. Smyth, and G. Jarvis

This chapter will focus on challenges anesthesiologists need to navigate as patients with life-limiting and life-threatening illness present to the operating room (ORm). This chapter will discuss:

- trajectories toward death, challenges in identifying dying patients, decision making, and perioperative do-not-resuscitate (DNR) status
- the use of neuraxial analgesia, in partnership with palliative care (PC), as an interventional option for patients with refractory pain at end-of-life

Dying is a phase of life

Dying is a normal phase of life and death is a social event, yet, the healthcare system has positioned dying and death, as a failure of the patient or acute care, to prevent death. Preventing death is an impossible task to live up to and sets up unmet expectations and experiences of suffering for all involved.

As the baby boomers age, more patients approaching the end of their lives require surgery and anesthesiology care. Acknowledging this reality and creating an approach to care may improve the quality of their care and the flow of ORm practices.

Trajectories toward death

Trajectories toward death describe how patients approach the end of their lives.

Three trajectories [1] toward death include terminal illness, chronic illness, and frailty. These trajectories can occur in combination as well.

- Terminal illness: patients tend to have a steady predictable decline over a relatively short period of time, usually with a clear terminal phase of illness such as advanced cancer.
- Chronic illness: patients have a gradual decline over a prolonged period of time; this decline is punctuated with sudden events of serious illness with some recovery, and the patient often dies suddenly during one of these events. Patients with organ failure such as liver, heart, or lung disease tend to die along a chronic illness trajectory.
- Frailty: patients have prolonged gradual decline and dwindling.

Individual patients die along his/her unique trajectory often blending these general pathways toward death. Consider the patient's trajectory toward death as it provides a more comprehensive assessment and it may influence the goals and plan of care [2].

Anesthesia and Perioperative Care of the High-Risk Patient, Third edition, ed. Ian McConachie. Published by Cambridge University Press.

Challenges in identifying dying patients

Patients being followed by a PC service can be at risk of dying. However, traditional PC services have been developed for patients with terminal illness [3] that only serve a proportion of dying patients.

Dying patients not being followed by PC in the perioperative period may be more difficult to identify:

- It is difficult to apply population-based mortality data to individuals.
- PC is often not involved with patients dying along the chronic illness or frailty trajectories, even as they approach death.
- Referrals to PC often occur late, if at all, even for patients with terminal illness.

Prognostic uncertainty verses risk of dying

- Predictions regarding prognosis are more reliable when a patient is likely to do well, or very poorly [4].
- It can be difficult to determine prognosis with certainty, and providers tend to offer over-optimistic predictions [4].
- Attempts that are being made to predict a patient's risk of dying, using risk stratification from biochemical data, recognize patients at increased risk of dying with limited precision [5].
- Clinical skills are important in prognostication [4].

In practice, the unexpected death is often harder to cope with than the death occurring after substitute decision makers (SDMs) and providers acknowledge the patient is at risk of dying.

Decision making

- Patients may experience sudden serious acute events with some recovery or may die during the event.
- It is difficult to predict with certainty when an event will occur, its severity, the healthcare choices, the patient's response to therapy, and the unique individual decision making regarding care.
- Decision making affects healthcare use as patients approach death.
- If a patient is known to be at risk of dying, acute, chronic, and palliative issues may influence his/her goals of care and the care plans [2].
- Consider the influence of both the patient's trajectories toward death and also his/her acute presenting issues when discussing goals of care and care plans.

Surgery

- Palliative surgery is provided for symptom management for patients with life-limiting illness; for example, patients with known metastatic illness may require bypass of a malignant bowel obstruction.
- Urgent surgery is provided in an attempt to reverse life-threatening illness, such as ruptured aortic aneurysm repair.
- Patients may or may not have a pre-existing DNR documentation prior to arriving in the ORm.

Perioperative DNR status

Resuscitation began in the ORm in the 1960s to manage witnessed arrests. By the mid 1970s the American Medical Association recommended documentation of the decision not to resuscitate and that it was intended for prevention of sudden, unexpected death and not for the treatment of terminal illness [6]. By the mid 1980s it was determined that attempting resuscitation was favored in the majority of situations and therefore patients were presumed to give consent unless otherwise stated as a DNR [6].

Suspending DNR orders in ORm

- U.S. law requires life-sustaining treatments to be continued if the documentation is not clear, or if the physician is unable to validate alternate instructions [6].
- When resuscitation occurs despite DNR orders, the courts resist awarding "wrongful life" damages [7]. Therefore, aggressive resuscitation often becomes the default practice in the ORm [6].

The debate over patient autonomy

In the 1990s, the debate over patient autonomy instigated the American Society of Anesthesiologists (ASA) policy guideline development. The ASA guidelines called for discussions with the patient/SDM to determine the intraoperative DNR status.

The DNR status options include:

- suspending DNR status
- establishing a patient's goals and objectives, allowing the anesthesiologist to provide intraoperative care in keeping with these
- detailing a list of interventions that may and may not be allowed in the ORm [6]

Applying the DNR order in the ORm guideline, in practice, creates challenges [6,7]. Practical considerations are influenced by the:

- ORm environment
- lack of common understanding of the meaning of the DNR among the patient, SDM's, and all providers in the ORm
- role of the anesthesiologist, which is to maintain airway and cardiovascular stability

Therefore, it is confusing where the line would be drawn to apply a DNR order [6,7].

Death in the ORm

- The ORm is isolated from the rest of the healthcare system and the patient's family. ORm policy and procedures after a death do not honor the dying patient; therefore, it is not a location designed for good end-of-life care [6].
- Death that is supported by a medical palliative approach to care is typically expected and accepted. In contrast, surgical deaths are shrouded in a "shame and blame" culture [8].
- Allowing intraoperative DNR instigates cognitive dissonance as individuals (patients/SDMs, ORm providers) and healthcare cultures grapple with divergent contradictory beliefs requiring the simultaneous respect for patient autonomy right to determine his/her resuscitation status [7], with the goal of ORm being safety and survival.

Patient's understanding of DNR status in the ORm

To complicate the understanding of patient expectations, a recent study demonstrated:

- 57% of physicians providing care for patients with a prior DNR thought the DNR should be suspended in the ORm.
- In contrast, only 24% of patients expected the physician to follow the request for DNR intraoperatively [7].

Patients may request the DNR to continue during surgery for a variety of reasons that include their fear of debility post-arrest, or hope an intraoperative death would be a peaceful death [7]. However, the patient does still expect a safe anesthetic standard of practice [9].

Ignoring the issue

Anesthesiologist and surgeons cannot ignore this issue because of social pressures, including:

- increasing rights of autonomy
- aging population
- increasing availability of interventions for life-limiting and life-threatening illness
- usual ORm policy and procedures after intraoperative death
- contradictory notion that death is normal and simultaneously shame and blame surgical culture [8]
- the possible necessity to determine the cause of an intraoperative death as either the result of illness or if it would be blamed on an intraoperative event

Growth in perioperative DNR orders

Perioperative DNR orders are becoming increasingly common [6,7,9] and need to be considered by the patient/SDM, anesthesiologist, surgeon, and others involved in the surgery.

Most importantly, discussions regarding code status between the ORm physicians and patients should always happen [7,9]. However, it has been a source of confusion and tension.

- Time and space are required to have appropriate collaborative conversations that determine whether the DNR order will be suspended, or under what circumstances it will be respected during the ORm, and how this will be communicated in the ORm [9].
- If the DNR is suspended, it is necessary to discuss when or if it will be reinstated [10].
- Providing an anesthetic for patients with prognostic uncertainty and precarious life-limiting and life-threatening illness is commonplace; therefore, skills regarding intraoperative DNR are important.
- Care for patients with a DNR requires an approach that permits discussions, a common understanding, changing ORm policies and procedures on death, etc. to be developed.

Prediction of death and scoring systems

- Frail patients are presenting for surgery and proactive surgical teams for the geriatric populations are being created [10].

- Preoperative scoring systems for emergency surgery that predict death have been reviewed [11]. Age alone does not predict mortality; however, age plus severity of acute illness and comorbidities does predict mortality [11]. Scoring systems do not replace good clinical judgment [11,12].
- Sickness assessment identifies three important variables prior to emergency surgery: hypotension, severe chronic disease, and patients' independent ability to care for themselves [11].
- Most importantly, population-based scoring systems discuss the likelihood of survival, but they do not determine the individuals outcome [11].
- Meaningful bedside preoperative decision making incorporates available resources, patients' lived experiences, patients'/SDMs' decision making and goals, outcome expectations, and ethical issues. These can only be integrated using experienced clinical judgment [11].

Palliative approach

There is a likely role for a palliative approach to be integrated in a systematic way in the perioperative setting to:

- identify patients at risk of dying in the perioperative period [13]
- clarify discussions regarding goals of surgical care as curative, maintenance, or palliative [10]

Palliative medicine certification programs are developing for anesthesiologists and surgeons [14].

Conversations that address end-of-life decision making are edging into anesthesia practice [6,7,9]. Physicians would benefit from a skill set in having end-of-life discussions to understand the goals of care and to ensure an appropriate care plan follows the goals of care [8].

Management of refractory cancer pain

Pain is still a common and feared symptom [15] of cancer with prevalence rates of 64% in patients with advanced disease and more than one third of these rating their pain as moderate or severe [16]. Unfortunately, conventional medical management informed by guidelines and expert opinion might still leave 10%–15% of patients with inadequate pain control at end-of-life [17]. Anesthesiologists can play an essential role in the care of the dying by providing analgesia to cancer patients with intractable pain using such interventional pain management techniques as neuraxial analgesia.

Neuraxial analgesia

Neuraxial analgesia has proven to be effective and is often employed as a "last chance" for pain relief in patients who have failed to gain relief from numerous other treatment modalities [18,19]. The European Society of Medical Oncology published a practice guideline for cancer pain denoting that "intraspinal techniques monitored by a skilled team should be included as part of a cancer pain management strategy, but widespread use should be avoided" [20].

When to consider interventional techniques

The main indications for interventional pain management options in cancer patients are:

- intractable pain that has not responded to conventional pharmacological approaches
- dose-limiting side effects from conventional analgesics [21]

These indications are general, making it challenging for teams to decide when a patient is refractory to treatment. This can be overcome by:

- developing a robust collaboration between Oncology, Palliative Care, and Anesthesiology and providing more analgesic choices to cancer patients at end-of-life [22]
- developing a patient-centered treatment plan early in the patient's disease trajectory that includes as many analgesic tools that interdisciplinary teams have at their disposal; including conventional analgesics, interventions, and a psychosocial-spiritual approach

Although oral, transdermal, and parenteral analgesics still play the principal role in managing cancer pain, there is no good reason that interventional techniques should not be considered when effective analgesia for a cancer patient remains elusive.

Interdisciplinary teams, policies, and procedures

Interventional pain management techniques should be offered in the context of an organized multidisciplinary approach to patient care [23].

Ideally, teams should be made up of anesthesiologists (interventionalists), PC physicians, nurse specialists, pharmacists, social workers, physical therapists, and psychologists [24]. Minimum standards for establishing an interventional cancer pain program [25] include the following:

- institution-specific policies and procedures for the acute care hospital, hospice, and home-care setting
- multidisciplinary team support
- effective communication between team members and clear definition of team members' roles and responsibilities
- continuing education for staff, patients, and families
- clear discharge and follow-up plans for the patient
- provision of 24-hour on-call coverage for patients receiving interventional pain management options

Patient assessment

A thorough medical history, physical examination, and appraisal of laboratory work and diagnostic imaging are necessary prior to interventional pain management [26]. Palliative cancer patients are complex and a thorough understanding of their medical and psychosocial issues will inform a risk–benefit analysis for the individual patient. The necessary components of the assessment include:

- pain history
- completion of the Brief Pain Inventory (BPInv) and/or Edmonton Symptom Assessment Scale (ESAS) to allow comparison pre- and post-intervention
- cancer history, including:

  - diagnosis
  - prognosis
  - metastases (paying particular attention to the spine and central nervous system)
  - previous treatments (surgery, radiation, chemotherapy)
  - planned treatments
  - associated conditions (e.g., hypercalcemia, paraneoplastic syndromes, organic failure, deep vein thrombosis, or pulmonary embolism)
  - ECOG (Eastern Cooperative Oncology Group) performance status
- past medical history
- past psychiatric history (including substance dependence)
- social history (including place of residence and planned disposition following discharge)
- DNR status
- medications (current and past)
- allergies and sensitivities
- physical examination, including:
  - vitals
  - mental status and level of consciousness
  - location of stoma and catheters
  - examination of skin (radiation, ulceration, infection)
- laboratory work (rule out coagulopathy, organ dysfunction, infection)
- diagnostic imaging

Relative and absolute contraindications to intrathecal analgesia

Relative contraindications to intrathecal analgesia in patients with refractory cancer pain are weighted differently in the risk–benefit analysis than relative contraindications to spinal anesthesia in patients requiring elective or emergency surgery. There are many relative contraindications to intrathecal analgesia that commonly occur in cancer patients, including chronic infection, spinal metastases, anticoagulation, and thrombocytopenia. With planning and communication between medical services, many of these issues can be suitably managed, mitigating complications. In cancer patients with refractory pain at end-of-life, the risk of complications may be superseded by goals of care and palliative needs for the individual patient.

Absolute contraindications to intrathecal anesthesia [27]

- lack of informed consent
- evidence of raised intracranial pressure or unstable neurological findings
- untreated local or systemic infection
- untreated coagulopathy

Obtaining patient consent at end-of-life can be challenging, particularly when the patient has an altered level of consciousness from pain, pain medications, or systemic illness. Whenever possible, it is important to involve the family or legal representatives in the consent discussion with the patient, and allow time for consideration and deliberation rather than expediting the consent process.

Treatment planning

Once the decision to proceed with an intrathecal catheter has been made, an individualized treatment plan should be developed. A variety of approaches to the neuraxis can be utilized in a safe manner and will vary depending on clinician expertise, team support, and funding models. There is no consensus in the literature as to whether to proceed with a trial prior to permanent implantation. The interventional treatment plan, however, should be well established in advance and include the following components [26]:

- choice of neuraxial intervention: intrathecal or epidural
- type of catheter infusion system to implant

Pre-procedure:

- management of anticoagulants and antiplatelet agents
- transfusion as required
- patient disposition post-discharge from hospital

Procedure:

- anesthetic for intervention: general anesthetic or conscious sedation
- patient position: prone, lateral decubitus, or sitting
- interlaminar level and approach to enter the spine: midline, left versus right paramedian
- interlaminar level to place the catheter tip
- location to tunnel catheter and/or implant port or intrathecal drug delivery system (IDDS)

Post-procedure:

- neuraxial infusion orders
- titration plan for oral or parenteral analgesics

Epidural versus intrathecal approach

Although both epidural and intrathecal options have been shown to be effective in reducing severe cancer pain [28], the intrathecal approach is preferred for several reasons. These include:

- need for small drug dose and volume
- faster onset of analgesia
- lower risk of catheter occlusion or failure due to fibrosis
- allows for sampling of the cerebrospinal fluid

The disadvantages of an intrathecal approach include:

- increased risk of postdural puncture headache
- small risk of meningitis
- small risk of developing an intraspinal granuloma

Neuraxial infusion systems

There are three [3] types of infusion system utilized in neuraxial analgesia for refractory cancer pain.

- completely implanted system (intrathecal catheter and infusion pump; IDDS)

- partially implanted system (subcutaneous port and intrathecal catheter with external pump)
- percutaneous catheter (with external pump)

There is wide variability in the cost of the different systems. Usage will depend greatly on funding and clinician experience.

Choice of medication

Consensus-based algorithms exist to guide drug therapy for neuraxial analgesia in both chronic pain [29] and cancer pain [30]. The availability of analgesics that can be applied to the neuraxis varies widely depending on the treating center.
The most common and widely used analgesic is morphine.

- Morphine is a hydrophilic opioid that ascends rostrally in the cerebrospinal fluid and acts at the level of the brain and brainstem.
- Morphine has a slow onset of action.
- Morphine is associated with delayed respiratory depression (12–24 hours).
- Pruritus and urinary retention are common side effects of intrathecal morphine.
- 1 mg of intrathecal morphine is equivalent to 100 mg of intravenous morphine or 300 mg of oral morphine.

Fentanyl can also be used in a continuous intrathecal infusion.

- Fentanyl is a lipophilic compound that acts in the spinal cord in close proximity to the dermatome it is infused.
- Fentanyl has a rapid onset of action.
- There is less dose sparing in the conversion of intravenous to intrathecal fentanyl than seen with morphine.

These medications can be used alone or in combination with other analgesics, such as local anesthetics or clonidine.

Effectiveness of intrathecal drugs

There are many factors contributing to the effectiveness of an intrathecal infusion for cancer pain. Some of these factors are modifiable while others are static or out of our control. They can be subdivided into medication, and patient and catheter considerations (modified from Wagemans et al. [31]).
Medication

- dose or mass of drug
- hydrophilic or lipophilic opioid
- hypobaric, hyperbaric, or isobaric solution

Patient

- anatomy of the spine
- intra-abdominal pressure
- age
- weight
- cancer invasion of the spine or neural elements

Catheter

- interlaminar level of catheter tip

Complications and side effects

Neuraxial analgesics are reported to cause less drug toxicity and sedation than conventional medical management [31]. Despite this beneficial effect, there are medication-, patient-, and equipment-related complications specific to neuraxial infusions [32].

Medication-related

- sedation
- respiratory depression
- hypotension
- pruritus
- urinary retention
- constipation
- hypogonadism
- peripheral edema
- drug toxicities
- intraspinal granuloma

Patient-related

- nerve injury and paralysis
- postdural puncture headache
- meningitis
- local infection or cellulitis over implant
- wound dehiscence
- hematoma or seroma

Equipment-related

- catheter dislodgement or migration
- catheter obstruction
- catheter tears
- mechanical failure
- pump or subcutaneous port flipping

In summary, the benefit of neuraxial analgesia in cancer patients is clear but must be juxtaposed against the potential for serious complications and the need for complex specialized care. Despite this, neuraxial analgesia provided by anesthesiologists and organized through a multidisciplinary team can play a significant role in relieving suffering and improving quality of life for cancer patients.

References

1. Murray SA, Kendall M, Boyd K, et al. Illness trajectories and palliative care. *BMJ* 2005; **330**: 1007–11.
2. Streat SJ. Illness trajectories are also valuable in critical care. *BMJ* 2005; **330**: 1272.
3. Fassbender K, Fainsinger RL, Carson M, et al. Cost trajectories at the end of life: the Canadian experience. *J Pain Symptom Manage* 2009; **38**: 75–80.
4. Stiel S, Bertram L, Neuhaus S, et al. Evaluation and comparison of two

prognostic scores and the physicians' estimate of survival in terminally ill patients. *Support Care Cancer* 2010; **18**: 43–9.

5. Brabrand M, Knudsen T, Hallas J. Identifying admitted patients at risk of dying: a prospective observational validation of four biochemical scoring systems. *BMJ Open Access* 2013; **3**: e002890.

6. Ewanchuk M, Brindley PG. Ethics review: perioperative do-not-resuscitate orders–doing 'nothing' when 'something' can be done. *Crit Care* 2006; **10**: 219.

7. Burkle CM, Swetz KM, Arnstrong MH, et al. Patient and doctor attitudes and beliefs concerning perioperative do not resuscitate orders: anesthesiologists' growing compliance with patient autonomy and self determination guidelines. *BMC Anesthesiol* 2013; **13**: 2.

8. Novick RJ, Schulz V. The distinct role of palliative care in the surgical intensive care unit. *Semin Cardiothorac Vasc Anesth* 2013; **17**: 240–8.

9. Brindley PG. Perioperative do-not-resuscitate orders: it is time to talk. *BMC Anesthesiology* 2013; **13**: 1.

10. Hardin RE, Le Jemtel T, Zenilman ME. Experience with dedicated geriatric surgical consult services: meeting the need for surgery in the frail elderly. *Clin Interv Aging* 2009; **4**: 73–80.

11. Rix TE, Bates T. Pre-operative risk scores for the prediction of outcome in elderly people who require emergency surgery. *World J Emerg Surg* 2007; **2**: 16.

12. Horwood J, Ratnam S, Maw A. Decisions to operate: the ASA grade 5 dilemma. *Ann R Coll Surg Engl* 2011; **93**: 365–9.

13. Neary WD, Foy C, Heather BP, et al. Indentifying high-risk patients undergoing urgent and emergency surgery. *Ann R Coll Surg Engl* 2006; **88**: 151–6.

14. Physician Certification. Physician Board Certification in Hospice and Palliative Medicine (HPM). Available from: http://www.nhpco.org/palliative-care/physician-certification

15. Lemay K, Wilson KG, Buenger U, et al. Fear of pain in patients with advanced cancer or in patients with chronic noncancer pain. *Clin J Pain* 2011; **27**: 116–24.

16. van den Beuken-van Everdingen MHJ, de Rijke JM, Kessels AG, et al. Prevalence of pain in patients with cancer: a systematic review of the past 40 years. *Ann Oncol* 2007; **18**: 1437–49.

17. Fallon M. When morphine does not work. *Support Care Cancer* 2008; **16**: 771–5.

18. Pasutharnchat K, Tan KH, Hadi MA, et al. Intrathecal analgesia in patients with cancer pain–an audit in a tertiary institution. *Ann Acad Med Singapore* 2009; **38**: 943–6.

19. Kim JH, Jung JY, Cho MS. Continuous intrathecal morphine administration for cancer pain management using an intrathecal catheter connected to a subcutaneous injection port: a retrospective analysis of 22 terminal cancer patients in Korean population. *Korean J Pain* 2013; **26**: 32–8.

20. Ripamonti CI, Santini D, Maranzano E, et al. Management of cancer pain: ESMO Clinical Practice Guidelines. *Ann Oncol* 2012; **23**: vii139–54.

21. Myers J, Chan V, Jarvis V, et al. Intraspinal techniques for pain management in cancer patients: a systematic review. *Support Care Cancer* 2009; **18**: 137–49.

22. Anghelescu DL, Faughnan LG, Baker JN, et al. Use of epidural and peripheral nerve blocks at the end of life in children and young adults with cancer: the collaboration between a pain service and a palliative care service. *Paediatr Anaesth* 2010; **20**: 1070–7.

23. Hawley P, Beddard-Huber E, Grose C, et al. Intrathecal infusions for intractable cancer pain: a qualitative study of the impact on a case series of patients and caregivers. *Pain Res Manag* 2009; **14**: 371–9.

24. Farquhar-Smith P, Chapman S. Neuraxial (epidural and intrathecal) opioids for intractable pain. *Br J Pain* 2012; **6**: 25–35.

25. Myers J, Chan V, Jarvis V, et al. Intraspinal techniques for pain management in cancer patients. *Support Care Cancer* 2010; **18**: 137–49.

26. Smyth CE, Jarvis V, Poulin P. Brief review: neuraxial analgesia in refractory malignant pain. *Can J Anesth* 2013 [Epub ahead of print]

27. Deer TR, Smith HS, Burton AW, et al. Comprehensive consensus based guidelines on intrathecal drug delivery systems in the treatment of pain caused by cancer pain. *Pain Physician* 2011; **14**: E283–312.

28. Burton AW, Rajagopal A, Shah HN, et al. Epidural and intrathecal analgesia is effective in treating refractory cancer pain. *Pain Med* 2004; **5**: 239–47.

29. Deer T, Krames ES, Hassenbusch SJ, et al. Polyanalgesic consensus conference 2007: recommendations for the management of pain by intrathecal (intraspinal) drug delivery: report of an interdisciplinary expert panel. *Neuromodulation* 2007; **10**: 300–28.

30. Stearns L, Boortz-Marx R, Du Pen S, et al. Intrathecal drug delivery for the management of cancer pain: a multidisciplinary consensus of best clinical practices. *J Support Oncol* 2005; **3**: 399–408.

31. Wagemans MFM, Zuurmond WWA, de Lange JJ. Long-term spinal opioid therapy in terminally ill cancer pain patients. *Oncologist* 1997; **2**: 70–5.

32. Mercadante S, Porzio G, Gebbia V. Spinal analgesia for advanced cancer patients: an update. *Crit Rev Oncol Hematol* 2012; **82**: 227–32.

The high-risk or critically ill patient in the operating room

I. McConachie

Anesthetic management of the critically ill patient requiring operative intervention remains a significant challenge. This chapter will review selected aspects of anesthesia for the high-risk patient with relevance to the critically ill patient.

The patient with multiple injuries

- Traumatic injury is the leading cause of death under the age of 40 years and the third leading cause overall.
- Many patients are intoxicated.
- Injuries are often multisystem in nature.

Deaths from trauma follow a trimodal distribution:

- Immediate deaths in the first minutes at the scene are either due to massive hemorrhage or crush injuries, massive central nervous system trauma or (potentially avoidable) airway obstruction.
- Early deaths are often due to the effects of hemorrhage or hypoxia and may be preventable.
- Late deaths are chiefly due to sepsis and organ failures. Many of these may be preventable by prompt recognition of injuries and their physiological significance and definitive intervention.

Assessment of the trauma patient

- A system for evaluation of trauma victims results in faster, more effective resuscitation, fewer life threatening injuries missed, and a greater appreciation of priorities.
- The Advanced Trauma Life Support system, as promoted by the American College of Surgeons since 1979, is one such system that has gained widespread acceptance.
- Assessment, diagnosis, and initial treatment should be carried out simultaneously.
- This is facilitated by a team approach with a "team leader."
- The patient needs to be completely undressed and examined thoroughly as blunt, high-velocity trauma can result in injury to virtually any part of the body.
- The first priorities are to detect and treat life threatening conditions immediately while second priorities are to detect other injuries (none should be missed).
- Radiological investigations should not take priority over resuscitation.

Anesthesia and Perioperative Care of the High-Risk Patient, Third edition, ed. Ian McConachie.

- Relevant specialists should be involved at an early stage.
- The abdomen should be evaluated. Focused abdominal ultrasound or computerized tomography (CT) scanning have their advocates. Diagnostic peritoneal lavage may be performed where doubt exists regarding the presence of an intra-abdominal injury.
- One must not forget to administer appropriate antibiotics and tetanus toxoid.
- All dislocations and fractures should be splinted and reduced if possible. This eases nursing, reduces pain and bleeding, and may reduce the incidence of acute respiratory distress syndrome (ARDS).

Airway and cervical spine protection

- The airway must be clear or permanent neurological damage or death may occur within minutes. If the patient cannot be intubated then a surgical airway should be created.
- The cervical spine should be assumed to be at risk and protected from further damage until proven to be intact. A hard cervical collar is mandatory.
- Cervical spine injuries are not uncommon in multiply injured patients and may be missed or the radiography misinterpreted.
- Aspects of perioperative care of the patient with suspected cervical spine injury are covered in the chapter on neurotrauma.
- Most critically ill patients presenting to the operating room (ORm) will already have some form of definitive airway control in place. Under most circumstances, it would be prudent to leave this airway alone for fear of losing control in a patient who may have acquired abnormalities with their airway due to tissue swelling or trauma. If the airway is not secure, one should assume a full stomach and take appropriate precautions.

Breathing/ventilation

- High-flow O_2 should be administered to all patients. In animal models, increased oxygen inspired concentrations prolong survival in hemorrhagic shock [1].
- Clinically obvious pneumothoraces should be drained.
- There should be a low threshold for immediate tracheal intubation on clinical grounds – even before the result of arterial blood gases analysis.
- Indications for immediate intubation and ventilation include gross respiratory distress, obvious hypoventilation, and severe shock.
- Delayed ventilation by promoting tissue hypoxia results in an increased incidence of organ failures.

Circulation

- External hemorrhage must be controlled.
- Large-bore catheters (× 2) are inserted and volume infused.
- All multiple-injured patients should have large volumes of warmed IV fluids, administered quickly (see later for more detail on fluid therapy).
- One is far more likely to run into problems of inadequate infusion than problems of excess infusion.
- As soon as possible, blood should be sent for arterial blood gases analysis and cross-matching of blood.

Differences between hemorrhagic shock and traumatic shock

Hemorrhage results in well-known physiological changes. Traumatic shock includes these responses but they are modified by the tissue injury and its associated inflammatory response. This has several practical effects:

- Heart rate responds to hemorrhage by an initial tachycardia followed eventually by a progressive bradycardia – the heart slowing in the absence of adequate venous return in an attempt to maintain stroke volume. With tissue injury there is no late slowing of the heart and tachycardia continues.
- Blood pressure is maintained by vasoconstriction until more than one third of blood volume has been lost. With tissue injury, blood pressure is maintained to a greater degree by the surge in catecholamines and other nociceptive stimuli, but this is at the expense of tissue perfusion due to excessive vasoconstriction.

Operative intervention in the trauma patient

- Many trauma patients will need surgery.
- In general, all the required surgical procedures should be performed acutely, that is, during one anesthetic, providing the patient has been appropriately resuscitated and is hemodynamically stable.
- The rationale is that, once the patient is resuscitated, s/he may be in the best condition that s/he will be in for some time, before the development of sepsis, tissue edema, malnutrition, and metabolic complications, for example.
- Delayed fixation of long bone fractures may increase the incidence of ARDS [2]. The mechanisms are uncertain but probably include ongoing bleeding, increased pain and the physiological stress response, and possible fat embolus.
- Conversely, if the patient undergoing surgery is unstable, with developing hypothermia, coagulopathy, and acidosis, prolonged surgery has a high mortality. Many surgeons now accept that the best way to manage these patients is to "bail out," for example, to pack the abdomen to stop bleeding, bring out bowel ends on to the abdominal wall, etc., and take the patient to ICU for stabilization and further resuscitation. Further surgical intervention is deferred to a later date. This has been described as "damage control surgery" [3].
- Blood clots, packing the abdomen, ileus, and tissue edema, however, all contribute to the development of an abdominal compartment syndrome where the increase in pressure literally squeezes the kidneys. This causes a reduction in renal blood flow, glomerular filtration rate, direct compression of the renal parenchyma, and increased release of antidiuretic hormone and aldosterone from stimulation of abdominal wall stretch receptors. In general, intra-abdominal pressures of 15–20 mmHg are associated with oliguria while pressures greater than 30 mmHg may be associated with anuria. Interestingly, the use of large volumes of fluids in an attempt to achieve resuscitation goals has been shown to be associated with an increased incidence of abdominal compartment syndrome [4].

Management of the critically ill or injured patient in the ORm

Patient transfer to and from the ORm

The safe transfer of any patient within a hospital requires organization and planning. Even the most urgent of transfers to the ORm must not be undertaken until all steps to ensure that the patient will not be harmed by the transfer have been addressed. One needs to guard against complacency because one is "only going down the corridor."

The principles of safe patient transfer are the same, regardless of the distance involved. These include:

- Patient's airway must be adequately secured.
- Beware of occult injuries in multiple trauma patients.
- Ventilation must be adequate, either spontaneous or mechanical. It has been shown that manual ventilation with a bag is unpredictable and unreliable compared with a portable mechanical ventilator. Intensive care unit (ICU) patients should be ventilated with the same mode as in ICU, if possible. Modern portable ventilators can apply positive end expiratory pressure (PEEP) and vary the inspiration to expiration (I:E) ratio.
- Lifting of patients on and off stretchers is a cause of inadvertant extubation. It is probably safest to disconnect the ventilator temporarily for a few seconds during movement.
- Blood pressure must be maintained with a combination of fluids and inotropic agents. Stabilize the patient before transfer, if possible.
- Patient monitoring must be appropriate to ensure safe transfer.
- Consideration should be given to pharmacological sedation and muscle relaxation as indicated by the clinical condition.
- Communication between transferring and receiving staff should ensure safe receipt of the patient.
- Inexperienced medical or nursing staff should not be used for transferring critically ill patients.
- One must avoid last minute panic and rush. Planning should be such as to minimize delays and waiting in ORm reception areas. Check the availability of equipment in the X-ray department before the transfer commences. Check that adequate porter services are available.
- Appropriate equipment required during the transfer includes a portable ventilator, full oxygen cylinder, equipment for reintubation, drugs (for sedation, paralysis, cardiac resuscitation), self inflating bag or equivalent for the event of ventilator/oxygen supply failure, and battery-powered syringe pumps, if required. There is no excuse for battery-powered equipment becoming exhausted, oxygen cylinders emptying, or drug syringes running out.

As important as ensuring the safety of the patient to be transferred is the importance of not delaying the transfer to the ORm by undertaking procedures that can be performed later during the operation. For example, if a patient is exsanguinating and needs a laparotomy for abdominal trauma, there is little to be gained by spending time in the emergency department inserting an arterial line. This procedure can be performed during the laparotomy when the surgeon has begun to effect hemostasis. There is no merit in delivering a corpse with an arterial line to the operating table.

Patient positioning

When positioning the critically ill patient, there are a number of points that merit emphasis.

- The number of lines, tubes, and bags increases with the severity of the patient's condition. Every piece of equipment inserted into the patient is there for a reason (or time should not have been wasted inserting it), and therefore it must be accessible during an operative procedure.

- Patients who have come to the ORm as a result of trauma may well not have had a full primary and secondary survey. In such cases, it is vital that the presence of as yet undiagnosed fractures to any part of the spine is taken into account when moving and positioning the patient. In particular, the cervical spine should stay fixed with head blocks and strapping and the patient should not be moved without a formal log-rolling technique being used.
- Patients who have been critically ill in the ICU and have a significant sequestration of fluid into the extra-vascular compartments will have edematous skin that is weakened and is prone to tearing and bruising, and vulnerable to pressure injury. Every effort should be made to minimize any damage done to the skin in such cases by providing adequate support and padding to the patient's exposed extremities.

Perioperative hypothermia

Maintenance of body temperature is important, but it is common for the trauma patient to present to the ORm cold and peripherally "shut down." The reasons for this are as follows:

- Following acute blood loss, the cardiovascular response is profound peripheral vasoconstriction resulting in maintained perfusion of vital organs – brain, heart, lungs, and kidneys – at the expense of other vascular beds.
- During acute traumatic injury, central mechanisms of thermoregulation are disrupted. Thus, shivering is diminished or absent. Whether this is secondary to reduced oxygen delivery or a response to altered hormonal activity in the thermoregulatory center in the brainstem is unclear.
- In order to assess the extent of injury in the traumatized patient fully, it is necessary to remove clothing and leave the patient exposed during repeated examination. This is compounded by the infusion of unwarmed intravenous (IV) fluid and blood worsening the hypothermia.

In addition to these problems in trauma patients, all patients undergoing major surgery are at risk of becoming hypothermic (core temperature <36 °C). Reasons include:

- reduced metabolic rate associated with anesthesia
- vasodilation under anesthesia
- abolished subclinical shivering
- exposure
- cold fluids used for skin preparation, which are usually allowed to evaporate
- heat loss from open body cavities
- inadequately warmed IV fluids

Thus, steps should be taken to maintain body temperature perioperatively.

Adverse effects of perioperative hypothermia

Postoperative hypothermia has become recognized in recent years as a significant and common problem:

- Delayed awakening may occur due to decreased clearance of anesthetic agents.
- Most organ function is depressed by hypothermia.

- Hemodynamic instability during rewarming – increased fluids are often needed as the patient vasodilates during rewarming. The hypotension thus produced can be confused with continued bleeding.
- Oxygen consumption is increased by about 140% by shivering during rewarming. If oxygen delivery to the tissues is not able to match this increase, the oxygen debt is prolonged.
- Wound infection rates may be increased by reductions in skin blood flow.
- Cell mediated immune function may be reduced.
- Hypothermia causes increased bleeding by several mechanisms [5] such as cold-induced defects in platelet function and number and depression of temperature-dependent enzymes in the coagulation cascade. Fibrinolysis may also be increased. Even mild hypothermia increases blood loss and risk of transfusion [6]. Normalization of coagulation problems may require normalization of temperature as well as giving coagulation factors.
- Adrenergic responses are increased postoperatively in hypothermic patients, and are responsible for increased cardiac morbidity. There is a 55% less relative risk of adverse cardiac events when normothermia is maintained [7]. Unintentional hypothermia is associated with increased incidence of myocardial ischemia in the postoperative period.
- However, postoperative hypothermia after non-cardiac surgery has not been shown to independently predict increased mortality [8].

Note: laboratories perform coagulation studies at 37 °C, regardless of the temperature of the patient at the time the sample was taken. Thus, these studies may underestimate the degree of impairment of coagulopathy in the hypothermic patient what is, after all, a dynamic problem in vivo rather than in vitro.

Prevention of hypothermia

All practical measures should be undertaken to minimize heat loss and maintain the patient's body temperature:

- circle system ventilation with carbon dioxide absorber and heat and moisture exchanger in the patient circuit
- fluid warmer for all IV fluids
- warmed patient mattress
- insulation of all areas of the patient that do not need to be exposed for either surgical or anesthetic access
- use of a forced air warming system – use of heat-retaining insulating materials is less effective at maintaining patient temperatures than forced air warming systems [9], which add energy to the system

Ventilatory management

In severe shock, the reduced blood flow to the diaphragm coupled with the increased minute volume and respiratory energy expenditure causes respiratory failure – even in normal lungs. This is demonstrated convincingly in animal studies – much of the lactic acid accumulating in shock comes from the respiratory muscles [10]. Controlled ventilation, by reducing the work of breathing, lessens the blood lactate levels compared with spontaneous breathing. Thus, controlling ventilation during anesthesia will be essential in the shocked patient.

Ventilation of the critically ill patient should always be controlled using appropriate drugs for anesthesia and muscle relaxation. There is no place for spontaneous ventilation because the patient's work of breathing is usually increased, causing "rapid, shallow breathing," which will result in the development of atelectasis.

Ideally, the mode of ventilation in the ORm and, indeed, in transit to and from the ICU or emergency department should be of the same standard as can be delivered in the ICU. Pressure-control ventilation with the ability to alter (reverse) the I:E and to apply PEEP is ideal. Lack of ongoing ventilation with PEEP and the other lung recruitment maneuvers taken in the ICU will result in loss of recruitment of alveoli and hypoxia.

Occasionally, to ensure minimal deterioration in respiratory physiology, it may be necessary to move a static ICU ventilator to the ORm and ventilate the patient with it throughout the procedure. Under this circumstance, it may be necessary to adopt a total IV anesthetic technique.

Further discussion of intraoperative ventilation of the high-risk patient is given in the chapter on intraoperative ventilatory management.

Cardiac effects of ventilation

- Decreased venous return and therefore decreased cardiac output with intermittent positive pressure ventilation (IPPV) is the major hemodynamic effect of ventilation in most patients. As it is related to intrathoracic pressure (ITP), it is worse if the ventilator is set to provide either a high tidal volume (high peak ITP) or a prolonged inspiratory time (high mean ITP). PEEP also exacerbates the fall in venous return.
- Venous return and cardiac output can be restored by either fluid infusion or sympathetic drugs, both of which restore the gradient for venous return despite further increases in right atrial pressure.
- With IPPV, the increased ITP decreases the gradient across the left ventricle (LV) that the LV has to work against – one aspect of afterload. In other words, decreased transmural pressure decreases LV afterload. Any beneficial effect on afterload in the normal heart is limited by the fall in venous return. In the failing heart, the cardiac output is relatively insensitive to changes in preload but exquisitely sensitive to small reductions in afterload. Thus, in patients with heart failure undergoing surgery, there may be beneficial effects on cardiac output from increases in ITP with ventilation.
- Conversely, at the end of surgery, patients with failing hearts may deteriorate during attempts to wean off IPPV rapidly for extubation. This is as a result of increased LV afterload and increased venous return due to the fall in ITP with spontaneous ventilation, and also the tachycardia, myocardial ischemia, and release of catecholamines during spontaneous breathing and awakening.
- Therefore, patients with heart failure undergoing surgery may require a period of postoperative respiratory support and a more gentle return to spontaneous ventilation.

Anesthetic agents

Every available technique and drug combination has been used to anesthetize the critically ill patient. To some extent, the practitioner must distil his/her own technique. The way a drug is used, that is, dose, speed of injection, etc., may be more important in many patients than the absolute choice of drug.

Induction agents

1. Thiopental (thiopentone): a rapidly effective drug for the induction of general anesthesia. Many believe that thiopental is still the best choice of induction agent for rapid sequence induction for the purposes of securing the airway due to a slightly faster onset than propofol, for example. Thiopental is the induction agent that most reduces the brain's metabolic requirement for oxygen and hence is neuroprotective. It produces depression of myocardial contractility together with vasodilation, resulting in a fall of blood pressure. It is noteworthy that in the hypovolemic or shocked patient, the sleep dose of thiopental is greatly reduced as compared to that for the healthy patient. Thiopental has become less available in many countries in recent years.
2. Etomidate (carboxylated imidazole): etomidate shares many common properties with other anesthetic induction agents, namely a predictable, rapid onset of anesthesia, relatively short emergence time, and falls in cerebral blood flow, cerebral metabolic rate, and intracranial pressure. Cerebral perfusion pressure is usually maintained. Etomidate is discussed in detail later in this chapter.
3. Propofol (di-isopropyl phenol): has a rapid onset (although a little slower than thiopentone) and obtunds pharyngeal and glottal reflexes to a greater extent than thiopentone. Widely used for total IV anesthesia and ICU sedation. The hypotension produced is chiefly secondary to vasodilation rather than myocardial depression.
4. Ketamine (phencyclidine derivative): its sympathomimetic effects maintain blood pressure but the increases in heart rate and stroke volume increase myocardial work. Profoundly analgesic and an effective analgesic agent at subanesthetic doses. Despite its sympathomimetic effects, ketamine may cause cardiac depression, myocardial ischemia, and collapse in shocked patients in whom catecholamine stores may be exhausted. Ketamine increases intracranial pressure and is often considered contraindicated in head injuries. However, it is argued that these undesirable effects are countered by the beneficial effects of IPPV [11]. A novel combination of ketamine and propofol (nicknamed ketofol) has been used by physicians in some emergency departments and may be worth exploring further in the ORm [12].

Opioids

1. Remifentanil: the cautious use of short-acting agents is important in critically ill patients unless, of course, postoperative ventilation is planned or anticipated. The shortest available is remifentanil, which is metabolized by esterases. Remifentanil produces no postoperative analgesia and additional measures must be taken for postoperative analgesia, such as use of epidural anesthesia.
2. Fentanyl: has a minimal effect on the cardiovascular system in the stable, calm, patient undergoing cardiac surgery. In shocked patients exhibiting high sympathetic tone, abolition of this with fentanyl results in a fall in blood pressure (BP).
3. Morphine: should be used with great care in the critically ill patient as it has pharmacologically active metabolites and is reliant on the liver and kidneys for its elimination. Morphine is still a very useful drug for postoperative analgesia in the critically ill patient and is widely used for sedation of the postoperative ventilated patient.

Muscle relaxants

There are four main factors governing the choice of muscle relaxant for anesthesia.

1. Onset: all critically ill patients are assumed to have a full stomach. Despite recent introduction of faster onset non-depolarizing drugs such as rocuronium, succinylcholine (suxamethonium) remains the "gold standard" for rapidly securing the airway. If cardiac instability is a major concern, rocuronium may be a better choice.
2. Cardiovascular effects: rocuronium has the least cardiac effects of the relaxants, followed by vecuronium. However, the vagolytic and sympathomimetic effects of pancuronium may make it an appropriate choice in shocked patients.
3. Termination of effect and excretion: agents not dependent on the kidney or liver for termination of effect sound attractive in the critically ill patient, but from a practical point of view, few critically ill patients are "reversed" at the end of the operation due to planned ongoing ventilatory support. Thus, an effect of reduced elimination of muscle relaxants is not a big problem.
4. Duration: in a similar manner, short or long duration is not usually an issue.

Inhalational agents

1. Enflurane: has the greatest degree of myocardial depression for equivalent minimum alveolar concentration (MAC) among all volatile agents. There is limited use now in many countries.
2. Sevoflurane: has less increase in cerebral blood volume, rapid onset, and rapid recovery.
3. Halothane: is rarely used nowadays. It is long acting with more active metabolites retained in the body than other volatile agents, with the potential for liver toxicity. It sensitizes the heart to endogenous and exogenous catecholamines, with the potential for arrhythmias.
4. Isoflurane: has an impressive safety profile in large numbers of patients. Hypotension is caused chiefly by vasodilation rather than myocardial depression. Early concerns as regards coronary steal are unfounded in conventional usage.
5. Desflurane: specialized delivery systems are required. It is very short acting, and there are some residual concerns regarding coronary steal.
6. Nitrous oxide (N_2O): due to low blood gas solubility, it has very fast uptake and onset, limited anesthetic efficacy due to low potency, but it speeds uptake of other volatile agents due to the second gas effect. In some countries its useful analgesic properties maintain its role in analgesia in the field when administered by paramedics, for example, extrication of trauma patients. It has the longest history of any inhalational anesthetic still in routine usage in the western world, but is under increasing scrutiny and controversy in recent years (see following).

Choice of anesthetic agent in the shocked patient

Controlled studies on shocked patients undergoing anesthesia are problematic due to:

- differences in severity of injury or shock
- differences in fluids administered
- adequacy of resuscitation prior to surgery

- hemodynamic state and degree of cardiovascular support
- previous health, most notably cardiac reserve

Thus, one must take guidance from basic anesthetic and pharmacological principles including guidance from the notes summarized earlier in this chapter. In addition, studies on animal models are available, case studies and series may be of interest, and there are reports on the use of anesthesia in military situations.

A major dilemma is how to provide any anesthesia for the profoundly shocked patient:

- Many patients suffering from an exsanguinating injury may be so "shocked" as to be thought to not require or be able to tolerate any anesthetic administration.
- While the intent to save life in this situation is laudable, the absence of recordable blood pressure does not guarantee lack of awareness. It is strongly recommended that, at the very least, small amounts of midazolam are given to the patient as this will reduce the incidence of recall [13].
- As the patient's condition improves, as when hemorrhage is controlled, judicious amounts of opioids and other anesthetic agents may be introduced.
- Ketamine may be a useful option in these circumstances, but the profoundly shocked patient whose endogenous catecholamine stores have been exhausted may still suffer significant falls in blood pressure on induction. Indeed, ketamine has negative inotropic effects on human heart muscle in vitro and reduces the heart's ability to respond to β stimulation.

There are animal studies to guide choice of anesthesia in the shocked patient:

- Ketamine was associated with significantly increased survival compared with other agents in a model of hemorrhagic shock [14]. In that study, the animals anesthetized with ketamine had better preservation of cell structure in splanchnic organs.
- An IV regime with ketamine, buprenorphine, and midazolam was associated with less hypotension than isoflurane anesthesia in pigs with hemorrhagic shock [15]. However, there was some evidence of better maintenance of organ blood flow in the isoflurane group.
- Ketamine was associated with increased cardiac output compared to thiopental in another animal hemorrhagic shock model [16]. Vital organ blood flow was also improved in the ketamine group. The percentage of blood volume loss required to cause significant hypotension was significantly less in the thiopental group.
- Hemorrhagic shock alters the pharmacokinetics and pharmacodynamics of propofol [17], suggesting that less propofol is required to achieve its desired effect in hemorrhagic shock.
- Conversely, animal studies suggest minimal adjustment in the dose of etomidate [18] to achieve the same drug effect in hemorrhagic shock.
- Hemorrhagic shock altered the pharmacokinetics of remifentanil [19], suggesting that less remifentanil would be required to maintain a target plasma concentration.

Choice of anesthetic agent in the septic patient

There are no controlled studies of septic patients from the ICU undergoing surgery in the ORm. What guidance is available comes from case reports and animal studies.

- The sympathetic stimulation associated with the use of ketamine may result in improved hemodynamics, diuresis, and reduction in the degree of cardiovascular support required in patients with septic shock [20].
- In animals with septic shock, volatile agents have been associated with increases in serum lactate while ketamine was associated with reductions in lactate. Ketamine preserved systemic vascular resistance and blood pressure best [21]. To summarize a complex paper, ketamine best preserved cardiac function and tissue oxygenation.
- Ketamine directly suppresses proinflammatory cytokine production [22].
- The beneficial effect of even low-dose ketamine on cytokine function has been shown in patients to persist into the postoperative period [23]. Thus, ketamine may be of value in preventing immune function alterations in the early postoperative period.
- Many anesthesiologists have experience of continuing propofol sedation from ICU into the ORm. Propofol, after endotoxin injection, reduced the mortality rate of rats and attenuated their cytokine responses [24]. These findings suggest that propofol administration may be advantageous during sepsis.
- The beneficial effects of propofol treatment may, in part, be due to reductions in the overproduction of nitric oxide in sepsis [25].
- Sevoflurane pretreatment decreased mortality rate, severity of hypotension, and acidosis, and inhibited cytokine responses in rats injected with endotoxin, suggesting that sevoflurane may also be an appropriate anesthetic choice in sepsis [26].

It seems that most anesthetic agents have potentially beneficial effects on the inflammatory response to sepsis and could be recommended for the septic patient – assuming that clinical studies corroborate these findings. Hemodynamic effects may favor ketamine over volatile agents.

Comparative studies of induction agents

Thus, animal studies, case reports, and reviews [11] support the use of ketamine in shocked and septic patients undergoing anesthesia, but caution is still advised. Falls in blood pressure and cardiac output may still occur. There are a few comparative studies in patients:

- A randomized trial of ketamine versus etomidate for acutely ill patients requiring rapid sequence intubation found no differences in adverse events between the two drugs [27].
- A comparison of thiopental, propofol, and etomidate for intubations in the emergency room found no difference in mortality when adjusted for age and risk, but more hypotension and vasopressor use in the propofol group [28].
- Retrospective analyses of ICU databases found no difference in eventual outcome with the use of various induction agents (including etomidate–see later) for anesthesia for emergency laparotomy [29]. Hypotension may have been less with etomidate.

Most anesthesiologists use the techniques they are most familiar with, either total IV anesthesia or inhalational anesthesia, for the critically ill patient in the ORm. Few have much experience of ketamine. Therefore, despite its strong theoretical advantages, it is not commonly used. Further clinical studies in this patient group are needed urgently.

The etomidate controversy

Although not widely used for routine anesthesia, many believe etomidate's properties enable it to occupy a specific niche in anesthetic practice for the high-risk and critically ill patient. Its use by non-anesthetists, for example in the emergency department in many countries, seems to be expanding and this, and its unique properties, have resulted in renewed interest (and controversy) in recent years.

The chief advantageous property of etomidate is its remarkable cardiovascular stability, even in patients with cardiac disease. However, other properties of etomidate are not so desirable, namely adrenal suppression, pain and thrombophlebitis, and myoclonus.

Etomidate hemodynamics

- Careful recent studies suggest that (at least in vitro) the effects of different induction agents on the heart are less different than previously believed. In isolated human atrial muscle, no significant inhibition of cardiac contractility is produced by propofol, midazolam, or etomidate, in contrast to thiopental which showed strong and ketamine weak negative inotropic properties [30].
- The cardiac effects in vivo will depend on more than the inotropic properties of agents, and it is of interest that animal studies suggest that etomidate may act as an agonist at α_2-adrenoceptors [31], perhaps contributing to its cardiovascular stability.
- Recent reviews still recommend etomidate for induction of anesthesia in the high-risk cardiac patient owing to its cardiovascular stability [32], and in the U.K., Mackay et al. [33] have suggested that etomidate is the agent of choice for trauma patients requiring a rapid sequence induction due to its lesser cardiovascular depression compared to other agents.
- It is not universally accepted, however, that etomidate is the safest agent in either high-risk or shocked patients. Many practitioners believe they can achieve equal hemodynamic stability in such patients by careful titration of the dose of other induction agents.

Current controversy in ICU

- It has long been accepted that etomidate infusions have a negative effect on the outcome of ICU patients, despite preservation of hemodynamics. The current issue is whether the potential for adrenal suppression from even a single dose of etomidate counterbalances the reduced hypotension possibly seen after induction and intubation.
- There have been numerous studies over the years convincingly demonstrating that even a single induction dose of etomidate has a reversible inhibitory effect on cortisol production, lasting potentially up to 48 hours [34]. It has always been assumed that the transient adrenal suppressant effect of a single etomidate bolus for intubation would not have a significant effect on overall ICU outcome and, indeed, it is even conceivable that modification by etomidate of the normal "stress response" to surgery (in part due to elevations in serum cortisol levels) may be desirable in some patients.
- In one study [35], adrenal depression in septic shock was, perhaps not surprisingly, associated with a worse outcome. The authors suggested, but by no means proved, that etomidate exposure could be a major risk factor for mortality in septic shock. Editorials in the anesthetic [36] and ICU literature [37] called for a moratorium on the use of

etomidate in ICU patients and patients who will be going to ICU. Others [38] suggested that each time etomidate is administered, hydrocortisone should be administered to prevent adrenal dysfunction. The pendulum of evidence swung further against the routine use of etomidate for intubation following a study suggesting that etomidate given in the previous 72 hours may increase the incidence of adrenal suppression in septic ICU patients, and may worsen outcome [39].

- After more recent studies, for example showing less requirement for vasopressors following induction with etomidate [40], it seems the pendulum of evidence may be swinging back in favor of the use of etomidate for induction and intubation. The use of hydrocortisone supplementation to protect against adrenal suppression in non-septic patients given etomidate has been questioned after a study found no differences in outcome apart from faster reduction in vasopressor requirements [41]. In septic patients, large retrospective studies found that use of etomidate at intubation was not associated with any notable differences in outcome [42,43]. Nor does the use of etomidate for intubation subsequently increase vasopressor requirements during the first 24 hours after admission to ICU [44].
- The most recent meta-analysis of patients with sepsis found convincing evidence of adrenal suppression and a weak association between etomidate use for intubation and increased mortality [45]. Countering this is the review of a large ICU database (741 036 patients with sepsis, including 2014 intubated in the ICU), which found that use of etomidate for intubation was not associated with any increase in adverse outcomes, including mortality [46].

Few of these studies are adequately powered to address the issue of mortality associated with use of etomidate in critically ill patients and many comprise analyses of database information. The best opinion at present is that caution may still be warranted around the use of etomidate for intubation in critically ill patients.

The nitrous oxide controversy

In normal patients, mild indirect sympathetic stimulation reduces any myocardial depressant actions of N_2O. Following hemorrhage, this protecting effect is lost and N_2O may have the same depressant effects on the heart as halothane.

With the additional concerns regarding resultant use of lesser inspired oxygen concentrations and the potential for expansion of air spaces like pneumothoraces, it is difficult to see a major role for N_2O in critically ill patients. In recent years, additional concerns have been raised:

- Is N_2O a neurotoxin in usual clinical circumstances? An increasing body of animal work supports the concept that N_2O is neurotoxic [47].
- Does N_2O cause myocardial ischemia? N_2O inhibits methionine synthase, which aids in the conversion of homocysteine to methionine. Homocysteine is a marker for coronary artery disease and is associated with endothelial dysfunction. Use of N_2O during carotid artery surgery has been shown to cause increases in postoperative plasma homocysteine concentration and increased postoperative myocardial ischemia [48]. Longer exposure to N_2O is associated with progressive increases in homocysteine, and these increases were independently associated with the risk of major complications after major surgery [49].

- Does N_2O impair endothelial function? N_2O has been shown indirectly to impair endothelial function temporarily, as indicated by flow-mediated dilation of the brachial artery [50]. In vitro animal studies suggest that N_2O may increase signs of endothelial dysfunction and inflammation in the brain [51] – the significance of which has yet to be determined.
- Does N_2O worsen outcome in high-risk patients? A large, multicenter randomized trial (ENIGMA) examined the effect of N_2O on outcome in major surgery. Unfortunately, the inspired oxygen levels in the two groups were widely different (80% in the N_2O-free group and 30% in the N_2O group). The N_2O group had an increased incidence of pulmonary complications after major surgery, but no significant difference in length of hospital stay [52]. Bizarrely, five-year follow-up of the enigma study patients [53] found that use of N_2O at that time was associated with a long-term increase in the risk of myocardial infarction but not of overall mortality or risk of a cardiovascular accident (CVA)!

The definitive answer to this last question may perhaps be provided by the ENIGMA 2 study, but many anesthesiologists no longer use N_2O in critically ill patients.

Practical conduct of anesthesia in the critically ill patient

- Conventional assessments of fitness for anesthesia and surgery may not be helpful. The bleeding patient may not be able to be stabilized until the bleeding is controlled.
- Many of these patients require ongoing resuscitation. The ABC system is widely followed :

  A = airway including cervical spine protection
  B = breathing
  C = circulation

The less well known system of VIP (ventilation, infusion, perfusion) is perhaps equally appropriate for surgical and trauma patients, as it emphasizes the interrelationship between ventilation and perfusion in overall oxygen transport, and because it reminds us that the cornerstone of resuscitation in these patients is fluid infusion.

- It is an important principle that inotropes and vasopressors should not be given as a substitute for fluids in the hypovolemic patient, but perfusion of the coronary and cerebral circulations must be maintained. It is therefore appropriate to use such drugs to maintain perfusion of the heart and brain in the short term while one "catches up" with blood loss. Many anesthesiologists routinely follow injection of propofol for induction, for example, with a phenylephrine "chaser" in order to prevent falls in blood pressure being precipitated by the induction agent. Although a useful approach to this problem, this should not result in over confidence!
- Many patients coming to the ORm from the ICU will already be receiving hemodynamic support with infusions of inotropes and/or vasopressors. These obviously should be continued and, indeed, usually require to be increased to compensate for the effects of the anesthetic agents.
- If invasive monitoring is not *in situ*, it may be prudent (time permitting) to establish this using local anesthesia prior to induction for beat-to-beat monitoring of this period of the anesthetic (see later).

- Ruptured aneurysms and other cases of massive hemorrhage should be "prepped" on the table prior to induction, as discussed in the chapter on vascular anesthesia.

Intraoperative monitoring

Full monitoring according to local and national protocols should be employed in all patients. In addition, many high-risk and all critically ill patients will require invasive monitoring with:

1. An indwelling arterial line is used for:
   - beat-to-beat monitoring of blood pressure
   - sampling of blood for blood gas measurement
   - control of inotrope and vasopressor infusions
2. A central venous catheter is required for:
   - measurement of central venous pressure (CVP) – a reflection of preload of the right ventricle (RV)
   - guide to fluid requirements
   - infusion of irritant drugs like inotropes, vasopressors, and IV nutrition
3. A urinary catheter is required for hourly urine volume measurement.
4. Temperature should be monitored for all long procedures because of the dangers of perioperative hypothermia, as discussed earlier.

Monitoring strategies in the high-risk surgical patient

Invasive monitoring of elderly surgical patients has revealed a high incidence of "hidden" abnormalities, reflecting their reduced physiological reserve even in patients "cleared" for surgery. Invasive monitoring during anesthesia and in the postoperative period may result in early recognition of problems, "fine tuning" of cardiovascular parameters and, in some studies, an improved outcome [54].

Preload monitoring

- CVP reflects right atrial pressure, which is usually taken to reflect RV end-diastolic pressure. It does not necessarily reflect LV preload and also correlates poorly with blood volume. CVP is often used as a guide to LV function. Directional changes in CVP may reflect alterations in LV performance. However, if either ventricle is depressed, or if there is severe pulmonary disease, changes in CVP may not reflect changes in LV function accurately.
- Recent studies suggest that the presence of arterial pulse pressure variation (PPV) during the respiratory cycle indicates a relative hypovolemia [55] and, indeed, predicts an increase in cardiac output with fluid. Most monitors can "freeze" the arterial trace and quantify this PPV, or one can simply view the "swing" on the arterial trace. Devices measuring cardiac output from arterial pulse contour analysis are available. These also measure the variation in pulse pressure or stroke volume during the inspiratory cycle. This has also been shown to accurately guide fluid therapy [56], but not all studies have been supportive of this monitoring modality [57].

Pulmonary artery catheter (PAC)

- The PAC is often known as the Swan Ganz catheter after its original inventors.
- It enables measurement of filling pressures of the left heart (estimated by the pulmonary capillary wedge pressure [PCWP]) as the inflated balloon at the catheter tip is "wedged" in the pulmonary artery. It can also measure thermodilution cardiac output and derived hemodynamic variables.
- The PAC may be used in patients with severe disease of either ventricle, but most commonly in patients with severe LV dysfunction, in order to optimize preload and guide the use of inotropes.
- In addition, the PAC may enable early diagnosis of cardiac ischemia if there are sudden increases in PCWP, guide hemodynamic management of septic patients, and monitor pulmonary artery pressures where these are elevated.
- Perioperative use of the PAC is controversial with studies casting doubt on the role of the PAC in elective high-risk surgery. Even in ICU patients, there is no convincing evidence of benefit (but no convincing evidence of harm either) arising from the use of the PAC [58]. The American Society of Anesthesiologists (ASA) has published guidelines for its perioperative use [59].

The esophageal Doppler

Stroke volume (and therefore cardiac output) may be measured by orally inserting an ultrasound probe with a Doppler ultrasound transducer on its tip into the esophagus until it reaches the mid-thoracic area. This measures blood flow velocity in the descending aorta. Numerous studies support the usefulness of this technique in perioperative management of the high-risk patient [60]. Fluid management may be guided and optimized to maximize cardiac output and organ blood flow. This is further explored in the chapters on gastro-intestinal surgery and perioperative optimization.

Transesophageal echocardiography (TEE)

In recent years, the intraoperative use of TEE has become routine for many patients undergoing cardiac surgery – and is becoming more common for other high-risk and emergency situations. It is used for:

- assessing preload and guiding IV fluid management
- assessing overall RV and LV function
- diagnosis of various cardiac complications perioperatively
- real-time cardiac valve assessment during repair or transcutaneous aortic valve implantations (information not readily obtainable by other means)

The equipment is expensive but individual examinations are relatively cheap. However, appropriate training is time consuming and expensive. The procedure itself is relatively noninvasive, and in general, is very safe – there are not the same complication concerns as for the pulmonary artery flotation catheter (PAFC), although reports have appeared of failure of the technique and trauma, including esophageal perforation.

Formal accreditation in its use is becoming increasingly mandatory for cardiac anesthesiologists. Most literature and guidelines are for cardiac surgery and less for non-cardiac surgery uses, but it is being adopted enthusiastically with little evidence base. There is little high-quality evidence of improved outcomes through the use of TEE.

Some authors have compared its use as a diagnostic tool with other standard monitors, for fluid status assessment, for example. However, other methods of preload assessment may be superior [61] for predicting fluid responsiveness. TEE is also used as a therapy – more accurately, the information gained is used to guide therapy [62].

Much of the TEE assessment is subjective. There are concerns regarding the potential for inappropriate interpretation and accuracy (as there were for interpretation of PAFC numbers), especially in occasional practitioners or poorly trained practitioners. In the U.K. in 2012, as few as 30% of members of the Association of Cardiothoracic Anesthesia were thought to be TEE accredited [63]. In North American, some centers require all cardiac anesthesia fellows to sit national certification examinations – a written examination plus case studies/TEE examinations.

Are there parallels between the PAFC and TEE? The introduction of TEE into anesthesia practice is similar to that for the PAFC. Both are diagnostic tools – in the case of TEE, its usefulness will depend on visualizing good images, interpretation of the images obtained, selection of appropriate therapy in response, and the titration of that therapy. Both became standard of care before proof of benefit was established fully (lack of such proof not preventing endorsement in official practice guidelines).

TEE is now a routine monitoring tool in cardiac anesthesia, leading to frequent changes in management (and also surgical decision making – its use is increasingly being driven by the cardiac surgeons) [64]. It is well established that changes in management are prompted by information obtained from TEE – this is exactly what PAC monitoring achieved [65] but ultimately was found not to improve outcome. Will TEE suffer the same fate?

TEE is probably here to stay (certainly for cardiac anesthesia) but the challenge is to develop its role appropriately. The ASA has produced guidelines for its suitable use [66].

Fluid therapy

The crystalloid versus colloid debate

- There has been controversy over the best type of fluid for resuscitation, such as crystalloids or colloids. There are problems with most of the available studies; for example, different species, fluids, injuries, illnesses, and complications studied.
- There has been significant debate since the 1970s regarding the superiority of colloids or crystalloids for fluid resuscitation.
- In more recent years, concerns have been expressed regarding the use of starch containing colloid solutions; for example, renal damage, impaired coagulation, pruritus after deposition in the tissues. The introduction of tetrastarches such as Voluven were thought to decrease the incidence of adverse effects. However, many studies were withdrawn after concerns raised regarding academic fraud of a prolific investigator [67].
- Recent large, well-conducted studies suggest that ICU patients do not benefit from colloids compared to crystalloids and may have increased risks of renal dysfunction requiring renal replacement therapy [68,69], and that patients with sepsis in particular have increased mortality following use of starch fluids for resuscitation [70].
- This is a complex, long-standing debate but the conclusion in recent reviews and meta-analyses [71,72] of no benefit and increased risk of harm from colloids

(especially starches), including increased bleeding and renal dysfunction, is best summed up by a recent Cochrane review[(73]: "There is no evidence from randomised controlled trials that resuscitation with colloids reduces the risk of death, compared to resuscitation with crystalloids, in patients with trauma, burns or following surgery. Furthermore, the use of hydroxyethyl starch might increase mortality."

- The position may be less clear regarding the use of colloids intraoperatively for resuscitation and/or maintenance of goal-directed therapy where a recent review found no evidence of increased harm, including bleeding risk and renal dysfunction [74].
- Nevertheless, IV colloids containing starches have been withdrawn from the market in some countries, as for example in the U.K. by the Medicines and Healthcare Products Regulatory Agency [75]. Ultimately, such decisions go a long way toward settling the colloid/crystalloid debate!

Saline induced metabolic acidosis and choice of crystalloid

- In a study of elderly surgical patients, the use of crystalloids and colloids containing balanced electrolyte solutions prevented the development of hyperchloremic metabolic acidosis and improved indices of gastric mucosal perfusion compared with saline-based crystalloid and colloid fluids [76].
- A study of saline versus Ringer's lactate in aortic aneurysm surgery showed higher perioperative blood loss in the saline group [77].
- In ICU patients, a chloride-restrictive strategy (chiefly by reducing the use of normal saline and saline containing colloids) decreased the incidence of kidney dysfunction and the need for renal replacement therapy [78].
- Hyperchloremia (from saline infusion) was independently associated with increased morbidity and mortality after non-cardiac surgery in a recent, large propensity matched cohort study [79].
- It has been suggested that normal saline should not be our routine choice of crystalloid for surgical patients [80].

Intraoperative fluid loading or fluid restriction?

- Some studies show benefits from fluid loading in the high-risk or critically ill patient. In one study, fluid loading after induction of anesthesia to a maximum stroke volume led to a reduction in the incidence of low pHi (an index of gastric mucosal perfusion) from 50% to 10% [81]. In a more recent study of patients undergoing major elective surgery, goal-directed volume loading resulted in earlier return of bowel function and a decreased length of hospital stay [82].
- This approach must be tempered with caution in the elderly or patients with known heart failure due to the potential risk of fluid overload precipitating pulmonary edema. Perioperative invasive monitoring may be indicated.
- However, inadequate fluid therapy is dangerous if resulting organ hypoperfusion leads to organ failure, such as renal failure.
- More recent studies have examined the role of fluid excess (primarily crystalloid) as a factor in outcome in high-risk surgical patients. Most of these studies have been performed on patients undergoing bowel surgery. This is discussed in the chapter on gastrointestinal surgery.

Endpoints of fluid therapy

The endpoints of fluid therapy may need to be chosen with care in high-risk or critically ill patients.

- Reduction in tachycardia and improvement in blood pressure and urine volumes are important albeit crude signs of response to fluids.
- CVP trends are more useful than absolute CVP numbers.
- PPV during the respiratory cycle may be useful as discussed earlier.
- Saturation of the central venous blood ($ScvO_2$) has been shown to be a useful sign of tissue hypoxia and guide to early resuscitation in patients presenting to the emergency room with septic shock [83]. Preliminary work suggests that a low $ScvO_2$ perioperatively is associated with an increased risk of postoperative complications in high-risk surgery [84]. The use of $ScvO_2$ as a guide to fluid therapy warrants further investigation.

Permissive hypovolemia in trauma patients

- An important study of penetrating trauma in 1994 showed an improved survival in those patients with "delayed" fluid resuscitation or minimal IV fluids given prior to definitive operative intervention [85]. This has been called permissive hypovolemia.
- The rationale, borne out by previous animal studies, is that full resuscitation results in:
  - higher BP, disrupting clot formation
  - hemodilution and decreased viscosity, disrupting clot formation
  - dilutional coagulopathy
- The recommendation, therefore, has been made in penetrating injury to limit fluids to maintain a mean arterial pressure of not >50 mmHg until bleeding has been controlled surgically, then to continue with full resuscitation.
- The biggest problem is that this study was performed in penetrating injuries. Patients with blunt trauma are not so likely to have definitive surgical interventions.
- This approach is inapplicable in head injured patients who require maintenance of cerebral perfusion pressure to reduce secondary brain injury.
- Further controlled trials are awaited, but it would be unfortunate if improvements in trauma management, related to an understanding of the importance of rapid resuscitation with volume infusion as a cornerstone of that resuscitation, were lost because fluid restriction was seen as appropriate in only a few specific (and uncommon) circumstances.

Blood transfusion

From the perspective of the anesthesiologist, certain points are worth emphasizing:

- The importance of communication with the surgeon regarding bleeding. On occasion the surgeon may need to be told to stop dissecting and control active bleeding to allow one to "catch up."
- Similarly, one must communicate early with the blood bank about requirements, especially for clotting factors.

- Many anesthesiologists only start to consider blood transfusion once approximately 10% of the patient's blood volume (based on 80 mL/kg body weight) has been lost. With ongoing brisk hemorrhage, one should not wait until 10% has been lost!
- Avoiding hypothermia will minimize coagulopathy as already described.
- Maintaining blood volume is probably more important in the short term than maintaining hemaglobin. However, with major hemorrhage, blood will be needed!
- Autologous transfusion systems like "cell savers" should be considered for appropriate "clean" operations.

Blood transfusion is discussed further in its own chapter.

Inotropes and vasoactive drugs

In addition to the normal anesthetic goals that pertain to all patients, one must pay especial attention to the maintenance of organ blood flow and function in the critically ill patient. This is obviously the case for all our patients, but fortunately the vast majority of low-risk patients present few problems and rarely need any form of circulatory support. In septic or shocked patients, this is the norm and the choice of inotropes and vasopressors and monitoring of the circulation are discussed as follows.

- Adequate filling pressures and intravascular volume are crucial prior to anesthesia and the use of inotropic agents. With hypovolemia, the vasdodilator effects of inotropic agents such as dobutamine predominate, leading to hypotension. The use of vasopressors in hypovolemia will reduce splanchnic and muscle blood flow.
- Cardiac function can be severely compromised in hemorrhagic shock so that an element of cardiogenic shock contributes to the shocked state. In such cases, the response to resuscitation may be compromised and invasive monitoring and/or inotropes required, as detailed here. As early as the 1950s, the contribution of the heart to progressive, irreversible shock was recognized and it was also demonstrated that the homeostatic mechanisms and vasoconstriction were not sufficient to maintain coronary perfusion in severe hemorrhage. Therefore, cardiac dysfunction needs to be detected and corrected as early after injury as possible.
- For myocardial support in the failing heart and low output states, dobutamine is probably the agent of choice.
- For vascular support, as with abnormal vasodilation, a vasopressor such as norepinephrine (noradrenaline) is probably the agent of choice.

References

1. Bitterman H, Reissman P, Bitterman N, et al. Oxygen therapy in hemorrhagic shock. *Circ Shock* 1991; **33**: 183–91.
2. Brundage SI, McGhan R, Jurkovich GJ, et al. Timing of femur fracture fixation: effect on outcome in patients with thoracic and head injuries. *J Trauma* 2002; **52**: 299–307.
3. Parr MJ, Alabdi T. Damage control surgery and intensive care. *Injury* 2004; **35**: 713–22.
4. Balogh Z, McKinley BA, Cocanour CS, et al. Supranormal trauma resuscitation causes more cases of abdominal compartment syndrome. *Arch Surg* 2003; **138**: 637–42.
5. Watts DD, Trask A, Soeken K, et al. Hypothermic coagulopathy in trauma: effect of varying levels of hypothermia on enzyme speed, platelet function, and fibrinolytic activity. *J Trauma* 1998; **44**: 846–54.

6. Rajagopalan S, Mascha E, Na J, et al. The effects of mild perioperative hypothermia on blood loss and transfusion requirement. *Anesthesiology* 2008; **108**: 71–7.

7. Frank SM, Fleisher LA, Breslow MJ, et al. Perioperative maintenance of normothermia reduces the incidence of morbid cardiac events: a randomised clinical trial. *JAMA* 1997: **227**: 1127–43.

8. Karalapillai D, Story D, Hart GK, et al. Postoperative hypothermia and patient outcomes after major elective non-cardiac surgery. *Anaesthesia* 2013; **68**: 605–11.

9. Berti M, Casati A, Torri G, et al. Active warming, not passive heat retention, maintains normothermia during combined epidural–general anesthesia for hip and knee arthroplasty. *J Clin Anesth* 1997; **9**: 482–6.

10. Aubier M, Vines N, Syllie G, et al. Respiratory muscle contribution to lactic acidosis in low cardiac output. *Am Rev Resp Dis* 1982: **126**: 648–52.

11. Morris C, Perris A, Klein J, et al. Anaesthesia in hemodynamically compromised emergency patients: does ketamine represent the best choice of induction agent? *Anaesthesia* 2009; **64**: 532–9.

12. Willman EV, Andolfatto G. A prospective evaluation of "ketofol" (ketamine/propofol combination) for procedural sedation and analgesia in the emergency department. *Ann Emerg Med* 2007; **49**: 23–30.

13. Bogetz MS, Katz JA. Recall of surgery for major trauma. *Anesthesiology* 1984; **61**: 6–9.

14. Longnecker DE, Sturgill BC. Influence of anesthetic agent on survival following hemorrhage. *Anesthesiology* 1976; **45**: 516–21.

15. Englehart MS, Allison CE, Tieu BH, et al. Ketamine-based total intravenous anesthesia versus isoflurane anesthesia in a swine model of hemorrhagic shock. *J Trauma* 2008; **65**: 901–8.

16. Idvall J. Influence of ketamine anesthesia on cardiac output and tissue perfusion in rats subjected to hemorrhage. *Anesthesiology* 1981; **55**: 297–304.

17. Johnson KB, Egan TD, Kern SE, et al. The influence of hemorrhagic shock on propofol: a pharmacokinetic and pharmacodynamic analysis. *Anesthesiology* 2003; **99**: 409–20.

18. Johnson KB, Egan TD, Layman J, et al. The influence of hemorrhagic shock on etomidate: a pharmacokinetic and pharmacodynamic analysis. *Anesth Analg* 2003; **96**: 1360–8.

19. Johnson KB, Kern SE, Hamber EA, et al. Influence of hemorrhagic shock on remifentanil: a pharmacokinetic and pharmacodynamic analysis. *Anesthesiology* 2001; **94**: 322–32.

20. Yli-Hankala A, Kirvela M, Randell T, et al. Ketamine anaesthesia in a patient with septic shock. *Acta Anaesthesiol Scand* 1992; **36**: 483–5.

21. Van der Linden P, Gilbart E, Engelman E, et al. Comparison of halothane, isoflurane, alfentanil and ketamine in experimental septic shock. *Anesth Analg* 1990; **70**: 608–17.

22. Kawasaki C, Kawasaki T, Ogata M, et al. Ketamine isomers suppress superantigen-induced proinflammatory cytokine production in human whole blood. *Can J Anaesth* 2001; **48**: 819–23.

23. Beilin B, Rusabrov Y, Shapira Y, et al. Low-dose ketamine affects immune responses in humans during the early postoperative period. *Br J Anaesth* 2007; **99**: 522–7.

24. Taniguchi T, Yamamoto K, Ohmoto N, et al. Effects of propofol on hemodynamic and inflammatory responses to endotoxemia in rats. *Crit Care Med* 2000; **28**: 1101–6.

25. Yu HP, Lui PW, Hwang TL, et al. Propofol improves endothelial dysfunction and attenuates vascular superoxide production in septic rats. *Crit Care Med* 2006; **34**: 453–60.

26. Kidani Y, Taniguchi T, Kanakura H, et al. Sevoflurane pretreatment inhibits endotoxin-induced shock in rats. *Anesth Analg* 2005; **101**: 1152–6.

27. Jabre P, Combes X, Lapostolle F, et al. Etomidate versus ketamine for rapid sequence intubation in acutely ill

patients: a multicentre randomised controlled trial. *Lancet* 2009; **374**: 293–300.

28. Baird CR, Hay AW, McKeown DW, et al. Rapid sequence induction in the emergency department: induction drug and outcome of patients admitted to the intensive care unit. *Emerg Med J* 2009; **26**: 576–9.

29. Ray DC, Hay AW, McKeown DW. Induction drug and outcome of patients admitted to the intensive care unit after emergency laparotomy. *Eur J Anaesthesiol* 2010; **27**: 481–5.

30. Gelissen HP, Epema AH, Henning RH, et al. Inotropic effects of propofol, thiopental, midazolam, etomidate, and ketamine on isolated human atrial muscle. *Anesthesiology* 1996; **84**: 397–403.

31. Paris A, Philipp M, Tonner PH, et al. Activation of alpha 2B-adrenoceptors mediates the cardiovascular effects of etomidate. *Anesthesiology* 2003: **99**; 889–95.

32. Budde AO, Mets B. Pro: etomidate is the ideal induction agent for a cardiac anesthetic. *J Cardiothorac Vasc Anesth* 2013; **1**: 180–3.

33. Mackay CA, Terris J, Coats TJ. Prehospital rapid sequence induction by emergency physicians: is it safe? *Emerg Med J* 2001; **18**: 20–4.

34. Vinclair M, Broux C, Faure P. Duration of adrenal inhibition following a single dose of etomidate in critically ill patients. *Intensive Care Med* 2008; **34**: 714–19.

35. den Brinker M, Hokken-Koelega AC, Hazelzet JA, et al. One single dose of etomidate negatively influences adrenocortical performance for at least 24 h in children with meningococcal sepsis. *Intensive Care Med* 2008; **34**: 163–8.

36. Morris C, McAllister C. Etomidate for emergency anaesthesia; mad, bad and dangerous to know? *Anaesthesia* 2005; **60**: 737–40.

37. Annane D. ICU physicians should abandon the use of etomidate! *Intensive Care Med* 2005; **31**: 325–6.

38. Stuttmann R, Allolio B, Becker A, et al. Etomidate versus etomidate and hydrocortisone for anaesthesia induction in abdominal surgical interventions. *Anaesthetist* 1988; **37**: 576–82.

39. Cuthbertson BH, Sprung CL, Annane D, et al. The effects of etomidate on adrenal responsiveness and mortality in patients with septic shock. *Intensive Care Med* 2009; **35**: 1868–76.

40. Ray DC, McKeown DW. Effect of induction agent on vasopressor and steroid use, and outcome in patients with septic shock. *Crit Care* 2007; **11**: R56.

41. Payen JF, Dupuis C, Trouve-Buisson T, et al. Corticosteroid after etomidate in critically ill patients: a randomized controlled trial. *Crit Care Med* 2012; **40**: 29–35.

42. Dmello D, Taylor S, O'Brien J, et al. Outcomes of etomidate in severe sepsis and septic shock. *Chest* 2010; **138**: 1327–32.

43. Ehrman R, Wira C, Lomax A, et al. Etomidate use in severe sepsis and septic shock patients does not contribute to mortality. *Intern Emerg Med* 2011; **6**: 253–7.

44. Elliot M, Brown G, Kuo IF. Does etomidate increase vasopressor requirements in patients needing mechanical ventilation? *Can J Hosp Pharm* 2012; **65**: 272–6.

45. Chan CM, Mitchell AL, Shorr AF. Etomidate is associated with mortality and adrenal insufficiency in sepsis: a meta-analysis. *Crit Care Med* 2012; **40**: 2945–53.

46. McPhee LC, Badawi O, Fraser GL, et al. Single-dose etomidate is not associated with increased mortality in ICU patients with sepsis: analysis of a large electronic ICU database. *Crit Care Med* 2013; **41**: 774–83.

47. Jevtovic-Todorovic V, Wozniak DF, Benshoff ND, et al. A comparative evaluation of the neurotoxic properties of ketamine and nitrous oxide. *Brain Res.* 2001; **895**: 264–7.

48. Badner NH, Beattie WS, Freeman D, et al. Nitrous oxide-induced increased homocysteine concentrations are associated with increased postoperative myocardial ischemia in patients undergoing carotid endarterectomy. *Anesth Analg* 2000; **91**: 1073–9.

49. Myles PS, Chan MT, Leslie K, et al. Effect of nitrous oxide on plasma homocysteine and folate in patients undergoing major surgery. *Br J Anaesth* 2008; **100**: 780–6.

50. Myles PS, Chan MT, Kaye DM, et al. Effect of nitrous oxide anesthesia on plasma homocysteine and endothelial function. *Anesthesiology* 2008; **109**: 657–63.

51. Lehmberg J, Waldner M, Baethmann A, et al. Inflammatory response to nitrous oxide in the central nervous system. *Brain Res* 2008; **1246**: 88–95.

52. Myles PS, Leslie K, Chan MT, et al. Avoidance of nitrous oxide for patients undergoing major surgery: a randomized controlled trial. *Anesthesiology* 2007; **107**: 221–31.

53. Leslie K, Myles PS, Chan MT, et al. Nitrous oxide and long-term morbidity and mortality in the ENIGMA trial. *Anesth Analg* 2011; **112**: 387–93.

54. Del Guercio LRN, Cohn JD. Monitoring operative risk in the elderly. *JAMA* 1980; **297**: 845–50.

55. Tavernier B, Makhotine O, Lebuffe G, et al. Systolic pressure variation as a guide to fluid therapy in patients with sepsis-induced hypotension. *Anesthesiology* 1998; **89**: 1313–21.

56. Derichard A, Robin E, Tavernier B, et al. Automated pulse pressure and stroke volume variations from radial artery: evaluation during major abdominal surgery. *Br J Anaesth* 2009; **103**: 678–84.

57. Lahner D, Kabon B, Marschalek C, et al. Evaluation of stroke volume variation obtained by arterial pulse contour analysis to predict fluid responsiveness intraoperatively. *Br J Anaesth* 2009; **103**: 346–51.

58. Harvey S, Harrison DA, Singer M, et al. Assessment of the clinical effectiveness of pulmonary artery catheters in management of patients in intensive care (PAC-Man): a randomised controlled trial. *Lancet* 2005; **366**: 472–7.

59. American Society of Anesthesiologists Task Force on Pulmonary Artery Catheterization. Practice guidelines for pulmonary artery catheterization: an updated report by the American Society of Anesthesiologists Task Force on Pulmonary Artery Catheterization. *Anesthesiology* 2003; **99**: 988–1014.

60. Schober P, Loer SA, Schwarte LA. Perioperative hemodynamic monitoring with transesophageal Doppler technology. *Anesth Analg* 2009; **109**: 340–53.

61. Belloni L, Pisano A, Natale A, et al. Assessment of fluid-responsiveness parameters for off-pump coronary artery bypass surgery: a comparison among LiDCO, transesophageal echochardiography, and pulmonary artery catheter. *J Cardiothorac Vasc Anesth* 2008; **22**: 243–8.

62. Schulmeyer MC, Santelices E, Vega R, et al. Impact of intraoperative transesophageal echocardiography during noncardiac surgery. *J Cardiothorac Vasc Anesth* 2006; **20**: 768–71.

63. Skinner H, Morgan-Hughes N, Swanevelder J, et al. Accreditation in transoesophageal echocardiography in the UK: the initial experience. *Br J Anaesth* 2012; **109**: 487–90.

64. Klein AA, Snell A, Nashef SA, et al. The impact of intra-operative transoesophageal echocardiography on cardiac surgical practice. *Anaesthesia* 2009; **64**: 947–52.

65. Mimoz O, Rauss A, Rekik N, et al. Pulmonary artery catheterization in critically ill patients: a prospective analysis of outcome changes associated with catheter-prompted changes in therapy. *Crit Care Med* 1994; **22**: 573–9.

66. American Society of Anesthesiologists and Society of Cardiovascular Anesthesiologists Task Force on Transesophageal Echocardiography. Practice guidelines for perioperative transesophageal echocardiography. An updated report by the American Society of Anesthesiologists and the Society of Cardiovascular Anesthesiologists Task Force on Transesophageal Echocardiography. *Anesthesiology* 2010; **112**: 1084–96.

67. Wise J. Boldt: the great pretender. *BMJ* 2013; **346**: f1738.

68. Bayer O, Reinhart K, Kohl M, et al. Effects of fluid resuscitation with synthetic colloids or crystalloids alone on shock reversal, fluid balance, and patient outcomes in patients with severe sepsis: a prospective sequential analysis. *Crit Care Med* 2012; **40**: 2543–51.

69. Myburgh JA, Finfer S, Bellomo R, et al. Hydroxyethyl starch or saline for fluid resuscitation in intensive care. *N Engl J Med* 2012; **367**: 1901–11.

70. Perner A, Haase N, Guttormsen AB, et al. Hydroxyethyl starch 130/0.42 versus Ringer's acetate in severe sepsis. *N Engl J Med* 2012; **367**: 124–34.

71. Zarychanski R, Abou-Setta AM, Turgeon AF, et al. Association of hydroxyethyl starch administration with mortality and acute kidney injury in critically ill patients requiring volume resuscitation: a systematic review and meta-analysis. *JAMA* 2013; **309**: 678–88.

72. Haase N, Perner A, Hennings LI, et al. Hydroxyethyl starch 130/0.38–0.45 versus crystalloid or albumin in patients with sepsis: systematic review with meta-analysis and trial sequential analysis. *BMJ* 2013; **346**: f839.

73. Perel P, Roberts I, Ker K. Colloids versus crystalloids for fluid resuscitation in critically ill patients. *Cochrane Database Syst Rev*. 2013; **2**: CD000567.

74. Van der Linden P, James M, Mythem M, et al. Safety of modern starches used during surgery. *Anesth Analg* 2013; **113**: 35–48.

75. Nolan JP, Mythen MG. Hydroxyethyl starch: here today, gone tomorrow. *Br J Anaesth* 2013; **111**: 321–4.

76. Wilkes NJ, Woolf R, Mutch M, et al. The effects of balanced versus saline-based hetastarch and crystalloid solutions on acid-base and electrolyte status and gastric mucosal perfusion in elderly surgical patients. *Anesth Analg* 2001; **93**: 811–16.

77. Waters JH, Gottlieb A, Schoenwald P, et al. Normal saline versus lactated Ringer's solution for intraoperative fluid management in patients undergoing abdominal aortic aneurysm repair: an outcome study. *Anesth Analg* 2001; **93**: 817–22.

78. McCluskey SA, Karkouti K, Wijeysundera D, et al. Hyperchloremia after noncardiac surgery is independently associated with increased morbidity and mortality: a propensity-matched cohort study. *Anesth Analg* 2013; **117**: 412–21.

79. Yunos NM, Bellomo R, Hegarty C, et al. Association between a chloride-liberal vs chloride-restrictive intravenous fluid administration strategy and kidney injury in critically ill adults. *JAMA* 2012; **308**: 1566–72.

80. Butterworth JF IV, Mythen MG. Should "normal" saline be our usual choice in normal surgical patients? *Anesth Analg* 2013; **117**: 290–1.

81. Mythen MG, Webb AR. Perioperative plasma volume expansion reduces the incidence of gut mucosal hypoperfusion during cardiac surgery. *Arch Surg* 1995: **130**: 423–9.

82. Gan TJ, Soppitt A, Maroof M, et al. Goal-directed intraoperative fluid administration reduces length of hospital stay after major surgery. *Anesthesiology* 2002; **97**: 820–6.

83. Rivers E, Nguyen B, Havstad S, et al. Early goal-directed therapy in the treatment of severe sepsis and septic shock. *N Engl J Med* 2001; **345**: 1368–77.

84. Pearse R, Dawson D, Fawcett J, et al. Changes in central venous saturation after major surgery, and association with outcome. *Crit Care* 2005; **9**: R694–9.

85. Bickell WH, Wall MJ Jr, Pepe PE, et al. Immediate versus delayed fluid resuscitation for hypotensive patients with penetrating torso injuries. *N Engl J Med* 1994; **331**: 1105–9.

Chapter 21

The elderly patient

C.H. Brown IV and F. Sieber

Physiology of aging

Aging is a progressive physiological process characterized by "declining end organ reserve, decreased functional capacity, increasing imbalance of homeostatic mechanisms and an increasing incidence of pathologic processes" [1]. The effects of aging are particularly manifest in discrete organ systems:

Central nervous system (CNS)

- Biochemical and structural changes have been described in the aging brain, but the exact mechanisms causing changes in functional reserve are unclear.
- Structurally, gray and white matter volume in the CNS decrease [2], but it is unclear whether the number of synapses present in the cortex is also altered.
- Older adults demonstrate increased sensitivity to anesthetic drugs, and increased risk of both perioperative delirium and postoperative cognitive dysfunction, likely due to decreases in brain reserve.
- Neuraxial structural changes include a reduced volume of cerebrospinal fluid, reduction of the epidural space, and increased dura permeability. The diameter and number of myelinated fibers in the dorsal and ventral nerve roots are reduced in older adults.

Cardiovascular

- Cardiac structure and function is altered in older adults. Structural changes include a decrease in number of myocytes and left ventricular (LV) hypertrophy. These structural changes result in decreased contractility, increased myocardial stiffness, and increased ventricular filling pressures.
- Impairment of diastolic relaxation, which can occur as a result of LV hypertrophy, also leads to diastolic dysfunction in the aging heart. With diastolic dysfunction, echocardiography may demonstrate preserved or hyperdynamic LV systolic function but show characteristic changes in the pattern of flow through the mitral valve. Systolic dysfunction may also be present.
- Increased vascular stiffness is common with advancing age and leads to important secondary responses in the heart. With increased resistance in the vasculature, the velocity of pulse wave conduction down the vascular tree increases, and reflected pulse

Anesthesia and Perioperative Care of the High-Risk Patient, Third edition, ed. Ian McConachie. Published by Cambridge University Press.

waves return to the heart at the end of ejection, resulting in increased cardiac afterload [3] and subsequent LV wall thickening, hypertrophy, and impaired diastolic filling [4].

- Decreased ventricular compliance and increased afterload combine to result in decreased early diastolic filling time, and thus the contribution of atrial contraction to ventricular filling becomes more important. For this reason, non-sinus cardiac rhythms are often poorly tolerated in the elderly and maintaining adequate preload is important.
- Calcification of aortic and mitral valves are common in the elderly, and can be easily seen echocardiographically.
- Changes in the autonomic system with aging include an increase in sympathetic nervous system activity [5]. Increased resting sympathetic nervous system activity may result in increased systemic vascular resistance and lead to more intraoperative hemodynamic lability.
- With aging, there is decreased β-receptor responsiveness, which is associated with decreased maximal heart rate and decreased peak ejection fraction. Thus, the metabolic demand for increased cardiac output is met primarily by preload reserve, rendering the heart more susceptible to cardiac failure [6].

Respiratory

- The elderly patient is at increased risk for perioperative pulmonary complications, due to alterations in control of respiration, lung structure, lung mechanics, and pulmonary blood flow.
- Important ventilatory responses to hypoxia, hypercapnia, and mechanical stress are attenuated, and the respiratory depressant effects of benzodiazepines, opioids, and volatile anesthetics are exaggerated [7]. Together, these changes reduce important protective responses against hypoxemia in the postoperative period.
- Structural changes in the lung with aging lead to an increase in lung compliance.
- Increased compliance leads to limited maximal expiratory flow, manifest by a progressive decrease in forced expiratory volume in one second (FEV_1) by 6%–8% per decade. Furthermore, loss of elastic elements within the lung is associated with enlargement of the respiratory bronchioles and alveolar ducts, and a tendency for small airway collapse during exhalation, with a subsequent increased risk of air trapping and hyperinflation.
- The functional results of these changes are increased anatomical dead space, decreased diffusing capacity, and increased closing capacity – all changes that result in impaired gas exchange.
- In terms of lung volumes, total lung capacity remains constant, while residual volume increases by 5%–10% per decade. As a result, vital capacity decreases. Closing capacity, the volume at which small airways close, also increases in the elderly. Importantly, when functional residual capacity is below closing capacity, increasing shunt results in a decrease in arterial oxygenation and an increase in the alveolar-arterial oxygen gradient.
- Pulmonary vascular resistance and pulmonary artery pressures increase with age, in part due to a reduction in the cross-sectional area of the pulmonary capillary bed.

Renal

- Renal blood flow decreases approximately 10% per decade after the age of 40 years [1].

- Although creatinine clearance falls, muscle mass also decreases with aging, hence serum creatinine is a poor predictor of renal function in older adults [8], and proper dosage adjustment for renally excreted medications is essential.
- Older adults have a diminished ability to handle salt loads as well as a diminished capacity to conserve sodium, thus putting them at higher risk for both dehydration and fluid overload.

Pharmacological

Factors that impact the pharmacological responses in older adults include changes in:

- Body content – older individuals have decreased lean body mass, increased body fat, and decreased total body water. Decreases in total body water may decrease the central compartment leading to increased peak serum concentrations after bolus administration of hydrophilic drugs. Body fat increases the volume of distribution and prolongs effects of lipophilic medications [9].
- Drug metabolism – hepatic and renal clearance decrease with aging and can affect pharmacokinetics.
- Pharmacodynamics – alterations in receptor numbers or sensitivity will determine the relative influence of pharmacodynamic alterations on anesthetic effect in elderly patients. Generally, the elderly are more sensitive to anesthetic agents, and drug effect is prolonged.

Anesthetic management

Consent

- Dementia, depression, hearing difficulties, and stroke all may interfere with the ability of older adults to make independent decisions, and obtaining true informed consent may be difficult in frail elderly patients.
- A surrogate must give consent for patients whose decision making is significantly impaired. Advance directives, when available, can be helpful.
- Increasing numbers of patients present to the operating room with "do not resuscitate" orders [10].

Assessment

Geriatric specific principles of preoperative evaluation include:

- Maintain a high index of suspicion for disease processes common in older adults, which may affect anesthetic management.
- Neurological, pulmonary, and cardiac events are the most common types of postoperative complications in the elderly [11], and thus require the most attention.
- Preoperative evaluation should assess the patient's overall physiological and functional reserve, in addition to a focus on pertinent organ systems. This combined approach will help the anesthesiologist gauge how the patient will fare following surgery and anesthesia.
- Accurate diagnosis of dementia is not always easy, but abbreviated screening tools are available [12].

- A commonly used screening tool for assessing functional level in the preoperative assessment is the activities of daily living (ADL) and instrumental activities of daily living (IADL). Daily self care activities are assessed through the ADL scale while IADLs assess more complex tasks. IADL and ADL assessments are important for their predictive ability for mortality and functional recovery [13], and serial measurements can document functional change.
- Frailty is an independent risk factor for major morbidity, mortality, protracted length of hospital stay, and institutional discharge [14,15]. Frailty is a clinical syndrome characterized by weight loss, fatigue, and weakness, and the specific components of the syndrome include mobility, muscle weakness, poor exercise tolerance, unstable balance, and body composition factors such as weight loss, malnutrition, and muscle wasting [16]. Frailty may be common in older adults presenting for surgery, with the incidence in a community dwelling population greater than 65 years of age estimated to be 7% [16]. Malnutrition and muscle wasting are discussed further in the chapter entitled *Obese or thin patient*.
- Acute illness in older adults may have an atypical presentation [17]. In particular, there may be significant differences in the presentation of disease in demented versus nondemented patients. The nonspecific presentation of disease in older people has been linked to accompanying dementia rather than a characteristic of the aging process intrinsically [18].
- Polypharmacy is common in hospitalized elderly patients [19], and the probability of an adverse drug reaction is proportional to the degree of polypharmacy. It is important to understand potential interactions between the medications a patient is taking, as well as the interactions with medications used in the perioperative period.
- Malnourishment is associated with increased morbidity and mortality as well as increased length of stay [20]. In the community dwelling aged population, the prevalence of malnutrition has been estimated to be 17% in females and 11% in males. Among acutely hospitalized older adults, the prevalence of malnutrition is 52% [19].
- Falls are the leading cause of unintentional traumatic injury and death in older adults [21]. Substance abuse, in particular alcohol, is often under-recognized as a factor [22].
- Chronic pain is under-appreciated, but prevalence estimates in community dwelling older adults range from 25% to 50%. Consequences of chronic pain include depression, sleep disturbance, and impaired ambulation [23]. In nursing home residents, arthritis is the most common indication for analgesics, followed by bone fracture and other musculoskeletal conditions. In the perioperative period, it is important to evaluate the baseline use of pain medication.
- Depression is asscociated with increased risk of major adverse cardiac events including death [24].

Anesthetic drug management

Inhaled anesthetics

Both the minimum alveolar anesthetic concentration (MAC) and MAC-awake decrease by approximately 6% per decade of age [25].

Intravenous anesthetics and benzodiazepines

Brain sensitivity to thiopental is unchanged with age [26]. The thiopental dose required for anesthesia decreases with age because of a reduction in the initial distribution volume of the drug. The decreased initial distribution volume is associated with higher serum drug levels following a given dose of thiopental in the elderly [26]. Etomidate dose requirements in the elderly are reduced secondary to both decreased clearance and initial volume of distribution [27]. There is a 30%–50% increased sensitivity to propofol in the elderly, secondary to the additive effects of increased brain sensitivity and decreased clearance [9]. The dose requirement of midazolam to produce sedation is reduced approximately 75% in elderly patients, secondary to both increased brain sensitivity and decreased drug clearance [28].

Opiates

Both morphine and its metabolite morphine-6-glucuronide have decreased clearance in the elderly [29]. Sufentanil, alfentanil, remifentanyl, and fentanyl are approximately twice as potent in elderly patients, primarily due to an increase in brain sensitivity to opioids rather than pharmacokinetic changes [30].

Muscle relaxants

Age does not significantly affect the pharmacodynamics of muscle relaxants, although the duration of action may be prolonged for drugs dependent on liver or renal metabolism. Pancuronium clearance is dependent on renal excretion, but the effect of aging on pancuronium clearance is controversial [31]. Atracurium is partially cleared through hepatic mechanisms and its elimination half-life is prolonged in the elderly. However, atracurium clearance is unchanged with age, implying that ester hydrolysis and Hofmann elimination pathways may be important in older adults [32]. Cisatracurium clearance is unaffected by age. Plasma clearance of vecuronium is lower in elderly patients, which may reflect decreases in renal or hepatic reserve [33]. Rocuronium is associated with a prolonged duration in elderly patients [33].

Neuraxial anesthesia and peripheral nerve blocks

Age does not alter the duration of motor blockade with bupivicaine spinal anesthesia or with epidural anesthesia using 0.5% bupivacaine [34]. However, the duration of motor and sensory blockade after peripheral nerve block using 0.75% ropivacaine is increased in older adults.

Anesthetic management – intra- and postoperative

- Shorter-acting anesthetic agents may be preferred for elderly patients. For example, there is an increased incidence of residual neuromuscular blockade as well as pulmonary complications in patients receiving longer-acting muscle relaxants.
- Optimal physiological management in the elderly has not been determined, although hemodynamic changes may be associated with poor outcomes. The severity and duration of intraoperative hypotension in elderly patients has been associated with one-year mortality, although controlled hypotensive anesthesia (mean arterial blood pressure range of 45–55 mmHg) during orthopedic procedures has been demonstrated

in one study to be safe in older adults [35]. Pulmonary artery catheterization has not been shown to be beneficial over standard care in elderly, high-risk surgical patients requiring intensive care [36].

In general, outcomes are not different between regional and general anesthesia in elderly patients [37]. Some specific effects of regional anesthesia that may provide benefit include:

- There may be a decrease in the incidence of deep vein thrombosis with regional anesthesia following total hip arthroplasty, but not following total knee arthroplasty [38].
- The incidence of postoperative graft thrombosis following lower extremity revascularization may be decreased with regional compared to general anesthesia [39].
- There may be decreased blood loss in pelvic and lower extremity surgery using regional anesthesia [40].
- There may be a lower risk of hypoxemia with regional anesthesia [41].
- Opiate usage is decreased following total joint arthroplasty under regional anesthesia.

There are no elderly-specific guidelines for post-anesthesia care unit (PACU) management, although elderly-specific issues include:

- Age is an important risk factor for postoperative pulmonary complications [42], and there is a greater reported incidence of postoperative desaturation in the PACU in the elderly.
- Impaired laryngopharyngeal sensory discrimination and dysfunctional swallowing may lead to a higher risk for aspiration among older adults [43].
- Urinary retention is more common in elderly males [44].

Several principles should be kept in mind when managing pain in frail, elderly patients:

- Multiple modalities of analgesia may be useful, especially in frail patients, who tolerate systemic narcotics poorly.
- Local nerve blocks may be a helpful adjunct.
- Non-steroidal anti-inflammatory drug preparations should be used to enhance analgesia and decrease inflammatory mediators, unless there is a contraindication or concern about hemostasis or peptic ulceration.
- Opioid-based postoperative pain management in the elderly must take into account the decreased dose requirements with age.
- Both experimental and clinical studies provide support for the notion of an age-related decrease in pain perception [45].
- Pain can be difficult to evaluate in the cognitively impaired. Although the sensory-discriminative component of pain is maintained in patients with Alzheimer's disease, pain tolerance increases with increasing dementia [46].

Complications

General

Major perioperative complications increase with age [47] and are associated with greater mortality [48]. The most important risk factors for perioperative complications in the elderly are:

- age
- physiological status and coexisting disease (ASA class) – older adults have decreased functional organ reserve and increased prevalence of chronic systemic diseases. In the setting of decreased physiological reserve and increased comorbidity, usual compensatory mechanisms for perioperative insults can be inadequate.
- The urgency of surgery – emergency surgery is an independent predictor of poor postoperative outcomes in older patients [49]. Patients who present for emergency surgery may have atypical presentations, thus delaying their diagnosis. Changes in pulmonary and circulatory systems and fluid and electrolyte imbalances require special attention.
- Type of procedure – surgical mortality in the elderly varies widely according to procedure [50]. The cardiovascular risk of surgeries may be categorized into low, intermediate, and high-risk, based on current American Heart Association (AHA) guidelines for cardiovascular evaluation of patients undergoing non-cardiac surgery [51].

Delirium

Postoperative delirium is an acute confusional state with changes in attention and consciousness, and is defined in the fourth edition of the *Diagnostic and Statistical Manual of Mental Disorders* (DSM-IV) as: "The essential feature of a delirium is a disturbance in consciousness that is accompanied by a change in cognition that cannot be better accounted for by a preexisting or evolving dementia" [52].

- The prevalence of postoperative delirium in older adults has been estimated to be 10%, although estimates vary depending on many factors including the type of surgery and intensive care unit (ICU) stay. Cardiac surgery and hip fracture repair may have the highest incidence of delirium [53].
- The Confusion Assessment Method (CAM) [54] is widely used to detect delirum, and is designed to be rapid, accurate, and able to be used by non-clinicians. The sensitivity of the CAM against the gold standard of psychiatric diagnosis is 94%–100% with specificity of 90%–95% [54]. The CAM–ICU has been developed for assessing delirium in ventilated ICU patients [55].
- The consequences of delirium are profound, and delirium is associated with prolonged hospital stay, increased incidence of nursing home placement, an increased incidence of postoperative complications [56], and in patients with dementia, an acceleration of cognitive decline [57]. Overall two to three million elderly patients per year develop delirium during hospitalization, and one-year health costs attributable to delirium are estimated to be higher than $100 billion in the U.S.
- The basic mechanisms of delirium are poorly characterized, but some investigators hypothesize that delirium may be associated with inflammatory mediators or alterations in one of several neurotransmitter systems [58].
- In the geriatrics paradigm, delirium represents an atypical presentation of disease [59], in which dysfunction in the most vulnerable organ system (in this case, the brain) results from acute illness.
- A validated risk model for delirium in medical and surgical patients includes advanced age, alcohol abuse, cognitive impairment, poor functional status, electrolyte abnormalities, and type of surgery [60].

- A foundation in perioperative management of delirium is prevention, and multimodal interventions have proven effective. Recent studies have shown that early proactive geriatrics consults [61] or protocols to manage known risk factors (e.g., cognitive impairment, sleep deprivation, immobility, visual impairment, hearing impairment, and dehydration) reduce the number and length of delirium episodes in hospitalized older adults [62].
- Prophylactic antipsychotic administration may be effective to reduce delirium in high-risk patients [63].

Anesthetic-specific interventions include optimization of electrolytes, perioperative continuation of drugs for neuropsychiatric disorders, and limiting known pharmacological triggering agents (e.g., opioids – particularly meperidine, benzodiazepines, dihydropyridines, and antihistamines) [64]. Type of anesthesia (regional versus general) has not been associated with delirium, although the incidence of postoperative delirium may be decreased by targeting lighter depth of sedation during regional anesthesia [65].

- Antidepressants should be continued during the perioperative period so that abrupt discontinuation does not cause an increase in symptoms of depression or confusion [66].
- Recent randomized controlled trials have demonstrated no impact of blood transfusion strategy on severity or incidence of delirium [67], although retrospective studies have reported an association between delirium and greater intraoperative blood loss and more postoperative blood transfusions.

For patients who develop delirium, supportive care should be provided with a focus on preventing complications, such as self-injury or dislodgement of catheters. Next, precipitating medical causes should be investigated and treated. Pharmacological intervention may be needed, and management algorithms are available [68].

Postoperative cognitive dysfunction (POCD)

- POCD is common in the first days to weeks following surgery and in most cases is reversible, although in approximately 1% of cases, POCD may be persistent.
- The etiology of POCD is likely multifactorial, but may include medications, type of surgery, or underlying comorbidity. Recent studies suggest that POCD may be independent of both surgery and anesthesia [69] and may be more related to underlying patient comorbidities, particularly pre-existing cognitive impairment or atherosclerotic disease [70]. The contribution of anesthesia to POCD is not well defined, and there is no best anesthetic practice to prevent POCD.
- There is no difference in POCD incidence between regional and general anesthetic techniques.
- There is no specific treatment for POCD.
- It is controversial whether general anesthesia accelerates the downward cognitive trajectory of dementia. Available human studies on anesthesia and Alzheimer's disease are inconclusive because they are under-powered or confounded by coincident illness, independent risk factors for dementia, and surgery [71] However, sevoflurane compared to propofol or epidural anesthesia is associated with an enhanced downward cognitive trajectory of patients with minimal cognitive impairment [72].

Outcomes

While the mortality risk associated with many procedures is low, functional recovery may require significant time for many high-risk elderly patients.

- For example, after major abdominal surgery in older adults, functional recovery has been estimated to take up to six months or longer [73].
- Many elders require assistance with IADLs up to one year post-discharge.
- For elderly patients requiring admission to ICU, survival to discharge is most closely related to severity of illness at the time of admission, while age and pre-hospital functional status correlate most closely with long-term survival [74].
- A significant number of patients undergoing vascular surgery experience a decline in capacity for independent function [75].
- Dementia is associated with a 2.18 (1.10–4.32) relative risk of developing a patient-related adverse event during an unplanned acute hospital admission [76]. In addition, the presence and severity of dementia is associated with increased long-term postoperative mortality [77].

References

1. Sieber FE, Pauldine R. Anesthesia for the elderly. In: *Miller's Anesthesia*, 7th edn. Philadelphia, PA: Elsevier Churchill Livingstone, 2010; 2261–76.
2. Ge Y, Grossman RI, Babb JS, et al. Age-related total gray matter and white matter changes in normal adult brain. Part I: Volumetric MR imaging analysis. *AJNR Am J Neuroradiol* 2002; **23**: 1327–33.
3. Steppan J, Barodka V, Berkowitz DE, et al. Vascular stiffness and increased pulse pressure in the aging cardiovascular system. *Cardiol Res Pract* **2011**; 2011: 263585.
4. Frenneaux M, Williams L. Ventricular-arterial and ventricular-ventricular interactions and their relevance to diastolic filling. *Prog Cardiovasc Dis* 2007; **49**: 252–62.
5. Rooke GA. Cardiovascular aging and anesthetic implications. *J Cardiothorac Vasc Anesth* 2003; **17**: 512–23.
6. Priebe HJ. The aged cardiovascular risk patient. *Br J Anaesth* 2000; **85**: 763–78.
7. Zaugg M, Lucchinetti E. Respiratory function in the elderly. *Anesthesiol Clin North America* 2000; **18**: 47–58.
8. Musso CG, Oreopoulos DG. Aging and physiological changes of the kidneys including changes in glomerular filtration rate. *Nephron Physiol* 2011; **119**: 1–5.
9. Shafer SL. The pharmacology of anesthetic drugs in elderly patients. *Anesthesiol Clin North America* 2000; **18**: 1–29.
10. Scott TH, Gavrin JR. Palliative surgery in the do-not-resuscitate patient: ethics and practical suggestions for management. *Anesthesiol Clin* 2012; **30**: 1–12.
11. Liu LL, Leung JM. Predicting adverse postoperative outcomes in patients aged 80 years or older. *J Am Geriatr Soc* 2000; **48**: 405–12.
12. Carpenter CR, Bassett ER, Fischer GM, et al. Four sensitive screening tools to detect cognitive dysfunction in geriatric emergency department patients: brief Alzheimer's screen, short blessed test, Ottawa 3DY, and the caregiver-completed AD8. *Acad Emerg Med* 2011; **18**: 374–84.
13. Inouye SK, Peduzzi PN, Robison JT, et al. Importance of functional measures in predicting mortality among older hospitalized patients. *JAMA* 1998; **279**: 1187–93.
14. Lee DH, Buth KJ, Martin BJ, et al. Frail patients are at increased risk for mortality and prolonged institutional care after cardiac surgery. *Circulation* 2010; **121**: 973–8.
15. Makary MA, Segev DL, Pronovost PJ, et al. Frailty as a predictor of surgical outcomes

in older patients. *J Am Coll Surg* 2010; **210**: 901–8.

16. Fried LP, Tangen CM, Walston J, et al. Frailty in older adults: evidence for a phenotype. *J Gerontol A Biol Sci Med Sci* 2001; **56**: M146–56.

17. Fletcher KFW. Acute symptom assessment: determining the seriousness of the presentation. *Lippincotts Prim Care Pract* 1999; **3**: 216–28.

18. Johnson JC, Jayadevappa R, Baccash PD, et al. Nonspecific presentation of pneumonia in hospitalized older people: age effect or dementia? *J Am Geriatr Soc* 2000; **48**: 1316–20.

19. Buurman BM, Hoogerduijn JG, de Haan RJ, et al. Geriatric conditions in acutely hospitalized older patients: prevalence and one-year survival and functional decline. *PLoS One* 2011; **6**: e26951.

20. Potter J, Klipstein K, Reilly JJ, et al. The nutritional status and clinical course of acute admissions to a geriatric unit. *Age Ageing* 1995; **24**: 131–6.

21. Injury Prevention and Control: Data and Statistics. Ten leading causes of death and injury. Available from: http://www.cdc.gov/injury/wisqars/LeadingCauses.html

22. Zautcke JL, Coker SB Jr, Morris RW, et al. Geriatric trauma in the state of Illinois: substance use and injury patterns. *Am J Emerg Med* 2002; **20**: 14–17.

23. AGS Panel on Persistent Pain in Older Persons. The management of persistent pain in older persons. *J Am Geriatr Soc* 2002; **50**: S205–24.

24. Blumenthal JA, Lett HS, Babyak MA, et al. Depression as a risk factor for mortality after coronary artery bypass surgery. *Lancet* 2003; **362**: 604–9.

25. Eger EI II. Age, minimum alveolar anesthetic concentration, and minimum alveolar anesthetic concentration-awake. *Anesth Analg* 2001; **93**: 947–53.

26. Homer TD, Stanski DR. The effect of increasing age on thiopental disposition and anesthetic requirement. *Anesthesiology* 1985; **62**: 714–24.

27. Arden JR, Holley FO, Stanski DR. Increased sensitivity to etomidate in the elderly: initial distribution versus altered brain response. *Anesthesiology* 1986; **65**: 19–27.

28. Maitre PO, Buhrer M, Thomson D, et al. A three-step approach combining Bayesian regression and NONMEM population analysis: application to midazolam. *J Pharmacokinet Biopharm* 1991; **19**: 377–84.

29. Baillie SP, Bateman DN, Coates PE, et al. Age and the pharmacokinetics of morphine. *Age Ageing* 1989; **18**: 258–62.

30. Minto CF, Schnider TW, Egan TD, et al. Influence of age and gender on the pharmacokinetics and pharmacodynamics of remifentanil. I. Model development. *Anesthesiology* 1997; **86**: 10–23.

31. Rupp SM, Castagnoli KP, Fisher DM, et al. Pancuronium and vecuronium pharmacokinetics and pharmacodynamics in younger and elderly adults. *Anesthesiology* 1987; **67**: 45–9.

32. Kent AP, Parker CJ, Hunter JM. Pharmacokinetics of atracurium and laudanosine in the elderly. *Br J Anaesth* 1989; **63**: 661–6.

33. Furuya T, Suzuki T, Kashiwai A, et al. The effects of age on maintenance of intense neuromuscular block with rocuronium. *Acta Anaesthesiol Scand* 2012; **56**: 236–9.

34. Veering BT, Burm AG, Spierdijk J. Spinal anaesthesia with hyperbaric bupivacaine. Effects of age on neural blockade and pharmacokinetics. *Br J Anaesth* 1988; **60**: 187–94.

35. Williams-Russo P, Sharrock NE, Mattis S, et al. Randomized trial of hypotensive epidural anesthesia in older adults. *Anesthesiology* 1999; **91**: 926–35.

36. Sandham JD, Hull RD, Brant RF, et al. A randomized, controlled trial of the use of pulmonary artery catheters in high-risk surgical patients. *N Engl J Med* 2003; **348**: 5–14.

37. Roy RC. Choosing general versus regional anesthesia for the elderly. *Anesthesiol Clin North America* 2000; **18**: 91–104.

38. Williams-Russo P, Sharrock NE, Haas SB, et al. Randomized trial of epidural versus general anesthesia: outcomes after primary total knee replacement. *Clin Orthop Relat Res* 1996; **331**: 199–208.

39. Christopherson R, Beattie C, Frank S, et al. Perioperative morbidity in patients randomized to epidural or general anesthesia for lower extremity vascular surgery. Perioperative ischemia randomized anesthesia trial study group. *Anesthesiology* 1993; **79**: 422–34.

40. Shir Y, Raja SN, Frank S, et al. Intraoperative blood loss during radical retropubic prostatectomy: epidural versus general anesthesia. *Urology* 1995; **45**: 993–9.

41. Moller JT, Wittrup M, Johansen SH. Hypoxemia in the postanesthesia care unit: an observer study. *Anesthesiology* 1990; **73**: 890–5.

42. Smetana GW. Postoperative pulmonary complications: an update on risk assessment and reduction. *Cleve Clin J Med* 2009; **76**: S60–5.

43. Aviv J. Effects of aging on sensitivity of the pharyngeal and supraglottic areas. *Am J Med* 1997; **103**: 74S–6.

44. Keita H, Diouf E, Tubach F, et al. Predictive factors of early postoperative urinary retention in the postanesthesia care unit. *Anesth Analg* 2005; **101**: 592–6.

45. Washington LLGS, Helme RD. Age-related differences in the endogenous analgesic response to repeated cold water immersion in human volunteers. *Pain* 2000; **89**: 89–96.

46. Benedetti F, Vighetti S, Ricco C, et al. Pain threshold and tolerance in Alzheimer's disease. *Pain* 1999; **80**: 377–82.

47. Polanczyk CA, Marcantonio E, Goldman L, et al. Impact of age on perioperative complications and length of stay in patients undergoing noncardiac surgery. *Ann Intern Med* 2001; **134**: 637–43.

48. Hamel MB, Henderson WG, Khuri SF, et al. Surgical outcomes for patients aged 80 and older: morbidity and mortality from major noncardiac surgery. *J Am Geriatr Soc* 2005; **53**: 424–9.

49. Leung JM, Dzankic S. Relative importance of preoperative health status versus intraoperative factors in predicting postoperative adverse outcomes in geriatric surgical patients. *J Am Geriatr Soc* 2001; **49**: 1080–5.

50. Finlayson EV BJ. Operative mortality with elective surgery in older adults. *Eff Clin Pract* 2001; **4**: 172–7.

51. Fleisher LA, Beckman JA, Brown KA, et al. ACC/AHA 2007 guidelines on perioperative cardiovascular evaluation and care for noncardiac surgery: a report of the American College of Cardiology/American Heart Association Task Force on Practice Guidelines (writing committee to revise the 2002 guidelines on perioperative cardiovascular evaluation for noncardiac surgery): developed in collaboration with the American Society of Echocardiography, American Society of Nuclear Cardiology, Heart Rhythm Society, Society of Cardiovascular Anesthesiologists, Society for Cardiovascular Angiography and Interventions, Society for Vascular Medicine and Biology, and Society for Vascular Surgery. *Circulation* 2007; **116**: e418–99.

52. Diagnostic and Statistical Manual of Mental Disorders, 4th edn. Text Revision (DSM-IV-TR), Vol 4. Washington, DC: American Psychiatric Publishing, Inc.; 2000.

53. Rasmussen LS, JT M. Central nervous system dysfunction after anesthesia in the geriatric patient. *Anesthesiol Clin North America* 2000; **18**: 59–70.

54. Inouye SK, van Dyck CH, Alessi CA, et al. Clarifying confusion: the confusion assessment method. A new method for detection of delirium. *Ann Intern Med* 1990; **113**: 941–8.

55. Ely EW, Inouye SK, Bernard GR, et al. Delirium in mechanically ventilated patients: validity and reliability of the confusion assessment method for the intensive care unit (CAM–ICU). *JAMA* 2001; **286**: 2703–10.

56. McCusker J, Cole MG, Dendukuri N, et al. Does delirium increase hospital stay? *J Am Geriatr Soc* 2003; **51**: 1539–46.

57. Fong TG, Jones RN, Shi P, et al. Delirium accelerates cognitive decline in Alzheimer disease. *Neurology* 2009; **72**: 1570–5.

58. Simone MJ, Tan ZS. The role of inflammation in the pathogenesis of delirium and dementia in older adults: a review. *CNS Neurosci Ther* 2011; **17**: 506–13.

59. Resnick NM, Marcantonio ER. How should clinical care of the aged differ? *Lancet* 1997; **350**: 1157–8.

60. Marcantonio E, Goldman L, Mangione C, et al. A clinical prediction rule for delirium after elective non-cardiac surgery. *JAMA* 1994; **271**: 134–9.

61. Marcantonio ER, Flacker JM, Wright RJ, et al. Reducing delirium after hip fracture: a randomized trial. *J Am Geriatr Soc* 2001; **49**: 516–22.

62. Inouye SK, Bogardus ST Jr, Charpentier PA, et al. A multicomponent intervention to prevent delirium in hospitalized older patients. *N Engl J Med* 1999; **340**: 669–76.

63. Kalisvaart KJ, de Jonghe JF, Bogaards MJ, et al. Haloperidol prophylaxis for elderly hip-surgery patients at risk for delirium: a randomized placebo-controlled study. *J Am Geriatr Soc* 2005; **53**: 1658–66.

64. Clegg A, Young JB. Which medications to avoid in people at risk of delirium: a systematic review. *Age Ageing* 2011; **40**: 23–9.

65. Sieber FE, Zakriya KJ, Gottschalk A, et al. Sedation depth during spinal anesthesia and the development of postoperative delirium in elderly patients undergoing hip fracture repair. *Mayo Clin Proc* 2010; **85**: 18–26.

66. Kudoh A, Katagai H, Takazawa T. Antidepressant treatment for chronic depressed patients should not be discontinued prior to anesthesia. *Can J Anaesth* 2002; **49**: 132–6.

67. Gruber-Baldini AL, Marcantonio E, Orwig D, et al. Delirium outcomes in a randomized trial of blood transfusion thresholds in hospitalized older adults with hip fracture *J Am Geriatr Soc* 2013; **61**: 1286–95.

68. Inouye SK. Delirium in older persons. *N Engl J Med* 2006; **354**: 1157–65.

69. Evered L, Scott DA, Silbert B, et al. Postoperative cognitive dysfunction is independent of type of surgery and anesthetic. *Anesth Analg* 2011; **112**: 1179–85.

70. Bekker A, Lee C, de Santi S, et al. Does mild cognitive impairment increase the risk of developing postoperative cognitive dysfunction? *Am J Surg* 2010; **199**: 782–8.

71. Baranov D, Bickler PE, Crosby GJ, et al. Consensus statement: first international workshop on anesthetics and Alzheimer's disease. *Anesth Analg* 2009; **108**: 1627–30.

72. Liu Y, Pan N, Ma Y, et al. Inhaled sevoflurane may promote progression of amnestic mild cognitive impairment: a prospective, randomized parallel-group study *Am J Med Sci* **201**; 345: 355–60.

73. Lawrence VA, Hazuda HP, Cornell JE, et al. Functional independence after major abdominal surgery in the elderly. *J Am Coll Surg* 2004; **199**: 762–72.

74. Hennessy D, Juzwishin K, Yergens D, et al. Outcomes of elderly survivors of intensive care: a review of the literature. *Chest* 2005; **127**: 1764–74.

75. Crouch DS, McLafferty RB, Karch LA, et al. A prospective study of discharge disposition after vascular surgery. *J Vasc Surg* 2001; **34**: 62–8.

76. Watkin L, Blanchard MR, Tookman A, et al. Prospective cohort study of adverse events in older people admitted to the acute general hospital: risk factors and the impact of dementia. *Int J Geriatr Psychiatry* 2012; **27**: 76–82.

77. Lee HB, Kasper JD, Shore AD, et al. Level of cognitive impairment predicts mortality in high-risk community samples: the memory and medical care study. *J Neuropsychiatry Clin Neurosci* 2006; **18**: 543–6.

The patient with cardiac disease undergoing non-cardiac surgery

Z. Zafirova

Coronary artery disease

Epidemiology of coronary artery disease (CAD)

CAD is the most common cause of mortality, causing approximately one of every six deaths in the U.S. Total CAD prevalence is 6.4% in U.S. adults of ≥20 years of age, 7.9% in men and 5.1% in women. The lifetime risk of developing CAD after 40 years of age is 49% for men and 32% for women. Epidemiological and family studies have shown repeatedly that genetic predisposition accounts for 40%–60% of the risk for CAD. Risk factors for CAD include hypertension (HTN), hypercholesterolemia, diabetes mellitus, cigarette smoking, and renal failure. Furthermore, 21% of the myocardial infarctions (MIs) are silent. The incidence of perioperative MI (PMI) is difficult to assess due to variability in the diagnostic methods of different studies, and is likely underestimated as many PMIs are silent. The estimate is between 1% and 3% for low-risk patients and 2.7%–4.1% for high-risk patients with CAD; however, some studies have suggested it is much higher [1,2].

Pathophysiology and clinical presentation

- Exposure of the endothelium to inciting factors such as dyslipidemia, hyperglycemia and glycoxidation, vasoconstrictor hormones in hypertension, smoking, and proinflammatory cytokines derived from excess adipose tissue contribute to oxidative stress and the inflammatory response. Atheromatous plaque develops as a result of endothelial dysfunction – transmigration of leukocytes, migration and proliferation of smooth muscle cells and extracellular matrix, calcification, cellular death, and accumulation of lipid-rich necrotic core [3]. Progressive reduction of coronary flow and gradual anginal symptoms ensue. The clinical presentation is stress-induced chest pain and other anginal equivalents such as dyspnea, diaphoresis, nausea or vomiting, fatigue, and dizziness; hypotension, pallor, signs of congestive heart failure (CHF) or shock, and arrhythmia are more likely to be associated with acute coronary syndrome (aCS). Elecrocardiographic (ECG) changes of T-wave inversion and ST-segment depression can be identified.
- Inflammatory pathways and T-cell-derived activation play a role in plaque instability; disruption of unstable plaque, exposure of a prothrombotic surface, platelet aggregation, activation of the coagulation cascade, and intracoronary thrombus trigger aCS, including unstable angina, non-ST-segment elevation and ST-segment elevation MI,

Anesthesia and Perioperative Care of the High-Risk Patient, Third edition, ed. Ian McConachie. Published by Cambridge University Press.

and sudden cardiac death [4]. The clinical symptoms of aCS are more severe, occur more frequently, are present at rest, last longer, and may not resolve easily with or without therapy. ST depression and elevation, bundle–branch block, and arrhythmia are demonstrated on ECG, as well as by elevated cardiac markers.

- In the perioperative period, the stress response from surgery with catecholamine and cortisol surge and increased chronotropy and inotropy leads to an increase in oxygen demand, and ischemia if the supply from the diseased arteries is inadequate. Additionally, the induction of the systemic proinflammatory and prothrombotic state with the increase in inflammatory mediators, vasoconstriction, increased platelet and coagulation factor activity, and decreased fibrinolysis further increases the risk of reduction of coronary blood supply, especially at vulnerable plaques. Plaque rupture and arterial thrombosis is the cause of perioperative MI in only 25%–50% of patients [5,6]. aCS does not necessarily involve the most stenotic plaques that would be identified by the positive stress test [7].

Perioperative management

- The preoperative evaluation includes identification of the presence and nature of symptoms of CAD, identification of significant risk factors for CAD such as smoking, HTN, vascular disease, diabetes mellitus (DM), and renal failure. These data help to assess the perioperative risk utilizing scoring systems such as the Revised Cardiac Risk Index (RCRI) and to plan further diagnostic and therapeutic interventions. ECG, the stress test, and myocardial perfusion studies may be indicated.
- The medical management of a patient with CAD or substantial risk factors should be instituted preoperatively and continued through the perioperative period. Along with life-style modifications, it includes β-blockers, HMG-CoA reductase inhibitors, and antiplatelet agents. The recent studies bring into question the benefit to risk ratio of the wide-spread use of β-blockers; nonetheless, for specific high-risk populations, they may be beneficial [8,9]. The timing and the specific agent used vary in the studies. The combined use of β-blockers and HMG-CoA reductase inhibitors confers further benefit; even preoperative initiation of therapy with HMG-CoA reductase inhibitors has effects within a short time [10].
- Antiplatelet therapy, specifically aspirin (acetylsalicylic acid), is used as a primary and secondary prevention in patients with risk factors and known disease. It should be continued in the perioperative period at a low dose of 81 mg, except in procedures with high-bleeding risk. This therapy is discussed in further detail later.
- The preoperative revascularization in preparation for surgery is likely to benefit only very select group of patients, such as those with left main disease. It remains a subject of controversy and further study [11].
- The anesthetic management of these patients should focus on maintenance of hemodynamic stability. Studies have attempted to identify certain agents and techniques as more cardioprotective and associated with a lesser degree of hemodynamic alterations, such as benzodiazepines, opiates, and etomidate. The choice of anesthetic technique is less relevant; the specific use of the agents and their combinations and the clinician's experience with them have more influence on outcomes. Reduction in mean arterial pressure (MAP), cardiac index (CI), and stroke volume index (SVI) ranging from 10% to 40% can be seen with most agents [12]. The use of volatile agents, with

their potential cardioprotective effects, remains a subject of study. The evidence in cardiac surgery indicates benefits; however, the benefits and risks in non-cardiac surgery need to be examined further [13]. The use of regional techniques may reduce the impact of anesthesia on patients with CAD, provided that the hemodynamic stability is maintained, especially with neuraxial modalities.

- Intraoperative monitoring with ECG with ST-segment analysis and non-invasive blood pressure (BP) is essential; 12-lead ECG is more accurate than five-lead ECG; however, it is often impractical in the intraoperative setting. Additional invasive hemodynamic monitoring such as central venous pressure (CVP), pulmonary artery catheter (PAC), and transesophageal echocardiography (TEE) may be utilized, depending on the patient's baseline risk and the procedural factors.
- Extended postoperative monitoring in the intensive setting and serial investigation with 12-lead ECG and cardiac biomarkers is guided by the patient's condition and the occurrence of intraoperative events.

The patient with a coronary stent

The use of percutaneous coronary intervention (PCI) revascularization to restore arterial patency and improve myocardial perfusion in CAD is widely used in emergency and non-emergency situations. Deployment of stents improves long-term arterial patency and is estimated to be used in 85%–95% of PCIs.

- Bare-metal stents (BMS) have an associated risk of stent restenosis and thrombosis. Drug-eluting stents (DES) have antiprolipherative properties, thus reducing the incidence of restenosis; however, they impair endothelialization and the blood is exposed to the denuded endothelium and the thrombogenic stent struts, resulting in increased risk of stent thrombosis (ST).
- The incidence of stent restenosis for BMS is 10%–67%, for DES 0%–11%. The overall incidence of ST is 0.3%–0.6% per year and 0.6%–3.5% for BMS and 1.2%–3.6% for DES [14].

Perioperative management

The patients with recent coronary stents present a particular challenge in the perioperative period due to the need for continuous antiplatelet therapy and the balance between risk of ST and bleeding.

- The preoperative evaluation should identify the stent type, placement date (<1 month, 1–12 months, or >12 months), as well as signs and symptoms of ischemia pre- and post-stent placement, their nature, resolution, and recurrence.
- The medical therapy should be documented, and ideally continued, including antiplatelet therapy (APT), β-blockers, HMG-CoA reductase inhibitors, and angiotensin-converting enzyme (ACE) inhibitors.
- The status of APT needs to be clarified – the agents used for single, dual (DAPT), or triple therapy, their dose, the duration of therapy, and the time of the last dose administration. The most recent American Heart Association (AHA) guidelines recommend at least one month of DAPT for BMS, followed by aspirin indefinitely, while DES require at least 12 months of uninterrupted DAPT, followed by aspirin [15]. These recommendations will likely require update as the advances in stent development continue, such as the

production of biodegradable and polymer-free stents, new metal stent platforms–platinum chromium, new coating–titanium-nitride oxide, CD34 antibodies.

- The risk of ST increases substantially with premature discontinuation of DAPT; the relative risk is as high as 57–161. The short-term mortality of ST is 20%–45%, but in the perioperative setting, it has been reported as high as 85% [16].
- The increase in the bleeding risk from aspirin and DAPT is difficult to assess. Many surgical procedures can be performed with low-dose aspirin, alternative antiplatelet agents, or even DAPT with acceptable bleeding risk; there may be a slight increase in bleeding and transfusions, but no major morbidity or mortality. Low bleeding risk procedures such as dental, endoscopic, minor general, plastic, orthopedic, ear–nose–throat (ENT) and anterior eye surgery, are the ones that normally do not require transfusion. Intermediate bleeding risk procedures require transfusion frequently, such as major orthopedic, ENT, general surgery, and cardiac and major vascular surgery. Significant morbidity and mortality from APT has been demonstrated in high bleeding risk surgeries, in which bleeding has major impact, such as bleeding in a closed space; for example, neurosurgical and neurointerventional procedures, spine surgery, and surgery on the posterior eye chamber [17–19).
- The perioperative management of APT in patients with stents requires a multidisciplinary approach to determine the optimal balance between bleeding and thrombosis risk. Patients at high ST risk are those with PCI or BMS within four to six weeks and DES within 12 months. The intermediate risk period for ST consists of BMS placed between six and 24 weeks and DES possibly within six to 12 months, depending on the stent. The low ST risk period extends beyond six months for BMS and 12 months for DES; although occasional occurrence of ST with DES has been reported for up to 10 years after placement.
- DAPT should be continued during that high-risk period, and elective surgery should be postponed. Urgent or emergency surgery that has low or intermediate bleeding risk should be done with DAPT; high bleeding risk surgery can be done with aspirin or with bridging protocols (discussed later).
- Low bleeding risk procedures can be done with DAPT at any time.
- Table 22.1 summarizes recommendations for perioperative antiplatelet therapy in patients with coronary stents.

Table 22.1. Antiplatelet therapy for surgery in patients with recent coronary stents

ST risk \ Bleeding risk	Low	Intermediate	High
High	Emergency surgery with DAPT	Emergency surgery with DAPT (bridging and aspirin less optimal)	Emergency surgery – consider aspirin or bridging
Intermediate	Elective and emergency surgery with DAPT	Emergency surgery with DAPT or bridging	Emergency/urgent surgery – consider aspirin or bridging
Low	Elective and emergency surgery with DAPT or single agent	Elective and emergency surgery with single agent or DAPT (for higher-risk lesions)	DAPT can be held for 7 d

- If premature DAPT interruption is necessitated in the setting of major bleeding risk, transition with bridging protocol may provide protection from ST, while minimizing the bleeding complications. DAPT should be interrupted for as short a time as possible and consideration should be given to stopping the DAPT at three to four days preoperatively. If DAPT is interrupted for seven days preoperatively, the bridging protocol should be initiated two to four days preoperatively.
- Strong evidence to support a specific bridging protocol is lacking as the data come from single case reports or small case series. Bridging has been done with intravenous antiplatelet agents, direct thrombin inhibitors (DTI), anticoagulants, and combinations of these drugs.
- On the basis of pathophysiological mechanisms, utilization of intravenous platelet inhibitors such as eptifabitide or tirofiban is most suitable. Infusion of the agent can be initiated 48–72 hours preoperatively and continued until six to 12 hours before the procedure, depending on the half-life of the specific agent [20].
- Intravenous DTI bivalirudin and argatroban have also been used as bridging agents. Infusion is initiated 48–72 hours preoperatively. The timing for termination of the infusion should take into account the half-life of the agent and the adequacy of the elimination pathways [21].
- Intravenous anticoagulants such as low-molecular weight heparin have been used, but because they lack antiplatelet activity, their use as sole agents is not recommended. They have been used in combination with the aforementioned regimens.
- In the postoperative period, the oral DAPT should be restarted as soon as possible; if unsafe to resume promptly, the intravenous bridging agent may be used instead.

Valvular heart disease

Epidemiology

The assessment of the prevalence of valvular disease is challenging due to the variability in the definition used in epidemiological studies and in inclusion of specific lesions. In a large population-based study in the U.S., prevalence of valvular disease was 2.5% (95% confidence interval [CI_{95}] 2.2%–2.7%): aortic stenosis (AS) 0.4%, aortic regurgitation (AR) 0.5%, mitral stenosis (MS) 0.1%, and mitral regurgitation (MR) 1.7% [22]. Prevalence increases with age, from <2% before the age of 65 years to 13.2% >75 years, without substantial gender differences. In a study from Europe [23], among 3532 patients with valve disease AS was 34%, AR 10.5%, MS 9.5%, MR 25%, isolated right-sided valve disease 1%, and 20% had multiple valve lesions.

The etiology of the disease has changed, more evidently in the developed countries, where the most common cause is degenerative valve disease (DVD), accounting for 68%, followed by rheumatic heart disease (RHD) 22%; the remaining 10% comprise a heterogeneous group, including infective endocarditis (IE), inflammatory diseases, congenital heart diseases, and drug- and radiation-induced and connective tissue disorders. The annual incidence of IE has been estimated between 15 and 60 cases per million. In the developing countries, RHD is still the leading cause of valve disease.

Aortic stenosis

Pathophysiology and clinical presentation

- AS is a result of DVD, congenital valve abnormality, and less commonly, RHD. The risk factors are the same as those for atherosclerosis: increasing age, male gender, smoking, hypertension, and hypercholesterolemia.
- The severity is defined, according to AHA guidelines, as: mild (area 1.5 cm^2, mean transvalvular gradient <25 mmHg, jet velocity <3.0 m/s); moderate (area 1.0–1.5 cm^2, mean gradient 25–40 mmHg, jet velocity 3.0–4.0 m/s); severe (area <1.0 cm^2, mean gradient >40 mmHg, jet velocity >4.0 m/s). In severe AS, the mean gradient can be >40 mmHg when the cardiac function and cardiac output (CO) is normal, but as the cardiac function deteriorates, the gradient and velocity can be lower [24].
- The narrowing of the valve opening leads to increased resistance to flow and a high pressure gradient; chronic pressure overload results in compensatory concentric left ventricular hypertrophy (LVH) with greater intraventricular pressures generated with lower wall tension. Impairment of diastolic relaxation due to LVH results in increased isovolemic relaxation time and requires higher left atrial pressure for early diastolic filling to maintain adequate preload and CO. The ventricle is more dependent on the atrial contribution – atrial systole may account for up to 40% of ventricular filling. When the compensatory mechanisms fail, the CO decreases.
- The hypertrophic myocardium has increased oxygen demand, while the capillary vascularization is inadequate, leading to risk of myocardial ischemia due to supply–demand mismatch. Impaired coronary perfusion due to lower aortic diastolic pressure or increased left ventricular end-diastolic pressure (LVEDP) as well as to shortening diastole contributes to myocardial ischemia.
- The clinical presentation ranges from asymptomatic to the classical symptoms of severe AS, including angina, CHF, and syncope late in the disease.

Perioperative management

Perioperative complications, including major adverse cardiovascular events (MACE) and death, can be linked to the severity of AS, the presence of other comorbidities, and the type of surgery. A study comparing patients with AS to a control group, undergoing non-cardiac surgery, found that patients with a mean arteriovenous (AV) gradient of >25 mmHg had a higher incidence of perioperative mortality and nonfatal MI (14% versus 2%), and patients with severe AS (mean AV gradient of >50 mmHg) had more perioperative complications when compared with patients with moderate AS (31% versus 11%). After adjusting for cardiac risk factors, AS remained a strong predictor (odds ratio [OR]=5.2; CI_{95}, 1.6–17.0) [25]. Another study found AS to be an increased risk of perioperative MI (OR=1.55) but not of overall mortality [26].

- The preoperative evaluation should focus on the severity of AS and other comorbidities, and includes clinical signs and symptoms of AS; ECG demonstration of LVH or myocardial ischemia; pulmonary edema or pleural effusions on chest X-ray (CXR); recent two-dimensional and Doppler transthoracic echocardiography (TTE) or TEE to assess the valvular and cardiac function. Exercise or the chemical stress test and perfusion assessment in asymptomatic AS can assist in risk stratification and assessment of LV function and ischemia; in symptomatic AS, such testing carries substantial risk and is a grade III recommendation. Assessment of coronary anatomy, transvalvular gradient, LV function, and LVEDP can be achieved with angiography.

- The preoperative optimization includes treatment of the risk factors associated with AS such as HTN, hypercholesterolemia, and smoking, as well as medical management of heart failure, CAD, and rhythm abnormalities. Medications, including antihypertensive drugs, should be continued through the perioperative period, as long as the risk of hypotension is controlled. Valve interventions, such as balloon valvuloplasty, and percutaneous or open valve repair or replacement, should be considered, depending on the severity and symptoms of the disease, the associated comorbidities, and the urgency of the planned non-cardiac surgery.
- Cautious use of premedication should be done under monitoring of hemodynamic and respiratory status. Sedation may result in respiratory depression and hypotension, cardiac depression, and precipitation of ischemia. Inadequate anxiolysis and pain control can also potentiate ischemia. Anticholinergic drugs may precipitate detrimental tachycardia and should be avoided.
- The hemodynamic goals during anesthesia should focus on maintenance of adequate preload, sinus rhythm and atrial contribution to filling, control of heart rate (HR) and maintenance of contractility, and higher afterload. These patients are highly preload dependent, and the preoperative fasting and diuretic use place them at risk for a suboptimal preload state and resulting hemodynamic instability during induction and maintenance of anesthesia; fluids should be administered, in particular prior to neuraxial anesthesia. Tachyarrhythmia results in shortened diastolic filling time and systolic contraction, precipitating significant reduction in CO and risk of cardiac arrest. Treatment with β-blockers and amiodarone, especially in LVF, should be aggressive and cardioversion done early. Severe bradycardia can also reduce the CO. Afterload is maintained with vasopressors, phenylephrine, and vasopressin, to minimize tachycardia; however, norepinephrine, and in the setting of severely reduced contractility and CO, epinephrine, can be used as needed.
- The choice of anesthetic technique depends on the planned procedure and the feasibility of hemodynamic preservation with its execution.
- Peripheral nerve blockade can offer hemodynamic stability; the risks of local anesthetic toxicity and epinephrine in the anesthetic solution should be considered.
- Neuraxial anesthesia is not absolutely contraindicated, and can be performed safely in these patients, if adequate preload and afterload control is achieved and the level and extent of the block is gradual and controlled; in this scenario, consideration is given to epidural over spinal technique, or use of combined spinal/epidural or continuous spinal anesthesia to control the rate and degree of sympatholysis.
- General anesthesia can provide more stability; the choice of medications and the dose used have an impact on the hemodynamic parameters, and careful titration to effect, monitoring, and maintenance of systemic vascular resistance (SVR) and CO are essential. Induction agents with less hemodynamic depression theoretically may offer an advantage, such as etomidate, opioids, and short-acting benzodiazepines, while propofol and thiopental result in greater reduction of preload, contractility, and afterload; however, etomidate is the least effective in attenuation of the stress response and may result in undesirable tachycardia. Therefore, more important than the selection of a specific agent is the dose used, the rate of induction, the combination with other agents,

and the familiarity of the practitioner with its use. Neuromuscular agents devoid of significant cardiovascular effects are recommended, such as cisatracurium, vecuronium, and doxacurium. Drugs that lead to tachycardia such as ketamine, pancuronium, and rocuronium should be avoided.

- The perioperative monitoring should include standard American Society of Anesthesiologists (ASA) monitors – ECG (with leads II and V_5), pulse oximetry, $ETCO_2$, temperature, noninvasive BP. Continuous invasive arterial BP for most anesthetic procedures, particularly in severe AS, should be utilized and placed before induction of anesthesia. A CVP catheter to measure the right ventricular (RV) pressures can assist in directing preload management; however, its accuracy in assessing preload and in predicting fluid responsiveness in various clinical situations is poor. The utilization of PAC remains controversial and strong evidence to support its use to improve outcomes is lacking. While it can help the experienced practitioner to estimate the LVEDP and to alter management based on hemodynamic data interpretation, the potential benefits should be weighed against the risks of insertion, including arrhythmia, which can precipitate instability. TEE is valuable in the assessment of the cardiac function, including preload, contractility, and regional wall motion variability and carries a designation as a class IIA indication in the AHA guidelines [24].
- The postoperative recovery of these patients may require more extensive monitoring in telemetry or in the intensive care setting for prevention and prompt treatment of arrhythmia and hypotension, and for fluid management.

Aortic regurgitation

Pathophysiology and clinical presentation

The majority of the disorders result in chronic AR, such as congenital abnormalities of the aortic valve, Marfan syndrome, idiopathic dilatation of the aorta, calcific and myxomatous degeneration, HTN, RHD, inflammatory and autoimmune diseases, ventricular septal defects with prolapse of an aortic cusp, and anorectic drugs. The gradual progression of the disease leads to an initial asymptomatic state, followed by the manifestations of exertional and resting dyspnea, exercise-induced angina, tachycardia, and palpitations.

Some conditions such as IE, trauma, and aortic dissection lead to acute AR, with acute LV overload and presentation of cardiogenic shock, pulmonary edema, myocardial ischemia, and arrhythmia, which are emergency clinical situations.

- In chronic AR, the chronic LV overload as a result of diastolic regurgitation of the stroke volume triggers an increase in end-diastolic volume, LV dilatation with increased compliance, accommodating the increased volume without an increase in filling pressures, and eccentric and concentric hypertrophy. These compensatory changes maintain the stroke volume despite increased afterload; however, over time the preload reserve is exhausted and decreased ejection performance and elevated wall stress lead to symptoms.
- The normal ventricle in acute AR lacks the compensatory mechanisms and the increase in end-diastolic volume results in rapid LV end-diastolic and left atrial pressure elevation. The compensatory tachycardia is often insufficient to maintain CO, which can become severely reduced. The increase in the work load on the LV increases oxygen demand, while cardiac perfusion is reduced due to an increase in LVEDP and the low

diastolic aortic pressure. Myocardial ischemia, cardiogenic shock, and end-organ failure develop. The derangements are more pronounced in a heart with pre-existing pressure-overload concentric hypertrophy.

Perioperative management

The impact of AR on non-cardiac surgery is difficult to evaluate reliably due to a paucity of studies examining the connection of AR and perioperative outcomes. Asymptomatic patients with mild AR and preserved LV function are probably less likely to present a major perioperative risk. Patients with advanced AR, who are symptomatic and have impaired LV function, are at increased risk of perioperative major cardiac events and mortality; that risk is difficult to assess due to selection bias, as many of these patients likely have been precluded from undergoing elective non-cardiac surgery before valve-corrective surgery [27]. In the general nonsurgical population, more than 25% of the patients with AR who die or develop systolic dysfunction lack warning symptoms [28].

- The preoperative assessment of patients with AR should include evaluation of the degree of AR and LV dysfunction, in addition to documentation of symptoms and signs, evidence of volume overload, and pulmonary edema. ECG may reveal signs of LVH, ischemia, or arrhythmia. CXR may show cardiomegaly and pulmonary edema. The TTE or TEE is essential in the diagnosis of the severity of AR and assessment of LV function, as well as coexisting AS; a regurgitant fraction >0.6, a large regurgitant jet, and a holodiastolic flow reversal in the descending aorta suggest severe AR. The stress test and angiography can aid further in the evaluation of LV function and ischemia.
- The preoperative optimization with medical therapy or surgical intervention depends on the clinical status of the patient and the urgency of the non-cardiac procedure, as well as other comorbidities. The mainstay of medical therapy consists of long-term oral vasodilators and intravenous agents acutely; their use is recommended in the symptomatic patient with LV dysfunction and severe AR. Vasodilator therapy is not recommended for asymptomatic patients with mild or moderate AR and normal LV function in the absence of systemic hypertension. There are no strong data in support of systematic diuretic use, and if used in the pulmonary edema state, they should be administered judiciously as these patients rely on higher preload. β-blockers for ischemia and hypertension, including in the setting of aortic dissection, should be used cautiously, due to the attenuation of the compensatory tachycardia. In the acute setting, inotropes may be needed as well, such as dobutamine, dopamine, and epinephrine. The preoperative medications should be continued in the perioperative period; however, exaggerated hypotension under anesthesia is well recognized with ACE inhibitors and angiotensin receptor blocking (ARB), and a dosage adjustment may be needed. In severe symptomatic AR, corrective surgery may be indicated and the benefits and risks of cardiac surgery should be weighed against the risks of non-cardiac surgery with unrepaired severe AR.
- The hemodynamic goals of the perioperative management include decreasing regurgitant volume and optimization of forward flow and CO, which is achieved by maintenance of higher HR, normal to higher contractility, and afterload reduction. β-blockade and control of sympathetic tone in the setting of aortic aneurysm is indicated and should be done carefully, with strict monitoring. Hypotension should be treated with agents that support higher HR and contractility, such as ephedrine,

epinephrine, and dobutamine; phenylephrine and vasopressin increase the afterload and should be avoided.

- General and regional anesthesia can be used and the choice of anesthetic technique and specific medications should be tailored to the aforementioned hemodynamic goals. Medications resulting in significant cardiodepression and bradycardia, as well as increase in SVR, such as ketamine, should be avoided. Hypotension requiring therapy is best addressed with ephedrine and epinephrine, to augment HR and contractility; phenylephrine should be avoided due to a decrease in HR and increase in SVR.
- The perioperative monitoring, in addition to the basic anesthesia monitoring, depends on the severity and the symptoms of AR, as well as the anticipated hemodynamic alterations due to the surgery and anesthesia. Major surgical procedures in symptomatic patients or those with severe AR should include invasive arterial blood pressure measurement, before induction of anesthesia; a central venous line for pressure monitoring and administration of vasoactive agents should be considered. PAC may be helpful in monitoring of CO and estimation of SVR; however, the pulmonary artery occlusion pressure (PAOP) may overestimate the preload in severe AR due to premature mitral valve (MV) closure. TEE is valuable in assessment of the regurgitant flow, LV function and preload, and ischemia.
- In the postoperative period, patients with severe disease and those undergoing major fluid shifts should be monitored in a more intense setting, and pulmonary edema and ischemia prevented and treated accordingly.

Mitral stenosis

Pathophysiology and clinical presentation

MS is predominantly due to rheumatoid disease, and rarely, to congenital malformations, degenerative disease, severe annular calcification, left atrial myxoma, systemic inflammatory disease, ball valve thrombus, and mucopolysaccharidosis.

- The normal mitral orifice area is 4–6 cm^2 and the severity of the disease can be defined, according to the AHA guidelines as: mild (area >1.5 cm^2, mean gradient <5 mmHg, or pulmonary artery systolic pressure [PASP] <30 mmHg), moderate (area 1.0–1.5 cm^2, mean gradient 5–10 mmHg, or PASP 30–50 mmHg), and severe (area <1.0 cm^2, mean gradient >10 mmHg, or PASP >50 mmHg).
- The reduction in the valve area leads to impaired LV diastolic filling and necessitates a diastolic transvalvular gradient to flow blood across the valve, resulting in distention and pressure elevation of the left atrium (LAt) and the pulmonary venous circulation. As the severity of stenosis increases, CO decreases at rest and fails to increase during stress. The LV filling is dependent on the atrial contraction and is impaired by tachycardia and atrial fibrillation (AF).
- The elevation of the pulmonary vascular pressures is reversible early in the disease; however, the pulmonary vasculature develops vasoconstriction, intimal hyperplasia, and medial hypertrophy, leading to pulmonary hypertension (PHTN) and RV failure.
- Increased pressure and distension of the pulmonary veins and capillaries can lead to pulmonary edema as pulmonary venous pressure exceeds that of plasma oncotic pressure. In chronic MV obstruction, pulmonary edema may not occur even if pulmonary venous pressure is very high, due to a decrease in pulmonary microvascular permeability.

- LV contractility is generally preserved, but may be impaired by rheumatic damage to the papillary muscles and mitral annulus, as well as by the shift of the interventricular septum toward the LV in RV failure.
- The development of symptoms typically does not occur under stress until the valve area is $<2.5\text{cm}^2$, and at rest until the valve area is reduced to $<1.5\ \text{cm}^2$. The usual presenting symptoms are fatigue, dyspnea, orthopnea, syncope, and palpitations, and less frequently, onset of AF, an embolic event, hemoptysis, hoarseness, or dysphagia. The symptoms are precipitated initially by stress, AF with rapid ventricular response, sepsis, anemia, pregnancy, or thyrotoxicosis, but with progression of the disease, are produced at rest. The degree of pulmonary vascular disease is also an important determinant of symptoms.

Perioperative management

The incidence of perioperative adverse events in asymptomatic patients with mild MS is low, while patients with severe MS and PHTN are at high-risk for MACE and mortality. The exact risk is difficult to estimate from the limited data, most of which are in pregnant patients [29].

- The goals of the preoperative evaluation are to assess the severity of MS and PHTN, the presence of symptoms, and diagnosis of associated arrhythmia. In addition to the clinical examination, ECG can identify arrhythmia – specifically AF – and RV dysfunction, and CXR can demonstrate pulmonary edema. TTE/TEE assesses the severity of MS and pulmonary artery pressure, as well as the presence of thrombus in the LAt. Stress ECHO can aid further in the assessment and risk stratification of asymptomatic patients with more advanced disease, or symptomatic patients in whom the TTE fails to demonstrate moderate to severe MS. Invasive angiography is useful in cases where the noninvasive testing is inconclusive and to assess the degree of PHTN and identify responsiveness to medical therapy [30].
- The preoperative medical management focuses on symptomatic patients with advanced disease and includes drugs with negative chronotropic properties, such as β-blockers or HR-regulating calcium channel blockers (CCBs), especially in exertion-related symptoms. Those agents along with the anti-arrhythmics digoxin and amiodarone can be used to maintain normal sinus rhythm and control the HR in AF; electrical cardioversion may be attempted, but these patients are likely to present with chronic AF and will benefit from anticoagulation. The medications should be continued through the perioperative period and the anticoagulation regimen should be managed and transitioned to parenteral agents accordingly. Diuretics can assist in the treatment of pulmonary edema. Medical therapy for optimization of PHTN should be considered. Percutaneous valvotomy or MV surgery prior to elective surgery is advisable in symptomatic patients with moderate to severe MS, who are candidates for corrective intervention.
- Anxiolysis and control of pain and sympathetic tone are useful in these patients. Premedication with anticholinergics should be avoided due to risk of tachycardia.
- The hemodynamic goals in the perioperative period focus on control of HR and optimization of preload. Aggressive maintenance of sinus rhythm should be attempted. The preload should be maintained high to support LV filling, while avoiding fluid overload and precipitation of pulmonary edema. The higher afterload helps to support

perfusion in the setting of relatively fixed CO. The presence of significant PHTN requires additional hemodynamic considerations, which are described in further detail in the subsequent section of this chapter. Hypotension should be treated with phenylephrine and vasopressin, while ephedrine and catecholamines should be avoided due to detrimental tachycardia and proarrhythmic effects.

- General and regional anesthesia can be performed safely, as long as the outlined hemodynamic goals are achieved. Anesthetic agents that do not increase heart rate or decrease preload or afterload are beneficial, such as etomidate, benzodiazepines, and opiates. Ketamine and pancuronium should be avoided due to their tachycardia effect. Propofol and thiopental reduce the preload, afterload, and contractility and are less suitable. Volatile agents should be used carefully in lower doses and selected according to the outlined goals.
- The utilization of invasive monitoring is recommended in patients with advanced disease. Invasive arterial blood pressure monitoring to detect and control hemodynamic alterations promptly, as well as CVP and PAC monitoring for direct measurement of pulmonary artery pressure, assessment of SVR and PVR, and guidance in the management of preload are beneficial.
- Postoperative recovery in an intensive monitored setting is advisable, with continued control of HR, management of the preload and PHTN, and treatment of arrhythmia and pulmonary edema.

Mitral regurgitation

Pathophysiology and clinical presentation

Ischemic heart disease and degenerative changes of the MV, from myxomatous degeneration, fibroelastic deficiency, and calcifications, are the most common etiologies of MR; rheumatic heart disease, infective endocarditis, dilated annulus from dilation of the LV, drugs, collagen vascular disease, trauma, and congenital abnormalities are other etiologies. The disease can progress slowly or present as acute MR as a result of ruptured chordae tendineae or papillary muscle, or infective endocarditis.

- Gradual increase in mitral orifice area results in chronic regurgitation of the stroke volume and increase in volume overload. Functional MR occurs in the setting of a structurally normal valve and dilated and impaired LV and LA, while in organic MR there is a structural valve abnormality, but generally normal LV size and function initially.
- The development of compensatory eccentric cardiac hypertrophy leads to increased left ventricular end-diastolic volume (LVEDV), preload, and total stroke volume, accommodating the regurgitant volume at a lower filling pressure, and to the maintenance of the forward CO.
- As the disease advances, systolic dysfunction arises, although it may be masked by unloading into the highly compliant LA. Diastolic dysfunction occurs as the LV becomes less compliant and filling pressures increase. The forward flow is reduced and pulmonary congestion ensues; the development of PHTN is associated with a worse prognosis.
- In acute MR, a sudden volume overload in the LA and LV occurs. While small augmentation in the total stroke volume may be present due to the increased LV

preload, the absence of compensatory dilation and hypertrophy results in reduction of the forward stroke volume and CO. The LA and LV cannot accommodate the regurgitant volume and acute elevation of the pulmonary vascular pressures and pulmonary congestion develop.

- The asymptomatic compensated phase of chronic MR is followed by gradual development of symptoms initially under stress, and as the disease progresses, at rest. The patients present with dyspnea, fatigue, orthopnea, palpitations, and chest pain, and have increased mortality and risk of sudden death [31]. Acute MR presents with dyspnea, chest pain, acute pulmonary edema, and cardiogenic shock.

Perioperative management

The impact of mild asymptomatic MR on perioperative outcomes is likely low. However, in observational, nonrandomized studies, patients with moderate to severe MR were at significantly increased risk of 30-day mortality, myocardial infarction, heart failure, and stroke compared to matched controls (22.2% versus 16.4%, P=0.02); those with ischemic mitral regurgitation had significantly more events than those with non-ischemic mitral regurgitation (39.2% versus 13.3%, P<0.001). Another similar study identified the risk of morbidity at 27.4% and mortality at 11.9%; AF was identified by multivariate logistic regression analysis as a predictor of in-hospital death (OR 11.579, P=0.003) [32].

- The preoperative evaluation includes clinical examination, ECG to assess the rate and rhythm, and CXR for demonstration of cardiomegaly or pulmonary edema. TTE and TEE evaluation of the severity of MR and LV systolic and diastolic function and pulmonary artery pressure is essential. The stress test, a perfusion study, or angiography may be indicated for the diagnosis of CAD and further assessment of LV function and cardiac and pulmonary vascular pressures.
- The benefits of medical therapy for patients with MR depend on the stage of the disease. Asymptomatic patients with preserved LV function may obtain only limited benefits from afterload-reducing agents in the absence of systemic HTN. Vasodilators may have clinical utility in functional or ischemic MR; when significant LV dysfunction is present, ACE inhibitors, ARBs, β-blockers (specifically carvedilol), and biventricular pacing diminish the severity of the functional MR. β-blockers, HR-regulating CCBs, digoxin, and amiodarone are used to control tachycardia and AF. Anticoagulation for AF is used and should be transitioned to shorter-acting parenteral agents preoperatively. Corrective surgery is indicated in symptomatic patients with advanced MR for long-term therapy. However, before non-cardiac surgery, the potential risks and benefits of such correction in the setting of organic MR should be assessed carefully. In ischemic MR, revascularization in addition to medical management of CAD may be indicated.
- Preoperative premedication with anxiolytics and anticholinergics can be used as indicated; in ischemic MR, the tachycardia limits the use of anticholinergics. All cardiovascular medications should be continued in the perioperative period; ACE inhibitors and ARBs may precipitate significant hypotension under anesthesia, and should be used with caution.
- The hemodynamic goals for patients with MR focus on maintenance of relatively high HR to decrease diastolic time and the volume of regurgitation, as well as afterload reduction to increase the effective CO by decreasing resistance to LV flow and the

regurgitant fraction. The treatment of hypotension is best achieved with positive chronotropic and inotropic agents such as ephedrine, epinephrine, or dobutamine, while the bradycardia and elevation of the afterload with phenylephrine should be avoided. Ischemic MR poses additional challenges, as the outlined hemodynamic objectives may worsen the ischemia and thus the MR; a higher HR increases the myocardial oxygen consumption, while the lower afterload decreases myocardial perfusion. Judicious preload administration to support the CO, while balancing the risk of pulmonary congestion is important. The presence of significant PHTN further complicates the hemodynamics management.

- Various anesthetic techniques can be used safely. Neuraxial anesthesia and most intravenous and inhaled agents may offer the benefit of afterload reduction in most cases of MR, with the exception of ischemic MR. Etomidate and opiates offer more hemodynamic stability in this latter situation. Anesthetic-induced cardiodepression should be avoided, particularly when LV dysfunction is present.
- The basic anesthesia monitors are sufficient in asymptomatic patients with mild disease, undergoing minor procedures. For more advanced disease and major surgery, invasive arterial BP monitoring and central pressure monitoring via CVL or PAC is indicated frequently, particularly when significant PHTN is present. The right-sided thermodilution measurement of CO may overestimate the effective LV CO. TEE offers more accurate evaluation of LV function, preload, and regurgitant flow.
- The persistent risk of fluid overload, pulmonary edema, arrhythmia, and ischemia in the postoperative period often necessitates recovery in the intensive care setting.

Table 22.2 summarizes anesthetic hemodynamic goals for major valvular pathologies.

Table 22.2. Hemodynamic goals during anesthesia for valvular surgery

Disease	Preload	Rate	Contractility	Afterload	Hemodynamic agents	Specific considerations
AS	NL/↑	NL/↓	NL/↑	↑	Phenylephrine Norepinephrine Vasopressin	Maintain sinus rhythm Caution with regional anesthesia
AR	↑	↑	NL/↑	↓	Ephedrine Epinephrine Dobutamine	β-blockade for aortic aneurysm IABP contraindicated
MS	NL/↑	NL/↓	NL	↑	Phenylephrine Norepinephrine Vasopressin	Maintain sinus rhythm Anticoagulation management
MR	↑	↑	NL/↑	↓	Ephedrine Epinephrine Dobutamine	IABP can be used

NL, normal; IABP, intra-aortic ballon pump.

Hyperthrophic obstructive cardiomyopathy (HOCM)

HOCM is a heterogenic group of cardiomyopathies with asymmetric thickening of the LV wall, and LV outflow tract (LVOT) obstruction. The prevalence of the disease is 1:500 [33].

- The etiology of HOCM lays in genetic predisposition with diverse phenotypic expression, is influenced by genetic and environmental factors, and results in a variable clinical presentation and onset of symptoms.
- The underlying pathophysiology of HOCM is asymmetric hypertrophy of the ventricular septum, which causes narrowing of the LV outflow. Systolic anterior motion (SAM) of the MV leaflets is the cause of LVOT obstruction. The SAM causes a dynamic subaortic pressure gradient and leads to hypertrophy of the LV and reduced LV compliance. High filling pressures are required to maintain adequate LV end-diastolic volume (LVEDV) and CO, and the atrial contraction has a higher contribution to the preload. The severity of LVOT obstruction is exacerbated by reduced preload and afterload, and increased contractility and HR, as during exercise, anesthesia, and major surgery.
- The clinical presentation ranges from asymptomatic to exertional dyspnea, angina, dizziness, syncope, palpitations, AF, severe heart failure, cardiovascular accident (CVA), and sudden death.
- Increased risk of perioperative adverse cardiac events, such as myocardial ischemia, CHF, arrhythmia, and death is identified in several retrospective studies, indicating that 40%–60% of the patients with HOCM undergoing non-cardiac surgery experience complications, with an estimated OR=2.82; CI_{95}=2.59–3.07 [34].
- The preoperative evaluation should identify the presence of symptoms and signs, by taking a complete history and performing a thorough physical examination, including utilization of provocative maneuvers. The valsalva maneuver, rising from squatting to the standing position, and peripheral vasodilators decrease preload, LV filling, and afterload, thus increasing the LVOT obstruction. ECG frequently reveals LVH, arrhythmia, or ST changes. TTE, TEE, and magnetic resonance imaging (MRI) are used to identify the type and severity of HOCM, location and pattern of hypertrophy, site and degree of left LVOT obstruction, presence of SAM, and the resting gradient, as well as to assess and differentiate other valvular abnormalities. Provocative maneuvers and stress testing may aid further in the evaluation of HOCM, especially when the resting gradient is normal.
- The medical therapy of HOCM consists of β-blockers and CCBs with negative inotropic and chronotropic activity, such as verapamil and diltiazem; CCBs with peripheral vasodilating properties should be avoided. Disopyramide, an anti-arrhythmic agent with negative inotropic and peripheral vasoconstrictive properties can be used in poorly controlled disease. These agents, along with amiodarone, can be utilized to control the arrhythmias as well. The interventional treatment options include septal myomectomy, percutaneous alcohol ablation, and permanent dual-chamber pacemaker/ACD placement.
- The premedication includes continuation of the aforementioned drugs, as well as anxiolytics for HR control; anticholinergic agents should be avoided.
- The hemodynamic goals in the perioperative period focus on maintenance of high preload and afterload, and control of HR and contractility to reduce the LVOT

obstruction. Hypotension should be treated promptly with preload and direct vasopressors that do not increase contractility or HR, such as phenylephrine and vasopressin; ephedrine and catechols should be avoided. Blood loss and postural changes that decrease preload should be controlled and corrected. Control of sympathetic stimulation and tachyarrhythmia is essential.

- Regional, neuraxial, and general anesthesia can be performed safely; the more gradual modality of neuraxial anesthesia should be used as an epidural, combined spinal-epidural, or continuous spinal technique. Etomidate, opiates, and benzodiazepines are the preferred induction agents; thiopental and propofol can be used as long as reduction in preload and afterload are prevented and corrected promptly. Ketamine, which has sympathomimetic effects, and morphine and atracurium, with their histamine-releasing properties, should be avoided. Inhalation agents with the least reduction of afterload and increase in HR should be selected – sevoflurane in preference to isoflurane or desflurane.
- Invasive monitoring for major procedures, in addition to the basic anesthesia monitoring, is recommended; invasive arterial BP monitoring should be initiated before induction of anesthesia. CVP and PAC monitoring are helpful, especially when major fluid shifts are anticipated. TEE provides the most useful dynamic assessment of preload, LV filling and contractility, and LVOT obstruction.
- Recovery after major procedures is best done in an intensive care setting to control hemodynamics and prevent and treat complications.

The patient with a prosthetic valve

The patients with a prosthetic valve may continue to have hemodynamic alterations as a result of their prior valve disease, which are dependent on the stage and severity of the valvular pathology and cardiac pathophysiology prior to the valvular intervention, as well as on the post-operative rate and ability of cardiac remodeling and recovery. Additional considerations relate to the risks of IE, thrombosis, and recurrence of valvular pathology.

Prevention of IE

The AHA guideline update on prevention of IE, published in 2007, indicates that preprocedural anti-microbial prophylaxis is not routinely advised for many cardiac conditions and identifies the following high-risk lesions, in which the use of IE prophylaxis is indicated due to the high-risk of adverse outcomes [35]:

- previous IE
- prosthetic cardiac valve or prosthetic material used for cardiac valve repair
- congenital heart disease (CHD)
- unrepaired cyanotic CHD, including palliative shunts and conduits
- completely repaired congenital heart defect with prosthetic material or device, whether placed by surgery or by catheter intervention, during the first six months after the procedure
- repaired CHD with residual defects at the site or adjacent to the site of a prosthetic patch or prosthetic device
- cardiac transplantation recipients who develop cardiac valvulopathy

Table 22.3. Summary of recommendations for anti-microbial prophylaxis for IE

Procedures for which IE prophylaxis or anti-microbial therapy are indicated	Procedures for which IE prophylaxis is NOT indicated
All dental procedures involving manipulation of gingival tissue, or the periapical region of teeth, or perforation of the oral mucosa	Routine anesthetic injections through noninfected tissue, taking dental radiographs, placement of removable prosthodontic or orthodontic appliances, adjustment of orthodontic appliances, placement of orthodontic brackets, shedding of deciduous teeth, and bleeding from trauma to the lips or oral mucosa
Invasive procedure of the respiratory tract that involves incision or biopsy of the respiratory mucosa (tonsillectomy and adenoidectomy) *Invasive respiratory tract procedure to treat an established infection, such as drainage of an abscess or empyema	Bronchoscopy unless it involves incision of the respiratory tract mucosa
*Established GI or GU tract infection or for those who receive antibiotic therapy to prevent wound infection or sepsis associated with a GI or GU tract procedure *Elective cystoscopy or other urinary tract manipulation with pre-existing enterococcal urinary tract infection or colonization – *antibiotic therapy to eradicate enterococci from the urine*	GU or GI tract procedures, including diagnostic esophagogastroduodenoscopy or colonoscopy
*Infected skin, skin structure, or musculoskeletal Tissue – *therapeutic regimen administered for treatment of the infection*	Clean skin incisions

* The anti-microbial therapy goals for these procedures include treatment of the infection with agents directed at the specific organisms – identified or suspected high-risk organisms; GI, gastrointestinal; GU, genitourinary.

The administration of anti-microbial prophylaxis in patients with high-risk lesions undergoing procedures is determined by the nature of the procedure, and is summarized in Table 22.3. Table 22.4 outlines an anti-microbial regimen for IE prophylaxis.

Anti-thrombotic prophylaxis

The indications and goals of antithrombotic prophylaxis depend on the specific prosthetic valve and the presence of risk factors, such as AF, previous thromboembolism, LV dysfunction, and a hypercoagulable condition.

- After aortic valve replacement (AVR) or mitral valve replacement (MVR) with a bioprosthesis and no risk factors, aspirin is indicated at 75–100 mg daily. If risk factors are present, warfarin is indicated with an international normalized ratio (INR) goal of 2.0 to 3.0.

Table 22.4. Antimicrobial regimen for IE prophylaxis

Situation	Agent	Single dose 30–60 min before procedure	
		Adult	Pediatric
Oral	Amoxicillin	2 g	50 mg/kg
Unable to take PO	Ampicillin Cefazolin or ceftriaxone	2 g IM or IV 1 g IM or IV	50 mg/kg IM or IV 50 mg/kg IM or IV
Allergic to PCN – PO	Cephalexin Clindamycin Azithromycin/clarithromycin	2 mg 600 mg 500 mg	50 mg/kg 20 mg/kg 15 mg/kg
Allergic to PCN parenteral	Cefazolin or ceftriaxone Clindamycin	1 g IM or IV 600 mg IM or IV	50 mg/kg IM or IV 20 mg/kg IM or IV

PO, per os; PCN, penicillin; IM, intramuscular; IV, intravenous.

- After AVR with Starr-Edwards valves or mechanical disk valves (other than Medtronic Hall prostheses), and no risk factors, warfarin is indicated with an INR goal of 2.5 to 3.5.
- After AVR with bileaflet mechanical or Medtronic Hall prostheses, without risk factors, warfarin is indicated for an INR of 2.0 to 3.0; if risk factors are present, the INR goal is 2.5 to 3.5.
- Aspirin at 75 to 100 mg daily, in addition to therapeutic warfarin, is recommended for all mechanical valves and for bioprosthetic valves in the presence of risk factors.
- If patients are unable to take warfarin, aspirin is indicated at 75 to 325 mg daily. If patients are unable to take aspirin, clopidogrel may be considered at 75 mg daily.
- In the preoperative period, in high-risk patients, transition is indicated from warfarin to parenteral unfractionated or low-molecular weight heparin.

Heart failure

Heart failure (HF) is a complex clinical syndrome that results from any cardiac disorder that impairs the ability of the ventricle to fill with or eject blood. It ranges from chronic compensated or decompensated HF to acute HF and cardiogenic shock. In the U.S., an estimated 5.1 million people of $\geq$20 years of age have HF [36].

Pathophysiology and clinical presentation

- Systolic HF is impaired myocardial contractility with reduced LV ejection fraction and systemic hypoperfusion. The normal Starling response to increased preload is lost, and increasing cardiac volumes and pressures result in symptoms of congestion.
- Diastolic HF is characterized by impaired ventricular filling of a noncompliant ventricle and reduced CO, caused by reduced relaxation or compliance. Elevated LV filling pressure leads to rise in LAt, pulmonary artery, and RV pressures. The myocardial contractility is generally preserved.
- The underlying processes include neurohormonal activation and ventricular remodeling. Elevation in the circulating catecholamines and sympathetic activity leads to an increase in HR, contractility, and CO; peripheral vasoconstriction results in

increased afterload and myocardial oxygen consumption. The activation of the renin–angiotensin–aldosterone system, elevated natriuretic peptides, and endothelin, the hormonal response, causes salt and water retention and increased cardiac afterload. Elevated local neurohormonal factors angiotensin II, norepinephrine, and endothelin lead to ventricular dilation.

- Supraventricular arrhythmias, particularly AF, often herald the onset of HF. Abnormal myocardial conduction can also lead to delays in ventricular conduction and bundle–branch block. Left bundle–branch block is a significant predictor of sudden death and a common finding in patients with myocardial failure.
- It also causes abnormal ventricular activation and contraction, ventricular dyssynchrony, delayed opening and closure of the mitral and aortic valves, and abnormal diastolic function. Hemodynamic sequelae include a reduced ejection fraction, decreased CO and arterial pressure, paradoxical septal motion, increased LV volume, and MR.
- The clinical presentation of HF is with dyspnea on exertion and rest, orthopnea, pulmonary and peripheral edema, arrhythmia, and sudden death.
- Therapy goals focus on correcting the underlying problem, optimizing preload, improving cardiac contractility, reducing afterload, restoring normal cardiac synchrony, and treating rhythm abnormalities. Therapeutic interventions include treatment of HTN, DM, dyslipidemia, dietary sodium restriction; diuretics, ACE inhibitors and ARBs, β-blockers, digoxin, aldosterone antagonist, nesiritide, calcium sensitizers, inotropes; cardiac resynchronization, implantable cardioverter-defibrillators (ICD) implantation; revascularization, MV surgery, ventricular assist device (VAD), and transplantation.

Perioperative management

- The preoperative evaluation focuses on identification of the etiology, symptomatology, and stage; arrhythmia, LVH, chamber dilation, ischemic changes on ECG, and CXR documentation of cardiomegaly and pulmonary edema are sought. TTE, TEE, stress testing, and angiography help further with the staging of the disease and the underlying conditions.
- Preoperative medications need to be continued. Interventional therapeutic procedures as outline previously may be indicated before major non-cardiac surgery.
- The hemodynamic goals include optimization of preload, control of afterload, and augmentation of contractility. Intravenous inotropes may be required, including catecholamines, dobutamine, dopamine, milrinone, vasodilators, and diuretics.
- Regional anesthesia, if feasible, offers the benefits of the least amount of hemodynamic perturbation. Neuraxial anesthesia can be used safely, as long as preload is not abruptly reduced. The choice and dose of intravenous and inhaled agents aim to minimize the cardiodepression and abrupt preload changes.

Management of the patient with mechanical circulatory assist devices

A variety of VADs are available for short-term or long-term, partial or complete mechanical support to the failing ventricle. They can be used as a short-term salvage therapy, as a bridge to recovery, for transplantation, or as a destination therapy.

- These devices have mechanical pumps that can be placed inside the body (intracorporeal) or outside the body (extracorporeal), are inserted percutaneously or via sternotomy, and provide pulsatile or nonpulsatile flow. Extracorporeal pulsatile devices are Abiomed and Thoratec VAS, and intracorporeal devices are with pulsatile flow (Novacor, HeartMate) or nonpulsatile flow (HeartMate II, Thoratec; Jarvik 2000, DeBakey VAD), or complete heart support (AbioCor, CardioWest, SynCardia). Percutaneous VADs such as TandemHeart and Impella Recover LP System provide temporary partial or total circulatory support; they are inserted through the femoral artery and recirculate oxygenated blood from the left heart into the systemic circulation.
- Patients with these devices may present for emergency, urgent, and less frequently, elective surgery, and present unique challenges in the perioperative period [37].
- The continued presence of a healthcare professional, who is familiar with the specific device and can manage the device and take corrective actions in case of malfunction, is essential in the perioperative period.
- The thrombotic risk is high with some variability between the devices, but generally, therapeutic anticoagulation is indicated. Accordingly, thrombotic and bleeding complications are a frequent source of morbidity and mortality for these patients.
- For most surgical interventions, the transition from long-term oral anticoagulation to short-acting parenteral agents and complete or partial reversal of the anticoagulation in the immediate perioperative period are indicated. The risk of operative bleeding should be weighed against the thrombotic risk of the specific device to determine the timing and the exact method of reversal. Therapeutic anticoagulation should be restarted as soon as the bleeding risk has reduced.
- Neuraxial anesthesia may be contraindicated by the presence of residual anticoagulation, and the normalization of the coagulation parameters should be documented by laboratory results. The patients should be informed of the added risks of bleeding and complications.
- Infections are also a significant concern and appropriate antibiotic prophylaxis and treatment, as indicated, should be strictly adhered to.
- RV failure can present a substantial challenge after insertion of a LV VAD.
- The hemodynamic goals depend on the device. Generally, maintenance of adequate preload is an important determinant of pump effectiveness and forward flow. The interplay between venous return, RV function, pulmonary vascular resistance, and LV preload determines the device output and organ perfusion. Low device output may be a product of RV failure, intravascular volume depletion, or tamponade. In continuous-flow pump devices, the amount of CO support is affected by the afterload and it is essential to maintain a normal SVR and afterload. Sudden increases in afterload could result in sudden pump failure. Control of tachyarrhythmia generally has less importance than in the native heart; however, the individual device and clinical situation may vary and may require anti-arrhythmia therapy [38,39].
- Outflow obstruction by a kinked cannula is a potential reason for malfunction and should be diagnosed and relieved promptly. Thrombosis in the device presents with high power and estimated flow, and decreased pulsatility index. Echocardiography and catheterization may be required to confirm the diagnosis.
- The monitoring in the perioperative period can be challenging due to the diminished pulse pressure. Pulse oximetry, if obtainable, may be unreliable; cerebral oximetry can

be used. Noninvasive BP monitoring may be unreliable and a Doppler ultrasound machine and sphygmomanometer may be helpful. Invasive arterial BP monitoring and sampling of paO_2 for oxygenation should be utilized. CVP and PAC can be useful in the management of preload and pulmonary pressures.

- Regional and general anesthesia can be performed safely when the outlined hemodynamic goals are achieved under the appropriate monitoring.

References

1. Kumar R, McKinney WP, Raj G, et al. Adverse cardiac events after surgery: assessing risk in a veteran population. *J Gen Intern Med* 2001; **16**: 507–18.
2. Landesberg G, Mosseri M, Zahger D, et al. Myocardial infarction following vascular surgery: the role of prolonged, stress-induced, ST-depression-type ischemia. *J Am Coll Cardiol* 2001; 7: 1839–45.
3. Mahmoudi M, Curzen N, Gallagher PJ. Atherogenesis: the role of inflammation and infection. *Histopathology* 2007; **50**: 535–46.
4. Li JJ, Jiang H, Huang CX, et al. Elevated level of plasma C-reactive protein in patients with unstable angina: its relations with coronary stenosis and lipid profile. *Angiology* 2002; **53**: 265–72.
5. Duvall WL, Sealove B, Pungoti C, et al. Angiographic investigation of the pathophysiology of perioperative myocardial infarction. *Catheter Cardiovasc Interv* 2012; **80**: 768–76.
6. Devereaux PJ, Goldman L, Cook DJ, et al. Perioperative cardiac events in patients undergoing noncardiac surgery: a review of the magnitude of the problem, the pathophysiology of the events and methods to estimate and communicate risk. *Can Med Assoc J* 2005; **173**: 627–34.
7. Poldermans D, Boersma E, Bax JJ, et al. Correlation of location of acute myocardial infarct after noncardiac vascular surgery with preoperative dobutamine chocardiographic findings. *Am J Cardiol* 2001; **88**: 1413–14.
8. Devereaux PJ, Yang H, Yusuf S, et al. Effects of extended release metoprolol succinate in patients undergoing non-cardiac surgery (POISE TRIAL): a randomized controlled trial. *Lancet* 2008; **31**: 1839–47.
9. Fleisher LA, Beckman JA, Brown KA, et al. ACCF/AHA focused update on perioperative beta blockade incorporated into the ACC/AHA 2007 guidelines on perioperative cardiovascular evaluation and care for noncardiac surgery. *J Am Coll Cardiol* 2009; **54**: e13–118.
10. Dunkelgrun M, Boersma E, Schouten O, et al. Bisoprolol and fluvastatin for the reduction of perioperative cardiac mortality and myocardial infarction in intermediate-risk patients undergoing noncardiovascular surgery: a randomized controlled trial (DECREASE-IV). *Ann Surg* 2009; **249**: 921–6.
11. Jeremias A, Kaul S, Rosengart TK, et al. The impact of revascularization on mortality in patients with nonacute coronary artery disease. *Am J Med* 2009; **122**: 152–61.
12. Singh R, Choudhury M, Kapoor PH, et al. A randomized trial of anesthetic induction agents in patients with coronary artery disease and left ventricular dysfunction. *Ann Card Anaesth* 2010; **13**: 217–23.
13. Zangrillo A, Testa V, Aldrovandi V, et al. Volatile agents for cardiac protection in noncardiac surgery: a randomized controlled study. *J Cardiothorac Vasc Anesth* 2011; **25**: 902–7.
14. Simsek C, Magro M, Boersma E. The unrestricted use of sirolimus- and paclitaxel-eluting stents results in better clinical outcomes during 6-year follow-up than bare-metal stents. *J Am Coll Cardiol Cardiovasc Interv* 2010; **3**: 1051–8.
15. Wright RS, Anderson JL, Adams CD, et al. ACCF/AHA focused update of the guidelines for the management of patients with unstable angina/non-st-elevation myocardial infarction (updating the 2007

guideline): a report of the American College of Cardiology Foundation/ American Heart Association Task Force on Practice Guidelines. *J Am Coll Cardiol* 2011; **57**: 1920–59.

16. Pfisterer M, Brunner-La Rocca HP, Buser PT, et al. Late clinical events after clopidogrel discontinuation may limit the benefit of drug-eluting stents: an observational study of drug-eluting versus bare-metal stents. *J Am Coll Cardiol* 2006; **48**: 2584–9.
17. Cerfolio R, Minnich DJ, Bryant AS, et al. General thoracic surgery is safe in patients taking clopidogrel (Plavix). *J Thorac Cardiovasc Surg* 2010; **140**: 970–6.
18. Wang J, Zhang C, Tan G, et al. Risk of bleeding complications after preoperative antiplatelet withdrawal versus continuing antiplatelet drugs during transurethral resection of the prostate and prostate puncture biopsy: a systematic review and meta-analysis. *Urol Int* 2012; **89**: 433–8.
19. Qureshi AI, Saad M, Zaidat OO, et al. Intracerebral hemorrhages associated with neurointerventional procedures using a combination of antithrombotic agents including abciximab. *Stroke* 2002; **33**: 1916–19.
20. Broad L, Lee T, Conroy M, et al. Successful management of patients with a drug-eluting coronary stent presenting for elective, non-cardiac surgery. *Br J Anaesth* 2007; **98**: 19–22.
21. Wessely R. Initial experience with an institutional bridging protocol for patients with recent coronary stent implantation requiring discontinuation of dual antiplatelet therapy resulting from urgent surgery. *Am J Ther* 2011; **18**: e280–2.
22. Nkomo VT, Gardin JM, Skelton TN, et al. Burden of valvular heart diseases: a population-based study. *Lancet* 2006; **368**: 1005–11.
23. Iung B, Baron G, Butchart EG, et al. A prospective survey of patients with valvular heart disease in Europe: the Euro Heart Survey on Valvular Heart Disease. *Eur Heart J* 2003; **24**: 1231–43.
24. Bonow RO, Carabello BA, Chatterjee K, et al. 2008 focused update incorporated into the ACC/AHA 2006 guidelines for the management of patients with valvular heart disease: a report of the American College of Cardiology/American Heart Association Task Force on Practice. *Circulation* 2008; **118**: e523–661.
25. Kertai MD, Bountioukos M, Boersma E, et al. Aortic stenosis: an underestimated risk factor for perioperative complications in patients undergoing noncardiac surgery. *Am J Med* 2004; **116**: 8–13.
26. Zahid M, Sonel AF, Saba S, et al. Perioperative risk of noncardiac surgery associated with aortic stenosis. *Am J Cardiol* 2005; **96**: 436–8.
27. Lai H-C, Lai H-C, Lee W-L, et al. Impact of chronic advanced aortic regurgitation on the perioperative outcome of noncardiac surgery. *Acta Anaesthesiol Scand* 2010; **54**: 580–8.
28. Dujardin KS, Enriquez-Sarano M, Schaff HV, et al. Mortality and morbidity of aortic regurgitation in clinical practice: a long-term follow up study. *Circulation* 1999; **99**: 1851–7.
29. Silversides CK, Colman JM, Sermer M, et al. Cardiac risk in pregnant women with rheumatic mitral stenosis. *Am J Cardiol* 2003; **91**: 1382–5.
30. Reis PD, Motta MS, Barbosa MM, et al. Dobutamine stress-echocardiography for noninvasive assessment and risk-stratification of patients with rheumatic mitral stenosis. *J Am Coll Cardiol* 2004; **43**: 393–401.
31. Enriquez-Sarano M, Avierinos JF, Messika-Zeitoun D, et al. Quantitative determinants of the outcome of asymptomatic mitral regurgitation. *N Engl J Med* 2005; **352**: 875–83.
32. Bajaj NS, Agarwal S, Rajamanickam A. Impact of severe mitral regurgitation on postoperative outcomes after noncardiac surgery. *Am J Med* 2013; **126**: 529–35.
33. Maron BJ, McKenna WJ, Danielson GK, et al. Task Force on Clinical Expert Consensus Documents. American College of Cardiology; Committee for Practice

Guidelines. European Society of Cardiology. American College of Cardiology/European Society of Cardiology clinical expert consensus document on hypertrophic cardiomyopathy: a report of the American College of Cardiology Foundation Task Force on Clinical Expert Consensus Documents and the European Society of Cardiology Committee for Practice Guidelines. *J Am Coll Cardiol* 2003; **42**: 1687–713.

34. Hreybe H, Zahid M, Sonel A, et al. Noncardiac surgery and the risk of death and other cardiovascular events in patients with hypertrophic cardiomyopathy. *Clin Cardiol* 2006; **29**: 65–8.

35. Wilson W, Taubert KA, Gewitz M, et al. Prevention of infective endocarditis: guidelines from the American Heart Association: a guideline from the American Heart Association Rheumatic Fever, Endocarditis, and Kawasaki Disease Committee, Council on Cardiovascular Disease in the Young, and the Council on Clinical Cardiology, Council on Cardiovascular Surgery and Anesthesia, and the Quality of Care and Outcomes Research Interdisciplinary Working Group. *Circulation* 2007; **116**: 1736–54.

36. Go AS, Mozaffarian D, Roger VL, et al. Heart disease and stroke statistics–2013 update: a report from the American Heart Association. *Circulation* 2013; **127**: e6–245.

37. Kartha V, Gomez W, Wu B, et al. Laparoscopic cholecystectomy in a patient with an implantable left ventricular assist device. *Br J Anaesth* 2008; **100**: 652–5.

38. Stone ME, Soong W, Krol M, et al. The anesthetic considerations in patients with ventricular assist devices presenting for noncardiac surgery: a review of eight cases. *Anesth Analg* 2002; **95**: 42–9.

39. Garatti A, Bruschi G, Colombo T, et al. Noncardiac surgical procedures in patient supported with long-term implantable left ventricular assist device. *Am J Surg* 2009; **197**: 710–14.

Chapter

23 Vascular surgery

M. McFarling and I. Bruni

Anesthesia for surgical interventions of the aorta and its branches is known to be associated with high perioperative morbidity and mortality.

This chapter will highlight anesthetic and perioperative management principles for the following three vascular procedures:

- management principles for carotid endarterectomy
- anesthetic management of elective thoracic aneurysm repair
- peripheral vascular access for renal dialysis

The principles outlined for these procedures will include important principles of care of all vascular surgery patients.

The key problems encountered in vascular surgery include:

- impairment of organ perfusion by way of the disease process, or the exclusion of organs from the circulation by cross-clamping
- perioperative hemorrhage and emergency surgery
- consequences of massive transfusion (discussed elsewhere in this text)
- effects of thoracic and abdominal aneurysm resection

Carotid endarterectomy

Extracranial stenosis of the carotid artery accounts for 15%–20% of ischemic strokes; carotid endarterectomy (CEA) is the most common surgical intervention to prevent stroke and is unique among vascular surgeries in that it carries an intermediate risk of perioperative cardiac complications [1,2].

Atherosclerosis is a systemic disease and coronary artery pathology therefore is prevalent in patients presenting with carotid stenosis. Cardiac morbidity and mortality have not declined at a rate comparable to the improvements in neurological outcomes.

Symptomatic stenosis

Management options include:

- Symptomatic carotid stenosis of <50% is best managed medically as the risk of operative complication outweighs the risk of stroke over five years [3].
- Meta-analysis [4] suggests that the benefit of CEA is seen only in patients with >50% stenosis with two or more years of life expectancy, in agreement with current Society

Anesthesia and Perioperative Care of the High-Risk Patient, Third edition, ed. Ian McConachie. Published by Cambridge University Press.

for Vascular Surgery Guidelines. Patients with lesser degrees of stenosis may be harmed by the procedure.
- CEA is the first line of treatment for most patients with recent symptomatic stenosis (50%–99% occlusion) of the carotid bifurcation or proximal internal carotid artery associated with atherosclerosis [3].
- In patients with 100% occlusion suffering from recurrent neurological or ocular symptoms, CEA (plus oral anticoagulation) is advocated [5].
- The high morbidity of CEA should prompt consideration of carotid artery stenting (CAS).

Features of "high-risk for CEA" include adverse vascular and local anatomic features [6]:
- contralateral laryngeal nerve palsy
- previous radical neck dissection
- cervical irradiation
- restenosis of prior CEA
- high bifurcation or intracranial lesion

CAS, although arguably less invasive, has not achieved outcomes comparable to those of CEA. The rate of stroke at 30 days is 5.6%, myocardial infarct 0.9%, and death 1.1%. Combined stroke and death rates (6%–9.6%) in symptomatic patients is unacceptably high to recommend it over medical therapy alone.

Asymptomatic patients

Management options include:
- CEA should be considered in asymptomatic stenosis of 60%–99% if life expectancy exceeds five years and complication rates (stroke or death) are <3% [3]. Stroke/death rates at two to 2.7 years follow-up were 20.9% for CEA plus medication therapy and 30.4% for medical therapy alone [7].
- At two and 3.4 years follow-up, stroke/death rates are 29.7% and 28.3% for CEA and medical therapy, respectively. In asymptomatic stenosis of <50%, intervention is unnecessary due to lack of benefit and potential for harm [7].
- Periprocedural stroke or death in asymptomatic patients included in the CREST trial was not significantly different: 2.5% in CAS versus 1.4% in CEA. Likewise, there was no significant difference in the rate of myocardial infarction (MI) (1.2% versus 2.2%), any periprocedural stroke (2.5% versus 1.4%), or composite primary endpoint (any periprocedural stroke, MI, or death: 3.5% versus 3.6%) [6].

CAS is not recommended in the absence of symptoms.

Anesthetic and perioperative management of CEA

Improved patient selection in conjunction with increasing surgeon and hospital surgical experience, improved surgical techniques, and an array of evolving cerebral monitoring modalities have combined to reduce some of the complications associated with carotid endarterectomy.

The greatest benefit of surgery is achieved when neurologically stable patients undergo non-emergent surgery less than two weeks from the most recent symptoms; surgical benefit is quickly lost thereafter [8] although patients symptomatic within six months may still derive stroke and death benefits from CEA [7]. The patient care team therefore should strive to get suitable patients to the operating theater as expeditiously as possible, with appropriate workup and preparation including:

- documentation of pre-surgery neurological examination
- blood pressure (BP) optimization determined from the higher of bilateral arm measurements
- continuation of anti-hypertensive and anti-anginal medications, targeting BP ≤140/80 mmHg and heart rate (HR) 60–80 bpm
- antiplatelet therapy; aspirin (81–325 mg daily) (Grade 1 A evidence) [3] with clopidogrel considered on an individual basis (Grade 2, B level of evidence). Aspirin therapy should continue lifelong (Grade 1, C level of evidence) [5]. Perioperative dual agent antiplatelet therapy with aspirin and a second agent (ticlopidine or clopidogrel) is indicated in patients undergoing CAS, and should be initiated three days or more before the procedure and continued for one month
- statin therapy (LDL ≤100 mg/dL) (Grade 1, level of evidence B) reduces the five-year stroke rate (fatal and nonfatal) by 1.4% (to 4.3%) and any death by 1.8% (to 12.9%) after five years [9]
- extensive preoperative cardiac investigation: not warranted in the absence of unstable angina, recent MI/ongoing ischemia, decompensated congestive heart failure, or serious valvular disease [1,2]

Intraoperative management

General (GA) or regional anesthesia (RA), or a combination thereof, provides adequate conditions for completion of the procedure via cervical incision. Several reviews have failed to show significant benefit of any one technique relative to another; patient expectations and anesthesiologist and surgeon experience therefore inform the decision regarding technique [10–13].

Anesthetic and intraoperative goals simply stated are:

- maintenance of cerebral and cardiac perfusion to minimize ischemic and metabolic insult
- management of hemodynamic instability; maintenance of BP comparable to those recorded preoperatively prior to the day of surgery
- controlled transitions to and from anesthesia; reducing perioperative physiological stress
- rapid return to the non-anesthetized state facilitating early neurological assessment of intraoperative complications

Regional anesthesia

Completion of CAE under RA requires significant commitment and cooperation from the patient, as well as the surgeon and anesthesiologist. It may, however, provide the best opportunity to identify neurological injury early and the need for shunt insertion via direct assessment of cerebral function during initial cross-clamping. Identification of patients who require shunting (sensitivity) under RA is 59%–91%, and those who do not (specificity) is 57%–99% [14].

- Superficial cervical plexus blocks are safe and suitable for CEA, but are insufficient; additional local infiltration is required, especially at the superior aspect of the cervical incision approaching the mandibular ramus.
- The addition of deep cervical plexus blocks does not add to patient comfort during CEA and has attendant risks.
- Deep cervical blocks are associated with both higher incidence of serious complications and conversion to GA than superficial or intermediate depth blocks [15].
- Manipulation of the carotid sinus can produce profound changes in hemodynamics, namely bradycardia and hypotension. Aggressive intervention is often necessary and may include conversion to GA in non-ideal circumstances. Hemodynamic stability appears better under RA.
- A regional technique provides the cheapest and most sensitive cerebral perfusion monitor. No combination of monitors has proved superior in reducing serious outcomes [16].
- Sedative and analgesic interventions should be short acting to permit timely evaluation of the patient at any time during the operation.
- In the GALA trial, there was no definite advantage to local or RA over GA; fewer patients under RA required blood pressure manipulation, but were more hypertensive; shunt insertion was significantly reduced (14% under RA and 43% under GA) [17].
- Failure of RA is common (2%–6%) and may result from issues of patient cooperation, positioning, neurological deterioration, and hemodynamic instability – rapid conversion to GA in these circumstances may be complicated, and dependent on swift communication and coordination with the surgeon.
- In the GALA trial, more than 4% of patients receiving local anesthesia experienced complications necessitating cancellation of surgery, or conversion to GA [17].

General anesthesia

If organ perfusion is adequately maintained during anesthesia, a skilled anesthetist may consider most techniques of GA. Advantages of GA include:

- controlled ventilation (normocapnia)
- secured airway
- reduction in cerebral metabolic and oxygen demand
- avoidance of intraoperative conversion from RA

The prime disadvantage is the increased use of temporary carotid shunts and their associated risks. Serious shunt complications include:

- insertion problems or inability
- embolization of air or atheroma
- vessel dissection
- thrombosis
- malfunction or malposition

Stroke rates are similar in routine and selective shunting [18].

Furthermore, GA inherently results in the inability to monitor for neurological decline with sensitivity equivalent to RA or local anesthetic [16].

Monitoring modalities for cerebral perfusion include:

- observation of the awake patient
- electroecephalography (EEG)
- carotid stump pressure
- transcranial Doppler (TCD)
- near infrared spectroscopy (NIRS)
- jugular venous oxygen
- jugular venous lactate
- somatosensory evoked potentials (SEP)
- regional cerebral blood flow using xenon-133

No monitor can match the sensitivity of an awake patient under RA [16]. A recent meta-analysis by Guay and Kopp suggests a multi-monitor combination of stump pressure, and TCD or EEG provides optimal monitoring. Limitations of this approach include the lack of suitable boney windows for TCD (10%), and the technical and analytical resources required to use multi-channel real-time EEG in the operating room for clinical decision making. A firm recommendation for the monitoring modality is not possible at this time.

Postoperative management

The high rate of complications related to hemodynamic derangement in both early and late periprocedural periods cannot be overstated. The risk of death is significantly higher in those patients experiencing stroke or myocardial infarction perioperatively. Frequent assessment and monitoring for signs and symptoms of the following are recommended:

- periprocedural stroke
- hemodynamic instability, hypertension, or hypotension
- intracranial hemorrhage
- reperfusion/hyperperfusion syndrome
- myocardial ischemia/infarction
- other: neck hematoma, anastomotic failure, seizures, cranial nerve injury

Patients should be monitored intensively for early complications, especially in the early postoperative period, making use of monitored areas, invasive BP monitoring, and clinical examination. Early, aggressive treatment of hemodynamic abnormalities may reduce both neurological and cardiac complications. Specific complications include:

- Hypertension is the most common postoperative complication and occurs in 30%–50% of patients and may result in cerebral edema or hemorrhage, myocardial ischemia, and/or congestive heart failure; it is worse in patients with pre-existing, poorly controlled hypertension. It often presents two to four hours postoperatively and may persist for 24 hours. Aggressive treatment with short-acting drugs is suggested, for example with sodium nitroprusside or nitroglycerin. β-blockers may reduce isolated systolic hypertension and control HR.
- Hypotension is nearly as common as hypertension, and may be more problematic in those having RA. Aggressive treatment with short-acting vasopressor drugs minimizes cerebral exposure to hypoperfusion.

- Hyperperfusion syndrome is postulated to result from elevated blood flow through vessels with residual impairment of autoregulation. Flow in excess of metabolic demand may cause ipsilateral frontal headache, seizures, and intracranial hemorrhage.
- Periprocedural strokes are typically ischemic (90%), in the anterior circulation (94%), and ipsilateral to the treated vessel (88%) [19]. Three imaging patterns are seen in these strokes: scattered (arteroembolic), cortical wedge (artero- or cardioembolic), and small subcortical patterning. Early investigation of neurological deterioration with Doppler ultrasound or rapid computerized topographical (CT) angiography is required to prove vessel patency; reoperation may be required.
- Intracranial hemorrhage after CEA or CAS is rare, but catastrophic and independent of the procedure undertaken.
- Hyperperfusion syndrome and autoregulatory impairment are suggested by the timing of presentation following the procedure.

Anesthesia for thoracic aortic aneurysm repair

Historically, open repair of the thoracic aorta has been regarded as extremely challenging, requiring multidisciplinary expertise for successful completion. There is insufficient evidence from randomly controlled trials (RCTs) to date to determine whether endovascular or open repair for descending thoracic aorta aneurysm (TAA) is associated with proven better outcomes [20,21].

Endovascular repair of thoracic aortic disease is becoming increasingly frequent and often undertaken in hospitals without cardiac surgery on site. As such, understanding of the proposed procedure with its inherent risks, limitations, and potential complications allows the anesthesiologist to provide complex perioperative care.

Unlike abdominal aortic aneurysms (AAAs) that are amenable to screening examinations (with resultant reduction in incidence of acute rupture and need for emergency surgery), TAAs remain difficult to screen for, and are associated with high morbidity and mortality. Endovascular techniques may provide a risk-reduced option for those patients at particularly high operative risk.

Discussion will be limited to disease of the descending thoracic aorta. Repair in the region of the aortic valve to the distal arch requires an experienced cardiac surgeon as well as cardiopulmonary bypass, and is beyond the scope of this chapter.

Epidemiology

- The majority of TAAs are due to atherosclerotic degeneration (80%) or chronic dissection (17%); the remainder are due to a host of conditions [22].
- Incidence is 5.9–10.4 per 100 000 person–years (descending aorta).
- Enlargement is progressive; rate of rupture 3.5/100 000 person–years and increases abruptly at 6 cm diameter – intervention is indicated.
- Most TAAs are asymptomatic, although some present with chest, back, or abdominal pain; discovery is often incidental during an investigation for other diseases. Symptoms, if present, are due to pressure on adjacent structures: left recurrent laryngeal nerve (hoarseness); trachea (stridor, cough); esophagus (dysphagia), lung (dyspnea), or aortic insufficiency, resulting in aortic regurgitation and congestive heart failure.
- Synchronous aneurysms (~10% of patients) involve the ascending aorta or arch.

- The chief risk factor is family history of aneurysmal disease, followed by hypertension, atherosclerosis, age, male gender, and smoking.
- 20%–40% of patients with chronic dissection will develop aneurysmal dilation.

Assessment

Careful identification of vascular anatomy is usually performed by a contrast-enhanced CT angiogram (CTA) or magnetic resonance angiogram (MRA). The thoracic aorta is best divided segmentally into aortic root, ascending aorta, arch, descending aorta, with aneurysms classified by Crawford et al. [22] as follows:

I. all or most of the descending thoracic aorta and upper abdominal aorta
II. all or most of the descending thoracic aorta and of the abdominal aorta (at greatest risk for paraplegia)
III. lower descending thoracic aorta and most of the abdominal aorta
IV. all or most of the abdominal aorta and visceral segment

Perioperative morbidity and mortality is principally associated with MI, respiratory failure (worsened by smoking and chronic obstructive pulmonary disease [COPD]), renal failure, and stroke. Postoperative pulmonary complications are frequent, approaching 50%, with a significant number requiring tracheostomy.

Preoperative investigations should be used to identify any modifiable risk factors and to quantify risk [20]. Investigations should include:

- pulmonary function testing
- identification and quantification of important coronary artery disease (CAD) with 12-lead ECG, echocardiography, and 24-hour Holter monitor
- aortography
- noninvasive carotid artery screening
- brain imaging
- neurocognitive testing
- preoperative laboratory investigations including complete blood count, coagulation, electrolytes, renal functions, arterial blood gases, blood group, and reserve
- to assist in developing an understanding of baseline function and to develop a risk profile, some centers additionally request noninvasive carotid artery screening (Doppler), brain magnetic resonance imaging (MRI), and neurocognitive testing. Importantly, efficacy in treating significant carotid disease prior to aortic surgery has not been studied in a systematic way [20]

Contemporary mortality is reportedly 5%–14%, but may be higher for open and emergency procedures.

Anesthetic planning

The surgical approach and exposure of the thoracic aorta is dependent on whether the procedure is emergent or elective and if repair or replacement of the descending aorta is intended. The procedure may be undertaken with an open, endovascular, or hybrid technique.

Consultation with the attending surgeon is important with regard to:

- vascular anatomy and planned surgical repair
- ventilation strategy
- planned shunts/bypass
- physiological monitoring (distal aortic or femoral pressure, spinal cord function)
- renal and spinal (via lumbar drain) protection strategies are mandatory

Anesthetic preparation and monitoring

- Use a minimum of two large-bore intravenous cannulae – the larger the better.
- Central venous access; a 9Fr introducer facilitates rapid infusion of fluids or vasoactive drugs and insertion of a pulmonary artery catheter.
- Blood products must be readily available. One should anticipate a potential massive blood transfusion.
- Routine monitoring, for example five-lead ECG monitoring, noninvasive BP, capnography, oxygen saturation via pulse oximetry (SpO_2), temperature, should be done.
- Use an arterial line (right radial) and additional sites if necessary.
- Neuromuscular blockade monitor is necessary.
- Lung isolation; left-sided double lumen endotracheal tube is preferable.
- Transesophageal echo should be available for intraoperative monitoring of cardiac function.
- Epidural site is preferable for postoperative analgesia.
- Intrathecal drain (class I, level B) is inserted if there is high-risk of injury.
- Cardiac Perfusion and Cell Salvage facilities may be required.
- Active patient warming and cooling devices should be available.
- Spinal cord monitoring is essential.

Spinal cord monitoring

The goals of spinal cord monitoring are conceptually simple:

- improve spinal cord oxygen delivery
- improve tolerance of ischemia
- reduce reperfusion injury

Attention to these goals forms the basis for pharmacological and intravascular volume management to maintain spinal cord perfusion pressure and oxygen delivery, while functional monitoring with SEP and/or motor evoked potentials (MEP) permits early identification of potentially reversible perfusion issues [23].

Anesthetic management

- No technique has proved superior with regard to long-term morbidity and mortality.
- Titrated inductions that avoid hypertension (increases wall stress and risk of rupture) and tachycardia (concurrent cardiac disease, myocardial oxygen demand) are advised.
- HR and BP should be actively managed throughout.

Maintenance of anesthesia

- If spinal monitoring with MEP or SEP is to be used, total intravenous anesthesia should be considered. All classes of anesthetic medications are known to affect MEP and SEP monitoring. Relative to inhaled volatile anesthetics, intravenous agents have significantly less effect on both amplitude and latency of signal. Techniques using propofol, opiates, ketamine, and etomidate have been well described during evoked response monitoring, and are supported in the literature [24].
- Volatile agents or propofol infusion and opiates should be titrated to maintain cardiovascular stability and ensure adequate anesthesia/analgesia.
- Non-depolarizing muscle relaxants should be titrated to maintain 50% reduction of train-of-four responses to prevent unexpected movement or breathing.
- One-lung ventilation (if required) should be instituted with the goal of maintaining normal hypoxic pulmonary vasoconstriction, normocarbia, and normal pH, while avoiding hyperoxemia, pain, hypothermia, and excess sympathetic stimulation.
- Avoidance of nitrous oxide prevents bowel and endotracheal tube cuff distention.

Postoperatively, patients should be transported to the intensive care unit where a period of hemodynamic, metabolic, and ventilatory stability is desirable prior to awakening and extubation.

Cross-clamping of the proximal descending aorta

Cross-clamping of the aorta results in severe, acute increases in afterload, with resultant stresses on the patient's cardiovascular system, potentially resulting inleading to myocardial ischemia, ventricular wall motion abnormalities, and arrhythmias. The effects are exaggerated compared to those seen with abdominal aortic surgery as the potential run-off vessels are greatly reduced.

- Left ventricle afterload is increased, simultaneously increasing proximal BP and decreasing stroke volume, ejection fraction, and cardiac output.
- Myocardial oxygen demand is increased by elevated wall stress and increased ventricular intracavitary pressure. Myocardial ischemia is common but may be ameliorated by nitroprusside (reduces systemic vascular resistance) and nitroglycerin (can reduce preload).
- Hyperperfusion may result from using nitroprusside as a sole agent for BP control.
- Transesophageal echocardiography (TEE) allows monitoring of myocardial and valvular performance during cross-clamping, and assessment of cardiac preload prior to reperfusion.
- Close communication with the surgeon allows pre-emptive treatment with appropriate vasodilators and/or negative inotropes.
- During clamp time, all organs perfused distally may be ischemic including spinal cord, kidneys, liver, and gut.

In select cases, cardiopulmonary bypass from the left atrium to the femoral artery may provide some advantage. The reduction in left ventricle preload may help to limit the hemodynamic stress of cross-clamping while simultaneously providing distal aortic perfusion to the spinal cord, kidney, and gut. The excluded segment of aorta remains hypoperfused to facilitate surgical repair or replacement but may still include spinal cord perfusing vessels.

Similarly, extensive hemodynamic changes can be expected when aortic cross-clamps are released. Hypotension due to the addition of relatively underfilled vascular space to the circulation as well as the myocardial depressant effect of cold, acidic, hypercarbic, hyperkalemic venous blood must be anticipated and treated with additional vascular volume, calcium, inotropes, and vasopressors – all of which must be prepared beforehand.

Spinal cord protection

- Spinal cord protection must be considered in every case.
- Paraplegia or paraparesis occurs in 2%–10% of elective TAA repairs and up to 40% of emergency surgical cases [20] secondary to interruption of spinal cord blood supply (principally at the radicular artery of Adamkiewicz).
- Paraplegia is associated strongly the with duration of aortic cross-clamping.
- Several methods for protection are described; intrathecal drain, vessel reimplantation (see next point), proximal-to-distal limited bypass, epidural cooling, SEP monitoring.
- Some patients undergoing thoracic endovascular aortic repair (TEVAR) have pathology necessitating stent placement over the origin of the left subclavian artery, which normally supplies the vertebral artery, anterior spinal artery, and ipsilateral arm. Endovascular occlusion in patients with a dominant left vertebral artery, solitary vertebral artery, carotid disease, or incomplete circle of Willis may compromise spinal cord or posterior circulation perfusion. The Society for Vascular Surgery recommends revascularization by connection to the left carotid artery pre- or perioperatively in patients at high-risk, based on individual assessment [25].
- Neuroprotection and maintenance of spinal cord blood flow can be challenging due to the anatomical and hydrodynamic variability in spinal cord perfusion.
- Conceptually, improvement of spinal cord perfusion pressure can be achieved by reduction of compartment pressure through cerebrospinal fluid (CSF) drainage and maintenance of spinal cord perfusion pressure (SCPP).
- Additionally, reduction of oxygen demand by cooling or pharmacology may reduce the incidence of cord ischemia and paraplegia further.

Thoracic endovascular aortic repair

Thoracic aortic disease remains a source of significant mortality and morbidity with a death rate of 10.4/100 000 person–years – the fifteenth most common cause of death in those patients over 65 years of age. Medical treatment alone is associated with dismal survival (13% at five years) while the majority of surgically treated patients (60%–80%) are alive at the same interval. Intervention typically is indicated when the aortic diameter exceeds 5.5 cm [26].

- Endovascular repair of TAA was described nearly 20 years ago [27], extending the concept of endovascular AAA repair proposed by Parodi et al. [28].
- In recent years, TEVAR has become commonplace for management of both elective and emergency TAA.
- Endovascular AAA repair and TEVAR result in improved outcome for repair of aortic dissection as a first-line treatment, with lower mortality and morbidity compared to open surgery [21,29,30].
- Jonker and colleagues published a meta-analysis comparing the outcomes of TEVAR and open repair in patients with ruptured descending TAA [31]. Early mortality was

reduced (19% versus 33%) as were cardiac and neurologically poor outcomes; however, late aneurysm-related deaths remained a concern.

- In a retrospective analysis of more than 12 000 Medicare claims, patients undergoing TEVAR had lower perioperative mortality. However, at one and five years, survival was significantly worse in propensity-matched cohorts, suggesting that higher-risk patients are being offered this surgery but long-term benefits are not being realized [29].
- Nonrandomized, retrospective, and database analysis data predominate the literature in this area – randomized trials are needed.

Suggested benefits include:

- less invasive procedure
- no need for cardiopulmonary bypass or differential lung ventilation
- reduced blood loss
- shorter hospital stay and lower perioperative morbidity and mortality

The lack of aortic cross-clamping and better hemodynamic stability may be associated with a reduced risk of spinal cord injury (SCI), although randomized trials currently are lacking [20][21].

Patient selection

- Generally, patients are considered preferentially for TEVAR due to their poorer overall health status; CAD, hypertension, diabetes, COPD, and renal dysfunction. These patients are considered to be at high-risk of complications such as stroke, myocardial infarction, acute renal insufficiency, infection, and failure to wean from the ventilator.
- Preoperative assessment of the elective patient should focus on cardiac, respiratory, and renal systems, as these account for the most perioperative morbidity and mortality [2,20,32].
- Considerations favoring TEVAR include: anatomy with appropriate landing zones (the non-aneurysmal portion of the proximal and distal diseased vessel where the stent fabric can seal the device to the vessel wall, thereby excluding the aneurysmal portion) and arterial access, advanced age, and increased medical risk. Thoracic aneurysms often impinge on important vascular branches, the occlusion of which must be carefully weighed when considering TEVAR over open repair.
- Contraindications include: aortic size beyond graft size, severely tortuous aorta, inaccessible access vessels, circumferential thrombus at the landing site, severe aortoiliac disease, significant renal insufficiency, and lack of available follow-up.
- Perioperative assessment should focus on documentation of cardiorespiratory, renal, and spinal cord function.
- In elective cases, coronary angiography and revascularization may be appropriate prior to thoracic aortic surgery.

The decision for surgery should be based on a discussion between the patient and surgeon based on the associated risk–benefit ratio. The decision to proceed implies acceptance of significant risks of complications, including death.

Complications

Perioperative mortality is related largely to failure of the cardiac, respiratory, and renal systems and to pre-existing disease.

Complications related directly to TEVAR include:

- SCI (infarction)
- left subclavian artery occlusion
- neurological injury/cerebrovascular accident (CVA)
- iliofemoral vascular injury
- endoleak
- aneurysm sac enlargement
- device migration

Endoleaks comprise a group of graft and aneurysm-sac-related complications. Five types are recognized, based on the origin of blood flow and patient care implications:

I. attachment site leak – proximal (Ia), distal (Ib), aorto-uni-iliac stents (Ic)
II. collateral vessel leak through aortic branches
III. graft failure – mid-graft leak, junction leak, or disconnect
IV. graft-wall porosity
V. endotension (expansion of aneurysm without conspicuous endoleak)

Spinal cord ischemia is potentially reversible and is a recognized complication of TAA repair, occurring in 2%–15% (5% is permanent) of cases, and is not reduced by endovascular repair [19,33].

Reported risks for SCI include:

- previous AAA repair
- intraoperative hypotension. A lowest mean arterial pressure (MAP) of <70 mmHg represented a significant predictor of SCI
- atherosclerosis of the thoracic aorta
- external iliac artery injury
- extensive aortic coverage by the graft
- Additionally involved: age, COPD, hypertension, dyslipidemia, cerebrovascular disease

The EUROSTAR study revealed an independent correlation with the number of stent grafts used, left subclavian artery coverage (without revascularization), renal impairment, and simultaneous AAA repair [34].

Paraplegia is a devastating complication of the treatment of thoracoabdominal aneurysms that has not decreased in parallel with overall complication rates in TEVAR. Early identification of neurological deficits intraoperatively allows the opportunity to modify both physiological (MAP, SCPP, hemoglobin, etc.) and surgical factors (endoleak creation, conversion to staged procedures, arterial bypass/reimplanation) with the aim of improving spinal cord outcomes. Ideally, all patients should be afforded due consideration for monitoring, especially in those centers where resources and skill permit modification of the intervention to reduce poor outcomes.

The incidence of stroke is approximately 3%–5% and for stroke with paraplegia ~5% [34]. Risk factors include:

- female gender
- long duration of procedure
- left subclavian artery origin coverage in patients with cerebrovascular disease or an incomplete circle of Willis. Management of the left subclavian artery may require transposition, shunt, or vascular bypass in a staged fashion (Grade 2b) to reduce the risk of stroke or SCI in patients with poor collateralization and/or an incomplete circle of Willis

Postoperative renal dysfunction is predicted by preoperative degree of insufficiency and the anatomy repaired – occurring in 30% of thoracic and 3% of abdominal repairs. Avoidance of hypoperfusion, hypotension, and nephrotoxic drugs may reduce the risk of acute renal failure.

Perioperative management principles

- withhold antihypertensive therapy (with the exception of β-blockers) due to the likelihood of difficult-to-treat postoperative hypotension
- preoperative placement of CSF drains or early placement on recognition of delayed onset SCI postoperatively
- active management of hemodynamic stress to minimize the risk of perioperative rupture, and appropriate to coexisting disease(s)
- hypertension is preferred to hypotension (mean of <70 mmHg is associated with increased SCI risk), except briefly during stent deployment

Anesthetic management

In contrast to open repair, the anesthetist may consider local anesthesia, RA, or GA as a means to facilitate TEVAR. However, TEVAR is performed most commonly under GA because of:

- reduced patient movement
- facilitating physiological monitoring
- ability to employ TEE
- ease of vessel cannulation
- ability to convert to open procedure if necessary

No difference in mortality or SCI was observed between techniques in the EUROSTAR study [34].

Monitoring for GA

- Routine monitors such as five-lead ECG, capnography, SpO_2, noninvasive BP, temperature, urinary catheter are used.
- Arterial line is inserted – right radial for proximal pressure monitoring and left hand to detect unintended subclavian occlusion.
- Intraoperative TEE is done.
- Central venous access should be available if myocardial performance is poor preoperatively.

- Evidence for use of the pulmonary artery catheter is lacking and increasingly unsupported in the general literature.
- Two large-bore intravenous cannulas (14G) are used.
- Lumbar CSF drain is a class I recommendation in patients at risk for SCI [20].

Intraoperative strategies to reduce SCI [20,26,35]

Increase spinal cord perfusion pressure

- lumbar CSF drainage (CSF pressure ≤10 mmHg)
- arterial blood pressure augmentation (MAP ≥85 mmHg)
- intravascular volume expansion
- vasopressor medications
- reduce central venous pressure

Increase oxygen delivery

- increase cardiac output
- transfusion to increase hemoglobin concentration
- supplemental oxygen

Deliberate hypothermia

- mild to moderate systemic hypothermia (32–35 °C)
- selective spinal cord hypothermia (epidural cooling, 25 °C)

Early detection of spinal cord ischemia

- spinal cord monitoring. Specificity and negative predictive value for SEP and MEP are >97% only when deficits are irreversible. Consensus on a preferred modality (SEP versus MEP) is lacking [35]. Patients without signal loss are unlikely to suffer neurological deficits
- transcranial MEPs
- serial neurological examinations

Neuropharmacological protection

- Various drugs have been utilized but are largely experimental (such as glucocorticoids, naloxone, barbiturates, or other central nervous system depressants, magnesium sulfate, mannitol, intravenous lidocaine, intrathecal papaverine).

Postoperative management

- Admission to an intensive care unit experienced in neurologic/spinal cord monitoring is done routinely.
- Continued invasive monitoring of hemodynamic parameters is essential.
- Postoperative respiratory, cardiac, and renal failure are common.
- Hypertension is common; aggressive management with vasodilators and/or β-blockers is appropriate to reduce systolic hypertension.
- However, one must maintain adequate perfusion pressures and avoid relative hypotension for end-organ preservation – most patients have atherosclerotic disease.

- Analgesia by intravenous or neuraxial techniques is given, depending on the surgical technique.
- Resume antihypertensive therapy cautiously.
- One should monitor for SCI resulting from operative occlusion of intercostal and lumbar arteries.
- Neurological assessment for early detection of delayed-onset SCI is important.

Suspected SCI

For suspected SCI, the following approach is suggested [26]:

1. Optimize oxygen delivery
   - Optimize the cardiac index.
   - Maintain hematocrit at 30% or greater.
2. Maximize SCPP
   - Maintain MAP above 90–110 mmHg by volume expansion and use of α-agonists (e.g., norepinephrine, phenylephrine, vasopressin).
   - CSF drainage to maintain intrathecal pressure <10 cmH_2O should be employed.
   - This is necessary whenever SCI is suspected, even if not inserted preoperatively. Complications of CSF drainage occur in approximately 1% of patients. These may include neuraxial or subdural hematoma, meningitis, spinal headache, intracranial hypotension, and catheter fracture [20,26].
   - This should be initiated when CVP is <10 mmHg.
3. Reduce neurotoxic excitatory neurotransmitters by naloxone infusion at 1 mcg/kg/h, continued for 48 hours postoperatively.
4. Carry out serial neurological examination to assess change in neurological deficit.
5. MRI is used to exclude spinal hematoma or other spinal cord abnormalities.

Arteriovenous fistula formation

- In Canada, patients with end-stage renal disease nearly tripled to 39 352 between 1991 and 2010 [36]. More than 23 000 of these cases were on dialysis.
- More than 5600 Canadians began renal replacement therapy in 2010 as compared to 2614 in 1991.
- Patients can receive dialysis via catheter access (70.4%–79.9%), arteriovenous fistulas (AVFs) (15.6%–19.8%), or grafts (AVGs) (1.1%–2.5%) [36].
- Creation of fistulas for long-term dialysis requires sedation and/or anesthesia.
- The Kidney Disease Outcomes Quality Initiative guidelines suggest that the first option for AVF construction is via the radiocephalic vessels, although the primary failure rate is high.
- AVFs require more than four to six weeks for maturation prior to their use. Thus, patients should undergo elective fistula creation only after they are euvolemic and comorbid conditions are optimized; dialysis shortly before surgery in those already dialysis-dependent is advised.

Anesthetic Management

Anesthetic management of patients undergoing AVF creation

- This procedure can be performed under local anesthesia or RA, with or without sedation, or under GA.
- There is no definitive evidence to support routine selection of a given technique to reduce cardiovascular and other complications, although some evidence exists for improved patency rates in highly selected patients receiving regional anesthesia.

The main principles of anesthetic management should be:

- protection of heart and brain from ischemia and metabolic upset
- recognition that BP may differ in the upper limbs due to atherosclerotic plaque
- control of heart rate
- management of sympathetic tone
- maintenance of normothermia
- maintenance of high blood flows through the fistula during surgery and postoperatively – may lead to improved patency and maturation rates [37].

Local anesthesia or RA

Fistula creation under infiltration of local anesthetic is possible when operating on both the arm and forearm. Superficial and deep infiltration throughout the operative field by the surgeon during the dissection requires patience and co-operation of the patient.

The obvious advantages include the avoidance of GA, enhanced venodilation, and excellent analgesia for the duration of the local anesthetic effect [38].

Unfortunately, arm dissections and prosthetic conduit grafting are less easily managed with local field infiltration due to the increased complexity and duration of surgery. Patients will have difficulty remaining still safely for prolonged periods of time despite the addition of generous sedation. Sedation will be associated with potential risks such as airway obstruction.

Regional anesthesia

- Bier's technique of RA can be used for creation of fistulas suitable for dialysis.
- In contemporary practice, brachial plexus block is a suitable technique. The failure rate of regional blocks in this context may be lower with the routine use of ultrasound imaging.
- For distal forearm procedures, targeted peripheral nerve blocks can be used.

Potential advantages include:

- sympathetic block with decreased surgical stress
- improved vasodilation
- reduced thrombosis of graft and vessels
- hemodynamic stability
- avoidance of prolonged GA and shorter recovery time

Potential risks are associated with needle trauma (hematoma and nerve injury), especially for anticoagulated patients or those with uremic platelet dysfunction.

General anesthesia

GA is the most commonly delivered anesthetic in many centers. Any technique of GA can be provided, as long as the principles of homeostasis are applied:

- Support of organ perfusion is paramount.
- Avoid hemodynamic instability and hypoperfusion.
- Avoid high circulating catecholamines, increases in sympathetic tone/pain, and hypothemia (vasoconstriction of graft vessels).
- A balanced, titrated anesthetic technique is appropriate and addresses the issue of cardiac comorbid disease insofar as oxygen demand is minimized and delivery is optimized.
- Of course, anesthetic plans must be tailored further to the individual patient.
- Anesthetic implications of patients with endstage renal failure are discussed fully elsewhere in the text.

Postoperative management

- Hemodynamic instability is common in this population and should be treated and stabilized before discharge from the recovery area.
- Prevention of undue stress/anxiety, hypothermia, shivering, and respiratory distress will reduce myocardial oxygen demand and the risk of developing myocardial ischemia.

References

1. Fleisher LA, Beckman JA, Brown KA, et al. ACCF/AHA focused update on perioperative beta blockade incorporated into the ACC/AHA 2007 guidelines on perioperative cardiovascular evaluation and care for noncardiac surgery. *J Am Coll Cardiol* 2009; **54**: e13–118.
2. Poldermans D, Bax JJ, Boersma E, et al. Guidelines for pre-operative cardiac risk assessment and perioperative cardiac management in non-cardiac surgery: the Task Force for Preoperative Cardiac Risk Assessment and Perioperative Cardiac Management in Non-Cardiac Surgery of the European Society of Cardiology (ESC) and European Society of Anaesthesiology (ESA). *Eur Heart J* 2009; **30**: 2769–812.
3. Chaturvedi S, Bruno A, Feasby T, et al. Carotid endarterectomy–an evidence-based review: report of the therapeutics and technology assessment subcommittee of the American Academy of Neurology. *Neurology* 2005; **65**: 794–801.
4. Guay J, Ochroch EA. Carotid endarterectomy plus medical therapy or medical therapy alone for carotid artery stenosis in symptomatic or asymptomatic patients: a meta-analysis. *J Cardiothorac Vasc Anesth* 2012; **26**: 835–44.
5. Ricotta JJ, Aburahma A, Ascher E, et al. Updated society for vascular surgery guidelines for management of extracranial carotid disease. *J Vasc Surg* 2011; **54**: e1–31.
6. Kakisis JD, Avgerinos ED, Antonopoulos CN, et al. The European Society for Vascular Surgery Guidelines for Carotid Intervention: an updated independent assessment and literature review. *Eur J Vasc Endovasc Surg* 2012; **44**: 238–43.
7. Guay J. Endovascular stenting or carotid endarterectomy for treatment of carotid stenosis: a meta-analysis. *J Cardiothorac Vasc Anesth* 2011; **25**: 1024–9.
8. Rerkasem K, Rothwell PM. Carotid endarterectomy for symptomatic carotid stenosis. *Cochrane Database Syst Rev* 2011; **4**: CD001081.
9. Heart Protection Study Collaborative Group. MRC/BHF heart protection study of cholesterol lowering with simvastatin in 20,536 high-risk individuals: a randomised placebo-controlled trial. *Lancet* 2002; **360**: 7–22.

10. Rerkasem K, Rothwell PM. Local versus general anaesthesia for carotid endarterectomy. *Cochrane Database Syst Rev* 2008; **4**: CD000126.

11. Marcucci G, Siani A, Accrocca F, et al. Preserved consciousness in general anesthesia during carotid endarterectomy: a six-year experience. *Interact Cardiovasc Thorac Surg* 2011; **13**: 601–5.

12. Menyhei G, Björck M, Beiles B, et al. Outcome following carotid endarterectomy: lessons learned from a large international vascular registry. *Eur J Vasc Endovasc Surg* 2011; **41**: 735–40.

13. Guay J. Regional anesthesia for carotid surgery. *Curr Opin Anaesthesiol* 2008; **21**: 638–44.

14. Sideso E, Walton J, Handa A. General or local anesthesia for carotid endarterectomy–the "real-world" experience. *Angiology* 201; **62**: 609–13.

15. Pandit JJ, Satya-Krishna R, Gration P. Superficial or deep cervical plexus block for carotid endarterectomy: a systematic review of complications. *Br J Anaesth* 2007; **99**: 159–69.

16. Guay J, Kopp S. Cerebral monitors versus regional anesthesia to detect cerebral ischemia in patients undergoing carotid endarterectomy: a meta-analysis. *Can J Anaesth* 2013; **60**: 266–79.

17. Lewis SC, Warlow CP, Bodenham AR, et al. General anaesthesia versus local anaesthesia for carotid surgery (GALA): a multicentre, randomised controlled trial. *Lancet* 2008; **372**: 2132–42.

18. Aburahma AF, Mousa AY, Stone PA. Shunting during carotid endarterectomy. *J Vasc Surg* 2011; **54**: 1502–10.

19. Hill MD, Brooks W, Mackey A, et al. Stroke after carotid stenting and endarterectomy in the carotid revascularization endarterectomy versus stenting trial (CREST). *Circulation* 2012; **126**: 3054–61.

20. Hiratzka LF, Bakris GL, Beckman JA, et al. ACCF/AHA/AATS/ACR/ASA/SCA/SCAI/SIR/STS/SVM guidelines for the diagnosis and management of patients with thoracic aortic disease: a report of the American College of Cardiology Foundation/American Heart Association Task Force on Practice Guidelines, American Association for Thoracic Surgery, American College of Radiology, American Stroke Association, Society of Cardiovascular Anesthesiologists, Society for Cardiovascular Angiography and Interventions, Society of Interventional Radiology, Society of Thoracic Surgeons, and Society for Vascular Medicine. *Circulation* 2010; **121**: e266–369.

21. Cheng D, Martin J, Shennib H, et al. Endovascular aortic repair versus open surgical repair for descending thoracic aortic disease: a systematic review and meta-analysis of comparative studies. *J Am Coll Cardiol* 2010; **55**: 986–1001.

22. Crawford ES, Crawford JL, Safi HJ, et al. Thoracoabdominal aortic aneurysms: preoperative and intraoperative factors determining immediate and long-term results of operations in 605 patients. *J Vasc Surg* 1986; **3**: 389–404.

23. Ullery BW, Wang GJ, Low D, et al. Neurological complications of thoracic endovascular aortic repair. *Semin Cardiothorac Vasc Anesth* 2011; **15**: 123–40.

24. Banoub M, Tetzlaff JE, Schubert A. Pharmacologic and physiologic influences affecting sensory evoked potentials: implications for perioperative monitoring. *Anesthesiology* 2003; **99**: 716–37.

25. Matsumura JS, Lee WA, Mitchell RS, et al. The society for vascular surgery practice guidelines: management of the left subclavian artery with thoracic endovascular aortic repair. *J Vasc Surg* 2009; **50**: 1155–8.

26. Nicolaou G, Ismail M, Cheng D. Thoracic endovascular aortic repair: update on indications and guidelines. *Anesthesiol Clin* 2013; **31**: 451–78.

27. Dake MD, Miller DC, Semba CP, et al. Transluminal placement of endovascular stent-grafts for the treatment of descending thoracic aortic aneurysms. *N Engl J Med* 1994; **331**: 1729–34.

28. Parodi JC, Palmaz JC, Barone HD. Transfemoral intraluminal graft

implantation for abdominal aortic aneurysms. *Ann Vasc Surg* 1991; **5**: 491–9.

29. Goodney PP, Travis L, Lucas FL, et al. Survival after open versus endovascular thoracic aortic aneurysm repair in an observational study of the medicare population. *Circulation* 2011; **124**: 2661–9.
30. Bavaria JE, Appoo JJ, Makaroun MS, et al. Endovascular stent grafting versus open surgical repair of descending thoracic aortic aneurysms in low-risk patients: a multicenter comparative trial. *J Thorac Cardiovasc Surg* 2007; **133**: 369–77.
31. Jonker FH, Trimarchi S, Verhagen HJ, et al. Meta-analysis of open versus endovascular repair for ruptured descending thoracic aortic aneurysm. *J Vasc Surg* 2010; **51**: 1026–32,
32. Fleisher LA, Beckman JA, Brown KA, et al. ACC/AHA 2007 guidelines on perioperative cardiovascular evaluation and care for noncardiac surgery: A report of the American College Of Cardiology/American Heart Association Task Force on Practice Guidelines (Writing Committee to revise the 2002 guidelines on perioperative cardiovascular evaluation for noncardiac surgery) developed in collaboration with the American Society of Echocardiography, American Society of Nuclear Cardiology, Heart Rhythm Society, Society of Cardiovascular Anesthesiologists, Society for Cardiovascular Angiography and Interventions, Society for Vascular Medicine and Biology, and Society for Vascular Surgery. *J Am Coll Cardiol* 2007; **50**: e159–241.
33. Desart K, Scali ST, Feezor RJ, et al. Fate of patients with spinal cord ischemia complicating thoracic endovascular aortic repair. *J Vasc Surg* 2013; **58**: 635–42.
34. Buth J, Harris PL, Hobo R, et al. Neurologic complications associated with endovascular repair of thoracic aortic pathology: incidence and risk factors. A study from the European Collaborators on Stent/Graft Techniques for Aortic Aneurysm Repair (EUROSTAR) registry. *J Vasc Surg* 2007; **46**: 1103–10.
35. Bobadilla JL, Wynn M, Tefera G, et al. Low incidence of paraplegia after thoracic endovascular aneurysm repair with proactive spinal cord protective protocols. *J Vasc Surg* 2013; **57**: 1537–42.
36. Canadian Institute for Health Information. *Canadian Organ Replacement Register Annual Report: Treatment of End-Stage Organ Failure in Canada, 2002 to 2011.* Ottawa, ON: CIHI, 2012.
37. Malinzak EB, Gan TJ. Regional anesthesia for vascular access surgery. *Anesth Analg* 2009; **109**: 976–80.
38. Hingorani AP, Ascher E, Gupta P, et al. Regional anesthesia: preferred technique for venodilatation in the creation of upper extremity arteriovenous fistulae. *Vascular* 2006; **14**: 23–6.

Chapter 24

Gastrointestinal surgery

S. Patel

This chapter will discuss several topics of relevance to anesthesia for gastrointestinal (GI) surgery, with especial reference to colorectal surgery.

Colorectal surgery

Colorectal surgery secondary to colorectal cancer, diverticular disease, inflammatory bowel disease and (less commonly) trauma, ischemic colitis, volvulus, and iatrogenic perforation is performed commonly in both an elective and emergency setting.

- Typical mortality following colorectal surgery in western countries is around 5% – higher than adult cardiac surgery.
- The incidence of complications after colorectal surgery varies from 13% to 37% in most studies [1]. In a recent retrospective study, the risk for incurring at least one postoperative complication was 24.0% in non-emergency and 48.2% in emergency patients [2].
- The 30-day in-hospital mortality during emergency surgery is three to four times higher in comparison to elective surgery [3]. The overall morbidity (medical or surgical complications) after emergency colorectal surgery is 3 to 10 times higher than morbidity after elective surgery.
- Several factors influence morbidity and mortality, such as functional status, nutrition, American Society of Anesthesiologists (ASA) grade, and perioperative optimization of physiology and clinical care.

Anesthesia for colorectal surgery is often poorly represented in major anesthesia textbooks. Indeed, publications related to enhanced recovery protocols and perioperative fluid therapy are frequently found in non-anesthesia journals.

Aspiration, rapid sequence induction, and cricoid pressure

In the U.K., a national audit of "Major complications of airway management" (NAP4) [4] has highlighted aspiration of stomach contents as a major contributory factor for anesthesia-related morbidity and mortality. In this audit, 55 serious airway-related incidents during general anesthesia were reported. Of these, 26 involved aspiration, and of all the anesthetic-related deaths reported to NAP4, 50% were due to aspiration.

Anesthesia and Perioperative Care of the High-Risk Patient, Third edition, ed. Ian McConachie. Published by Cambridge University Press.

Risk factors

In the NAP4 audit [4], risk factors were present in 90% of 23 cases in whom aspiration was the primary event. During the preoperative period, assessment of risk factors and of their modification are fundamental aspects for prevention of aspiration. This is particularly important for urgent or emergency surgery. However, failure to assess/recognize risk factors for aspiration and to adjust the anesthetic technique accordingly were strikingly evident in the NAP4 audit and other large studies. Factors which predispose patients to aspiration include:

- Stomach and lower GI: feeding or lack of adequate fasting and delayed gastric emptying due to structural or functional causes such as pain, trauma, pyloric stenosis, intestinal obstruction, diabetes mellitus, and chronic renal failure.
- Esophagus: reduced lower esophageal tone, reflux, hiatus hernia, motility disorders, and previous surgery.
- Impaired reflexes: head injury, stroke, loss or impaired consciousness due to drugs or diseases, and neuromuscular diseases such as myasthenia gravies and Guillain Barré syndrome.
- Other factors: emergency surgery, pregnancy of >20 weeks, obesity, raised intra-abdominal pressure (e.g., abdominal laparoscopic surgery), multiple laryngoscopy, difficult intubation, and the lithotomy position.
- Supraglottic airway devices (SGDs), such as the laryngeal mask airway (LMA), may also be a risk factor, although when aspiration occurs with the use of an SGD, other risk factors for aspiration are almost always present. In one case series, identified risk factors were present in 19 of 20 patients who aspirated while an LMA was in place [5]. Second generation devices (e.g., proseal LMA or igel), with a channel for the passage of regurgitated material, may be helpful. Other practical points to consider with the use of an SGD are careful selection of cases, assurance of proper placement, avoidance of high inflation pressures and a lighter plane of anesthesia during the maintenance phase, and adequate reversal if paralytic agents were used.

Prevention

- Use of regional anesthesia, fasting as per standard guidelines, premedication in indicated cases with prokinetics drugs, antacids, H2-blockers, and proton pump inhibitors for high-risk cases, and rapid sequence induction and intubation (RSII) may prevent aspiration or minimize consequences [6]. In selected cases, insertion of a nasogastric tube and drainage of stomach contents should be done, as with intestinal obstruction or a paralytic ileus.
- Awareness, education, and training of staff are also important to reduce the incidence of aspiration [7].

Diagnosis

- Presence of gastric contents in endotracheal tube, LMA, or suction catheter should raise suspicion of aspiration. Symptoms vary depending on the nature of aspirated material (volume, particles, and pH), its sterility, and whether the patient is awake or anesthetised. Hypoxia and airway obstruction may be mild to severe. Fever, coughing, tachypnea, presence of wheeze, and crepitations on auscultation are also common features. Aspiration should be included in the differential diagnosis of airway obstruction, laryngospasm, bronchospasm, cyanosis, and pulmonary edema during the perioperative period.

Management

- Depending on the urgency and patient's clinical condition, surgery may proceed. In one study, 42 (64%) patients who aspirated but did not develop a cough, wheeze, decrease in arterial hemoglobin oxygen saturation while breathing room air of >10% less than the preoperative value, or radiographic abnormalities within two hours of aspiration had no further respiratory sequelae [8].
- Management depends on severity and may include chest physical therapy, bronchodilators, intubation and mechanical ventilation, and antibiotics.

Rapid sequence induction and intubation

RSII is performed to minimize the time interval between loss of protective airway reflexes and tracheal intubation with a cuffed endotracheal tube to prevent the risk of aspiration in at-risk patients. NAP4 [4] has identified several cases where the omission of RSII, although there were strong indications for its use, was followed by patient harm or death from aspiration. RSII has evolved and it consists of: optimal positioning of the patient, pre-oxygenation, injection of an opioid and a hypnotic intravenous (IV) injection of a fast-acting neuromuscular blocking agent, cricoid pressure (CP), and tracheal intubation. However, most of these components have not been standardized to form a universal protocol [9]. Induction and neuromuscular blocking drugs, timing of their administration, position of the patient during RSII, whether to do manual positive pressure mask ventilation, suppression of the intubation response, and application of CP during RSII are all debatable issues. The use of CP is probably the most debated aspect of RSII.

Cricoid pressure

To apply CP or not has remained controversial five decades since its introduction in clinical practice by Sellick in 1961. There are arguments for and against its use, which are outlined in Table 24.1 [10]. Despite lack of strong supporting evidence, CP is still considered an integral part of RSII.

For its optimal use, knowledge of anatomy, training, and use of the correct force with correct timing at the correct site are all important. The technique is as follows:

- After identifying the cricoid cartilage, pressure of 10 to 20 N for an adult patient (1 N equals approximately 10 kg) should be applied while the patient is awake before induction.
- Force should be increased to 30 to 40 N when the patient is unconscious.
- Excessive or lighter force is often applied by anesthesiologists and other healthcare professionals.
- CP should be released if the glottic view is obscured.

Simulated demonstration and application, use of mechanical devices or models to "feel" the correct force, and frequent retraining are some of the measures to increase its successful use. In pediatric populations, CP is used less frequently. Smaller anatomical structures,

Table 24.1. Pros and cons of cricoid pressure

	Arguments in favor	Arguments against
Evidence	Time-tested technique and has been a standard component of rapid sequence induction to prevent aspiration in at-risk patients. In the U.K., it is standard	Level D evidence No RCTs are available Evidence is from study on cadavers
Benefits	Prevents aspiration of gastric contents in high-risk cases at induction	Regurgitation of esophageal contents and aspiration can occur at the time of extubation
Technical aspects	Simple procedure and easy to learn Easy to teach and apply in clinical circumstances Devices can be used to teach and monitor force applied	Knowledge of CP and force necessary among clinicians is poor Difficult to judge how much force is applied Usually variable force is applied and there is no monitoring It is difficult to sustain force if intubation takes time
Efficacy	If correctly applied, prevents aspiration	Regurgitation and aspiration has been reported despite applying CP
Anatomical basis	CP substitutes for the loss of tone in the cricopharyngeus, which forms the upper esophageal sphincter Cricoid ring is a complete cartilage and effectively occludes esophagus to prevent regurgitated material to enter into the trachea Esophagus position is irrelevant as CP occludes hypopharynx with which it constitutes an anatomical unit	Reduces the lower esophageal sphincter tone up to 50% depending on the degree of the force applied Esophagus is not in the central position in nearly 50% of patients. CP may further displace esophagus laterally and does not occlude it in all cases CP flexes the neck and head, which may cause a suboptimal intubating position
Risks	Safe to apply and has been used in millions of patients No difference in visualization of larynx and does not increase the risk of difficult intubation There is no evidence that CP leads to failed intubation Airway risks are because of lack of training in use of CP	Interferes with mask ventilation, changes laryngoscopy grade, and may increase the intubation time or make it difficult, particularly if excessive force is applied. The incidence of these risks varies depending on the degree of force, and may occur in 50% of cases with recommended 30–40 N force Make insertion of LMA and intubation via LMA difficult Glotic view with fiberoptic endoscope, and other video laryngoscopes may also be impeded Esophageal rupture if vomiting occurs while CP is applied

Table 24.1. *(cont.)*

	Arguments in favor	Arguments against
Other	Prevents gastric insufflation during mask ventilation, which can be beneficial particularly in pediatric patients Effective in the presence of nasogastric tube	Causes patient discomfort and may provoke retching and vomiting

unknown effective force, and practical difficulty in application with an adult hand are some limiting factors to the use of CP in these cases. The force required may be as low as 5 N in infants and up to between 15 and 25 N in teenagers [11].

Fluid therapy

There is evidence that the type of fluid, its volume and timing of administration, and the patient's baseline physiology and response to fluid therapy influence GI functional recovery and complications (Figure 24.1). Many colorectal surgical patients have cardiorespiratory, renal, and endocrine problems. This high-risk group of patients may be more at risk for fluid overload.

Intestinal fluid dynamics

- Intestinal capillaries are fenestrated. The intestines have a large extracellular compartment and are more susceptible to edema formation in comparison to lung tissue. Alterations in microvascular permeability, portal venous pressure, plasma albumin level, and intestinal lymphatic function or flow result in imbalance of intestinal capillary Starling forces.
- Diseases (e.g., inflammatory bowel, peritonitis, bowel obstruction), technical factors (e.g., bowel preparation, bowel exposure and manipulation), and luminal factors (e.g., nutrients, toxins) are some of the potential factors that interfere with GI fluid balance.
- Systemic hypovolemia or hypervolemia may lead to intestinal edema, ischemia, hypoxia, acidosis, impaired healing, reduced nutrient delivery, and bacterial translocation. Clinical GI complications, like delayed oral intake, anastomosis leak, and delayed hospital discharge, may develop if fluid therapy is not optimal.

Choice of fluid: crystalloid or colloid

The crystalloid/colloid debate has existed since the 1980s. The debate shall be summarized with special relevance to GI surgery.

Experimental studies

- Goal-directed (GD) colloid therapy is associated with a significant increase in microcirculatory blood flow and oxygen tension in the small intestine, and in healthy and perianastomotic colonic tissue [12].
- GD crystalloid therapy, although increasing cardiac index and mean blood pressure (BP) by 15%, did not improve intestinal macro- and microcirculatory blood flow and oxygenation.

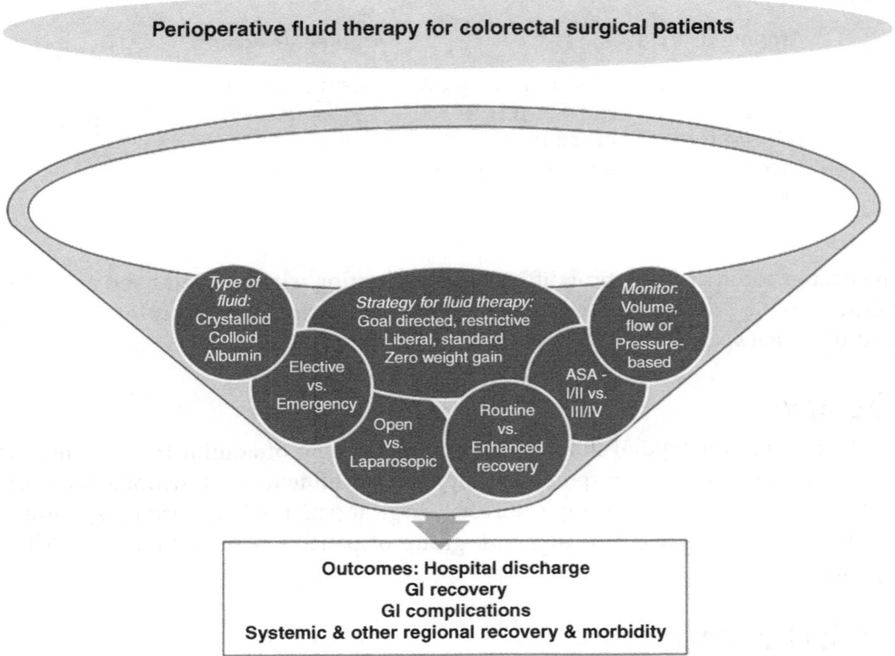

Figure 24.1. Influences of fluid therapy.

- Liberal crystalloid administration, even in large amounts (20 mL/kg), did not improve oxygen pressure in the small and the large intestine [13]. In fact, large-volume crystalloid therapy has been found to decrease bursting pressure, and also impaired healing at the anastomotic site with increased weight gain in experimental animals [14].
- In various septic models, colloids have been reported to have positive microcirculatory effects in the intestines, such as improved microcirculatory flow, decreased inflammatory markers, increased perfused capillary density, blockage of capillary leakage, reduced leukocyte adherence to endothelium, inhibition of platelet and erythrocyte aggregation.

Clinical crystalloid studies

- In a study by Prien et al. [15], colloid osmotic pressure decreased by 25% and water content in the jejunum increased significantly in patients receiving Ringer's lactate during Whipple's procedure. In contrast, both these parameters remained unchanged in the 10% hydroxyethyl starch group.
- In a retrospective review by Schnüriger et al. [16], high volume crystalloid resuscitation was found to be an independent risk factor for anastomotic leak (AL) following repair of traumatic colon injuries. The authors found a five-fold increased risk of anastomotic breakdown if the volume of crystalloid was more than 10.5 L in the first three postoperative days.

Clinical colloid Studies

- Recent large randomized controlled trials (RCTs) have raised concerns for the use of hydroxyethyl starch in severely septic patients, mainly because of increased renal complications, and recent guidelines recommend avoiding hetastarches [17]. Such clinical circumstances may arise in complicated colorectal surgical patients undergoing emergency surgery for severe peritonitis or a major AL, and in patients with abdominal sepsis.
- However, during elective abdominal surgery and in trauma patients, use of tetrastarches, particularly waxy maize-derived hydroxyethyl starch (130/0.4) is not associated with an adverse outcome [18,19]. There was no increased incidence of renal impairment or failure, or blood loss.

Recently, Chappell et al. [20] suggested the use of crystalloid to replace urinary loss and insensible loss via perspiration while iso-oncotic colloid should be used to replace plasma loss from the circulation due to pathological fluid shift and acute blood loss of up to a liter. They questioned the existence of a fluid-consuming "third space" whereby fluids are sequestered in the tissues.

Type of fluid therapy

Standard (routine), restrictive (low-volume), liberal (high-volume), goal-directed (targeted), and zero-weight gain are fluid management strategies studied in colorectal surgical patients. There is a lack of uniform definitions of the terms standard, restrictive, and liberal fluid administration [21].

- Standard (routine) fluid therapy is based on a fixed mL/kg/h calculation, which counts the period of perioperative fasting, maintenance, and replacement requirements. This approach may lead to fluid deficit or excess.
- Unmonitored restrictive (low-volume) and liberal (high-volume) fluid administration may also lead to hypovolemia or hypervolemia, respectively.
- There is evidence that liberal fluid therapy has been associated with weight gain, splanchnic edema, and pulmonary complications.
- In an RCT, Brandstrup et al. [22] reported a reduction in the rate of complications in a group of patients whose fluid therapy was designed to maintain unchanged body weight compared to a group receiving more liberal intravenous fluids.
- Restrictive fluid therapy may lead to increased sympathetic activation and may cause systemic hypotension, leading to increased use of vasopressors.

Restrictive fluid therapy

- In one RCT, intraoperative fluid restriction was associated with reduced perioperative central venous blood oxygen saturation ($ScvO_2$), even when using goal-directed boluses to correct hypovolemia [23]. The authors observed associations between reduced $ScvO_2$, hypovolemia, and postoperative complications in fluid restricted patients.
- Hubner et al. [24] studied restricted fluid therapy in patients undergoing fast-track open abdominal surgery in the presence of epidural analgesia. There was increased use of colloid boluses and vasopressors (to achieve a mean arterial pressure [MAP] of >60 mmHg and urine output of >0.5 mL/h) in fast-track patients, although this did not

reach statistical significance. The use of vasopressors during restrictive fluid therapy may raise concerns about intestinal oxygenation and metabolic function.
- Wenkui et al. [25] suggested monitoring serum lactate in fluid-restricted patients during fast-track surgery. In this study, colloid fluid boluses were needed in 25% of patients during the postoperative period to maintain the serum lactate level at the preoperative level.

Balanced fluid therapy

- Varadhan and Lobo [26] have analyzed studies using "fixed"-fluid volume therapy during major open abdominal surgery. Patients were considered in "fluid balance" if they received 1.75–2.75 L/d during the intraoperative and postoperative period. If patients received <1.75 L/d (restrictive) or >2.75 L/d (liberal), they were considered in "fluid imbalance" status. There was a 59% reduction in risk of developing complications and significant reduction in hospital stay in the fluid-balance group.

Goal-directed fluid therapy

- Stroke volume (SV) optimization is the common goal targeted in several studies. Fluid boluses are repeated until the increase in SV is less than 10% following the bolus. Colloids are frequently used to achieve a sustainable fluid bolus response.
- Other specific hemodynamic goals, such as SV variation or data derived from arterial pressure waveform analysis (stroke volume variation and pulse pressure variation) and central venous saturation, have also been used.
- Choice of the specific monitoring modality is still debated and there is no overwhelming evidence supporting the use of any particular tool.
- In the U.K., use of esophageal Doppler ultrasound has been recommended. However, it has generated controversy and it has been pointed out that initial clinical benefits with Doppler-guided fluid therapy might not be evident when compared with laparoscopic surgery together with enhanced recovery protocols [27].
- Early GI functional recovery and shorter hospital stay (average, two days) are frequently reported positive outcomes with GD fluid therapy [28]. This meta-analysis also reported a 30% reduction in the incidence of pneumonia and renal complications in a mixed surgical population.

Specific clinical circumstances (Figure 24.1)

Emergency surgery

- Emergency-complicated colorectal surgical patients are often fasted for days, poorly monitored for fluid balance, and have large concealed or revealed fluid losses.
- Inadequate resuscitation-associated systemic consequences and pre-existing medical problems makes fluid therapy more complex and challenging.
- Aggressive fluid therapy may be required to achieve optimal systemic perfusion.

Enhanced recovery protocols

- Patients on fast-track enhanced recovery protocols are expected to have no mechanical bowel preparation (except in left colon or rectal surgery), a short fasting period, oral

carbohydrate drink, no nasogastric tube, early postoperative oral intake, and reduced stress response (see later).
- As a result, fluid shift and duration of intravenous fluid therapy are likely to be small and short, respectively. Therefore, liberal use of fluid may not be justified. However, GD fluid therapy and fluid restriction are also controversial for patients on enhanced recovery protocols.

Laparoscopic surgery

- Bowel exposure and handling is minimal and recovery faster for patients undergoing laparoscopic colon surgery.
- Using transesophageal echocardiography, Concha et al. [29] found that patients undergoing laparoscopic colon surgery required 50% less crystalloid to maintain baseline left ventricular end-diastolic volume index and cardiac index when compared with open surgery: 3 mL/kg/h compared to 6 mL/kg/h.

In summary, a standard or formulaic approach is not possible because of the dynamic nature of the fluid shift and various fluid compartments. Frequent careful evaluations of the clinical condition and clinical contexts, and a review of fluid loss are essential and should not be overlooked because of overemphasis on technology and the search for optimized "numbers."

Anesthesia and the intestinal circulation

- The intestinal circulation is important for absorption of nutrients, formation and excretion of feces, and preservation of peristalsis. Protection of gut mucosal barrier function is pivotal during the perioperative period and certain critical conditions such as hemorrhage and sepsis.
- Normal superior and inferior mesenteric arterial blood flow is approximately 700 and 500 mL/min. There is an extensive collateral circulation. However, in some areas of the colon it is sparse, leading to a susceptibility to ischemia. The mucosa and submucosa receive 75% of the blood supply. A unique microcirculation permits transmural redistribution of blood flow. The mucosa is susceptible to hypoxia and hypoperfusion because of the counter current flow arrangement of the arteriole and venule in a villus.
- Several intrinsic (myogenic, metabolic, endothelium-derived factors, GI hormones, etc.) and extrinsic (sympathetic activity, circulatory vasoactive substances, systemic hemodynamic status) factors control intestinal blood flow [30].

Effects of anesthetic agents and techniques

Inhalational anesthetic agents may change intestinal blood flow (IBF) by direct cardiovascular effects like BP, cardiac output, redistribution of blood flow, or direct effects on mesenteric vascular smooth muscle. Effects on circulatory catecholamines, central sympathetic discharge, and splanchnic nerve activity influence mesenteric vascular resistance.

- In a human study [31], isoflurane increased pO_2 in the near resection and anastomotic site in comparison to desflurane. The authors suggested isoflurane preserved reactive hyperemia better following local tissue injury or manipulation.

- In another human study [32], use of one minimum alveolar concentration (MAC) desflurane increased jejunal blood flow compared to 1 MAC isoflurane, without significant changes in systemic hemodynamics.
- Thus, local mechanisms can play a crucial role during inhalational anesthesia. Isoflurane and sevoflurane also reduce mesenteric vascular resistance. The use of inhalational anesthetics may blunt the stress-induced increase in splanchnic vascular resistance.
- In addition, Kim et al. [33] recently demonstrated multiple protective effects of isoflurane postconditioning against intestinal ischemia–reperfusion injury.
- Propofol decreases mesenteric vascular resistance and increases IBF in a dose-dependant manner despite a decrease in MAP [34]. The increase in IBF is more in the small intestine than colon.
- Ketamine maintains capillary circulation and reduces leak following hemorrhagic shock and resuscitation [35].

Epidural analgesia

The level of epidural block (e.g., number of segments and region of block), baseline sympathetic activity in mesenteric and systemic blood vessels, volume status, and concentration of local anesthetic are important determining factors for intestinal circulatory effects of epidural anesthesia/analgesia. Theoretically, if the block is limited to mesenteric sympathetic activity (T8-L1), arteriolar dilation and venodilation would increase both macro- and microcirculation.

- Johannson et al. [36] observed an increase in intestinal microcirculatory blood flow despite a decrease in systolic BP in patients undergoing colon resection. Authors attributed this effect to decreased mean venous resistance.
- In contrast, Gould et al. [37] found a reduction in inferior mesenteric artery flow by 20% and colon serosal flow by 35% – both strongly correlated with reduction in MAP. In this study, blood flow was not related to cardiac output and did not respond to fluid alone but required vasopressor to restore MAP, inferior mesenteric artery flow, and colon serosal blood flow. The authors suggested maintaining the MAP with vasopressor during the perioperative period, in the presence of epidural block.
- In both these studies, 0.5% bupivacaine bolus was used during the intraoperative study period. Continuous infusion of lower concentrations of local anesthetic might have produced different results.

Recently, there has been interest in intestinal circulatory effects of epidural anesthesia during critical conditions such as sepsis and hemorrhage. There is a potential for redistribution of IBF to other organs or away from the ischemic or anastomotic site to normal intestine (longitudinal steal), or from mucosa to the muscularis region (horizontal steal). These effects are not well researched.

IBF in critical conditions

Hemorrhage

- The effect of angiotensin II and vasopressin on mesenteric vascular resistance may increase systemic vascular resistance significantly during shock [38].

- However, autoregulation of mucosa is better preserved in hemorrhagic shock in comparison to septic shock.
- Restoration of IBF and oxygenation, with fluid and blood resuscitation, usually lags behind improvements in systemic hemodyamic parameters [39].

Sepsis

- Stage of sepsis (early or late), volume status, and systemic hypotension are important clinical factors that determine the magnitude of intestinal circulatory and oxygenation disturbances.
- Redistribution of blood flow from muscularis to mucosa tends to maintain mucosal blood flow [40].
- However, in advanced septic shock, microcirulatory blood flow may be reduced by 50% due to endothelial swelling and microvascular thrombosis.

Increased intra-abdominal pressure (IAP)

- Direct effects lead to increased local vascular resistance.
- Mucosal perfusion is affected at lower pressures, but at higher pressures (>20 mmHg) mesenteric artery flow is also reduced [41].
- Persistent IAP causes intestinal hypoperfusion despite normal systemic BP. Decreased cardiac output and hypovolemia further exaggerate the effects. Bacterial translocation, intestinal edema, impaired intestinal motility, and breakdown of the anastomosis are serious consequences of moderate to severe IAP [42].

Effect of therapeutic strategies

Nutrition

With enteral feeding, macro- and micro-IBF is increased two to three times. Lipids followed by glucose are mostly responsible for the increase in blood flow. In contrast, total parenteral nutrition decreases intestinal blood flow [43].

Fluid therapy

Experimental studies suggest that goal-directed fluid therapy improves the small and large intestine macro- and microcirculation.

Vasopressors/inotropes

Effects of inotropes/vasopressors on the intestinal circulation are complex and may not follow systemic changes. Several reviews have addressed this subject [44,45].

- Norepinehrine (NE) may be the first choice for patients with septic shock who have received fluid resuscitation.
- NE may also be safe to use in fluid restricted patients undergoing abdominal surgery. Administration of 0.12±0.05 μg/kg/min NE was required to reach the target BP of 75 mmHg in fluid restricted (3 mL/kg/h) animals [46]. There were no adverse effects on the small intestine or colon blood flow and oxygenation.
- Anesthetic agents may modulate effects of vasopressors and inotropes. Dose-dependant increases in gastric mucosal oxygen saturation were observed with NE in the presence of sevoflurane [47]. Neither NE nor epinephrine changed gastric mucosal oxygen

saturation in the presence of propofol anesthesia despite doubling systemic oxygen delivery in the case of epinephrine.

In summary, the intestinal circulation is not well studied during the perioperative period in humans. There is very little information about the effects of anesthetic agents and techniques on intestinal macro- and microcirculation, or how anesthesia interacts with vasopressors or may modify the intestinal circulation in the presence of sepsis, hemorrhage, or other ischemic conditions.

Anesthesia and the anastomosis

AL is a major complication following GI surgery. AL occurs more frequently following esophagectomy and low rectal resection. For colorectal surgery, the incidence ranges from 2% to 4% for intraperitoneal and 6% to 12% for extraperitoneal anastomosis. It may lead to abdominal and systemic sepsis and increases the risk of mortality two to five times. The diagnosis is mainly clinical and/or radiological.

Risk factors

Risk factors have not been consistent in the various studies [48] because of heterogeneity of data (e.g., diagnosis, site of anastomosis, exclusion criteria) and different definitions used [49]. AL could occur due to patient, operative, or technical factors.

- Malnutrition (hypoalbuminemia and anemia), smoking, use of steroids, and an American Society of Anesthesiologists (ASA) score of >3 are frequently reported patient-related risk factors.
- Infraperitoneal anastomosis, prolonged surgery (>4 hours), amount of blood loss (>300 mL), blood transfusion, and intraoperative septic conditions may also predispose to AL.
- Male gender, obesity, location of tumor within 12 cm from anal verge, use of abdominal drains, and emergency surgery are also implicated in some studies.
- Mechanical bowel preparation, laparosopic surgery, surgical technique for anastomosis (e.g., hand sewn or stapled), and intraoperative testing of anastomosis does not seem to influence AL incidence.

Systemic and intestinal oxygenation

Tissue oxygenation

The oxygen supply to intestinal and abdominal wounds is critical for prevention of infection and promotion of healing at both ends of the anastomosis.

- In an experimental model, all intestinal anastomoses developed a major leak below a critical perianastomotic level of 25 mmHg pO_2 [50].
- In a human study [51], low tissue pO_2 levels were found to be of value in the prediction of an AL.
- However, Schietroma et al. [52] reported 46% lower anastomosis leak in an 80% inspired oxygen concentration (FiO_2) group (relative ratio [RR], 0.63; 95% confidence interval [CI_{95}], 0.42–0.98) compared to a 30% FiO_2 group, and suggested that 80% FiO_2 should be administered routinely during surgery and for up to six hours in the postoperative period.

Hemodynamic optimization

The blood supply at the anastomotic site may depend on blood volume status, cardiac output and its distribution, local capillary perfusion, and several pathological and technical factors (e.g., mobilization of tissue and suture tension). GD fluid therapy or GD hemodynamic management (fluids and or inotropes) have been suggested to reduce major GI complications including AL [53]. However, caution is necessary with regards to the use of vasopressors.

- Zakiroson et al. [54] found intraoperative use of intermittent boluses of vasopressors (phenylephrine and ephedrine) was not associated with increased AL. In contrast, NE infusion in an intensive care setting during the postoperative period increases the risk of AL three times. The authors suggested that it could be due to hypovolemia during the use of the vasopressor infusion.

Non-steroidal anti-inflammatory drugs (NSAIDs)

Inhibition of cyclooxygenase (COX) enzymes by NSAIDs affects leukocyte function, induces apoptosis, and decreases crypt survival. It also reduces production of vascular endothelial growth factor and angiogenesis, and interferes with collagen formation and cross-linking.

- Klein et al. [55] reported higher AL patients treated with diclofenac in comparison to ibuprofen and controls ($P<0.001$ for diclofenac versus controls; $P=0.004$ for ibuprofen versus controls). After multivariate logistic regression analysis, only diclofenac treatment was a risk factor for leakage (odds ratio [OR] 7.2, CI_{95} 3.8–13.4, $P<0.001$).
- There are contradictory reports with regard to selective COX-2 inhibitors. In one recent retrospective study [56], increased AL was found with the use of mainly non-selective NSAIDs such as diclofenac but not with selective COX-2 inhibitors such as meloxicam and celecoxib.

Large RCTs are needed to resolve the controversy surrounding NSAIDs and AL.

Neostigmine

- Neostigmine increases intraluminal pressure and colonic and rectal motor activity which, in theory, may cause excessive traction on anastomotic suture lines, resulting in leakage.
- However, animal studies do not suggest an increased incidence of AL associated with the use of neostigmine, but clinical evidence for such an effect is lacking.

N_2O

N_2O causes bowel distension. However, there are no reports of increased incidence of AL with its use.

Epidural analgesia

Epidural anesthesia increases intestinal motility and tone by interrupting nociceptive pain afferents and blockade of thoracolumbar sympathetic efferents. This could lead to anastomosis dehiscence. However, epidural analgesia may improve intestinal blood flow directly by mesenteric vasodilation.

- Holte and Kehlet [57] analyzed RCTs and concluded that there was no statistical difference in AL between:
  - epidural analgesia versus systemic opioid
  - epidural opioid versus systemic opioid
  - epidural analgesia – opioid mixture versus systemic opioid
- Thus epidural analgesia does not seem to have harmful effects on intestinal anastomosis and this has been confirmed by a recent large study [58].

Oxygen and surgical site infection (SSI)

SSI is one of the most common causes of hospital-acquired infection in surgical patients. The incidence of wound infection following colorectal surgery varies from 5% to 25% in different studies. Surgical (e.g., open versus laparoscopic, elective versus emergency, technique, duration, blood transfusion, etc.), host (e.g., nutritional immune status, obesity), clinical practice (e.g., administration of antibiotics, temperature, glycemic control, hand hygiene), and environmental (e.g., clean air, local infection control policy) factors may all influence the rate of SSI.

Rationale for perioperative hyperoxia

- Hyperoxia increases the rate of local phagocytosis and decreases systemic inflammatory mediators such as tumor necrosis factor (TNF)-α. Reactive oxygen species (ROS) are critical mediators required for oxidative intracellular killing of micro-organisms by leukocytes and macrophages.
- Wound hypoxia is common in the early postoperative period due to local tissue trauma leading to vasoconstriction, thrombosis and edema, and increased oxygen demand by defensive immune cells and healing tissue. Higher FiO_2 has been demonstrated to increase the pO_2 in subcutaneous tissue and the colon [59].
- The differing effects of moderate hyperoxia (e.g., FiO_2 40%–60%) or higher FiO_2 for long postoperative periods on SSI are not known.

Perioperative studies:

- Most studies have compared 30% with 80% FiO_2 during the intraoperative period and for a brief time in the immediate postoperative period. Both the concentration and duration of oxygen administration studied are arbitrary choices.
- In the first major study to examine this issue, Greif et al. [59] reported a 50% reduction in SSI with the use of 80% FiO_2 in elective colorectal surgical patients.
- Other studies have been performed, which vary in their methodology, exclusion criteria, definition of SSI, type of surgery, duration of surgery, bowel preparation, and fluid and pain management.
- Seven meta-analyses have examined the effectiveness of hyperoxia on SSI, the most recent being published in 2013 [60].
- For colorectal surgery, high FiO_2 reduced the risk of SSI (RR 0.78, CI_{95} 0.6–1.02). They found no increased risk of postoperative atelectasis and a reduction in postoperative nausea and vomiting in patients receiving inhalational anesthesia without prophylactic antiemetics [60].

In summary, hyperoxia may have a modest benefit in reduction of SSI in patients undergoing elective colorectal surgery. It is included in some institutions' "colorectal care bundle" to reduce SSI.

Enhanced recovery protocols

- Major surgical trauma disturbs homeostatic function and may result in organ dysfunction. In addition, several factors exaggerate the stress response or delay the return of normal physiological functions. These include inadequate nutrition, fluid and temperature imbalance, and pain.
- Kehlet and Wilmore [61] suggested that early recovery and hospital discharge could be achieved by adopting a multidisciplinary "bundle of care" protocol to achieve enhanced recovery after surgery (ERAS).
- Much of the focus has been on colorectal surgery.
- Each part of the protocol is potentially beneficial but the best results should be obtained by combining them into an overall package of care.
- The concept of fast-track surgery continues to evolve and is now well established in many countries to accelerate physiological and functional recovery following colorectal surgery.

Aims of the ERAS approach

Enhanced recovery protocols (ERP) incorporate and deliver evidence-based elements of clinical care in an integrated pathway (Figure 24.2). The aims of ERP for colorectal surgery are:

- to maintain or achieve early return of systemic and gastrointestinal functions
- to accomplish stress (e.g., hemodynamic, metabolic, inflammatory, and immune) and pain free surgery
- to rehabilitate patients from associated pathophysiological changes toward independence

Advantages

Length of stay

Length of the stay in hospital has been the primary outcome of many studies evaluating the usefulness of ERPs. Most RCTs and meta-analyses have demonstrated significant reduction of hospital stay by two to three days [62,63], when compared to conventional care after open colorectal surgery. However, there was significant heterogeneity among the RCTs for the effect of ERP on the length of hospital stay.

- In a Cochrane review [64] of four RCTs (119 ERAS patients versus 118 conventional recovery patients) including at least seven items in the ERAS group and no more than two in the conventional arm found that length of stay was significantly reduced in the ERAS group (mean difference, −2.94 d; CI_{95}, −3.69 to −2.19), and readmission rates were equal in both groups. However, the quality of RCTs was low.

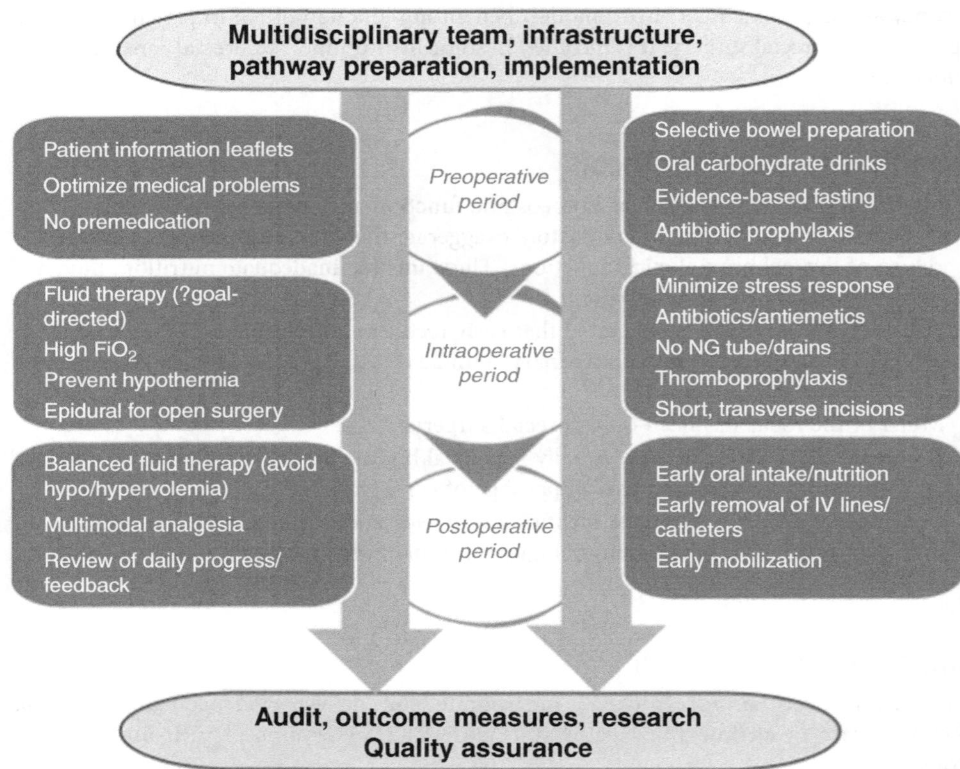

Figure 24.2. Enhanced recovery after surgery pathways.

Furthermore, hospital discharge criteria are not uniform.

- Massen et al. [65] suggested to use functional outcomes (first day tolerance of food, good pain control on oral analgesics, defecation, and independence in activities of daily living to preoperative care level) to judge the success of ERP.

Note: ERP may not reduce length of stay for patients undergoing laparoscopic surgery.

Effect on morbidity

In a meta-analysis of 453 patients (226 in the ERAS group and 226 in the traditional care group) from six RCTs, Vadradan et al. [63] found a 50% reduction in complication rates in the ERAS group after open surgery. However, the method of reporting complications and their severity was not uniform among studies.

Stress response

Ren et al. [66] reported lower insulin resistance, cortisol, and cytokine levels, and negative nitrogen balance and higher albumin in the ERP group compared to standard care. They suggested that lower stress and inflammatory responses and better metabolic and nutritive indices are responsible for the lower morbidity and early recovery with ERP.

Postoperative ileus

- Tolerance of a normal diet and time of first bowel movement were decreased by >1 day in all randomized trials.
- Elements of ERP such as avoidance of nasogastric (NG) tubes, optimal fluid therapy, use of epidural analgesia for open surgery, and emphasis on opiate-free analgesia are beneficial for early GI function recovery.
- Laparoscopic surgery may add advantage to ER protocols in minimizing postoperative paralytic ileus.

Safety

Most studies have found that ERP is safe and does not lead to increased rate of readmissions. It does not increase the rate of either medical or surgical complications. However, there is no difference in mortality compared to standard care.

Implementation

- Multidisciplinary teams, which include surgeons, anesthetists, nursing staff, pain team, physical therapists, and nutrition experts, are essential for implementing ERP. Patient education and counseling is also important. Depending on local structure, managerial or community support may be required.
- Acceptance of protocols, organization of structured perioperative care (e.g., to facilitate nutrition, mobilization, and other nursing care), training and retraining of staff (e.g., new junior doctors and other staff), and monitoring of protocol compliance are important for successful implementation.

ERP components and its compliance, deviation, and failure

Compliance

Comprehensive compliance for all components may not be possible and always practical. Even partial compliance is found to be beneficial but improving compliance results in more benefits.

- Gustafsson et al. [67] studied over 900 patients between 2002 and 2004, and 2005 and 2007. The adherence to ERP was 43% and 74%, respectively. Overall, moving from 50% to 90% compliance with ERP led to improvement in outcomes such as reduced complications, fewer symptoms causing delayed discharge, and shorter length of stay.
- In a systematic review, Ahmed et al. [68] found that compliance of ERP in the postoperative period was the most problematic. This may be due to multiple individuals being involved in care, lack of motivation to accept changes, and unawareness of ERP elements among staff.

Importance of individual components

- Recent guidelines have reviewed the evidence for each component [69].
- The influence of individual components of ERP on outcome is difficult to judge.
- The numbers of components used are variable in studies evaluating ERP and ranged from 4 to 12.
- Preoperative counseling, avoidance of NG tubes, postoperative enforced enteral nutrition, and early mobilization were included in all studies. Preoperative carbohydrate

loading, no mechanical bowel preparation, epidural analgesia, no abdominal drains, and morphine-sparing analgesia were also employed in most of the RCTs.

- Vlug et al. [70] found that two postoperative phase elements (normal diet and enforced mobilization in the first three postoperative days) were independent predictors for early discharge from hospital.

Deviation and failure

- In a retrospective study [71] of 385 patients who underwent laparoscopic colorectal surgery, the compliance rate was 85% for pre- and intraoperative elements; 41% deviated from one or two postoperative elements. In a univariate analysis, delayed discharge (31%) was associated strongly with deviation of all five postoperative elements – continued IV fluids after day 1, lack of functioning epidural analgesia, failure to mobilize on day 1, insertion of the NG tube for vomiting, and reinsertion of the urinary catheter.
- Intraoperative complications and failure to mobilize are important causes of deviation [72]. It has been suggested that failure to mobilize should be considered as a red flag sign following laparoscopic colorectal surgery and should be investigated. Failure to mobilize may occur due to postoperative complications (e.g., gut dysfunction), poor pain relief, or orthostatic hypotension due to various causes.
- ERP can be modified as per local need and if a complication occurs.
- ERP also depends on the individual surgery. For example, rectal surgery/pelvic surgery may require mechanical bowel preparation, stoma formation, longer urinary catheterization, etc.
- ERP may also be influenced by the patient's choice. For example, failure to consent for epidural analgesia.

Therefore, although the principles of ERP are generalized, an individualized approach is desirable.

References

1. Alves A, Panis Y, Mathieu P, et al. Association Française de Chirurgie: Postoperative mortality and morbidity in French patients undergoing colorectal surgery: results of a prospective multicenter study. *Arch Surg* 2005; **140**: 278–83.
2. Ingraham AM, Cohen ME, Bilimoria KY, et al. Comparison of hospital performance in nonemergency versus emergency colorectal operations at 142 hospitals. *J Am Coll Surg* 2010; **210**: 155–65.
3. Sjo OH, Larsen S, Lunde OC, et al. Short term outcome after emergency and elective surgery for colon cancer. *Colorectal Dis* 2009; **11**: 733–9.
4. Cook TM, Woodall N, Frerk C. Major complications of airway management in the UK: results of the 4th National Audit Project of the Royal College of Anaesthetists and the Difficult Airway Society. Part 1: Anaesthesia. *Br J Anaesth* 2011; **106**: 617–31.
5. Keller C, Brimacome J, Bittersohl J, et al. Aspiration and the laryngeal mask airway: three cases and a review of the literature. *Br J Anaesth* 2004; **93**: 579–82.
6. Ng A, Smith G. Gastresophageal reflux and aspiration of gastric contents in anesthetic practice. *Anesth Analg* 2001; **93**: 494–513.
7. Kluger MT, Short TG. Aspiration during anaesthesia: a review of 133 cases from the Australian Anaesthetic Incident Monitoring Study (AIMS). *Anaesthesia* 1999; **54**: 19–26.
8. Warner MA, Warner ME, Weber JG. Clinical significance of pulmonary

aspiration during the perioperative period. *Anesthesiology* 1993; **78**: 56–62.

9. Neilipovitz DT, Crosby ET. No evidence for decreased incidence of aspiration after rapid sequence induction. *Can J Anaesth* 2007; **54**: 748–64.
10. El-Orbany M, Connolly L. Rapid sequence induction and intubation: current controversy. *Anesth Analg* 2010; **110**: 1318–25.
11. Walker RWM, Ravi R, Haylett K. Effect of cricoid force on airway calibre in children: a bronchoscopic assessment. *Br J Anaesth* 2010; **104**: 71–4.
12. Kimberger O, Arnberger M, Brandt S, et al. Goal-directed colloid administration improves the microcirculation of healthy and perianastomotic colon. *Anesthesiology* 2009; **110**: 496–504.
13. Hiltebrand LB, Pestel G, Hager H, et al. Perioperative fluid management: comparison of high, medium and low fluid volume on tissue oxygen pressure in the small bowel and colon. *Eur J Anesthesiol* 2007; **24**: 927–33.
14. Marjanovic G, Villain C, Juettner E, et al. Impact of different crystalloid volume regimes on intestinal anastomotic stability. *Ann Surg* 2009; **249**: 181–5.
15. Prien T, Backhaus N, Pelster F, et al. Effect of intraoperative fluid administration and colloid osmotic pressure on the formation of intestinal edema during gastrointestinal surgery. *J Clin Anesth* 1990; **2**: 317–23.
16. Schnüriger B, Inaba K, Wu T, et al. Crystalloids after primary colon resection and anastomosis at initial trauma laparotomy: excessive volumes are associated with anastomotic leakage. *J Trauma* 2011; **70**: 603–10.
17. Dellinger RP, Levy MM, Rhodes A, et al. Surviving sepsis campaign: international guidelines for management of severe sepsis and septic shock: 2012. *Crit Care Med* 2013; **41**: 580–637.
18. Martin C, Jacob M, Vicaut E, et al. Effect of waxy maize-derived hydroxyethyl starch 130/0.4 on renal function in surgical patients. *Anesthesiology* 2013; **118**: 387–94.
19. Van Der Linden P, James M, Mythen M, et al. Review article: safety of modern starches used during surgery. *Anesth Analg* 2013; **116**: 35–48.
20. Chappell D, Jacob M, Hofmann-Kiefer K, et al. A rational approach to perioperative fluid management. *Anesthesiology* 2008; **109**: 723–40.
21. Rahbari NN, Zimmermann JB, Schmidt T, et al. Meta-analysis of standard, restrictive and supplemental fluid administration in colorectal surgery. *Br J Surg* 2009; **96**: 331–41.
22. Brandstrup B, Tønnesen H, Beier-Holgersen R, et al. Effects of intravenous fluid restriction on postoperative complications: comparison of two perioperative fluid regimens: a randomized assessor-blinded multicentre trial. *Ann Surg* 2003; **238**: 641–8.
23. Futier E, Constantin JM, Petit A, et al. Conservative vs restrictive individualized goal-directed fluid replacement strategy in major abdominal surgery: a prospective randomized trial. *Arch Surg* 2010; **145**: 1193–200.
24. Hubner M, Schafer M, Demartines N, et al. Impact of restrictive intravenous fluid replacement and combined epidural analgesia on perioperative volume balance and renal function within a fast track program. *J Surg Res* 2012; **173**: 68–74.
25. Wenkui Y, Ning L, Jianfeng G, et al. Restricted perioperative fluid administration adjusted by serum lactate level improved outcome after major elective surgery for gastrointestinal malignancy. *Surgery* 2010; **147**: 542–52.
26. Varadhan KK, Lobo DN. A meta-analysis of randomised controlled trials of intravenous fluid therapy in major elective open abdominal surgery: getting the balance right. *Proc Nutr Soc* 2010; **69**: 488–98.
27. Srinivasa S, Taylor MH, Sammour T, et al. Esophageal Doppler-guided fluid administration in colorectal surgery: critical appraisal of published clinical trials. *Acta Anesthesiol Scand* 2011; **55**: 4–13.

28. Corcoran T, Rhodes JE, Clarke S, et al. Perioperative fluid management strategies in major surgery: a stratified meta-analysis. *Anesth Analg* 2012; **114**: 640–51.

29. Concha MR, Mertz VF, Cortinez LI, et al. Pulse contour analysis and transesophageal echocardiography: a comparison of measurements of cardiac output during laparoscopic colon surgery. *Anesth Analg* 2009; **109**: 114–18.

30. Matheson PJ, Wilson MA, Garrison RN. Regulation of intestinal blood flow. *J Surgi Res* 2000; **93**: 182–96.

31. Müller M, Schindler E, Roth S, et al. Effects of desflurane and isoflurane on intestinal tissue oxygen pressure during colorectal surgery. *Anaesthesia* 2002; **57**: 110–15.

32. O'Riordan J, O'Beirne HA, Young Y, et al. Effects of desflurane and isoflurane on splanchnic microcirculation during major surgery. *Brit J Anaesth* 1997; **78**: 95–6.

33. Kim M, Park SW, Kim M, et al. Isoflurane postconditioning protects against intestinal ischemia-reperfusion injury and multi-organ dysfunction via transforming growth factor-beta1 generation. *Ann Surg* 2012; **255**: 492–503.

34. Carmichael FJ, Crawford W, Khayyam N, et al. Effect of propofol infusion on splanchnic hemodynamics and liver oxygen consumption in the rat: a dose-response study. *Anesthesiology* 1993; **79**: 1051–60.

35. Brookes Z, Brown L, Reilly C. Differential effects of intravenous anaesthetic agents on the response of rat mesenteric microcirculation in vivo after haemorrhage. *Brit J Anaesth* 2002; **88**: 255–63.

36. Johansson K, Ahn H, Lindhagen J, et al. Effect of epidural anaesthesia on intestinal blood flow. *Br J Surg* 1988; **75**: 73–6.

37. Gould TH, Grace K, Thome G, et al. Effect of thoracic epidural anaesthesia on colonic blood flow. *Brit J Anaesth* 2002; **89**: 446–51.

38. Reilly PM, Wilkins KB, Fuh KC, et al. The mesenteric hemodynamic response to circulatory shock: an overview. *Shock* 2001; **15**: 329–43.

39. Knotzer H, Pajk W, Maier S, et al. Comparison of lactated Ringer's, gelatine and blood resuscitation on intestinal oxygen supply and mucosal tissue oxygen tension in haemorrhagic shock. *Brit J Anaesth* 2006; **97**: 509–16.

40. Hiltebrand LB, Krejci V, Banic A, et al. Redistribution of microcirculatory blood flow within the intestinal wall during sepsis and general anesthesia. *Anesthesiology* 2003; **98**: 658–69.

41. Olofsson PH, Berg S, Ahn HC, et al. Gastrointestinal microcirculation and cardiopulmonary function during experimentally increased intra-abdominal pressure *Crit Care Med* 2009;, **37**: 230–9.

42. Faisal AM, Abell LM, Chawla LS. Understanding intra-abdominal hypertension from the bench to the bedside. *J Intensive Care Med* 2012; **27**: 145–60.

43. Marcel G, Macfie J, Anderson A, et al. Changes in superior mesenteric artery blood flow after oral, enteral, and parenteral feeding in humans. *Crit Care Med* **37**: 171–6.

44. Boerma EC, Ince C. The role of vasoactive agents in the resuscitation of microvascular perfusion and tissue oxygenation in critically ill patients. *Intensive Care Med* 2010, **36**: 2004–18.

45. Gelman S, Mushlin PS. Catecholamine-induced changes in the splanchnic circulation affecting systemic hemodynamics. *Anesthesiology* 2004; **100**: 434–9.

46. Hiltebrand LB, Koepfli E, Kimberger O, et al. Hypotension during fluid-restricted abdominal surgery: effects of norepinephrine treatment on regional and microcirculatory blood flow in the intestinal tract. *Anesthesiology* 2011; **114**: 557–64.

47. Schwarte LA, Schwartges I, Schober P, et al. Sevoflurane and propofol anesthesia differentially modulate the effects of epinephrine and norepinephrine on microcirculatory gastric mucosal oxygenation. *Br J Anesth* 2010; **105**: 421–8.

48. Kingham TP, Pachter HL. Colonic anastomotic leak: risk factors, diagnosis, and treatment. *J Am Coll Surg* 2009; **208**: 269–78.

49. Bruce J, Krukowski ZH, Al-khairy G, et al. Systematic review of the definition and measurement of anastomotic leak after gastrointestinal surgery. *Br J Surg* 2001; **88**: 1157–68.

50. Sheridan WG, Lowndes RH, Young HL. Tissue oxygen tension as a predictor of colonic anastomotic healing. *Dis Colon Rectum* 1987; **30**: 867–71.

51. Karliczek A, Benaron DA, Baas PC, et al. Intraoperative assessment of microperfusion with visible light spectroscopy for prediction of anastomotic leakage in colorectal anastomoses. *Colorectal Dis* 2010; **10**: 1018–25.

52. Schietroma M, Carlei F, Cecilia E, et al. Colorectal infraperitoneal anastomosis: the effects of perioperative supplemental oxygen administration on the anastomotic dehiscence. *J Gastrointest Surg* 2012; **16**: 427–34.

53. Giglio MT, Marucci M, Testini M, et al. Goal-directed haemodynamic therapy and gastrointestinal complications in major surgery: a metaanalysis of randomized controlled trials. *Br J Anaesth* 2009; **103**: 637–46.

54. Zakrison T, Nascimento BA Jr, Tremblay LN, et al. Perioperative vasopressors are associated with an increased risk of gastrointestinal anastomotic leakage. *World J Surg* 2007; **31**: 1627–34.

55. Klein M, Gogenur I, Rosenberg J. Postoperative use of non-steroidal anti-inflammatory drugs in patients with anastomotic leakage requiring reoperation after colorectal resection: cohort study based on prospective data. *BMJ* 2012; **345**: e6166.

56. Gorissen KJ, Benning D, Berghmans T, et al. Risk of anastomotic leakage with non-steroidal anti-inflammatory drugs in colorectal surgery. *Br J Surg* 2012; **99**: 721–7.

57. Holte K, Kehlet H. Epidural analgesia and risk of anastomotic leakage. *Reg Anesth Pain Med* 2001; **26**: 111–17.

58. Halabi WJ, Jafari MD, Nguven VQ, et al. A nationwide analysis of the use and outcomes of epidural analgesia in open colorectal surgery. *J Gastrointest Surg* 2013; **13**: 1130–7.

59. Greif R, Akca O, Horn EP, et al. Supplemental perioperative oxygen to reduce the incidence of surgical-wound infection. *N Engl J Med.* 2000; **342**: 161–7.

60. Hovaguimian F, Lysakowski C, Elia N, et al. Effect of intraoperative high inspired oxygen fraction on surgical site infection, postoperative nausea and vomiting, and pulmonary function: systematic review and meta-analysis of randomized controlled trials. *Anesthesiology* 2013; **119**: 303–16.

61. Kehlet H, Wilmore DW. Multimodal strategies to improve surgical outcome. *Am J Surg* 2002; **183**: 630–41.

62. Gouvas N, Tan E, Windsor A, et al. Fast-track vs. standard care in colorectal surgery: a meta-analysis update. *Int J Colorectal Dis* 2009; **24**: 1119–31.

63. Varadhan KK, Neal KR, Dejong CH, et al. The enhanced recovery after surgery (ERAS) pathway for patients undergoing major elective open colorectal: a meta-analysis of randomized controlled trials. *Clin Nutr* 2010; **29**: 434–40.

64. Spanjersberg WR, Reurings J, Keus F, et al. Fast track surgery versus conventional recovery strategies for colorectal surgery. *Cochrane Database Syst Rev* 2011; **2**: CD007635.

65. Maessen JMC, Dejong CHC, Kessels AGH, et al. Length of stay: an inappropriate readout of the success of enhanced recovery programs. *World J Surg* 2008; **32**: 971–5.

66. Ren L, Zhu D, Wei Y, et al. Enhanced Recovery After Surgery (ERAS) Program attenuates stress and accelerates recovery in patients after radical resection for colorectal cancer: a prospective randomized controlled trial. *World J Surg* 2012; **36**: 407–14.

67. Gustafsson UO, Hausel J, Thorell A, et al. Adherence to the Enhanced Recovery After Surgery Protocol and outcomes after colorectal cancer surgery. *Arch Surg* 2011; **146**: 571–7.

68. Ahmed J, Khan S, Lim M, et al. Enhanced Recovery after Surgery Protocols: compliance and variations in practice

during routine colorectal surgery. *Colorectal Dis* 2012; **14**: 1045–51.

69. Gustafsson U, Scott MJ, Schwenk W, et al. Guidelines for perioperative care in elective colonic surgery: Enhanced Recovery After Surgery (ERAS) society recommendations. *World J Surg* 2013; **37**: 259–84.

70. Vlug MS, Bartels SA, Wind J, et al. Which fast track elements predict early recovery after colon cancer surgery? *Colorectal Dis* 2012; **14**: 1001–8.

71. Smart NJ, White P, Allison AS, et al. Deviation and failure of enhanced recovery after surgery following laparoscopic colorectal surgery: early prediction model. *Colorectal Dis* 2012; **14**: e727–34.

72. Boulind CE, Yeo M, Burkill C, et al. Factors predicting deviation from an enhanced recovery programme and delayed discharge after laparoscopic colorectal surgery. *Colorectal Dis* 2012; **14**: e103–10.

Chapter 25

Anesthesia and cancer surgery

M. Koutra and A. McLeod

Introduction

Cancer is estimated to be the second leading cause of death in the U.S., and approximately 1.6 million new diagnoses will be made in 2013 [www.cancer.org]. Surgery remains the principal treatment for most solid tumors, and will represent a significant proportion of operations performed in high-risk patients. This chapter focuses on the impact of cancer and cancer treatment on patients undergoing surgery, and how this influences their management. Cancer is a heterogeneous disease affecting all age groups, and patients may be encountered during cancer resections, reconstructions, or as survivors of past malignancy undergoing surgery. Adequate assessment is vital but often time constrained by the risk of tumor progression. Delays for further investigation and optimization should be justified in terms of their likely benefit, and discussed with the multidisciplinary team in advance. Patients may be very motivated to undergo surgery, even if the risks are high. However, these risks must be balanced against the potential benefits of surgery, particularly where other therapies exist.

Assessment and optimization

Cancer is more common in older patients, who are more likely to have associated comorbidities and be unfit. In addition, known risk factors for cancer such as smoking, excess alcohol consumption, and obesity are more likely to be present. The following effects of malignancy or cancer treatment should be considered when assessing patients for surgery, and reasonable steps taken to optimize them before surgery.

Physical effects of tumor mass

- Airway obstruction may occur due to head and neck tumors, lymph node enlargement, and mediastinal masses. Airway compression due to mediastinal masses can be life threatening, yet may only develop under anesthesia. Laryngeal nerve palsy with vocal cord dysfunction may also be present.
- Major vessels such as the superior vena cava (SVC) can be obstructed by tumor masses, such as from lung cancer, and may influence the placement of central venous lines. SVC obstruction may require urgent treatment for the obstructing tumor, usually radiotherapy or, alternatively, endoluminal stenting.

Anesthesia and Perioperative Care of the High-Risk Patient, Third edition, ed. Ian McConachie. Published by Cambridge University Press.

- Abdominal masses can cause bowel dysfunction and obstruction, leading to malnutrition, dehydration, and increased aspiration risk. Supine hypotensive syndrome has been described with massive abdominal tumors.
- Pelvic and retroperitoneal masses may cause ureteric obstruction and renal dysfunction, and preoperative stent or nephrostomy placement may be required to relieve obstruction.
- Pelvic masses may cause bowel obstruction, ureteric obstruction, or neurological symptoms due to nerve compression, and can greatly increase the risk of venous thromboembolic (VTE) disease occurring.
- Spinal cord compression arises from metastatic tumor deposits, and may require urgent treatment. Neuraxial techniques may be contraindicated.

Systemic effects of cancer

Pleural effusions and ascites are common in mesothelioma, ovarian cancer, and metastatic disease. Effusions will often resolve with chemotherapy, but when symptomatic, they should be relieved by drainage accompanied by hemodynamic monitoring, and fluid replacement if indicated. Peripheral edema is also common due to reduced mobility, hypoalbuminemia, or lymphatic obstruction.

Paraneoplastic syndromes can be present in one in 10 cancer patients (especially tumors of the lung, breast, prostate, ovary, and pancreas, as well as lymphoma). Mechanisms are usually hormone overproduction, or autoantibody generation.

- Lambert–Eaton myasthenic syndrome is common in small cell lung cancer (SCLC) and thymus, breast, and gastrointestinal (GI) tract tumors. Patients may be especially sensitive to non-depolarizing muscle relaxants, and other problems include autonomic dysfunction, respiratory complications, and esophageal dysmotility. The syndrome usually resolves with treatment of the malignancy, although steroids and plasma exchange are also used.
- Cushing's syndrome occurs in lung, pancreas, thymus, and ovarian malignancy, via excess secretion of adrenocorticotropic hormone (ACTH). Drugs such as metyrapone or octreotide may be used if the syndrome persists after treatment of the malignancy.
- Hypercalcemia is caused by bony metastases or parathyroid-like compounds, and commonly occurs in tumors of the lung, kidney, pancreas, and head and neck. Usual treatment includes intravenous hydration, and pamidronate.
- Hyponatremia and syndrome of inappropriate antidiuretic hormone (SIADH) may be caused by SCLCs and also lymphoma, leukemia, and carcinoid and pancreatic tumors. Elective surgery should be postponed if serum $[Na^+]$ is <120 mmol/L, or patients are symptomatic. Usual treatment would include fluid restriction, and possibly democlocycline.
- Neurological syndromes mediated by auto-antibodies can produce diverse symptoms including myopathy, peripheral neuropathy, encephalopathy, and cerebellar degeneration. These syndromes may respond poorly to treatment, and may also compromise recovery from surgery.

Blood disorders

Cancer patients frequently are anemic due to blood loss, chronic illness, bone marrow suppression, erythropoietin (EPO) deficiency, and other effects of chemotherapy

Preoperative correction of anemia is important, but may be limited by time constraints or ongoing blood loss. In cancer patients, the following considerations also apply:

- Perioperative transfusion of blood products has been associated with increased cancer recurrence risk. Allogeneic transfusion modulates the immune system, enhances the inflammatory response, and may alter tumor surveillance. A recent meta-analysis confirmed the association of perioperative blood transfusion and colorectal cancer recurrence [1], although this relationship may be confounded by a greater propensity for blood loss and anemia in advanced cancers. Autologous blood transfusion following preoperative self-donation does not appear to decrease cancer recurrence when compared with allogeneic blood transfusion.
- Many cancer patients are iron deficient, due to chronic blood loss or a functional deficiency related to inflammation and chronic disease. Oral iron treatment often has poor patient adherence due to GI side effects, and also has unreliable absorption in patients with GI cancers. Intravenous iron can treat iron deficiency anemia effectively, and also enhances the effects of erythropoiesis stimulating agents (E-SAs). Preoperative iron supplementation has been shown to reduce the need for perioperative blood transfusion and there is increasing interest in its use, but it has yet to be shown to improve overall outcomes from cancer surgery [2].
- EPO and other E-SAs are widely used to treat anemia in patients undergoing chemotherapy, and improve their quality of life. However, data from a recent meta-analysis in colorectal cancer surgery indicated that currently there is insufficient evidence to recommend the perioperative use of EPO [3]. There are also concerns regarding the increased risk of VTE and promotion of tumor development in cancer patients. The U.S. Federal Drug Agency recommends limiting E-SA use for treatment of anemia in advanced cancer. The U.K. National Institute for Health and Clinical Excellence (NICE) has also indicated that E-SAs should only be used in patients with a hemoglobin concentration of $<$80 g/L, or where blood transfusions are inappropriate [4].

Chemotherapy can cause reduced white cell counts and low neutrophil counts in particular, which may render patients at greater risk of poor surgical wound healing and postoperative infections. A neutrophil count below 1×10^9/L is typically a contraindication for all but lifesaving surgery. Granulocyte colony-stimulating factor (G-CSF) is widely used in oncology practice to boost neutrophil levels, and has also been given to non-neutropenic patients undergoing cancer surgery [5]. In neutropenic surgical patients, G-CSF may improve blood counts, but the extent to which this contributes to defenses to infection is uncertain.

Thrombocytopenia is common, usually as a consequence of chemotherapy (discussed later). Sufficient time should be allowed for patients' platelet counts to recover. Conventional guidance would recommend platelet counts to be $>100 \times 10^9$/L before major surgery, but this assumes that platelet function is adequate. Platelet function analyzers or devices such as the thromboelastogram may be of value in establishing the need for platelet transfusion.

Malnutrition and cachexia

Malnutrition is widespread in cancer patients, particularly in GI tract tumors and ovarian malignancy, and causes include poor appetite, bowel dysfunction, or chemotherapy-induced vomiting. Malnutrition may progress to cachexia, which is the catabolic loss of muscle mass and adipose tissue associated with advanced cancer. Mechanisms of cachexia remain incompletely understood, but may be related to tumor metabolism, and inflammatory cytokines such as tumor necrosis factor (TNF)-α and interleukin (IL)-6· [6].

- Weight loss alone may not be a reliable marker of poor nutrition as it can be confounded by ascites accumulation or tumor mass. A number of scoring systems have been developed to assess malnutrition risk, and markers such as hypoalbuminemia (<35 g/L) are also useful indicators.
- Preoperative nutrition strategies should be employed where indicated, and instituted as early as possible. Preoperative nutrition, either enteric or as total parenteral nutrition, has been shown to be of value, although established cachexia responds less well to nutrition and may also indicate that surgery is inappropriate.

Venous thromboembolism

- VTE disease affects at least 15% of cancer patients, and is strongly associated with chemotherapy. Prophylactic measures are mandatory, while patients with current blood clots or recent pulmonary embolus may have an inferior vena cava filter inserted before surgery. Continued postoperative prophylaxis of VTE disease should be routine.

Effects of cancer treatment

Table 25.1 lists the commonly used chemotherapy drugs and their principal side effects. Those most relevant to anesthesia are as follows:

- Cardiotoxicity can be caused directly by some agents, or by the stress of chemotherapy on a compromised heart. Anthracycline-induced cardiac failure may be irreversible and has a mortality >30%, while trastuzamab-induced injury can be reversible. Echocardiography and a cardiology review are required preoperatively, and angiotensin-converting enzyme (ACE) inhibitors give symptomatic benefit.
- Pulmonary toxicity occurs in approxiamtely 10% of patients who receive bleomycin, classically consisting of an acute followed by chronic fibrosing alveolitis. Patients at greatest risk are those over 40 years of age, with poor renal function (GFR <80 mL/min), and those who have received doses exceeding 300 000 IU [7]. Patients exposed to bleomycin continue to be at risk of pulmonary complications following surgery. Avoidance of excessive oxygen exposure is recommended routinely, as oxygen-free radicals are probable mediators, but careful fluid balance, protective ventilation strategies, prompt treatment of chest infections, and treatment of acid reflux are probably also important.
- Renal impairment from chemotherapy occurs with platinum drugs and alkylating agents, and can be exacerbated by dehydration. Renal dysfunction is of particular importance prior to nephrectomy surgery, where the remaining kidney must provide sufficient function to avoid renal failure. Tests of differential function are important to establish this, and liaison with a nephrologist is recommended when postoperative renal insufficiency is likely.
- GI side effects are very common, but vomiting and diarrhea may lead to dehydration, malnutrition, and electrolyte disturbance. Mucositis triggered by chemotherapy or radiotherapy is an intensely painful inflammation of the oropharyngeal mucosa, leading to difficulties in eating and infection. Colitis or bowel perforation may also occur,

Table 25.1. Commonly used chemotherapy drugs and principal side effects

Drug or group	Typical oncology use	Important toxicities (not exhaustive)
Anthracyclines – daunorubicin, doxorubicin, idarubicin	Hodgkin's lymphoma, leukemia, and breast, bladder, stomach, lung, ovary, thyroid cancer	Cardiotoxicity, myocarditis, "hand–foot syndrome," low white cell count
Alkylating agents – cyclophosphamide, ifosfamide	Lymphoma, leukemia, solid tumors	Immunosuppression, hemorrhagic cystitis, left ventricle dysfunction, hyponatremia
Alkylating agents – melphelan	Multiple myeloma, ovarian cancer	Bone marrow suppression, interstitial pneumonitis
Asparaginase	Acute lymphocytic leukemia	Anaphylaxis, posterior reversible encephalopathy syndrome
Bleomycin	Hodgkin's lymphoma, squamous cell cancers, testicular cancer	Pneumonitis, pulmonary fibrosis
Cyproterone	Prostate cancer	Hepatotoxicity
Fluoracil, capecitabine	Colorectal, stomach, pancreas, and breast cancer	Angina, myocardial infarction, neurodegeneration, hyperbilirubinemia
Methotrexate	Acute lymphocytic leukemia, choriocarcinoma	Mucositis, pulmonary fibrosis, hepatitis, immunosuppression, nephrotoxicity
Platinum analogs, e.g., carboplatin, cisplatin oxaliplatin	Lymphoma, sarcoma, and ovarian, testicular, small cell lung cancer	Bone marrow suppression, nephro/oto/neurotoxicity, electrolyte disturbance
Procarbazine	Hodgkin's lymphoma, glioblastoma multiforme	Bone marrow suppression, hypersensitivity rash
Monoclonal antibodies – alemtuzumab (Campath®)	B-cell lymphoma	Chronic lymphocyte suppression
Monoclonal antibodies – bevacizumab (Avastin®)	Colon and non-small cell lung cancer	Bone marrow suppression bleeding, bowel perforation
Monoclonal antibodies – cetuximab (Erbitux®)	Colorectal, squamous cell, and head and neck cancers	Hypersensitivity reactions
Monoclonal antibodies – rituximab (Rituxan®)	Leukemia, lymphoma	Cytokine release syndrome/ anaphylaxis, acute interstitial pneumonitis
Monoclonal antibodies – trastuzumab (Herceptin®)	Breast cancer	Cardiotoxicity, hypersensitivity
Steroids – dexamethasone	Leukemia	Tumorlysis syndrome, Cushing's syndrome diabetes, hypertension

Table 25.1. *(cont.)*

Drug or group	Typical oncology use	Important toxicities (not exhaustive)
Sunitinib	Kidney, pancreatic neuroendocrine, and GIstromal tumors	Low blood counts, especially thrombocytopenia, hypothyroidism, seizures
Tamoxifen	Breast cancer	Venous thromboembolism, endometrial cancer, strokes
Taxanes, e.g., docetaxel, paclitaxel	Breast, prostate, and non-small cell lung cancer	Cardiac conduction defects, peripheral neuropathy, hypersensitivity
Thalidomide	Multiple myeloma	Teratogenicity, peripheral neuropathy
Topoisomerase inhibitors, e.g., irinotecan, topotecan	Colon cancer	Acute cholinergic syndrome
Vinca alkaloids – vincristine, vinblastine	Non-Hodgkin's lymphoma, acute lymphocytic leukemia, nephroblastoma	Hypernatremia, neuropathic ileus, peripheral neuropathy

requiring emergency laparotomy. Hepatic veno-occlusive disease is a progressive obliteration of venous channels in the liver, typically occurring after liver radiotherapy or a bone marrow transplant. Patients usually present with jaundice, ascites, and hepatomegaly or abdominal pain. Fulminant hepatic failure is usually fatal, and in this situation, anesthesia is contraindicated for anything except lifesaving surgery.

- Neurological symptoms such as peripheral neuropathy from paclitaxel and related drugs do not contraindicate neuraxial analgesia or anesthesia, but should be documented before surgery.
- Tumorlysis syndrome can occur when chemotherapy is initiated, typically in lymphoma and leukemias. Mass cell death can lead to renal failure with hyperkalemia, hyperphosphatemia, and hypocalcemia. This syndrome is uncommon in surgical patients, but requires correction of electrolyte imbalance and fluid overload, potentially with hemofiltration, before surgery can occur. The syndrome may be precipitated by dexamethasone, which should be used with great caution in oncology patients.

Radiotherapy

Many patients will have had prior radiotherapy for their current tumor or a separate malignancy. This can cause a progressive fibrotic reaction in the irradiated field, and the following complications should be considered:

- Radiotherapy to the upper airway will cause fibrosis and decreased compliance in the tongue and pharynx, and this effect will progress through time. Prior radiotherapy is a strong predictor of difficult laryngoscopy.

- Radiotherapy to the left chest field (e.g., for lymphoma, breast or lung cancer) may cause cardiac injury, and impaired function.
- Radiotherapy may cause loss of natural tissue plains, leading to difficulties in surgical dissection, and increased blood loss.

Fitness for surgery

Many cancer patients experience fatigue and have impaired physical fitness, while inactivity has been proposed conversely as a risk factor for the development of malignancy. Causes of low fitness include non-cancer comorbidities, the debilitating effects of cancer such as muscle wasting, anemia, and deconditioning through inactivity. Chemotherapy may also induce myocardial or lung injury, and the effects on oxygen utilization within the muscle are possible additional mechanisms [8].

- A number of studies have demonstrated that cardiopulmonary exercise testing (CPET) with measurement of anaerobic threshold and ventilatory equivalent for CO_2 can identify the risk of postoperative complications from cancer surgery more accurately than the use of clinical risk scores or activity assessments [9], although in some operations such as esophagectomy, the relationship is less clear cut [10].
- The detrimental effects of neoadjuvant chemoradiotherapy (NARC) or chemotherapy (NAC) on patients' fitness are increasingly recognized. NAC and NARC reduce physical activity and also objective measures of exercise capacity assessed by CPET, typically by 10%–20% at the end of a course [11]. The cause of this effect is complex and multi-factorial, and further research is required to establish its full effect on perioperative outcomes.
- The benefits of exercise training in cancer patients are receiving increasing interest. Patients report improved physical activity, fatigue, muscular strength, and emotional wellbeing [12]. These findings have led to the idea of physical training as a preoperative intervention to improve surgical outcomes. A recent systematic review concluded that preoperative aerobic exercise training improves at least one measure of fitness and benefits broader quality of life in these patients [13]. However, the response is variable among patients, and it remains to be proven that "prehabilitation" is effective in improving actual clinical outcomes for cancer patients, particularly if surgery must be delayed for training. In addition, there have been concerns that exercise effects could alter rates of angiogenesis or attenuate some of the cytotoxic effects of chemotherapy [8]. On balance, however, it is likely that many cancer patients stand to gain from exercise training, particularly if started early in their treatment pathway.

Risk assessment and decision making

Patients vary greatly as to the level of surgical risk they are prepared to face, but need reliable data to help them decide. Outcome risks can be calculated, for example the POSSUM (Physiological and Operative Severity Score for the Enumeration of Mortality and Morbidity) model can predict postoperative mortality and includes malignancy as one of its fields [14]. Derivative models have been developed for upper GI and colorectal surgery. These models, however, usually require intraoperative parameters such as blood loss and malignant spread to be entered, and therefore are less useful when trying to advise patients of risk prior to surgery. Thirty-day mortality risks may be of limited use for patient decision making however, as they often appear low. Outcomes such as 90-day mortality or one-year disability-free survival are probably more relevant measures to consider when discussing the risks of surgery, particularly if these can be presented alongside the outcomes from chemotherapy, radiotherapy, or palliative treatment.

Intraoperative management issues

Vascular access may be problematic for any of the following reasons:

- Past chemotherapy may have reduced the number of patent peripheral veins.
- Tunneled lines and other access devices may already be *in situ* but are often not ideal for intraoperative use.
- Patients who have had prior axillary lymph node clearances are advised routinely against peripheral lines sited in that arm.
- Cancer patients have a higher likelihood of thrombus or obstruction to their great vessels; ultrasound should be used for assessment and line placement.

Fluid balance may be challenging to manage during major cancer surgery. The following factors indicate the use of invasive arterial and central venous pressure monitoring, together with a monitor of cardiac output and fluid status.

- Fluid loss may be increased by ongoing ascitic production.
- Urine output may not be measurable during surgery to the bladder, or where ureters have been divided.
- Blood loss may be excessive during major resections, due to loss of natural tissue plains, vascularity of the tumor, or invasion of major blood vessels.
- Estimates of blood loss may be confounded by ascitic drainage and serosal fluid loss.
- Cancer patients appear more likely to develop systemic inflammatory response syndrome (SIRS) type phenomena and postoperative sepsis due to cytokine release [15]. This may require additional fluid therapy and vasopressors.

Analgesia

Analgesic needs may be influenced by the following factors in cancer patients:

- Many patients will already be receiving strong opioid analgesics for pain due to tumor expansion, nerve compression, or the side effects of chemotherapy or radiotherapy. Tolerance may develop after one to two weeks, putting patients at risk of increased pain after surgery, or withdrawal phenomena if their basal needs are not continued. Patients should be assessed to establish their total opioid requirement, which generally should be continued perioperatively.
- Pain after surgery may be unpredictable and even diminished due to the relief of tumor pain or nerve compression. Short-acting opioid drugs are usually needed for breakthrough pain, and patient-controlled analgesia devices allow background and breakthrough doses to be adjusted accordingly.
- Regional analgesic and anesthetic techniques are all of potential value in reducing opioid requirements, although the response to epidural or intrathecal opioids may be reduced. Assessment should take note of any pre-existing neurological deficits due to chemotherapy or nerve compression by tumor.
- Other analgesic drugs such as paracetamol and non-steroidal anti-inflammatory drugs are all valuable in the absence of contraindications.

Effects of anesthesia on cancer outcomes

Recent research has raised the question of whether anesthetic technique and other perioperative factors may influence tumor recurrence after surgery [16].

- Tumor metastasis can be triggered by surgery due to seeding of cancer cells into the circulation, lymphatic system, or adjacent cavity.
- Components of the immune system, particularly cytotoxic T-cells and natural killer (NK) cells are believed to play an important role in preventing the progress of cancer and the development of metastases, but their activity is suppressed by surgical stress and pain [17].
- Anesthetic techniques can attenuate the stress response but may also suppress the immune system, and the balance of these two actions may influence the likelihood of cancer recurrence. Some anesthetic agents, and morphine in particular, have been shown to suppress cell-mediated immunity (CMI) [18,19].
- A number of studies have shown reduced cancer recurrence rates associated with the perioperative use of regional anesthetic or analgesic techniques [20], although it is unclear whether it is the analgesic action or the morphine-sparing effect that is responsible. Clinical evidence from human subjects is largely retrospective, and those studies that were randomized prospectively (albeit for a different original purpose) have mostly failed to show similar positive results [21]. At the time of writing, results from two large prospective randomized studies investigating this question are awaited.
- Cancer cells express multiple receptors, such as adrenoreceptors and the opioid-μ3 receptor, while prostaglandin metabolism is important for tumor development. Animal models have shown potentially beneficial roles for COX-2 inhibitors and β-blockers [22].
- Metastases must develop a blood supply to grow beyond 2 mm, mediated by compounds such as vascular endothelial growth factor (VEGF). Levels of VEGF are altered by general anesthesia, and morphine in particular has been shown to be proangiogenic in animal models [23].

Despite the positive results from many animal studies, the mechanisms affecting recurrence in humans undergoing cancer surgery are likely to be complex. Many other perioperative factors may be relevant, such as hypothermia, hypoxia, and blood transfusion [16]. Present evidence suggests that good analgesia, minimizing the stress response, and limiting transfusion are all prion-sensible strategies. If there is an equal choice between two techniques, it would seem rational to choose that which is least likely to suppress CMI. At present, however, the role of interventions such as β-blockade or COX-2 antagonists is promising but speculative.

Intraoperative blood management

Reduction of intraoperative blood loss and transfusion should be natural aims in cancer surgery, but the following issues may arise in trying to achieve this:

- Cell salvage during cancer surgery carries concerns of introducing tumor cells to the systemic circulation, with dissemination of malignancy. Leukodepletion filters may reduce the load of tumor cells returned to the patient, although these cells are often already present in significant numbers in the circulation. In studies of cell salvage in hepatic resection and urological cancer surgery, no increase in metastasis or mortality was seen [24]. Routine use of intraoperative cell salvage has been approved for radical prostatectomy and cystectomy surgery in the U.K. by NICE [25]. Its use could also be justified in some specific instances, such as Jehovah's Witness patients undergoing other major cancer surgery, but this would require specific consent with an acknowledgment of the uncertainties.

- The routine use of irradiated blood during cancer surgery is not recommended. Exceptions are bone marrow transplant recipients, Hodgkin's lymphoma patients, and following certain chemotherapy agents (purine analogs) [26]. Leukodepleted blood has a theoretical advantage of reducing the release of inflammatory mediators, but currently there is no evidence to demonstrate improvement in recovery or cancer outcomes.
- The perioperative use of anti-fibrinolytic agents such as tranexamic acid (TXA) can reduce overall transfusion rates in surgical patients [27]. Concerns regarding thrombotic risk in cancer patients have been raised, however, although TXA has been shown to reduce transfusion during radical prostatectomy without increase in thrombotic complications [28]. Most studies of TXA in surgical patients did not examine this complication specifically, or include cancer patients. Thus on present evidence, anti-fibrinolytic agents should probably be used selectively rather than routinely in cancer patients until their safety is confirmed.

Ethical issues

Cancer patients may present for some operative procedures with an advance directive in place [29]. Where their stipulations conflict with safe anesthetic principles, it is reasonable to request that the directive is modified or suspended perioperatively, and guidance from a number of anesthesia bodies supports this. Surgery represents circumstances that patients may not have considered when they made their directives. The instability of anesthesia is distinct from the natural process of dying, yet many anesthesia techniques or drugs can overlap with resuscitation protocols. Patients should be helped to consider their broader goals as to the outcomes they hope to avoid, and the measures they would and would not accept, hopefully allowing a more pragmatic directive to cover the time of surgery.

References

1. Amato A, Pescatori M. Perioperative blood transfusions for the recurrence of colorectal cancer. *Cochrane Database Syst Rev* 2006; **1**: CD005033.
2. Aapro M, Osterborg A, Gascon P, et al. Prevalence and management of cancer-related anaemia, iron deficiency and the specific role of i.v. iron. *Ann Oncol* 2012; **23**: 1954–62.
3. Devon KM, McLeod RS. Pre and peri-operative erythropoeitin for reducing allogeneic blood transfusions in colorectal cancer surgery. *Cochrane Database Syst Rev* 2009; **1**: CD007148.
4. National Institute for Clinical Excellence. Epoetin alfa, epoetin beta and darbepoetin alfa for cancer treatment-induced anaemia 2008. Available from: http://www.nice.org.uk/nicemedia/live/11990/40744/40744.pdf (Accessed August 19, 2013.)
5. Bauhofer A, Plaul U, Torossian A, et al. Perioperative prophylaxis with granulocyte colony-stimulating factor (G-CSF) in high-risk colorectal cancer patients for an improved recovery: a randomized, controlled trial. *Surgery* 2007; **141**: 501–10.
6. Tisdale MJ. Cancer cachexia. *Curr Opin Gastroenterol* 2010; **26**: 146–51.
7. O'Sullivan JM, Huddart RA, Norman AR, et al. Predicting the risk of bleomycin lung

toxicity in patients with germ-cell tumours. *Ann Oncol* 2003; **14**: 91–6.

8. Jones LW, Eves ND, Haykowsky M, et al. Exercise intolerance in cancer and the role of exercise therapy to reverse dysfunction. *Lancet Oncol* 2009; **10**: 598–605.

9. Hightower CE, Riedel BJ, Feig BW, et al. A pilot study evaluating predictors of postoperative outcomes after major abdominal surgery: physiological capacity compared with the ASA physical status classification system. *Br J Anaesth* 2010; **104**: 465–71.

10. Forshaw MJ, Strauss DC, Davies AR, et al. Is cardiopulmonary exercise testing a useful test before esophagectomy? *Ann Thorac Surg* 2008; **85**: 294–9.

11. West MA, Jack S, Kemp G, et al. *The Effect Of Neoadjuvant Chemoradiotherapy On Fitness In Patients Undergoing Rectal Cancer Surgery–Fit For Surgery?* American Thoracic Society 2012 International Conference. San Francisco, CA: American Thoracic Society, 2012; A6395–A.

12. Adamsen L, Quist M, Andersen C, et al. Effect of a multimodal high intensity exercise intervention in cancer patients undergoing chemotherapy: randomised controlled trial. *BMJ* 2009; **339**: b3410.

13. O'Doherty AF, West M, Jack S, et al. Preoperative aerobic exercise training in elective intra-cavity surgery: a systematic review. *Br J Anaesth* 2013; **110**: 679–89.

14. Copeland GP, Jones D, Walters M. POSSUM: a scoring system for surgical audit. *Br J Surg* 1991; **78**: 355–60.

15. Mokart D, Merlin M, Sannini A, et al. Procalcitonin, interleukin 6 and systemic inflammatory response syndrome (SIRS): early markers of postoperative sepsis after major surgery. *Br J Anaesth* 2005; **94**: 767–73.

16. Gottschalk A, Sharma S, Ford J, et al. Review article: the role of the perioperative period in recurrence after cancer surgery. *Anesth Analg* 2010; **110**: 1636–43.

17. Ben-Eliyahu S, Page GG, Yirmiya R, et al. Evidence that stress and surgical interventions promote tumor development by suppressing natural killer cell activity. *Int J Cancer* 1999; **80**: 880–8.

18. Melamed R, Bar-Yosef S, Shakhar G, et al. Suppression of natural killer cell activity and promotion of tumor metastasis by ketamine, thiopental, and halothane, but not by propofol: mediating mechanisms and prophylactic measures. *Anesth Analg* 2003; **97**: 1331–9.

19. Afsharimani B, Cabot PJ, Parat MO. Morphine use in cancer surgery. *Front Pharmacol* 2011; **2**: 46.

20. Exadaktylos AK, Buggy DJ, Moriarty DC, et al. Can anesthetic technique for primary breast cancer surgery affect recurrence or metastasis? *Anesthesiology* 2006; **105**: 660–4.

21. Myles PS, Peyton P, Silbert B, et al. Perioperative epidural analgesia for major abdominal surgery for cancer and recurrence-free survival: randomised trial. *BMJ* 2011; **342**: d1491.

22. Glasner A, Avraham R, Rosenne E, et al. Improving survival rates in two models of spontaneous postoperative metastasis in mice by combined administration of a beta-adrenergic antagonist and a cyclooxygenase-2 inhibitor. *J Immunol* 2010; **184**: 2449–57.

23. Gupta K, Kshirsagar S, Chang L, et al. Morphine stimulates angiogenesis by activating proangiogenic and survival-promoting signaling and promotes breast tumor growth. *Cancer Res* 2002; **62**: 4491–8.

24. Esper SA, Waters JH. Intra-operative cell salvage: a fresh look at the indications and contraindications. *Blood Transfus* 2011; **9**: 139–47.

25. National Insitute for Clinical Excellence. Intraoperative red blood cell salvage during radical prostatectomy or radical cystectomy, 2008. Available from: http://www.nice.org.uk/nicemedia/live/11891/40380/40380.pdf (Accessed August 19, 2013.)

26. Treleaven J, Gennery A, Marsh J, et al. Guidelines on the use of irradiated blood components prepared by the British Committee for Standards in Haematology

blood transfusion task force. *Br J Haematol* 2011; **152**: 35–51.

27. Ker K, Edwards E, Perel P, et al. Effect of tranexamic acid on surgical bleeding: systematic review and cumulative meta-analysis. *BMJ* 2012; **344**: e3054.

28. Crescenti A, Borghi G, Bignami E, et al. Intraoperative use of tranexamic acid to reduce transfusion rate in patients undergoing radical retropubic prostatectomy: double blind, randomised, placebo controlled trial. *BMJ* 2011; **343**: d5701.

29. McBrien ME, Heyburn G. 'Do not attempt resuscitation' orders in the peri-operative period. *Anaesthesia* 2006; **61**: 625–7.

Chapter 26

Neurotrauma and other high-risk neurosurgical cases

P. Cowie and P.J.D. Andrews

In this chapter we will describe the challenges of managing a patient after traumatic brain injury. Many of the anesthetic principles central to the care of patients following neurotrauma can be applied to all acute brain injury syndromes and other neurosurgical cases. These include invasive monitoring for the prevention or management of secondary insults.

Traumatic brain injury

Key points

- Traumatic brain injury (TBI) is a commonly encountered problem.
- Patients who have suffered TBI often require induction of anesthesia, endotracheal intubation, and transfer.
- Operative management includes hematoma evacuation and other decompressive surgery.
- Many principles of TBI anesthetic care can be applied to other high-risk neurological cases.

Epidemiology [1,2]

- TBI is the leading cause of mortality and morbidity worldwide in people under 45 years of age [3].
- Approximately two million episodes occur annually in the U.S., mostly mild or moderate, with 75 000 deaths per year.

Risk factors for TBI

- age
  - youth (take risks)
  - older adults (age-related degeneration and falls)
- gender: males more than females
- alcohol or drug use
- motor vehicle collisions

Anesthesia and Perioperative Care of the High-Risk Patient, Third edition, ed. Ian McConachie. Published by Cambridge University Press.

Classification

- Common approaches involve the Glasgow Coma Scale (GCS), mechanism of injury, and radiological information.
- The heterogeneity of TBI is considered one of the principal barriers to finding effective therapeutic interventions.
- The GCS is the primary criterion for classification of TBI in clinical trials.
- Using GCS, TBI can be classified into mild (≥13), moderate (9–12), and severe (≤8, with no eye opening).
- While the GCS is extremely useful in the clinical management and prognosis of TBI, it does not provide specific information about the pathophysiological mechanisms.

Neurotrauma can also be classified according to the mechanism of injury:

- Concussion – movement of brain tissue with changes in electrical activity; can occur with relatively minor trauma.
- Contusion – hemorrhage into brain tissue due to disruption of small blood vessels; usually associated with increased force.
- Diffuse axonal injury (DAI) – characterized by white matter changes with axonal separation, although appearances on computed tomography (CT) imaging vary; is due to shearing forces, typically acceleration or deceleration, or rotational forces.
- Extra-axial bleeding (either a subdural or extradural hematoma); usually follows blunt trauma.
- Penetrating injury – usually is contusion-like, at high or low speed.

Normal neurophysiology

It is important to understand neurophysiology when dealing with neurotrauma or other neurosurgical conditions.

- Intracranial pressure (ICP) is normally between 5 and 12 mmHg, although it can decrease to subatmospheric levels on standing.

  Cerebral perfusion pressure (CPP) is the driving pressure for blood flow to the brain; it is equal to: mean arterial pressure (MAP) minus ICP plus venous pressure at jugular bulb (normally equal to 0).

$$CPP = MAP - ICP (+VP)$$

- Normally cerebral blood flow (CBF) remains fairly constant over a range of blood pressures, at ~50 mL/100 g tissue/min – “pressure autoregulation.”
- Some individuals, such as those with hypertension, will require higher MAPs to maintain normal CBF, making it even more important to avoid hypotension.

Regulation of CBF [4]

- There is an almost linear relationship between arterial carbon dioxide tension (pCO_2) and CBF. An acute pCO_2 increase causes free hydrogen ions to diffuse freely across the blood–brain barrier and decrease the pH of the cerebrospinal fluid (CSF). This is thought to have a direct effect on arterial and arteriolar smooth muscle, causing cerebral vasodilation.

- Only significant hypoxemia, partial pressures of less than 50 mmHg, cause an increase in CBF. Further decreases in arterial oxygen content cause marked increases in cerebral blood flow and volume.
- Neurogenic regulation: sympathetic neurons (responsive to norepinephrine and serotonin) cause vasoconstriction, helping prevent damage of cerebral tissue during times of stress [5].

These factors regulate global CBF, but blood flow varies throughout the brain:

- White matter receives much less flow than gray matter. More blood is directed toward areas of greater neurological activity, so-called "flow-metabolism coupling." The mechanisms for these variations are not completely understood, but it is thought that increases in products of aerobic metabolism (H^+, K^+, and adenosine diphosphate [ADP]) are central.
- As elsewhere in the body, CBF is influenced by viscosity. A hematocrit of approximately 30% allows a balance between flow and oxygen-carrying capacity [5].

Pathophysiology

TBI can be categorized into the *primary* injury occurring at the time of impact and *secondary* injury processes that follow.

- The secondary process involves inflammation, free radical release, heterogeneity of CBF, excess intracellular calcium, and mitochondrial dysfunction. Release of the neurotransmitter glutamate may also be implicated.
- The blood–brain barrier suffers direct traumatic disruption then secondary dysfunction.
- These changes all contribute to edema and cell death.
- Importantly, there remains no treatment that is able to prevent the secondary cascade of physiological events that leads to neuronal cell death, resulting in poorer functional recovery.

The goal for physicians is to prevent further insults, which worsen the secondary injury. These include hypoxemia, hypotension, raised ICP, and possibly raised core temperature.

Immediate resuscitation

A structured "ABC" approach is required:

A = airway

- If there is any doubt over the airway or the patient's ability to either oxygenate or control pCO_2, intubation is a priority.
- We recommend using a reinforced endotracheal tube for all neurosurgery, given the surgical requirement for head positioning, including the prone position.
- However, postoperative critical care admission may influence this choice and this decision needs to be made on an individual basis.
- Endotracheal tubes should be taped securely in place and not tied, to reduce potential occlusion of venous drainage of the neck.

B = breathing

It is important to maintain adequate oxygenation and close control of pCO_2.

- There is clear evidence to show that episodes of hypoxia – oxygen saturations of <90% – lead to a worse outcome [6]. There is also some evidence to suggest hyperoxia may be harmful.
- If mechanically ventilated, a normal pCO_2 (33–35 mmHg) should be the goal, and mandates regular arterial blood gas sampling.
- Hyperventilation (causing hypocapnia and subsequent cerebral vasoconstriction) should be avoided unless to manage acute herniation syndromes.

C = circulation and CPP

- It is difficult to predict CBF, whether trauma, tumor, or ischemia is the pathology.
- An initial decrease in flow is often followed by a reactive hyperemia. These periods of hypo- and hyperperfusion vary in time and extent. Both can be damaging, hypoperfusion leading to ischemia and hyperperfusion contributing to edema and increased ICP. As previously mentioned, autoregulation is effected by both the initial injury and the secondary inflammatory cascade.
- Evidence-based guidelines recommend avoiding a CPP of <50 mmHg [6].
- Most TBI patients who proceed to the operating room emergently will not have monitoring of their ICP; in these cases, guidance from CT imaging may aid the anesthetist or neurosurgeon in deducing whether there is a significant rise in the ICP.

Raised intracranial pressure

- Treatment should take place when ICP is >20 mmHg [2,7].
- This level has been determined from observational studies, which have shown a worse outcome with ICPs of >20 mmHg [8].
- Limited evidence supports the use of hypertonic sodium chloride to reduce ICP, rather than mannitol or barbiturate treatment.
- These treatments should only be used once ICP monitoring has been established, unless there is progressive decline or signs of herniation.
- ICP monitoring is recommended for those with a GCS of <8 and when a reliable neurological examination is not possible, for instance, prolonged anesthesia or sedation in critical care.
- ICP monitoring should be considered for patients with TBI and a normal CT scan, if associated with significant hypotension, or older than 40 years of age, or if the mechanism increases the possibility of DAI.
- A Cochrane systematic review of steroids showed no evidence for their use after TBI, but an increase in harmful events [9].
- Therapeutic hypothermia in neurotrauma is not supported by trial data, and currently, should not be used outside a clinical trial [10,11].
- Current practice is maintenance of normothermia and active treatment of increased core temperature, using physical and pharmacological methods.
- There is evidence for use of antiepileptic medication to prevent early seizures, although there is no evidence that this decreases long-term seizure rate or mortality [12].

- Many potential neuroprotective agents have been tested; however, none have been shown to be effective [8].

Clinical signs

- Reduced conscious level is the main clinical sign.
- Any decrease in GCS of 2 points, or 1 motor point, is significant.

There are syndromes associated with particular anatomical changes that the anesthetist should be aware of. As ICP rises, brain tissue is distorted and can cause herniation and vascular distortion. In these situations, typical clinical findings can occur [13,14].

Subfalcine (or cingulate) herniation

- A mass pushes the cingulate gyrus under the edge of the falx cerebri. The ipsilateral frontal horn is usually displaced and the anterior cerebral artery may be compressed against the edge of the falx.
- CT scanning shows dilation of the contralateral ventricle secondary to occlusion of the foramen of Munro.
- Can present with leg weakness following occlusion of the anterior cerebral arteries.
- May progress to other types of herniation.

Transtentorial (or uncal) herniation

- Occurs with middle fossa lesions, such as temporal tumors or acute extra- or subdural hematomas.
- The uncus of the temporal lobe herniates round the tentorial edge and compresses the rostral brainstem, the cerebral peduncle.
- Causes contralateral hemiplegia and ipsilateral third cranial nerve compression with mydriasis or partial ptosis or a "down-and-out" pupil.
- Can affect the ascending reticular activating system, reducing conscious level.
- Occasionally, uncal herniation can cause compression of the incisura of the contralateral tentorium, which will lead to ipsilateral hemiplegia.
- Compression of the posterior cerebral artery can cause unilateral or bilateral occipital infarction.

Central herniation

- Large lesions can cause a pressure cone that forces the brainstem downward, causing stretching of small vessels of the brainstem with associated appearance on CT imaging.
- Signs and symptoms are not pathognomic but may include Cushing's triad (hypertension, respiratory abnormalities, and bradycardia), decreased conscious level, or miosis.

Cerebellar tonsillar herniation

- Posterior fossa masses (or lumbar puncture in the presence of raised ICP) can push the cerebellum through the foramen magnum.
- This presses on the medulla and causes respiratory changes (Cheyne–Stoke breathing) or Cushing's triad, wide pulse pressure, impaired consciousness, and death.

Anesthesia

The goal of anesthesia is to prevent secondary injury by:

- minimizing increases in ICP during induction and maintenance of anesthesia – by achieving rapid and smooth induction
- maintaining an adequate CPP of ≥60 mmHg
- preservation of cerebral autoregulation
- rapid and predictable emergence to facilitate clinical examination (where appropriate)

Anesthetic agents

Inhalational agents

- Sevoflurane probably has the least effect on cerebral autoregulation, especially at concentrations <1.0 minimum alveolar concentration (MAC).
- The other inhalational agents are thought to cause more uncoupling; however, all volatile agents affect cerebral autoregulation, particularly at concentrations of >1.0 MAC.

Intravenous agents

- Propofol exhibits a desired reduction in cerebral metabolic rate and oxygen consumption.
- Propofol is thought to be neuroprotective; however, there is limited evidence of clinical benefit [15].
- Propofol's almost ubiquitous use makes future research challenging.
- Thiopentone (thiopental) is often used for rapid induction, but as the trend for barbiturate-induced coma has decreased, its use has declined.
- Etomidate has the benefit of relative cardiovascular stability for induction, but suppresses adrenal cortical function.
- For maintenance of anesthesia, propofol is probably the safest and most widely used intravenous agent.
- The addition of an opioid infusion can decrease the amount of anesthetic agent required, reducing the adverse effects on cerebral autoregulation.
- Remifentanil is used extensively for its quick onset and easy titration.
- An opioid infusion can also decrease the likelihood of coughing or straining with associated rises in ICP. It is becoming increasingly common to run a low concentration of remifentanil (0.02–0.05 μg/kg/min) to smooth the extubation process.

Neuromuscular blocking drugs

- Some choose to run neuromuscular blocking drugs as an infusion; this requires careful monitoring of neuromuscular function and reversal prior to waking.
- The use of suxamethonium (succinylcholine) as part of a rapid sequence induction continues to be contentious.
- Suxamethonium does cause a transient rise in ICP but provides quick reliable intubating conditions, reducing the risk of hypoxia.

- There is no strong evidence to argue either for or against its use. Other side effects include a release of intracellular potassium. This can be striking, with occasional serious side effects such as arrhythmias, especially in patients after spinal cord injury.
- The increasing use of rocuronium, with its potential reversal with sugammadex, provides a viable alternative method to afford prompt muscle relaxation.

Practical conduct of anesthesia

It is imperative that an anesthetist uses a technique that is familiar, but that can be varied as dictated by the clinical scenario.

- We recommend using a propofol bolus (adjusted to the patient's American Society of Anesthesiologists [ASA] score) with remifentanil infusion (approximately 1 μg/kg body weight) and rocuronium (0.6 mg/kg or 0.9 mg/kg for RSI) prior to intubation.
- For maintenance, use sevoflurane, keeping end tidal concentration below 1.0 MAC, and adjusting the remifentanil infusion rate for surgical stimulation.

Positioning, fluids, and positive end expiratory pressure (PEEP)

- Positioning of the patient in theater is determined by the procedure.
- Whatever the surgery, ensure all pressure points are protected and there is no risk of nerve injury.
- The eyes should be protected; it is essential there is no external pressure on the globe.
- Careful positioning of the head and neck, as with taping of an endotracheal tube, can reduce the risk of venous congestion, with increases in ICP and bleeding.
- The neurotrauma patient should be kept euvolemic with the use of isotonic crystalloid.
- We support the replacement of fluid losses, but judicious use of fluid resuscitation plus vasoactive drugs, if required, should be used to maintain MAP and CPP, as opposed to large volumes of fluids [6].
- Ideally, preoperative hemoglobin should be >12 g/dL. Intraoperatively, hemoglobin should be maintained at or above 9 g/dL [16]. These are higher than the levels most anesthetists would accept in critically ill patients, but are used to reduce the risk of secondary injury and its final common pathway – ischemia.
- The use of PEEP in neurosurgical patients is controversial. Some anesthetists avoid PEEP to minimize increasing intrathoracic pressure, and consequently, cerebral blood volume [17].
- However, given the potential for on-going mechanical ventilation or a long period of rehabilitation, PEEP may reduce atelectasis and promote better respiratory function.
- Studies show that low levels of PEEP do not affect ICP.
- If ventilatory requirements demand higher PEEP, such as the lung protective strategies in acute respiratory distress syndrome (ARDS), then pressure levels and their effect on ICP have to be determined on an individual basis.

Operative procedures

Evacuation of an extradural hematoma (EDH)

- Usually due to arterial bleeding and often from injury to the middle meningeal artery.
- Requires urgent evacuation, particularly in the presence of pupillary changes, and is time sensitive (<4 h).

- Almost always associated with skull fractures, except in children.
- EDH evacuation requires a craniotomy.

Evacuation of a subdural hematoma (SDH)

- Typically bleeding from bridging veins between the dura and cortex.
- May be acute or chronic.
- Early evacuation is associated with an improved clinical outcome.
- Chronic bleeds are more frequent in the elderly population; they may come on slowly and often recur.

Decompressive craniectomy

- Decompressive craniectomy tends to be reserved for the most serious cases of raised ICP and is often used as a "rescue therapy" when other treatments fail.
- It is unclear whether decompressive craniectomy improves the functional outcome in patients with severe TBI and refractory raised ICP.
- A recent large multicenter trial found craniectomy reduces ICP but was associated with worse outcomes; there has been some conjecture over this trial, which had strict exclusion criteria [18]. On-going trials may give further information.

Outcome

Outcome following severe TBI can be divided into five categories from the Glasgow Outcome Scale [13].

Good recovery	25%–30%
Moderate recovery	15%–20%
Severe disability	15%
Vegetative state	5%
Death	30%–35%

The following are independent variables for a worse prognosis:

- increasing age
- decreasing GCS, especially motor component
- abnormal pupillary responses – bilateral absent reflexes
- traumatic subarachnoid hemorrhage (SAH)

Transfer [19]

- Many TBI patients present to centers without specialist neurosurgical services.
- These patients require initial assessment (as described) and resuscitation prior to transfer to a neurosurgical unit. The majority of cases require endotracheal intubation prior to transfer.
- The cervical spine should be imaged and immobilized for transfer if stability is uncertain.

- The transfer team should include a doctor with airway skills and a trained assistant.
- The transferring team is responsible for checking that adequate equipment, monitoring, and drugs are available.
- During transfer, and hemodynamic and clinical monitoring of the patient should continue. CPP should be maintained at >60 mmHg.
- We recommend using propofol and opioid infusions with neuromuscular blockade.

These principles can be used for intra-hospital transfers to theater, scanning, or intensive care.

Unstable cervical spine

Key points

- Cervical spine injury is commonly associated with other trauma
- Airway maintenance is paramount, but ensure there is no contributory damage to the spinal cord
- Cervical spine injury can be complicated by respiratory failure, neurogenic shock, or later autonomic hyperreflexia

Epidemiology [20][21]

- There are approximately 10 000 cases of acute spinal cord injury in the U.S. every year.
- These are often associated with other severe trauma with or without TBI.
- Risk factors are similar to those for TBI.

Patterns of injury

- Hyperflexion: due to a blow to the back of the head or deceleration; often stable with no neurological damage.
- Hyperflexion–rotation: disruption of posterior ligamentous complex; may cause cervical root injury, usually without spinal cord damage.
- Axial loading (vertical compression): causes loss of vertebral body height with disruption of the vertebral body; it may displace posteriorly causing cord damage although the spine remains relatively stable.
- Hyperextension: due to applied force to the front of the head or severe whiplash injury; more common than flexion injuries; often associated with cord injury (for example, a "hangman's fracture," fracture of both pedicles, or pars interarticularis of C2, the axis).
- Hyperextension–rotation: a very unstable combination, associated with a high incidence of cord damage.
- Lateral flexion: often associated with flexion or extension injuries.

Pathophysiology of injury

- Primary injury causes microscopic hemorrhages in gray matter and edema of white matter of the cord. The microcirculation is impaired by edema and hemorrhage, further compromised by vasospasm.

- Necrosis of gray and white matter occurs. Function of nerves through the injured area is lost.
- Acceleration and deceleration, as occurs in motor vehicle accidents and falls, is the most common mechanism of abnormal spinal column movements.
- Other causes include penetration by bullets or foreign objects.

Instability

Instability can be defined as "the loss of ability of the cervical spine under physiological loads to maintain relationships between the vertebrae in such a way that spinal cord or nerve roots are not damaged or irritated and deformity or pain does not occur" [22].

The spine consists of three columns:

- anterior: consisting the anterior longitudinal ligament and the anterior half of the vertebral body
- middle: comprising the posterior half of the vertebral body, disk, annulus, and the posterior longitudinal ligament
- posterior: made up of the facet joints, their ligaments, and the ligamentum flavum.

Loss of any of these columns can cause instability.

- The most commonly affected regions are cervical (C1, C2, and C4–C6) and thoracolumbar junction (T11–L2).
- Cervical spine instability may also be caused or exacerbated by chronic conditions – rheumatoid arthritis, ankylosing spondylitis, infection, tumors, or congenital conditions such as Klippell–Feil or Down's syndrome.

Assessment of level of injury

Manifestations of injury at the cervical level:

- paralysis or weakness of all limbs
- respiratory distress
- pulse <60 bpm; blood pressure <80 mmHg
- decreased peristalsis

Manifestations of injury at the thoracic or lumbar level:

- flaccid paralysis or weakness of legs
- spinal shock
- loss of skin sensation
- areflexia
- absent bowel sounds
- bladder distention
- loss of cremasteric reflex in males

The American Spinal Injury Association (ASIA) impairment scale, based on clinical examination of sensory and motor function, is widely used by neurosurgeons to aid assessment [23] (Figure 26.1).

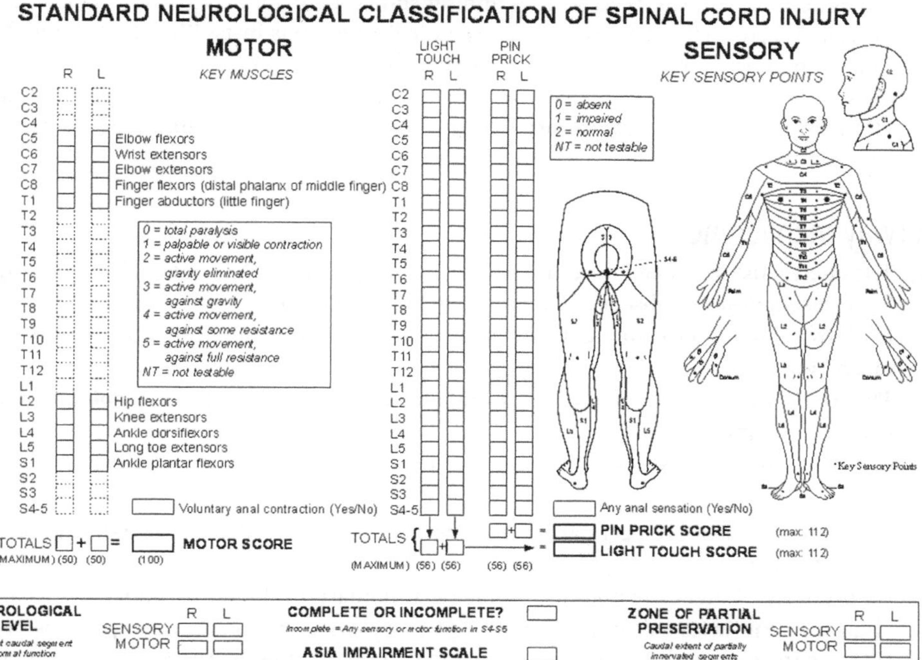

Figure 26.1. ASIA Impairment Scale.

Management

- All patients with major trauma should be considered to have a potential cervical spine injury unless proven otherwise.
- Care must start at the scene of injury to reduce injury and preserve function.
- It involves rapid assessment of ABC (airway, breathing, circulation). Immobilize and stabilize the head and neck, use a cervical collar before moving the patient onto the backboard.
- Take care with all transfers not to aggravate the original injury.
- Injuries at C1–C4 may result in respiratory paralysis but advances in trauma care allow patients to survive with ventilator assistance.
- Address other injuries that necessitate immediate care.

Clearing the cervical spine

- The cervical spine of awake and alert patients may be cleared by a history of a low-risk mechanism and a normal physical examination (using the Nexus criteria or Canadian cervical spine rule).

  Given the probability of head injury or other significant trauma, this is not always possible.

- For these patients, a multi-slice CT scan should be performed; this is most practical at the same time as a CT head scan. Scanning should be from occiput to T1 and allow sagittal and coronal reconstruction to exclude ligamentous instability. This should be as soon as practically possible, and is advisable within 72 hours.
- CT scanning has a very high sensitivity, therefore, unless there is a very strong suspicion of injury, a normal scan can be used to clear the cervical spine to minimize the potential complications from prolonged immobilization.

Airway management

- The anesthetist may need to secure an airway in a patient with an unstable cervical spine for resuscitation or subsequent surgery, including on other trauma injuries.
- It is advisable to perform a detailed assessment of the neurological deficit before intubation, if practical.
- The basic principle is to maintain a patent airway while minimizing any potential risk to the cervical spine.
- Every patient with a suspected cervical injury should be considered a potential difficult airway case [24], due to:
  - inability to achieve optimal positioning because of in-line manual stabilization or a collar
  - presence of blood, secretions, or edema secondary to the initial injury
- High spinal injuries cause significant respiratory dysfunction and these patients need airway control to maintain oxygenation and carbon dioxide clearance, even if there is no urgent operative intervention.
- Development of extra-junctional acetylcholine receptors results in the potential for significant hyperkalemia when using suxamethonium. It should not be used later than 72 hours after the injury.

The main choice for the anesthetist is between awake fiberoptic intubation (FOI) and intubation by direct laryngoscopy with in-line manual stabilization.

Awake FOI

Awake FOI should only be attempted by an experienced practitioner and is not advisable in situations where a patient cannot be cooperative (for example – intoxication or head injury).

- Careful use of sedation and appropriate use of local anesthetics can smooth the process and minimize any sympathetic response.
- An acceptable dose of lignocaine (lidocaine) is as high as 9 mg/kg, given the small amount of systemic absorption.
- This may be combined with cautious use of sedation, such as a remifentanil infusion.
- Awake FOI allows the anesthetist to assess neurology after intubation and prior to surgery.

Direct laryngoscopy

- Direct laryngoscopy should use a minimum amount of force.
- Many advocate the use of bougies to minimize the force required. Some studies have suggested no significant increase in complications, hypoxia, or time to intubation with bougie use [25].

- Video laryngoscopes may improve the view at laryngoscopy. They may require less force to obtain the view, although they should only be used by those experienced in its practice in this situation.
- There is still controversy regarding the role of video laryngoscopes in patients with cervical spine injury, with some studies suggesting that these devices do not reduce spine movement compared to conventional laryngoscopy. A fuller discussion of this topic may be found elsewhere [26].
- The use of cricoid pressure to minimize passive regurgitation of gastric contents may be necessary in unfasted patients but it may worsen intubating conditions and may possibly worsen cervical spine instability. Suction should be readily accessible.
- We recommend in-line manual stabilization, keeping in place the posterior part of the collar to reduce risk of movement.

Conduct of anesthesia

- While airway management is crucial, the anesthetist has to maintain a perfusion pressure to the damaged cord.
- Given the possibility of altered hemodynamics, we aim for a MAP of at least 80 mmHg. Invasive arterial blood pressure monitoring is mandatory for any spinal cord injury. As with other neurosurgical cases, large fluctuations in pressure are probably worse than a single brief episode.
- Ventilation should maintain pCO_2 within the normal range (33–35 mmHg).
- Large bore intravenous (IV) access is required, given the possibility of significant blood loss and central venous access to facilitate vasopressor infusion to manage spinal shock. Serial serum lactates can assess progression of shock.
- Careful intraoperative positioning can improve surgical access and decreases the risk of venous congestion, such as from compression of the inferior vena cava.
- Spinal surgery is high-risk for damage to vulnerable pressure areas, particularly the eyes. It is critical that the eyes are well protected with no external pressure.
- A review of those with visual loss following surgery found that obesity, male gender, Wilson frame use, increased duration, and greater blood loss were all risk factors [27]. We advocate the use of a skull fixation device to reduce morbidity.
- Analgesic requirements will depend on the nature of surgery – some patients will have lost sensation below the level of injury. When sensation remains, operations may be particularly painful due to the dissection of spinal muscles.
- All patients will need to go to a high-dependency area postoperatively.
- The level of injury may necessitate returning the patient to an intensive care unit prior to "waking up." Determining whether to extubate a patient will be a "case-by-case" decision.
- Doubt over the patient's ability to breathe adequately, prolonged extensive surgery, or significant blood loss increase the probability of postoperative ventilation. As an approximate guide, a vital capacity while intubated of >20 mg/kg would support early extubation.

Special situations

Neurogenic shock

- Cervical spinal injury, particularly transection, can cause profound cardiovascular instability.
- The loss of sympathetic vasoconstriction results in venous pooling of blood, while absence of sympathetic cardiac input prevents a compensatory tachycardia.
- Careful fluid resuscitation and early introduction of vasopressors can help counter hypotension.
- Invasive monitoring is mandatory and should include central venous cannulation.

Autonomic hyperreflexia

- In the weeks following a high spinal injury (above T6), stimulation of the autonomic nervous system can lead to profound systemic symptoms, including hypertension, tachycardia, flushing, sweating, and headaches.
- A stimulus, often from the bladder or bowel, causes nerve conduction up the spinal cord until terminated by the level of injury.
- A reflex is activated that increases activity of the sympathetic portion of the autonomic nervous system.
- This results in spasms and vasoconstriction, which causes a rise in the blood pressure. This is detected by the brain, which due to the injury, cannot respond.
- For these patients, spinal anesthesia may be useful although technically difficult.
- Otherwise, deep general anesthesia reduces the risk of complications.

Other spinal surgery

- Common surgical procedures involve decompression of the spinal cord, correction of spinal deformity, excision of spinal tumors, and trauma.
- Many of the general principles can be derived from cervical spinal surgery – use of reinforced tube, careful fluid balance, avoiding coughing, maintenance of normothermia, and particular attention to preventing pressure on vulnerable areas.
- Most patients will be prone and should be facilitated using a special spinal mattress or surgical frame.
- Turning should avoid twisting of the spine. If there is any risk of neurological damage, we advise formal log-rolling.
- Ensure there is no external pressure on the abdomen to allow ventilation and reduce venous compression, which can contribute to increased bleeding.
- Can be associated with significant blood loss especially those with large dissections, such as scoliosis surgery/tumors/pedicle screw insertion.
- Intraoperative assessment of neurology may be required; most commonly, somatosensory and motor evoked potentials are used.
- Neurophysiologists find a TIVA technique gives better electromyographic (EMG) recordings, but we feel that this should only be used if the anesthetist is comfortable with the technique and there are no other reasons for using volatile anesthesia. With any use of TIVA, we recommend using depth of anesthesia monitoring.
- Venous air embolism is a potential complication.
- Operations can be very painful especially if there is extensive muscle dissection.

Decompression of spinal cord

- Cauda equina syndrome is an indication for urgent intervention, within hours of symptom onset.
- Those with bladder symptoms or bilateral neurological changes have worse outcomes.

Spinal deformity surgery

- The most common is scoliosis surgery.
- There are two main patient groups – adolescents with idiopathic scoliosis or younger children with neuromuscular dysfunction.
- Surgery in the latter group is associated with higher blood loss.

Excision of spinal tumors

- May be extradural or intradural.
- Extradural tumors are commonly metastases from breast, prostate, or lung cancers.
- Most intradural tumors are benign (including hemangioma, ependymoma, or meningioma) and resection can be curative.

Trauma

- 45% of traumatic injuries involve the remainder of the spinal cord; approximately one third thoracic, one third thoracolumbar, and one third lumbosacral.
- Surgery may be during the initial period of spinal shock or hyperreflexia.

Subarachnoid hemorrhage and intracerebral aneurysms

Key points

- The majority of subarachnoid hemorrhages (SAH) are related to aneurysmal disease.
- There are significant differences in management of the condition among different centers.
- The main role of anesthetic care is in the treatment of complications and management of patients for coiling or clipping.
- Recovery can be complicated by rebleeding, hydrocephalus, or delayed cerebral ischemia.

Epidemiology

- Spontaneous SAH occurs in 10–20/100 000 persons per year.
- The peak incidence is around 50–55 years of age and there is a higher frequency in African American and Japanese populations.
- The majority are related to aneurysms (aSAH). This section will focus on this presentation, as these patients are most likely to require anesthetic input.
- The main risk factors for aneurysmal disease are smoking and hypertension.
- They are more common in women and those with an affected first-degree relative.
- A review in Scotland from 1986 to 2005 found 12 056 individuals with aSAH; 84% survived to reach hospital. Incidence rates were greater in women [14.8 (13.4–16.3)] than in men [9.4 (8.1–10.6)]; female to male ratio of 1.59.

- There is a poor prognosis with a 30-day mortality of approximately one third.
- Of the survivors, one third remain dependent; of the other two thirds, only 30% return to their premorbid quality of life at 18 months.
- aSAH accounts for nearly one third of all stroke-related years of potential life lost before the age of 65 years.

Diagnosis

- Classical presentation is a sudden "thunderclap" headache, often following exercise, but can be at rest. Vomiting, acute confusion, or seizures may occur.
- SAH is a medical emergency that is frequently misdiagnosed, so a high level of suspicion should exist in patients with acute onset of severe headache.
- CT scanning should be performed as soon as the diagnosis is suspected. Non-contrast CT changes may be subtle and lumbar puncture for analysis of CSF is strongly recommended when the CT scan is negative.
- Selective cerebral angiography should be performed in patients with SAH to document the presence and anatomical features of aneurysms.
- Magnetic resonance angiography (MRA) and CT angiography (CTA) may be considered when conventional angiography cannot be performed in a timely fashion.

There are different grading systems for SAH. Some of the common ones are detailed as follows:

The World Federation of Neurosurgical Societies (WFNS) grading system:

Grade	Glasgow Coma Scale	Mortality
I	15	
II	13–14 with no focal deficit	29%
III	13–14 with focal deficit	
IV	7–12	42%
V	3–6	70%

Hunt and Hess Scale:

Grade	Clinical	Mortality
I	Mild headache, minimal neck stiffness, oriented	Low <5%
II	Severe headache or neck stiffness; oriented and no focal deficit	<10%
III	Confusion, lethargy, mild neurological deficit	23%
IV	Significant neurological deficit	44%
V	Coma	91%

Fisher Scale:

Grade	CT appearance
1	No hemorrhage evident
2	Subarachnoid hemorrhage <1 mm thick
3	Subarachnoid hemorrhage >1 mm thick
4	Subarachnoid hemorrhage of any thickness with intra-ventricular hemorrhage or parenchymal extension

Management

For a disease process with such a high mortality, there is significant heterogeneity in clinical practice. This may be due to:

- differences in awareness and interpretation of the available data on SAH management
- absence of data to guide practice

Recent guidelines have been published to guide the treatment of patients following SAH [28,29].

Beneficial interventions include:

- coiling versus clipping. Endovascular coiling is superior to clipping if the aneurysm has favorable morphology. Coiling may have a higher rate of rebleeding [30]
- early aneurysm repair
- use of nimodipine
- heparin (unfractionated or low-molecular weight) for prophylaxis of venous thromboembolism
- lung protective ventilation, use of PEEP
- referral to high volume centers and admission to the neurological or neurosurgical intensive care unit

Complications

The main two complications are rebleeding and delayed cerebral ischemia (DCI). The risk of rebleeding with an untreated aneurysm is high.

- Initially the risk is 3%–4% in the first day, 1%–2% per day for the first month, and gradually decreasing to 3% per year at three months.
- To reduce the risk of rebleeding, early aneurysm repair should take place.
- A short course of antifibrinolytic therapy should be considered for these patients.

DCI is a syndrome of focal deficits with or without cognitive decline. It occurs in up to 30% of patients, even after seemingly successful treatment of the aneurysm, usually between the fourth and tenth day after aSAH.

- DCI has a high morbidity and mortality, approximately half of patients have a poor clinical outcome [31].
- DCI was felt to be due to arterial vessel narrowing secondary to the presence of oxyhemoglobin around the arteries at the base of the brain. This narrowing develops in 50%–70% of patients of which half will display clinical changes of DCI.

- This is now thought to be too simplistic a concept, with a multifactorial pathogenesis more likely.
- It would seem a combination of altered cerebral autoregulation, cerebral edema, altered ion channel function, similar to the pathological changes in TBI, plus vasoconstriction may be responsible [31].
- Multiple therapies have been tested, but in randomized controlled trials, only the calcium channel blocker nimodipine has been shown to reduce the risk. The precise mechanism of action is unclear, as nimodipine has been shown to be beneficial even without radiological evidence of vasodilation. It is therefore likely to have an intracellular calcium modulating effect.
- The classical triple-H therapy of hypertension, hemodilution, and hypervolemia has no evidence to support its use [32].
- Research has been unable to uncover predictive factors for DCI. There is also a substantial treatment "gap." This is the subject of many ongoing trials.
- Despite recent reductions in case fatality, DCI remains a major problem.

Coiling and clipping

Anesthesia for angiography and coiling [33,34]

Most patients do not need anesthesia for angiography but it may be requested for challenging cases.

- SAH can have multisystem effects so preassessment must be thorough.
- Catecholamine release can cause arrhythmias, electrocardiographic (ECG) changes, left ventricle dysfunction, and pulmonary edema.
- Decreased conscious level at the time of the ictus can lead to aspiration and pneumonia.
- There may be associated metabolic changes; particular attention needs to be paid to dysnatremias and blood glucose levels. These should be maintained within normal ranges.

Anesthetic goals and management are similar to those in patients with TBI, namely a careful induction and rapid, smooth emergence.

- We recommend reinforced endotracheal tubes, invasive blood pressure monitoring, remifentanil infusions, and monitored muscle relaxation.
- There are generally low analgesia requirements and no need for long-acting opioids – regular codeine and paracetamol is usually sufficient.
- Given the lack of surgical stimulation, we recommend use of depth of anesthesia monitors [35].

Clipping

- Since the advent of endovascular coiling, clipping is utilized less frequently in Europe and the U.K. Here, it is reserved for anatomically challenging cases, including middle cerebral artery aneurysms.
- As with other acute brain injury syndromes, attention to detail in neuroanesthesia is required.
- The need for brain "relaxation" is more common, achieved by using hypertonic solutions or CSF drainage. A lumbar CSF drain may be required.

- Burst suppression with thiopentone may be neuroprotective just prior to clipping of the aneurysm.
- The use of intraoperative hypothermia has been widely discussed.
- A Cochrane review from 2012, involving three trials with a total of 1100 patients, suggested slight benefit for those with good-grade aSAHs, but this was not statistically significant [36].
- There was insufficient evidence to determine the efficacy of hypothermia in a poor-grade group.
- Monitoring of neurological function may be required for these cases.

Intraoperative aneurysm rupture

- The risk of rupture is greater with giant aneurysms and those involving the basilar or anterior communicating artery.
- It can happen at any point but is more likely during dissection or clipping. It can lead to torrential bleeding. Both the surgical and anesthetic teams need to be prepared. All patients should have good IV access, two short wide-bore cannulae, and cross-matched blood available. For those who are at higher risk, some teams keep a rapid infuser device primed.
- As well as fluid resuscitation, the anesthetist may induce hypotension to aid control. There is obviously a difficult balance between maintaining cerebral perfusion and improving the surgical field. Increasing the end-tidal concentration of volatile agent is probably the easiest method to achieve a reduction in pressure.
- The surgeon can reduce local blood flow by temporary clipping the carotid artery or other proximal vessels.

Arteriovenous malformations

- Arteriovenous malformations are congenital abnormal connections between arteries and veins [21]. At least 70% of them are supratentorial, often arising from the middle cerebral artery.
- Most do not need surgical intervention unless causing pressure effects.
- Anesthetic management is similar to surgical clipping of an intracranial aneurysm, with risk of significant blood loss.

Special circumstances

Posterior fossa surgery

Posterior fossa surgery presents some unique challenges for the anesthetist.

- The majority of work involves tumor resection – acoustic neuromas, metastases, and meningiomas.
- The patient may have raised ICP due to hydrocephalus and cerebellar dysfunction, exhibiting ataxia, nystagmus, or abnormal gait.
- Tumor or edema compressing on the brainstem causes signs of ipsilateral cranial nerve palsies.
- Any respiratory changes are a clinical emergency and can progress to respiratory arrest.

- Altered conscious level or bulbar palsies can lead to loss of airway reflexes, thus pulmonary function and the possibility of aspiration need to be assessed.
- Patient positioning is important and will require discussion between the surgeon and anesthetist.
  - Where possible, it is sensible to avoid the sitting position due to the increased risk of venous air embolism and hypotension.
  - Alternatively, prone positioning or a lateral "park-bench position" should allow surgical access to most tumors.
- The proximity to the brainstem can cause intraoperative cardiovascular changes.
  - Stimulation of the fifth cranial nerve causes hypertension and reflex bradycardia, whereas stimulus to the tenth cranial nerve will cause hypotension and bradycardia.
  - These signs normally resolve with cessation of surgical stimulation.
  - Pharmacological intervention should be reserved for cases that do not resolve, as hasty administration of drugs can cause further hemodynamic instability.
- Anesthetic management is similar to that in other neurosurgical cases – use of a reinforced cuffed oral endotracheal tube (COETT), mandatory intra-arterial blood pressure monitoring, large bore IV access, and familiar agents.
- There is a high-risk for postoperative nausea and vomiting; we recommend using multimodal anti-emetics.

Acoustic neuroma

- Acoustic neuromas, or vestibular Schawnnomas, are tumors of the myelin shealth of the eighth cranial nerve [21].
- They arise in the internal auditory canal. As they grow, they extend into the cerebellopontine angle of the posterior fossa.
- Often they surround the facial nerve meaning lengthy surgical time due to painstaking dissection. Monitoring of the facial nerve is required, so the use of neuromuscular blockade is restricted to intubation.
- A remifentanil infusion should be used to reduce the risk of coughing or straining.

Venous air embolism

- Venous air embolism (VAE) occurs when there is a negative pressure gradient into an open venous structure [21]. Large veins, such as the dural sinuses or the emissary veins, that do not collapse easily, offer the greatest hazard for VAE.
- Neurosurgery is high-risk for VAE due to the frequency of head-up positioning and exposure of venous structures.
- The sitting position is associated with a vastly increased frequency (up to 45%) of VAE.
- Small volumes of air do not normally present a problem. However, large volumes can become entrapped in the RV, preventing ejection, leading to cardiovascular collapse.
- There are various monitoring tools, the most sensitive of which are precordial Doppler or transesophageal echocardiography.
- If there is a high-risk of VAE, a central venous catheter should be inserted preoperatively. Ideally, the tip should lie at the junction of the superior vena cava and the RAt to allow for easy aspiration of air.

- If VAE is suspected, the anesthetist should inform the surgical team to flood the surgical field, then aspirate the central venous catheter.
- The patient's position should be lowered and necessary hemodynamic support instituted.

Awake craniotomy

- Awake craniotomy is often used for epilepsy surgery and temporal lobe resections near to motor and speech areas [37]. This allows intraoperative functional testing or cortical mapping.
- Occasionally, significant patient comorbidity increases the risk of general anesthesia for other procedures, and in these cases, awake craniotomy may be considered.
- Different techniques have been described, including asleep–awake–asleep or awake with deep sedation for Mayfield pin insertion.
- There are different studies describing these techniques and show that they are well tolerated in experienced hands [38].
- Increasingly low levels of sedation are used alongside analgesics and local anesthetics.
- Premedication with clonidine or dexmedetomidine allows anxiolysis and good intraoperative blood pressure control without confusion or disinhibition.
- Remifentanil (using a low concentration of remifentanil of 10 μg/mL as opposed to 50 μg/mL to allow a reasonable rate in mL/min) and propofol infusions at low concentrations allow quick onset and offset of sedation.
- The aim of sedation is to achieve patient comfort while maintaining cooperation with the surgical team.
- Local anesthetic blocks to appropriate scalp nerves can provide anesthesia to allow surgery [37].
- Position the patient to permit interaction with the surgical team and anesthetist. Good communication will allow patient reassurance.
- Careful patient selection is vital in keeping complication rates low.

References

1. Coronado VG, McGuire LC, Sarmiento K, et al. Trends in Traumatic Brain Injury in the U.S. and the public health response: 1995–2009. *J Safety Res* 2012; **43**: 299–307.
2. Protheroe RT, Gwinnutt CL. Early hospital care of severe traumatic brain injury. *Anaesthesia* 2011; **66**: 1035–47.
3. Werner C, Engelhard K. Pathophysiology of traumatic brain injury. *Br J Anaesth* 2007; **99**: 4–9.
4. Cipolla MJ. Control of cerebral blood flow. In: *The Cerebral Circulation*. San Rafael, CA: Morgan & Claypool Life Sciences, 2009; 27–32.
5. Moss E. The cerebral circulation. *Br J Anaesth CEPD Rev* 2001; **1**: 67–71.
6. Bullock MR, Povlishock JT. Guidelines for the management of severe head injury, 3rd edn. Brain Trauma Foundation. *J Neurotrauma* 2007; **24**: S1–106.
7. White H, Venkatesh B. Cerebral perfusion pressure in neurotrauma: a review. *Anesth Analgesia* 2008; **107**: 979–88.
8. Wijayatilake DS, Shepherd SJ, Sherren PB. Update in the management of intracranial pressure in traumatic brain injury. *Curr Opin Anesthesiol* 2012; **25**: 540–7.
9. Roberts I. Aminosteroids for acute traumatic brain injury. *Cochrane Database Syst Rev* 2000; **4**: CD001527.
10. Sydenham E, Roberts I, Alderson P. Hypothermia for traumatic head injury. *Cochrane Database Syst Rev* 2009; **2**: CD001048.

11. Saxena M, Andrews PJD, Cheng A. Modest cooling therapies (35 °C to 37.5 °C) for traumatic brain injury. *Cochrane Database Syst Rev* 2008; **3**: CD006811.

12. Schierhout G, Roberts I. Antiepileptic drugs for preventing seizures following acute traumatic brain injury. *Cochrane Database Syst Rev* 2001; **4**: CD000173.

13. Samandouras G. *The Neurosurgeon's Handbook*. Oxford: Oxford University Press, 2010.

14. Greaves I, Porter K, Garner J, eds. Head injury. In: *Trauma Care Manual, 2nd edition*. London: Hodder Arnold, 2009; 99–112.

15. Tawfeeq NA, Halawani MM, Al-Faridi K, et al. Traumatic brain injury: neuroprotective anaesthetic techniques, an update. *Injury* 2009; **40**: 75–81.

16. El Beheiry H. Protecting the brain during neurosurgical procedures: strategies that can work. *Curr Opin Anesthesiol* 2012; **25**: 548–55.

17. Lowe GJ, Ferguson ND. Lung-protective ventilation in neurosurgical patients. *Curr Opin Crit Care* 2006; **12**: 3–7.

18. Cooper DJ, Jeffrey V, Rosenfeld JV, et al. Decompressive craniectomy in diffuse traumatic brain injury. *N Engl J Med* 2011; **364**: 1493–502.

19. Association of Anaesthetists of Great Britain and Ireland. *Recommendations for the Safe Transfer of Patients with Brain Injury*. London: Association of Anaesthetists of Great Britain and Ireland, 2006.

20. Greenburg MS, ed. Head trauma. In: *Handbook of Neurosurgery, 7th edition*. New York, NY: Thieme Medical Publishers, 2010; 850–929.

21. Schubert A, ed. *Clinical Neuroanesthesia*. Boston, MA: Butterworth-Heinemann, 1997.

22. Leemans M, Calder I. The unstable cervical spine. In: Johnston I, Harrop-Griffiths W, Gemmell L, eds. *AAGBI Core Topics in Anaesthesia.*. Chichester, UK: Wiley-Blackhall, 2012; 88–104.

23. American Spinal Injury Association. ASIA Exam Sheet for International Standards for Neurological Classification of Spinal Cord Injury. 2011. Available from: http://www.asia-spinalinjury.org (Accessed January 18 2013.)

24. Veale P, Lamb J. Anaesthesia and acute spinal cord injury. *Br J Anaesth CEPD Rev* 2002; **2**: 139–43.

25. Nolan JP, Wilson ME. Orotracheal intubation in patients with potential cervical spine injuries. *Anaesthesia* 2007; **48**: 630–3.

26. Robitaille A. Airway management in the patient with potential cervical spine instability: continuing professional development. *Can J Anaesth* 2011; **58**: 1125–39.

27. Postoperative Visual Loss Study Group. Risk factors associated with ischemic optic neuropathy after spinal fusion surgery. *Anesthesiology* 2012; **116**: 15–24.

28. Diringer MN, Bleck TP, Hemphill JC III, et al. Critical care management of patients following aneurysmal subarachnoid hemorrhage: recommendations from the Neurocritical Care Society's Multidisciplinary Consensus Conference. *Neurocrit Care* 2011; **15**: 211–40.

29. Bederson JB, Connolly ES Jr, Batjer HH, et al. Guidelines for the management of aneurysmal subarachnoid hemorrhage: a statement for healthcare professionals from a special writing group of the Stroke Council, *American Heart Association. Stroke* 2009; **40**: 994–1025.

30. Molyneaux AJ, Kerr RS, Yu LM, et al. International subarachnoid aneurysm trial (ISAT). *Lancet* 2005; **366**: 809–17.

31. Rowland MJ, Hadjipavlou G, Kelly M, et al. Delayed cerebral ischaemia after subarachnoid haemorrhage: looking beyond vasospasm. *Br J Anaesth* 2012; **109**: 315–29.

32. Dankbaar JW, Arjen JC, Slooter AJC, et al. Effect of different components of triple-H therapy on cerebral perfusion in patients with aneurysmal subarachnoid haemorrhage: a systematic review. *Crit Care* 2010; **14**: R23.

33. Dorairaj IL, Hancock SM. Anaesthesia for interventional radiology. *Br J Anaesth CEPD Rev* 2008; **8**: 86–9.

34. Priebe H-J. Aneurysmal subarachnoid haemorrhage and the anaesthetist. *Br J Anaesth* 2007; **99**: 102–18.

35. National Institute for Health and Clinical Excellence. *Depth of Anaesthesia Monitors (E-Entropy, BIS and Narcotrend) (DG6).* London: National Institute for Health and Clinical Excellence, 2012.

36. Li Luying R, You C, Chaudhary B. Intraoperative mild hypothermia for postoperative neurological deficits in intracranial aneurysm patients. *Cochrane Database Syst Rev* 2012; **2**: CD008445.

37. Costello TG, Cormack JR. Anesthesia for awake craniotomy: a modern approach. *J Clin Neurosci* 2004; **11**: 16–19.

38. de Monte A, Zorzi F, Saltarini M, et al. Anesthetic management in awake craniotomy. *Signa Vitae* 2008; **3**: 28–32.

Chapter 27

Anesthesia for end-stage renal and liver disease

S. Morrison and C. Harle

Patients with significant renal or hepatic disease present a daunting perioperative challenge in modern anesthesia practice. The multisystem consequences of these entities can escalate the complexity and risk of even the simplest surgical procedures significantly. Contemporary anesthesia practitioners must be well acquainted with the implications of chronic hepatorenal disease in order to deliver effective perioperative care safely.

The kidney

Overview of renal physiology

- The kidney is a complex organ, which performs multiple, diverse physiological functions necessary for the maintenance of homeostasis.
- It is the most highly perfused organ of the body, receiving 25% of cardiac output.
- Renal blood flow is not linked to metabolic demand and is consistently high in order to maintain rapid plasma filtration rates. Autoregulatory mechanisms exist to restrict renal blood flow at high pressures to protect the glomeruli from damage.
- The functional unit of the kidney is the nephron. It consists of a glomerulus and a tubule, which empties into a collecting duct. The collecting ducts empty into the renal pelvis, which drains urine into the bladder via the ureter.
- Each kidney, in health, contains approximately one million nephrons. Urine is formed by the combination of glomerular ultrafiltration and tubular reabsorption and secretion through a process called countercurrent exchange.
- A combination of active and passive diffusion along varying osmotic gradients produces urine appropriately concentrated for a given physiological state.
- The renal system regulates intravascular volume, osmolality, and acid–base and electrolyte balance and excretes end products of metabolism and drugs.
- Other key functions include the production of hormones that contribute to fluid homeostasis (renin, prostaglandins, kinins), bone metabolism (1,25-dihydroxycholecalciferol), and hematopoiesis (erythropoietin).

Anesthesia and Perioperative Care of the High-Risk Patient, Third edition, ed. Ian McConachie. Published by Cambridge University Press.

Chronic kidney disease (CKD)

Definitions

CKD is characterized by structural or functional abnormalities of the kidneys for three or more months, manifested as:

- Kidney damage – with or without decreased glomerular filtration rate (GFR). For example, presence of pathological abnormalities, markers of kidney damage such as urinary abnormalities (proteinuria), blood abnormalities (renal tubular syndromes) or imaging abnormalities, or following kidney transplant
- GFR of <60 mL/min/1.73 m^2, with or without kidney damage [1]

There are two principal outcomes of CKD: (1) the progressive loss of kidney function, and (2) the development and progression of cardiovascular disease (CVD) [2].

Kidney function

Persistent proteinuria is the principal marker of kidney damage. Other markers of damage include abnormalities in urine sediment, blood and urine chemistry, and imaging [2].

- GFR is the single best measure of overall kidney function. Normal variation occurs with gender, age, and body size. Normal GFR for healthy young adults is 120–130 mL/min/m^2 and declines with age [2].
- GFR of <60 mL/min/m^2 indicates loss of greater than 50% of normal adult level kidney function. Below this level, the prevalence of complications related to CKD increases [3].
- Level of kidney function determines the stage of CKD [2]:
  - stage 1 – kidney damage with normal or increased GFR (GFR>90 mL/min/m^2)
  - stage 2 – kidney damage with mildly decreased GFR (GFR=60–89 mL/min/m^2)
  - stage 3 – moderately decreased GFR (GFR=30–59 mL/min/m^2)
  - stage 4 – severely decreased GFR (GFR=15–29 mL/min/m^2)
  - stage 5 – kidney failure (GFR<15 mL/min/m^2 or on dialysis)
- Kidney failure is not synonymous with end-stage renal disease (ESRD). ESRD is an administrative term in the U.S. indicating that a patient is being treated with dialysis or a transplant, thus qualifying for coverage under the Medicare ESRD program. ESRD does not define kidney dysfunction precisely [2].

Prevalence

- CKD is an increasing health problem worldwide.
- In Canada, between 1.3 and 2.9 million people are estimated to have CKD.
- Approximately 12.5% of Canadian adults are living with CKD (any stage). The prevalence of adults with stages 3–5 CKD was 3%–4% [4].
- In the U.S., approximately 9.6% of non-institutionalized adults are estimated to have CKD [1].
- The prevalence of ESRD has increased by 20% since 2000 in the U.S. and stands at 1699 per million people [3].
- The annual incidence in the U.K. of new patients requiring renal replacement therapy (RRTh) is 108 per million people. The prevalence of patients alive requiring RRTh in the U.K. is 694 per million people [5].

- Most patients with CKD do not progress to renal failure or require RRTh. This is partly due to an increased mortality secondary to CVD as well as the advanced age at onset of many renal diseases, and the slow rate of decline of renal function, especially if treated [5].

Etiology

The etiology of CKD is often complex and heterogeneous. Common risk factors known to contribute to CKD include:

- hypertension
- diabetes
- systemic lupus erythematosis
- genetic (African American, Hispanic, Latino, Aboriginal heritage)
- age >60 years
- non-steroidal anti-inflammatory drug (NSAID) use [2]

Other important etiologies intrinsic to the kidney include glomerulonephritis, pyelonephritis, renovascular disease, and polycystic kidneys [5].

CKD can be divided into disorders of renal vasculature or interstitium.

- diabetic nephropathy – disease of the glomerulus. Most common cause of CKD in the U.S.
- hypertensive nephrosclerosis – bidirectional relationship between blood pressure and renal disease
- glomerular disease – nephrotic versus nephritic
- interstitial disease – drug reactions, allergy, NSAIDs, toxicity
- vascular disease of the kidney – inflammatory vasculitides
- inherited kidney disease, e.g., polycystic kidney disease [6]

Evaluation of CKD

- In addition to identifying patients at risk for CKD, that is, the presence of risk factors and associated comorbidities, laboratory measures are valuable in assessing CKD.
- Mathematical estimates of GFR using serum creatinine are the best overall indices of kidney function [2].
- Other variables such as age, gender, race, and body size should be taken into account when estimating GFR.
- Two commonly accepted formulae exist:
  - Cockcroft–Gault equation:

    $$C_{Cr}(\text{mL/min}) = (140 - \text{age} \times \text{weight}) / (72 \times S_{Cr}) \times 0.85 \text{ (if female)}$$

    where C_{Cr}= creatinine clearance, S_{Cr} = serum creatinine (mg/dL), age in years, weight in kg
  - modification of diet in renal disease:
- $\text{GFR} = 186 \times {S_{Cr}}^{-1.154} \times \text{age}^{-0.203} \times 0.74 \text{ (if female)} \times 1.21 \text{ (if African American)}$
- GFR must decline by approximately 50% before the S_{Cr} level rises above the upper limit of normal. Thus creatinine concentration itself is insensitive and should not be used as a sole means to evaluate kidney function [2].

- Several new biomarkers for the progression of CKD have been identified, including cystatin C, C-reactive protein, homocysteine, and asymmetric dimethyl arginine, but they require more validation in prospective clinical studies in different patient populations before their use in preoperative assessment can be generally recommended [6].

xtra-renal manifestations of CKD

ardiovascular disease

Ayocardial infarction (MI), heart failure, and stroke are the leading causes of death in atients with CKD [5]. CKD profoundly affects the cardiovascular system:

- salt and water retention, hypertension (HTN), left ventricular hypertrophy from pressure and volume overload
- congestive heart failure (CHF), cardiomyopathy, uremic pericarditis
- accelerated atherosclerosis due to dyslipidemia, inflammation, oxidative stress, and endothelial dysfunction, leading to MI, peripheral vascular disease, and stroke
- vascular calcification and myocardial fibrosis leading to conduction abnormalities, and valvular heart disease due to calcification [5,7]

n addition, pulmonary hypertension may be present in up to 40% of CKD patients equiring dialysis.

- ESRD or dialysis itself may be a trigger for the development of precapillary pulmonary hypertension in a predisposed patient, analogous to connective tissue disease, HIV, or portal hypertension.
- Hormonal and metabolic disturbances associated with CKD requiring dialysis might lead to pulmonary vascular constriction.
- Potential pathological mechanisms include nitric oxide (NO) abnormalities, impaired endothelial function, or increased levels of endothelin [8].
- This may reduce the ability of the pulmonary vasculature to accommodate the increase in cardiac output derived from the arteriovenous (AV) fistula [3].
- Arteriovenous access for dialysis results in pathologically elevated pulmonary artery pressure and cardiac output. Over time this may lead to permanent changes in pulmonic capillaries and the right heart, with increased morbidity and mortality [9].
- Another contributing factor may be injury resulting from chronic exposure to microbubbles originating in the dialyzer or its tubing [3].

lematological factors and coagulation

KD is associated with disorders of hemostasis resulting in an increased risk of both therothrombotic events and bleeding.

- Mild CKD is associated with a prothombotic tendency due to impaired release of tissue plasminogen activator (tPA), increased plasminogen activator inhibitor (PAI)-1, elevated fibrinogen and D-dimer, and increased tissue factor (TF)/FVIIa complex.
- This likely contributes significantly to major CVD events.
- With advancing CKD, prothombotic derangements persist as platelet dysfunction begins to manifest, presenting increased risk of hemorrhagic events.

- Platelet adhesion and aggregation is impaired leading to cutaneous, mucosal, and serosal bleeding. Patients with CKD are also at increased risk for gastrointestinal (GI) bleeding and intracranial bleeding, which might be partially attributable to platelet dysfunction [10].
- Interestingly, perioperative thromboelastography (TEG) data suggests all aspects of coagulation are increased in uremic patients, including initial fibrin formation, fibrin–platelet interaction, and qualitative platelet function. Decreased fibrinolysis was observed at one hour as well, suggesting imbalance with the accelerated coagulation [11].
- Normochromic/normocytic anemia typically develops when GFR falls below 60 mL/min/1.73 m^2, due to erythropoietin deficiency, hemolysis, presence of uremic inhibitors, blood loss (either occult or overt), and deficiency in iron, folate, or vitamin B12 [12].

Other systems

- Autonomic neuropathy is common in CKD
  - Can significantly effect arterial blood pressure perioperatively, especially with neuraxial anesthesia.
  - Peripheral sensory and motor neuropathy correlate with cardiac autonomic neuropathy.
  - High incidence of delayed gastric emptying occurs.
  - Reduced baroreceptor sensitivity, increased sympathetic activity, and parasympathetic dysfunction predispose to arrhythmia [5].
- Distal symmetrical mixed motor and sensory polyneuropathy (restless leg syndrome), sensory neuropathy, or distal weakness of the lower extremities (some uremic encephalopathy and peripheral neurological symptoms may be improved by dialysis)
- Musculoskeletal system – renal osteodystrophy, rhabdomyolysis after major surgery
- Endocrine system – secondary and tertiary hyperparathyroidism, vitamin D deficiency, diabetes mellitus
- Gastrointestinal system – delayed gastric emptying, anorexia, vomiting, reduced protein intake, malnutrition, reduced calcium absorption
- Immune system – immunosuppression due to uremia or drugs [5]

Fluids, electrolytes, acid–base

Sodium and volume status

- Sodium excretion is a function of GFR. With decreasing GFR, the ability to manage sodium loads leads to volume overload, edema, and hypertension [5,12].
- Sodium derangements are usually related to fluid shifts. Increased free water loss (diuresis) or reduced intake result in hypernatremia. Disproportional sodium and water losses or fluid retention lead to hyponatremia. Volume status becomes an important distinction when interpreting serum sodium levels [13].
- Despite traditional teaching that volume status is maintained until late in the course of CKD, volume overload may occur early in CKD and contributes to a chronic systemic inflammatory state. This likely promotes CVD and progression of CKD [14].

Potassium

- Plasma K^+ usually remains normal until stage 5 CKD [5].
- Severe renal dysfunction will cause K^+ retention and acidosis, leading to further hyperkalemia due to ion shifting. With acute acidosis K^+ will rise by ~0.5 mmol per drop in pH of 0.1 [13].
- Chronic hyperkalemia is better tolerated than the acute but K^+ >6.5 mmol/L can cause hypotension, weakness, and arrhythmias. K^+ >6.5 mmol/L or hyperkalemia associated with arrhythmias should be treated [13].

A number of medications can cause/exacerbate hyperkalemia perioperatively:

- β-blockers – reduce cellular uptake of K^+ and inhibit aldosterone secretion.
- Succinylcholine – transiently increases K^+ by 0.5–1.0 mmol/L.
- NSAIDs – decrease renal blood flow/GFR, inhibit aldosterone synthesis.
- Angiotensin-converting enzyme (ACE) inhibitors (ACE-i) or angiotensin receptor blockers (ARBs) – inhibit aldosterone synthesis, decrease renal blood flow/GFR.
- Digoxin – decrease Na^+–K^+ ATPase activity.
- K^+-sparing diuretics – are associated with aldosterone antagonism.
- Cyclosporin, tacrolimus – decrease aldosterone synthesis, Na^+–K^+–ATPase activity, K^+ channel activity [15].

Metabolic acidosis

- Metabolic acidosis develops in CKD due to an inability to excrete H^+ ions produced during metabolism of sulfur-containing amino acids and reduced synthesis of ammonia. As CKD advances, serum HCO_3 levels begin to fall (usually between 12 and 20 mEq/L) and the anion gap increases [5,15].
- Chronic acidemia is associated with worsening of hyperparathyroid-induced renal osteodystrophy and negative calcium balance, enhanced skeletal muscle breakdown and catabolism, growth retardation in children, and progression of GFR loss [12].
- Perioperative consequences of metabolic acidosis relate to an impaired ability to compensate for respiratory acidosis and altered anesthetic drug pharmacology [5].

Anesthetic management

Preoperative management

Due to the complexity of patients with ESRD and the associated systemic consequences, a multidisciplinary approach should be undertaken well in advance of any planned operative procedure. This may involve collaboration between surgery, anesthesia, cardiology, and nephrology services.

Assessment

- Thorough preoperative history, physical examination, and review of pertinent laboratory values are necessary.
- Review dialysis records including recency and type of dialysis.
- Carefully assess volume status:
  - Comparison between pre- and post-dialysis weight and preoperative weight can provide insight into volume status.
  - Examine vital signs including orthostatic changes.

- Assess for presence and severity of systemic complications of CKD, such as hypertension, CVD, pulmonary hypertension, anemia.
- Assess renal function using creatinine-based estimates of GFR.
- Vascular access may be either permanent or temporary. Options for permanent access include native AV fistulae, AV grafts, and long-term catheters [5].
- For temporary vascular hemodialysis catheters, the right internal jugular is the preferred site due to better blood flow and lower risk of complications such as venous stenosis. Venous stenosis is a concerning complication of dialysis catheter placement and may occur as frequently as 40%–50% in cannulated subclavian veins [5].
- Problems relating to vascular access are a leading cause of hospitalization, morbidity, and the need for anesthesia in patients with stage 5 CKD. These include infection, thrombosis, aneurysm, limb ischemia, and limb edema [5].
- As a general rule, hemodialysis catheters should not be used for purposes other than dialysis (e.g., blood sample, central venous monitoring, and drug administration) except in an emergency [3].
- Vascular access sites should be protected in the operating room.

Risk stratification

- CKD is a risk factor for serious postoperative complications, such as acute renal failure and cardiovascular complications, which are associated with an increased morbidity and mortality [5].
- The most universal risk factor for postoperative renal failure is poor preoperative renal function [16].
- Age and the cardiac risk factors of left ventricular dysfunction, increased left-sided heart pressures, and CHF may be predictive of postoperative renal failure [16].
- Creatinine of >2 mg/dL (177 μmol/L) has been identified as an independent predictor of cardiac complications, and was associated with major cardiac complications in 9% of cases [17].
- Renal dysfunction after coronary artery bypass grafting may be as high as 11% and is associated with increased length of stay in the intensive care unit (ICU) and hospital and an increased incidence of respiratory infections, sepsis, and GI or postoperative surgical bleeding [6].
- High-risk vascular procedures, such as thoracic aneurysm repair or suprarenal abdominal aortic aneurysm repair, are associated with a high-risk of renal dysfunction. However, laparoscopic procedures may also be implicated in transient renal dysfunction [6].

Optimization

- Treat anemia with iron supplementation and erythropoietic-stimulating agents to a target hemoglobin concentration of between 11 g/dL and 12 g/dL (hematocrit 33%–36%).
- Stablilize glycemic control.
- Dialytic correction of metabolic status
  - Patients with CKD undergoing elective surgery should receive hemodialysis (HD) the day before the planned surgery to optimize their electrolyte, metabolic, and volume status, and allow time for equilibration of electrolytes and volume [18].

  - Minimize intravenous fluid administration for minor surgery but maintain euvolemia during major surgery to preserve adequate preload, avoiding hypotension and potential organ hypoperfusion [19]. Hypovolemia contributes to intraoperative hemodynamic instability. Hypervolemia can lead to hypertension, pulmonary edema, and heart failure [3].
- Optimize blood pressure and heart failure medications.
  - Heart failure medication should be titrated to optimal effect prior to the operative date.
  - Consider holding ACE-i or ARB medications preoperatively in order to avoid refractory hypotension on induction of anesthesia [3].
- Nutritional status
  - A multifactorial malnutritional state is common and a contributing factor in patients with ESRD.
  - Poor nutritional status secondary to lack of appetite, dietary restrictions, medication-related impaired absorption of nutrients, loss of nutrients through HD, dialysis-induced catabolism, and chronic inflammation contribute to perioperative morbidity and mortality and should be optimized prior to proceeding to the operating room.

ntraoperative management

pecific goals of anesthesia in the CKD patient are:

- Ischemic heart disease – optimize the economy of myocardial oxygen supply and demand.
- Pulmonary hypertension – avoid increasing pulmonary vascular resistance and precipitation of right-sided heart failure.
- Note euvolemia.
- Monitor and treat electrolyte and acid–base disturbances – hyperkalemia, hypocalcemia, hyperphosphatemia, metabolic acidosis.
- Avoid inciting acute kidney injury – renal protection, avoiding nephrotoxins, hypotension, hypoxia.
- Prevent infection in an already immunocompromised patient.
- Protect existing vascular access sites from compressions, restriction, or injury.

Aonitoring

ntraoperative monitoring should be dictated by the pre-existing physical status of the patient and the scope of the planned surgical procedure. For minor procedures, standard Canadian Anesthesia Society/American Society of Anesthesiologists (ASA)/U.K. monitoring s likely adequate.

- Arterial line placement is valuable in major surgery for continuous blood pressure monitoring and rapid treatment of hypotension.
- Central venous access provides large caliber venous access, monitoring of central venous pressure (CVP) and a medication route for hemodynamic resuscitation. Consideration should be given for the possibility of existing venous stenosis and subclavian sites for central venous access should be avoided [3].

- Transesophageal echocardiography (TEE) and pulmonary artery catheterization may provide useful information in select patient populations. The routine use of these modalities is not supported in the literature.
- Point-of-care arterial blood gas testing can be a valuable tool for rapid assessment and management of metabolic and electrolyte abnormalities as well as anemia.

Renal protection

- Most common cause of perioperative acute tubular necrosis is hypovolemia and hypotension leading to hypoxic injury in the medullary region.This may result from over-aggressive correction of hypertension.
- Common toxic insults include: radiocontrast dye, amiglycoside antibiotics, and NSAIDs. Risk–benefit analysis should guide the use of nephrotoxic agents [6].
- Many interventions that were deemed successful in preclinical or early, small clinical trials were shown to be ineffective in larger studies that reflected realistic clinical scenarios.
- Renal protection is discussed further in the chapter on acute kidney injury in surgical patients.

Anesthetic pharmacology

Propofol

- The pharmacokinetics of bolus administration, and of maintenance infusion, do not seem to be markedly altered in patients with ESRD [3].
- Induction doses of propofol associated with a bispectral index score (BIS) of 50 are higher in renal failure. The time to eye opening following discontinuation of propofol infusion is shorter in renal failure as well [5].

Volatile anesthetics

- There has been concern with the biodegradation of potent volatile anesthetics resulting in elevated serum levels of nephrotoxic inorganic fluoride, but that is not a concern with modern agents (desflurane, sevoflurane, isoflurane).
- Sevoflurane can react with strong bases in CO_2 absorbents to form compound A, which has been shown to be nephrotoxic in animal studies. Human studies have not supported this concern.

Neuromuscular blocking drugs

- Succinylcholine – ESRD is associated with reduced plasma cholinesterase activity, which may prolong the action of succinylcholine. There is a transient increase in serum K^+ of 0.5–1.0 mmol/L associated with succinylcholine. Serum K^+ levels peak at three to five minutes and return to baseline 10 to 15 minutes later. There is a potential for myoglobinemia with succinylcholine, which can rarely cause rhabdomyolysis. Thus, if there are no airway indications for succinylcholine, it may be prudent to avoid its use [20].
- Non-depolarizing muscle relaxant initial dose required to produce a block is higher in ESRD. Atracurium and cis-atracurium onset and action are unaltered in renal disease Aminosteroids (pancuronium, vecuronium, and rocuronium) exhibit variable renal

clearance. Their duration of action is significantly prolonged in renal failure, with a high inter-individual variability [20].

- The reversal agent, neostigmine, undergoes 50% renal excretion, thus has a prolonged action and reduced renal clearance in patients with renal failure. Therefore, patients may be at risk of bradycardia and AV block [20].

Opioids

- Opioids do not have direct toxic effects on the kidney. Rare cases of rhabdomyolysis have been reported [5].
- Morphine is metabolized by the liver into several active metabolites, the most important being morphine-3-glucuronide (M3G) and morphine-6-glucuronide (M6G). Both M3G and M6G are excreted by the kidney and hence can accumulate in renal failure. M3G antagonizes the analgesic effect of morphine and can cause excitatory central nervous system (CNS) effects such as irritability and reduced seizure threshold. M6G has potent analgesic properties and can lead to delayed onset of respiratory depression [3].
- Fentanyl undergoes extensive hepatic metabolism with only approximately 7% being excreted unchanged by the kidney, making it a suitable and safe for short-term use in renal failure [21].
- The clearance and half-life of sufentanil are not significantly altered in renal dysfunction.
- Remifentanil is hydrolyzed by non-specific plasma and tissue esterases, and therefore, is not dependent on renal clearance for elimination. The principal metabolite is cleared by the kidney, but exerts an insignificant clinical effect due to its low potency [3].
- Oxycodone is metabolized to the liver into active metabolites that are excreted by the kidney. The parent compound and metabolites accumulate in renal failure, resulting in a prolonged elimination half-life. Dosing should be reduced and dose intervals increased in renal failure [5].

NSAIDs

- Are not recommended in CKD with residual kidney function due to nephrotoxicity.
- May exacerbate hypertension and precipitate edema, hyponatremia, and hyperkalemia. There is also an increased risk of GI bleeding and they may precipitate platelet dysfunction further [5].
- Require careful consideration prior to using in HD patients but potential risks are likely to outweigh potential benefits.

Intravenous fluids

- Non-potassium-containing fluids such as 0.9% saline have traditionally been recommended for kidney transplants and ESRD due to concerns with hyperkalemia.
- However, large volumes of normal saline have been recognized to cause hyperchloremic acidosis, which may precipitate hyperkalemia via intracellular H^+ ion shift.
- Recently, balanced salt-based solutions, such as lactated Ringers, have been demonstrated to be safe in ESRD, and potentially offer superior electrolyte and acid–base balance [22].

Regional anesthesia

- Numerous regional techniques have been used safely in patients with ESRD; for example, peripheral blocks for fistula formation, transversus abdominis plane blocks, paravertebral blocks, and neuraxial techniques [3].
- Platelet number/function and coagulation profile should be checked before any regional technique is performed.
- Patients undergoing spinal anesthesia should be assessed carefully for volume status and the presence of autonomic neuropathy. These patients are at increased risk for hemodynamic stability post-insertion of the block.

Postoperative management

- Admission to high dependency units or ICUs is often appropriate.
- Dialysis should be delayed ideally until the risk of fluid shifts and hemorrhage has declined; however, electrolyte, metabolic, and fluid status may dictate otherwise.
- Patients receiving opioid medications should have their doses reduced and need to be carefully monitored for narcotization.
- Medications for hypertension, heart failure, and ischemic heart disease should be restarted when feasible [3].

The liver

Overview of hepatic physiology

- The liver is the largest gland and internal organ in the body. It weighs approximately 1.5–1.7 kg in adults or 2% of total mass.
- It receives approximately 25% of the cardiac output, of which 75% is supplied by the portal vein and 25% by the hepatic artery. Each vessel delivers about 50% of the total hepatic oxygen supply. Regulation of this dual blood supply via the hepatic arterial buffer response (HABR) allows for preservation of hepatic perfusion when portal venous perfusion is reduced. Hepatic venous drainage is to the inferior vena cava via the hepatic veins.
- The liver lies at the hub of splanchnic circulation, receiving venous drainage from all splanchnic organs and vasculature. This represents the splanchnic reservoir, which may hold up to 20% of blood volume.
- Physiological functions of the liver include:
  - intermediary metabolism – carbohydrate, lipid, protein and bile metabolism
  - coagulation – synthesis of all procoagulant factors except III, IV, and VIII; production of anticoagulant factors such as protein S, protein C, protein Z, PAI, and antithrombin III
  - erythropoiesis and erythrocytosis – production of heme and metabolism of bilirubin
  - endocrine physiology – metabolism of hormones and production of endocrine substances such as angiotensinogen, thrombopoietin, and insulin-like growth factor I
  - immune and inflammatory response – specialized Kupffer cells filter splanchnic blood of antigens, bacteria, and toxins prior to entry into the systemic circulation, and also moderate inflammation

  - xenobiotic (drug) metabolism – the liver is the primary site of biotransformational reactions necessary for drug metabolism and elimination

Pathophysiology of liver disease

- Incidence and prevalence of liver disease (especially alcohol-related disorders and hepatitis C) is increasing in the developed world [23].
- Liver disease is often multifactorial and can be acute or chronic.
- Most common cause of acute hepatic failure is acetaminophen overdose (70%) in developed countries while worldwide it is viral hepatitis. Alcohol and other drugs including methyl-dopa, isoniazid, rifampicin, acetyl salicylic acid, and other NSAIDs are also implicated [23].
- Common causes of chronic liver disease are viral hepatitis (B and C), autoimmune hepatitis, non-alcoholic steatohepatitis (NASH), Laennec's cirrhosis, cryptogenic cirrhosis, and metabolic diseases such as hemachromatosis and Wilson's disease.
- Cholestatic causes of liver disease include primary biliary cirrhosis and primary sclerosing cholangitis.
- Liver cirrhosis occurs when fibrotic scar tissue or regenerative nodules replace normal hepatic tissue. With advancing hepatic fibrosis, there is progressive loss of liver function, and portal hypertension develops.
- Cirrhosis may occur in an indolent manner and may not be manifest clinically until 70% of hepatic tissue is compromised. This is due to the substantial physiological reserve of the liver. Portal hypertension is the predominant pathological manifestation of cirrhosis. Increased resistance to portal blood flow due to hepatic parenchymal scarring and fibrosis, and splanchnic hyperemia results in hypersplenism, thrombocytopenia, and the formation of varices.
- Normal portal pressures are usually in the range of 5–12 mmHg. Portal hypertension is generally defined by two of the following three criteria:
  - splenomegaly
  - ascites
  - esophageal varices

Portal pressures at this time are usually >20 mmHg [24].

Extra-hepatic manifestations of liver disease

CNS

- Hepatic encephalopathy (HE) is a neuropsychiatric syndrome that develops in 50%–70% of patients with cirrhosis.
- The spectrum of HE ranges from tremor, asterixis, and agitation to muscle rigidity, decerebrate posturing, and deep coma [23].
- Factors contributing to the pathophysiology include hepatobiliary dysfunction leading to the accumulation of various gut-derived chemicals, increased central inhibitory outflow due to false neurotransmitters, disruption of the blood–brain barrier, and defective cerebral energy regulation.
- Asterixis, a bilateral asynchronous flapping of outstretched, dorsiflexed hands, is frequently seen in patients with hepatic encephalopathy.

Cardiovascular

- Hyperdynamic circulation with high cardiac output and low systemic vascular resistance is typical of patients with liver disease.
- Advanced liver disease causes extensive, widespread AV communications (collateral vessels) within the splanchnic organs, lungs, muscle, and skin.
- High flow through these collateral vessels may result from increases in endogenous vasodilators, such as glucagon, NO, and vasoactive intestinal polypeptide, due to cirrhosis.
- A diminished response to physiological and pharmacological vasopressors is typical of cirrhosis.
- Cirrhotic cardiomyopathy, characterized by impaired ventricular response to stress, can result in relative cardiac depression and repolarization abnormalities, such as QT prolongation, heart block, and chronotropic incompetence [24].
- Patients with end-stage liver disease (ESLD) may also exhibit diastolic dysfunction.

Respiratory

- Ascites and pleural effusions can restrict ventilation, decrease FRC, promote atelectasis and lead to hypoxia [23].
- Hepatopulmonary syndrome results from significant pulmonary vascular shunting leading to orthodeoxia (hypoxia improving while supine), and can be diagnosed on echocardiography using a bubble study.
- Rarely, liver disease can lead to portopulmonary hypertension whereby increased resistance to pulmonary arterial flow occurs due to pulmonary endothelial/smooth muscle proliferation, vasoconstriction, and *in situ* thrombosis [24].

Gastrointestinal

- Hypoalbuminemia and portal hypertension results in the accumulation of ascites. Renal retention of sodium and water are contributory.
- Gastroesophageal varices can result in catastrophic gastrointestinal hemorrhage. Nearly one third of cirrhosis-related deaths are due to ruptured varices.
- Even mild GI bleeding results in digestion of blood, which grossly increases the hepatic bilirubin load and may precipitate or worsen encephalopathy.
- Splenomegaly leads to sequestration of platelets and thrombocytopenia.
- Massive ascites can raise intra-abdominal pressure with adverse effects on respiratory and renal function.
- Gastric emptying is also delayed and patients, therefore, are at increased risk of aspiration [23].

Renal and metabolic

- GFR steadily decreases, and renal tubules retain sodium, with no overt glomerular or tubular injury.
- Primary etiology of acute renal failure in decompensated cirrhosis is pre-renal failure and acute tubular necrosis.
- Hepatorenal syndrome (HRS) is acute renal failure in the absence of underlying kidney pathology, characterized by functional renal failure and intense renal vasoconstriction [25].

- HRS can be classified into Type I and II, based on onset and prognosis. Type I occurs rapidly and carries a worse prognosis than type II, which occurs over time and carries a more favorable prognosis.
- Salt and water retention associated with ESLD may lead to severe hyponatremia, which can precipitate seizures and decreased level of consciousness [23].

Hematological

- Anemia develops due to GI bleeding, hemolysis, hypersplenism, malnutrition, vitamin deficiencies, bone marrow depression, and plasma volume expansion.
- Hypersplenism, bone-marrow suppression, and immune-mediated platelet destruction lead to thrombocytopenia, which can be severe.
- Activation of fibrinolysis results in dysfibrinogenemia.
- The coagulation system is precariously rebalanced due to deficiencies in hepatic synthesis of both pro- and anticoagulant factors. The net result is unpredictable and standard coagulation measures may be less reliable in predicting perioperative bleeding risk.

Other stigmata of liver disease

- Spider angiomata or spider nevi – vascular lesions with a central arteriole surrounded by many smaller vessels due to increased estradiol, occur in approximately one third of patients.
- Palmar erythema – are exaggerations of normal speckled mottling of the palm secondary to altered sex hormone metabolism.
- Nail changes:
  - Muehrcke's nails – paired horizontal bands separated by normal color are due to decreased albumin.
  - Terry's nails – proximal two thirds of the nail plate appear white with the distal one third red, also due to decreased albumin.
  - Clubbing – angle between nail plate and proximal nail fold is $>180°$.
- Hypertrophic osteoarthropathy – chronic proliferative periostitis of long bones can cause considerable pain.
- Dupuytren's contracture – thickening and shortening of the palmar fascia that leads to flexion deformities of the fingers, is possibly due to fibroblastic proliferation and disorderly collagen deposition.
- Gynecomastia – benign proliferation of glandular tissue of male breasts presenting with a rubbery or firm mass extending concentrically from the nipples is due to increased estradiol and can occur in up to 66% of patients.
- Hypogonadism – manifested as impotence, infertility, loss of sexual drive, and testicular atrophy, is due to 1° gonadal injury or suppression of hypothalamic or pituitary function.
- Caput medusa – in portal HTN, the umbilical vein may open. Blood from the portal venous system may be shunted through periumbilical veins into the umbilical vein and ultimately to abdominal wall veins.
- Cruveilhier–Baumgarten murmur – a venous hum is heard in the epigastric region, due to collateral connections between the portal system and the remnant of the umbilical vein in portal HTN.

- Fetor hepaticus – there is a musty odor in the breath due to increased dimethyl sulfide.
- Jaundice – yellowish discoloration of skin, eye, and mucus membranes is due to increased bilirubin (at least 30 mmol/L). Urine is tea-colored.

Anesthetic management

Patients with ESLD require a multidisciplinary approach in order to optimize perioperative care and minimize risk. Collaboration between surgery, anesthesia, hepatology, and ICU services allow for multifaceted input into management of these complex patients. Elective surgery is generally contraindicated in: acute liver failure, acute viral hepatitis, alcoholic hepatitis, cardiomyopathy, hypoxemia, and severe intractable coagulopathy.

Preoperative assessment

Detailed history with particular attention to:

- etiology and chronology of liver dysfunction
- infectious status of the patient and risk to healthcare providers
- presence and severity of portal hypertension – presence of esophageal varices, previous GI bleeding, severity and management of ascites, prior transjugular intrahepatic portosystemic shunt (TIPS) procedure (see later)
- presence and severity of hepatic encephalopathy, hepatorenal and/or hepatopulmonary syndromes
- nutritional status – cirrhotic patients tend to be malnourished due to protein and other dietary restrictions

Physical examination with particular attention to:

- extrahepatic manifestations of liver dysfunction
- presence of cardiopulmonary embarrassment – hyperdynamic circulation, cirrhotic cardiomyopathy, pleural effusion, hypoxia, orthodeoxia
- severity of ascites and its consequences on respiratory function, positioning, and abdominal tension
- assessment of intravascular volume status

Laboratory studies and investigations:

- CBC to assess for anemia and thrombocytopenia
- baseline renal function studies and electrolytes
- liver enzymes (alanine transaminase, aspartate transaminase, γ-glutamyl transferase, alkaline phosphatase) can be important markers of active hepatocellular or cholestatic disease, but they are of limited value in preoperative assessment and should not be performed routinely [26]
- liver synthetic function, assessed through serum albumin, bilirubin and the international normalized ratio (INR), provides more meaningful information for perioperative risk stratification
- baseline arterial blood gases if suspected respiratory compromise
- chest X-ray to assess for pleural effusions
- blood type and cross-match
- baseline electrocardiograph

- all patients with ESLD should undergo preoperative echocardiography to assess ventricular size and function, valvular function, pulmonary artery pressure, and to exclude left ventricle outflow tract obstruction, or pericardial effusion
- selective use of further cardiac investigations based on history and screening investigations

Risk stratification

In a patient with liver disease, perioperative risk depends on the severity of liver disease, nature of the surgical procedure, and presence of comorbid conditions.

Child–Turcotte–Pugh Score

- Was initially formulated in 1964 to predict risk in patients undergoing portosystemic surgery and modified by Pugh in 1974, and used historically to risk stratify patients having hepatic and non-hepatic surgery.
- Patients were quantified based on five categories: serum albumin, serum bilirubin, prothrombin time, ascites, and encephalopathy. Each parameter scored from 1–3 and totaled out of 15.
  - class A (5–6) – low operative mortality risk (5%–10%)
  - class B (7–9) – moderate operative mortality (25%–30%)
  - class C (10–15) – high operative mortality (>50%)
- It is a well-validated tool – perhaps the best predictor of 30-day mortality [27].
- Short comings include subjectivity of the severity of ascites and encephalopathy, broad categories of risk, and limited discriminatory capacity [27].

Model for ESLD (MELD)

- Devised as a tool to predict mortality after TIPS, then broadly employed to allocate organs in liver transplantation.
- Is a linear regression model based on serum creatinine, INR, and bilirubin.
- There is an approximately 1% increase in mortality for each one point increase in the MELD score from 5 to 20 and a 2% increase in mortality for each one point increase in the MELD score above 20 [28].
- Advantages include objectivity, weighting of variables, and no reliance on arbitrary cutoffs.
- Good predictor of three-month mortality [27] but incorporation of serum sodium into MELD (MELD-Na) may be a superior predictor of one-year mortality [27].
- ASA classification and age contribute to perioperative risk. ASA IV adds the equivalent of 5.5 points to the MELD score whereas an age >70 years adds 3 points to MELD [29].

Type of surgery

- Emergency surgery is associated with higher morbidity and mortality than elective surgery [29].
- Morbidity and mortality are highest in patients undergoing cardiac and open abdominal surgeries including cholecystectomy, gastric resection, colectomy, and hepatic resection [29].
- Trauma patients with cirrhosis at laparotomy are also at increased risk for morbidity and mortality [29].

Optimization

Correct fluid/electrolyte abnormalities:

- Consider 5% albumin to correct intravascular volume depletion, to prevent intraoperative hypotension.
- Take caution with rapid correction of chronic hyponatremia.

Correct hematological abnormalities:

- TEG may provide more accurate assessment of clinical hemostasis than standard laboratory assays and should be used to guide coagulation management when possible
- Platelets of $>50 \times 10^9$ is generally regarded as safe for surgery [23].
- Cryoprecipitate is indicated if fibrinogen is <1 g/L [23].
- Treat anemia based on patient status and planned surgical intervention.

Consider therapeutic paracentesis in patients with tense ascites:

- Improve pulmonary function and reduce aspiration risk.
- Intravascular volume re-equilibration occurs six to eight hours after the removal of ascitic fluid, thus volume repletion will be necessary [26].

Consider timing of preoperative dialysis in patients with overt renal failure:

- Target moderate glucose control (blood glucose level of <180 mg/dL or <10 mmol/L)

Intraoperative management

Anesthetic goals

Avoid aspiration:

- Consider rapid sequence induction.
- This may be in conflict with hemodynamic goals (see following).
- Consider aspiration prophylaxis in the form of H2 receptor blocker or sodium citrate

Avoid exacerbation of encephalopathy:

- Avoid sedative premedication.

Maintain adequate hepatic blood flow and oxygen delivery:

- The cirrhotic liver relies predominantly on hepatic arterial blood flow for the bulk of it perfusion due to restricted portal venous drainage.
- Thus, it is extremely vulnerable to hypoxia and hypoperfusion with systemic arterial hypotension.
- Other intraoperative factors that can affect hepatic blood flow include surgical traction on the liver, positive pressure ventilation, hypocapnia, α-adrenoceptor agonists and laparoscopic surgery [23].

Minimize blood loss:

- Utilize goal-directed management of coagulation.
- Avoid hypothermia.
- There is documented reduction of blood loss in hepatic resection with CVP of $<6\ cmH_2O$ but potential increased risk of renal injury and hemodynamic instability [30].

- Avoid placement of unnecessary esophageal devices (TEE probe, naso-and orosgastric tube, esophageal stethoscope, etc.) in patients with esophageal varices.
- Pharmacological therapy for acute esophageal variceal bleeding includes the combination of vasopressin and nitroglycerin, somatostatin, or octreotide [26].

Monitoring

- Intraoperative monitoring should be dictated by the pre-existing physical status of the patient and the scope of the planned surgical procedure.
- Invasive arterial and central venous lines are recommended for major surgery.
- Large bore intravenous access is mandatory for major surgery with fluid warming and rapid infusion devices available.
- Esophageal devices are best avoided; however, mid-esophageal TEE monitoring can provide valuable information regarding right heart function and volume status. Its use in selective patients can be justified.
- Urine output should be monitored and maintained in longer surgeries.
- Intraoperative TEG should be used to guide transfusion when possible.

Anesthetic pharmacology

Liver disease impacts perioperative pharmacology in several important ways:

- alterations in protein binding
- reduced serum albumin and other drug-binding proteins
- altered volume of distribution due to ascites and increased total-body water
- reduced drug metabolism due to abnormal hepatocyte function [26]

Intravenous anesthetics

- There is limited clinical and experimental data.
- Intravenous agents have a modest impact on hepatic blood flow.
- There is no meaningful adverse influence on postoperative liver function when arterial blood pressure is maintained.
- Etomidate – clearance is unchanged in cirrhotic patients, but clinical recovery time can be unpredictable.
- Propofol – elimination is similar in cirrhotic patients as normal patients, mean clinical recovery times may be prolonged with infusions.
- Midazolam – there is a prolonged duration of action with an enhanced sedative effect, especially after multiple doses or prolonged infusions.
- Ketamine – has little impact on hepatic blood flow even in large doses.
- Dexmedetomidine – primarily metabolized in the liver. Dose adjustments are therefore indicated with significant hepatic dysfunction [26].

Volatile anesthetics

- All current volatile anesthetics decrease mean arterial pressure and portal blood flow.
- Sevoflurane, desflurane, and isoflurane have been shown to preserve hepatic blood flow and function better than halothane or enflurane.

- Halothane causes hepatic artery vasoconstriction and increased hepatic arterial resistance.
- Halothane appears to disrupt HABR, whereas it is preserved with sevoflurane or isoflurane [26].

Neuromuscular blocking drugs

- Succinylcholine – liver disease is associated with decreased plasma cholinesterase activity, thus prolonged neuromuscular block is possible [20].
- Neuromuscular blocking drugs require a larger initial dose due to increased volume of distribution in cirrhotic patients.
- Advanced liver disease will reduce the elimination of vecuronium, rocuronium, and mivacurium, and prolong the duration of neuromuscular blockade, especially after repeated doses or the use of prolonged infusions.
- Atracurium and cisatracurium are not dependent on hepatic elimination and can be used without modification of dosing [20].

Opioids

- Morphine – significantly reduced metabolism with increased bioavailability resulting in prolonged action and exaggerated effects. Reduced dose and prolonged administration interval is recommended.
- Fentanyl – primarily metabolized by the liver. A single dose retains short duration of action due to redistribution; however, accumulation occurs with multiple doses or infusions. Elimination does not appear to be altered significantly in cirrhosis.
- Sufentanil – single-dose pharmacokinetics are not altered significantly in cirrhosis, although the impact of continuous infusions and reduced protein binding is ill defined.
- Alfentanil – half-life is almost doubled and higher free fractions of the drug are observed in ESLD. This can potentially lead to a prolonged duration of action and enhanced effects.
- Remifentanil – elimination is unaltered in patients with severe liver disease or in those undergoing liver transplantation [26].

Postoperative management

Disposition

- Low threshold for high acuity monitoring is used in the ICU setting.
- Monitor for new or worsening hepatorenal dysfunction.
- Careful monitoring of coagulation is important.
- Ongoing assessment of volume status should occur because of postoperative fluid shift.
- Worsening encephalopathy, jaundice, and ascites are important clinical markers of decompensation of liver function.
- Hypoglycemia may occur in patients with decompensated cirrhosis or acute liver failure as a result of depleted hepatic glycogen stores and impaired gluconeogenesis. Serum glucose levels should be monitored closely.
- Remove invasive catheters, when no longer required, to reduce infection.

Analgesia

- Patient-controlled analgesic devices have been used successfully in patients with advanced liver diseases. Care must be taken to adjust doses and interval time appropriately. They will require close monitoring when in use.
- Acetaminophen is not contraindicated but should be used with caution in liver disease.
- NSAIDs are best avoided due to platelet dysfunction and the potential to exacerbate GI bleeding and renal dysfunction.
- Regional techniques such as TAP blocks and local infiltration can be done safely; however, hematoma formation is a potential complication.
- Due to concerns with coagulation and deteriorating liver function postoperatively, central neuraxial techniques should not be used without careful risk–benefit analyses. Guidelines provided by the American Society of Regional Anesthesia should be observed.

Liver-specific procedures

TIPS

- Used to decompress portal hypertension and attenuate symptoms associated with portal hypertension.
- Although it can be done with sedation alone, TIPS is typically performed under general anesthesia in the interventional radiology suite.
- A stent is placed under fluoroscopy via the jugular vein into the hepatic vein. It is then advanced through the liver parenchyma into the portal vein.
- It is not uncommon for TIPS to precipitate or worsen hepatic encephalopathy [24].

Transarterial chemoembolization (TACE)

- Transarterial microcatheters are used to inject anticancer agents selectively into hepatic tumors.
- Selected arteries are then embolized in order to minimize damage to collateral hepatic tissue.
- Indications for TACE include hepatic tumors inappropriate for resection or transplant due to tumor or patients factors [24].

Hepatic resection

- There is up to 25% mortality rate in cirrhotic patients post-resection.
- Preoperative MELD score correlates with postoperative liver dysfunction, as does the extent of liver resection, not surprisingly.
- A high-risk for significant intraoperative hemorrhage exists and should be anticipated in planning anesthesia management.

References

1. Levey AS, Atkins RR, Coresh JJ, et al. Chronic kidney disease as a global public health problem: approaches and initiatives– a position statement from Kidney Disease Improving Global Outcomes. *Kidney Int* 2007; **72**: 247–59.

2. Levey AS, Coresh J, Balk E, et al. National Kidney Foundation practice guidelines for chronic kidney disease: evaluation, classification, and stratification. *Ann Intern Med* 2003; **139**: 137–47.

3. Trainor D, Borthwick E, Ferguson A. Perioperative management of the

hemodialysis patient. *Semin Dial* 2011; **24**: 314–26.

4. Arora P, Vasa P, Brenner D, et al. Prevalence estimates of chronic kidney disease in Canada: results of a nationally representative survey. *Can Med Assoc J* 2013; **185**: E417–23.
5. Craig RGR, Hunter JMJ. Recent developments in the perioperative management of adult patients with chronic kidney disease. *Br J Anaesth* 2008; **101**: 296–310.
6. Eilers H, Liu KD, Gruber A, et al. Chronic kidney disease: implications for the perioperative period. *Minerva Anestesiol* 2010; **76**: 725–36.
7. Schiffrin EL, Lipman ML, Mann JE. Chronic kidney disease: effects on the cardiovascular system. *Circulation* 2007; **116**: 85–97.
8. Pabst S, Hammerstingl C, Hundt F, et al. Pulmonary hypertension in patients with chronic kidney disease on dialysis and without dialysis: results of the PEPPER Ssudy. *PLoS One* 2012; **7**: e35310.
9. Yigla MM, Nakhoul FF, Sabag AA, et al. Pulmonary hypertension in patients with end-stage renal disease. *Chest* 2003; **123**: 1577–82.
10. Jalal DI, Chonchol M, Targher G. Disorders of hemostasis associated with chronic kidney disease. *Semin Thromb Hemost* 2010; **36**: 34–40.
11. Pivalizza EG, Abramson DC, Harvey A. Perioperative hypercoagulability in uremic patients: a viscoelastic study. *J Clin Anesth* 1997; **9**: 442–5.
12. Obrador GT, Pereira BJ. Systemic complications of chronic kidney disease. Pinpointing clinical manifestations and best management. *Postgrad Med* 2002; **111**: 115–22.
13. Thomson H, Macnab R. Fluid and electrolyte problems in renal dysfunction. *Anaesth Intensive Care Med* 2009; **10**: 289–92.
14. Pecoits-Filho RR, Gonçalves SS, Barberato SHS, et al. Impact of residual renal function on volume status in chronic renal failure. *Blood Purif* 2004; **22**: 285–92.
15. Perazella MAM. Drug-induced hyperkalemia: old culprits and new offenders. *Am J Med* 2000; **109**: 307–14.
16. Novis BK, Roizen MF, Aronson S, et al. Association of preoperative risk factors with postoperative acute renal failure. *Anesth Analg* 1994; **78**: 143–9.
17. Fleisher LA, Beckman JA, Brown KA, et al. ACC/AHA 2007 guidelines on perioperative cardiovascular evaluation and care for noncardiac surgery: a report of the American College of Cardiology/American Heart Association Task Force on Practice Guidelines (Writing Committee to revise the 2002 guidelines on perioperative cardiovascular evaluation for noncardiac surgery). *Circulation* 2007; **116**: e418–500.
18. Ricaurte L, Vargas J, Lozano E, et al. Organ Transplant Group. Anesthesia and kidney transplantation. *Transplant Proc* 2013; **45**: 1386–91.
19. Wagener G, Brentjens TE. Anesthetic concerns in patients presenting with renal failure. *Anesthesiol Clin* 2010; **28**: 39–54.
20. Craig RG, Hunter JM. Neuromuscular blocking drugs and their antagonists in patients with organ disease. *Anaesthesia* 2009; **64**: 55–65.
21. Baxi VV, Jain AA, Dasgupta DD. Anaesthesia for renal transplantation: an update. *Indian J Anaesth* 2009; **53**: 139–47.
22. O Malley CMN, Frumento RJ, Hardy MA, et al. A randomized, double-blind comparison of lactated ringer's solution and 0.9% NaCl during renal transplantation. *Anesth Analg* 2005; **100**: 1518–24.
23. Vaja R, McNicol L, Sisley I. Anaesthesia for patients with liver disease. *Br J Anaesth CEPD Rev* 2010; **10**: 15–19.
24. Dalal A, Lang JD Jr. Anesthetic considerations for patients with liver disease. In: Abdeldayem H, ed. *Hepatic Surgery*. InTech, 2013. Available from: http://www.intechopen.com/books/hepatic-surgery/anesthetic-considerations-for-patients-with-liver-disease

5. Cardenas ASC. Hepatorenal syndrome: a dreaded complication of end-stage liver disease. *Am J Gastroenterol* 2005; **100**: 460–7.

6. Rothenberg DM, O'Connor CJ, Tuman KJ. Anesthesia and the hepatobiliary system. In: *Miller's Anesthesia, 7th Edition.* Elsevier Churchill Livingstone, 2010; 2135–53.

7. Causey MW, Steele SR, Farris Z, et al. An assessment of different scoring systems in cirrhotic patients undergoing nontransplant surgery. *Am J Surg* 2012; **203**: 589–93.

28. Pandey CK, Karna ST, Pandey VK, et al. Perioperative risk factors in patients with liver disease undergoing non-hepatic surgery. *World J Gastrointest Surg* 2012; **4**: 267–74.

29. Teh SH, Nagorney DM, Stevens SR, et al. Risk factors for mortality after surgery in patients with cirrhosis. *Gastroenterology* 2007; **132**: 1261–9.

30. Liu LL, Niemann CU. Intraoperative management of liver transplant patients. *Transplant Rev* 2011; **25**: 124–9.

Chapter 28

Transplant patients

A. Dhir and A. Suphathamwit

Introduction

Between 2002 and 2012, more than 25 000 solid organ transplants were performed annuall in the U.S. With current advances, survival of both the recipients as well as the transplante organs is improving continually. The number of people surviving solid organ transplant ation is higher than ever before. One-year and five-year survival rates are shown i Table 28.1.

Although organ transplantation has changed the management paradigm, it still remain a treatment rather than the cure for patients with end-stage organ disease. Immunosup pression is a necessary evil with significant side effects. The incidence of many disease requiring surgical interventions is increased in transplant patients [2]. To formulate specific plan for safe anesthetic, understanding of the altered physiology, effects c immunosuppression, and other risks such as infection and allograft rejection is essential.

Physiological changes in transplanted recipients

General health

- Although the majority of transplant recipients are able to lead a normal life, their functional reserves may be limited. Successful organ transplantation corrects most of the symptoms that were caused by the failing organ. This improvement persists until th graft starts to deteriorate. However, some functional abnormalities from the underlyin illness or from the transplantation itself may persist (e.g., diabetic autonomic neuropathy).
- Physical work capacity of most post-transplant patients is only 38%–64% of normal values. However, near normal values can be achieved by training. Lung transplant recipients have the lowest performance values.

Post-heart transplantation

Physiology of the denervated heart:

- Vagal tone is lost and the baseline heart rate is increased, typically at 90–100 beats/min Heart rate does not respond to the carotid sinus massage, Valsalva maneuver, or sympathetic stimulation caused by hypovolemia, laryngoscopy, or inadequate analgesia/anesthesia.

Anesthesia and Perioperative Care of the High-Risk Patient, Third edition, ed. Ian McConachie. Published by Cambridge University Press.

Table 28.1. Number of transplanted patients and survival (2012) (Adapted from [1].)

Organ	Number of recipients	1-yr graft survival	1-yr patient survival	5-yr graft survival	5-yr patient survival
Kidney	16487	87%–94%	91%–99%	58%–100%	64%–100%
Liver	6256	78%–84%	81%–92%	63%–75%	62%–85%
Heart	2378	82%–89%	83%–90%	66%–75%	65%–77%
Lung	1754	76%–88%	77%–88%	34%–50%	37%–52%

Cardiac output is preload dependent. Cardiac performance relies on the Frank–Starling mechanism as well as on circulating catecholamines.

Direct acting sympathomimetic drugs such as epinephrine, norepinephrine, isoproterenol, and dobutamine have augmented inotropic effects than indirectly acting agents like dopamine and ephedrine [3].

Inotropic effect of digoxin is preserved, but its effect on the heart rate is not.

Other drugs that act through the autonomic nervous system generally have minimal effects or side effects. These include anticholinergic agents, anticholinesterase agents, nifedipine, phenylephrine, and sodium nitroprusside [4]. However, neostigmine can still cause bradycardia by direct activation of cholinergic receptors on cardiac ganglionic cells [5,6].

Re-innervation has been reported to occur after heart transplantation but its timing may vary.

n biatrial anastomosis, there maybe two P-waves on the electrocardiograph (ECG), because f the intact native sinoatrial node. This has no hemodynamic importance. Right bundle–ranch block is also common. Spirometry-derived lung volumes normalize during the first ear, but carbon monoxide diffusion capacity remains reduced.

ost-lung transplantation

Denervation:

- Bilateral lung transplantation requires tracheal anastomosis, disrupting pulmonary innervation. This results in absence of the cough reflex and patients are prone to silent aspiration and retention of secretions. In single-lung transplantation, the cough reflex remains intact but the aspiration risk still exists.
- Rarely, bronchial hyper-responsiveness may occur.
- Denervation has minimal effects on respiratory rate or rhythm. Lung recipients tend to have increased tidal volume rather than respiratory rate.
- Airway tone, primarily controlled via parasympathetic efferents is preserved. Response to β_2-adrenergic agonists on airway tone and hypoxic pulmonary vasoconstriction is also preserved.
- Disruption of lymphatic drainage makes lung-transplant recipients susceptible to fluid overload and pulmonary edema [7].

There is dramatic improvement in lung function, gas exchange, and exercise tolerance. Arterial oxygenation usually returns to normal.

- Emphysematous patients after lung transplantation may still have prolonged hypercapnia for weeks, secondary to blunted ventilatory response to CO_2. Persistent hypercapnia suggests either allograft dysfunction or diaphragmatic dysfunction from phrenic nerve injury.
- Total lung capacity and FEV_1 tend to decrease in the first postoperative month with a gradual improvement over subsequent months.
- Mucociliary and bactericidal activity of alveolar macrophages are altered in the early post-transplant period. Perioperative chest physical therapy is of great importance.
- In patients with single-lung transplant, 60%–70% of pulmonary perfusion is directed toward the transplanted lung [8].

Post-liver transplant

- Normal physiological mechanisms that protect liver blood flow are blunted after liver transplantation. The liver is an important source of maintaining blood volume in shock states via a vasoconstrictive response, and this mechanism may be impaired after liver transplantation.
- Hyperdynamic state, a hallmark of end-stage liver disease, is reversed. Overall cardiac performance improves in the months following liver transplantation.
- Hypoxemia caused by ventilation/perfusion mismatch is usually reversed within the first month. There is complete resolution or significant improvement in gas exchange in the majority of patients with hepatopulmonary syndrome (HPS). However, recovery time in HPS is variable and may take more than one year. In pre-existing right-to-left shunts, hypoxemia takes even longer to recover or may never resolve.
- Recurrence of pre-transplant disease – hepatitis B and C – recur in more than 90% of cases. Other diseases known to recur in a transplanted liver are cholangiocarcinoma, hepatocellular carcinoma (HCC), and autoimmune liver disease. About 15% of patients revert back to alcohol intake (recidivism).

Post-kidney transplant

- Serum creatinine in patients with a functioning renal graft may be normal, but the effective renal plasma flow and the glomerular filtration rates are likely to be lower. Drug excretion activity may be prolonged.
- There is an increased incidence and severity of cardiovascular diseases especially in the diabetic and elderly patients.

Immunosuppression

With combinations of drugs targeting various pathways in recipients' immune system, rates of rejection have declined significantly.

Immunosuppressive agents can be classified simply as [9]:

- interleukin (IL)-2 inhibitors: calcinurin inhibitors (CNIs), mammalian target-of-rapamycin (mTOR) inhibitors
- nucleic acid inhibitors: azathioprine, mycophenolate mofetil (MMF)
- cytokine gene inhibitors: corticosteroids
- T-cell inhibitors: monoclonal antibodies

Table 28.2. Drugs altering blood levels of CNIs. (Adapted from [2].)

Drugs increasing CNI levels	Drugs decreasing CNI levels
Calcium channel blockers • Amlodipine • Nicardipine • Diltiazem • Verapamil	Anti-convulsive agents • Phenobarbital • Carbamazepine • Phenytoin • Valproic acid
Antibiotics and anti-fungal drugs • Clarithromycin/erythromycin • Imepenem/cilastatin • Fluconazole • Itraconazole • Ketonazole	Antibiotics • Nafcilin • Rifampicin • Sulfadimidine-trimethoprim
Others • Allopurinol • Acetazolamide • Bromocriptine • Colchicine • Danazol • Metoclopramide • Methyl testosterone • Oral contraceptives • Sulindac	Others • Ticlopidine • Octrotide

CNIs

- Cyclosporine A was the first CNI approved for clinical use in organ transplantation. It can be administered intravenously or orally, although enteral absorption is variable.
- Tacrolimus is a newer and more potent CNI with a 10–100-fold increased potency than cyclosporine in vitro. It has replaced cyclosporine for maintenance immunosuppression. It can be administered enterally, parentally, and sublingually.
- Both CNIs have a narrow therapeutic window and their levels must be closely monitored. They are metabolized via the hepatic cytochrome P-450 system, therefore are susceptible to drug interactions (Table 28.2).

mTOR inhibitors

- Sirolimus inhibits mTOR. Everolimus is a sirolimus derivative with a shorter half-life but similar adverse effects.
- Potential lack of nephrotoxicity and possible anti-cancer properties are the most favorable effects.

Nucleic acid inhibitors

- Azathioprine is the oldest drug in this category.
  - It can be administered orally or intravenously.

- Important drug interaction causing increased 6MP levels occurs with allopurinol, angiotensin-converting enzyme inhibitors, sulfasalazine, and 5-amino salicylic acid.
- MMF is another widely used anti-proliferative agent, hydrolyzed to mycophenolic acid.

Corticosteroids

- Unbound steroid diffuses passively through the cell membrane and binds to intracellular cytosolic receptors, resulting in decreased cytokine production, reduced lymphocyte proliferation, and changes in cellular trafficking [10].
- A general protocol is to administer fixed-dose intravenous methylprednisolone perioperatively. The maintenance dose is typically reduced to physiological doses.

T-cell inhibitors (monoclonal antibodies)

- Most commonly used agents are humanized or chimeric monoclonal antibody to CD 25, including daclizumab and basiliximab. These are well tolerated. Alemtuzumab is another humanized monoclonal antibody to CD 52, a cell surface marker (Table 28.3).

Table 28.3. Summary of adverse effects of immunosuppressive agents [10–12]

Immunosuppressive agents	Adverse effects
Calcineurin inhibitors	• Nephrotoxicity • Hypertension, hyperlipidemia • Diabetes • Electrolyte abnormalities • Neurotoxicity
mTOR inhibitors	• Impaired wound healing • Venous thromboembolism • Diarrhea, nausea • Cytopenia • Hyperlipidemia
Nucleic acid inhibitors	• Myelo-suppression • Pancreatitis and cholestatic hepatitis • Gastrointestinal disturbances (nausea, diarrhea, abdominal pain) • Neutropenia and anemia • Hypersensitivity reaction (rare)
Corticosteroids	• Weight gain, hyperglycemia, hypertension, and hyperlipidemia • Osteoporosis • Peptic ulcer and GI bleed • Adrenal insufficiency
T-cell inhibitors	• Anaphylaxis • Severe cytopenia • Aseptic meningitis • Nausea and vomiting

Infection

- Advanced immunosuppression increases the susceptibility of recipients to opportunistic infections. Early detection and specific treatment is essential to minimize anti-microbial therapy that frequently has toxic effects and usually interacts with immunosuppressive therapy.
- Detection of infection in post-transplant patients may be challenging because signs and symptoms of infection in an immune-compromised host are often diminished while fever may be present due to a non-infectious cause like allograft rejection.

Types of infection

- Donor-derived infections: screening for donor infection is limited by the present technology and time constraints. Unfortunately, negative results do not guarantee infection-free organs and some active infections may still remain undetected [13].
  - Latent infections in the donor organ, e.g., cytomegalovirus (CMV), tuberculosis, or *Trypanosoma cruzi* (*T. cruzi*).
  - Organ donors infected by drug-resistance organisms like vancomycin-resistant enterococcus (VRE) and azole-resistant candida species.
  - Rare central nervous system infections that are hardly recognized: West Nile virus, rabies, HIV, and Chagas disease.
  - Hepatitis B-infected liver donors are now used for some vaccinated or seropositive recipients. Use of hepatitis C-infected organs is limited to seropositive recipients only.
- Recipient-derived infections:
  - Common recipient-derived infections are tuberculosis, parasites (*Strongyloides stercoralis, T. cruzi*), viral (CMV, Epstein–Barr virus [EBV], varicella zoster virus, hepatitis B and C virus, and HIV), and some endemic fungi.
  - Some recipients can also be colonized with nosocomial and drug-resistance organisms while awaiting transplantation.
- Community-acquired infections: exposure to some environmental organisms may cause fatal infection after transplantation, including aspergillus, nocardia species (in soil), *C. neoformans* (in birds), and other respiratory viruses.

Graft rejection

Graft rejection often presents as deterioration in the graft function. Common signs and symptoms may include fever, chills, fatigue, and leukocytosis. Allograft tissue biopsy is always required for definitive diagnosis. Elective operations should be postponed due to higher morbidity and mortality [14].

Post-heart transplantation

- Almost 40% of heart-transplant recipients experience an episode of acute rejection. After the first year, acute rejection is rare.
- Signs and symptoms suggestive of acute rejection include bradycardia, atrial fibrillation or flutter, fatigue, fever, unexplained weight gain, peripheral edema, and dyspnea.

Myocardial biopsy should be performed to confirm the diagnosis, although negative results do not totally exclude rejection.

- Mild rejection does not affect cardiac contractility significantly; severe rejection causes systolic and diastolic dysfunction.
- Chronic allograft rejection usually presents as accelerated coronary artery disease (transplant vasculopathy), a leading cause of death in long-standing cardiac recipients. The disease is diffuse, involves distal coronary vessels, and is not amenable to revascularization. Significant silent myocardial ischemia may occur due to denervation [15].

Post-lung transplantation

- Acute rejection usually presents with dyspnea and hypoxemia. Prompt investigation with bronchoscopy, lung biopsy, and bronchoalveolar lavage should be performed.
- Bronchiolitis obliterans represents chronic rejection, is uncommon during the first six months, but affects up to 50%–60% of patients who survive five years after transplantation. It manifests as gradual-onset dyspnea, cough, and recurrent bouts of purulent tracheobronchitis, and it limits patient survival. Investigations show air trapping in the chest radiograph, evidence of inflammation, submucosal fibrosis, and luminal obliteration of the small airways. This can progress to chronic obstructive pulmonary disease [16].

Post-liver transplant

- Elevated bilirubin after three months of transplantation favors rejection, biliary obstruction, or hepatitis.
- Clinical manifestations of graft rejection include jaundice, dark urine, pale stools, pruritus, peripheral edema, ascites, asterixis, weight gain, increased prothrombin time, and decreased albumin.

Post-kidney transplant

- Important signs of graft rejection are reduced urine output, presence of uremic symptoms, progressive azotemia, proteinuria, hypertension, recent weight gain, and edema.
- Some patients with chronic graft rejection are dialysis dependent.
- Biopsy is often required to differentiate rejection from acute CNI nephrotoxicity. Fever and pain at the allograft site suggest rejection as these rarely occur with immunosuppression.

Post-transplantation malignancies

It is estimated that over the next 20 years, mortality from malignancy might exceed that from cardiovascular complications among transplanted patients [17]. Common post transplant malignancies include skin cancer, lymphoproliferative disorder, and other solid organ malignancies. Immunosuppressive agents are involved in carcinogenesis.

Post-transplant lymphoproliferative disorders (PTLDs)

- PTLDs are the second most common malignancy in renal transplant recipients, occurring in approximately 11% of recipients. Although overall frequency is less than 2%, they are the major cause of cancer-related mortality, ranging from 30% to 60% [17,18].
- Clinical manifestations can vary from mononucleosis or tonsillar hyperplasia in pediatric patients (benign form), to frank lymphomas.
- Reduction in immunosuppression improves survival in patients with PTLD. Use of systemic chemotherapy (CHOP regimen: cyclophosphamide, hydroxydaunorubicin, oncovin, and prednisolone) is a common practice, but not without significant morbidity and/or mortality [17].

Post-transplant skin malignancies

- Non-melanotic skin cancers are the most common. Squamous cell carcinoma (SCC) occurred 65–250 times more frequently than in the general population and basal cell carcinoma increased by a factor of 10 [19]. SCC in post-transplant population tends to be more aggressive than in the general population. Almost 15% of all SCC is associated with multiple recurrences or metastasis.
- Melanoma has also been a significant concern in post-transplant recipients due to distant metastasis. Whole body investigation and proper staging is essential.

Solid organ malignancies

- Post-transplant patients are at higher risk for developing malignancy not only from chronic immunosuppression, but also from their underlying chronic disease. Early detection and prompt treatment is critical.
  - Cardiac- and lung-transplant patients often have an extensive smoking history predisposing them to lung and esophageal cancer.
  - Duration of end-stage renal disease (ESRD) is the primary determinant for renal cell carcinoma in post-renal transplant patients, with an estimated incidence of 4.2% [20,21].
  - Both hepatitis B and C viruses are associated with HCC. Risk of malignant transformation is reported at 0.05% per year in the setting of a chronic hepatitis infection.
  - Patients with primary sclerosing cholangitis often have concurrent ulcerative colitis. The presence of both is associated with colorectal cancer and/or cholangio carcinoma. The incidence of colon cancer in post-transplant patients is higher than in the general population with a lower survival rate.
- Certain viral infections are also linked with particular malignancies: EBV with lymphoproliferative disorder, hepatitis B and C virus with HCC, human herpes virus-8 with Kaposi's sarcoma, and possibly papillomaviruses with squamous cell carcinoma.
- Some immunosuppressive agents possess antitumor effects and are widely used to reduce the incidence of post-transplant malignancy.
  - MMF has anti-proliferative activity against leukemias and lymphomas. It also demonstrates significant antitumor effects against colon, prostate, and skin cancers.
  - Utility of antitumor effects of sirolimus is limited due to impaired wound healing and hepatic artery thrombosis.

Table 28.4. Bone disorders in transplant patients (Adapted from [22].)

Persistent pre-transplant disorders	Post-transplant disorders
• Osteopenia/osteoporosis	• Epiphyseal impaction • Avascular bone necrosis • Reactive arthritis (post-antithymoglobulin administration, CMV infection) • Infectious arthritis • Renal tubular dysfunction • Crystal-induced arthritis

Post-transplant bone disorders

Bone disorders are not rare in post-transplant patients and are shown in Table 28.4.

Preoperative evaluation and preparation

No elective surgery should be performed during an episode of rejection due to high mortality [23]. Elective surgery should preferably be done one year post-transplant, or at least six months post-transplant, and it should ideally be conducted at a transplant center. There should be good communication between the transplant team and the perioperative care team. The basic principle of preoperative evaluation in the post-organ transplantation recipient is to assess all organ systems. One should assess physical activity, evaluate the functional state of the graft, and look for signs and symptoms of infection and rejection. Other comorbidities such as diabetes, hypertension, and ischemic heart disease should also be looked for and their severity assessed.

Cardiovascular system

- Cardiovascular disease (CVD) is the leading cause of morbidity and mortality in organ transplant patients, especially post-renal transplant.
- Patients should have an extensive cardiovascular evaluation before undergoing non-transplant surgery. An exercise tolerance test should be performed for at-risk patients. Cardiac catheterization is also suggested in patients where myocardial ischemia is suspected.
- One important question is: "How long can a negative result be relied upon?" This should be decided on an individual basis [24].
- In post-heart transplant patients, the ECG is assessed for rhythm, heart rate variability QT-interval, and signs of ischemia. Right bundle–branch block is common. A second P-wave generated from the recipient's remnant atrium (if the surgical technique was biatrial anastomosis) is functionally insignificant and disappears with time. Up to 5% of post-heart transplant patients will present with a pacemaker requiring confirmation of proper function [25].

Pulmonary system

- In general, chest auscultation and chest X-ray should be performed routinely in the search for infection and intra-thoracic PTLDs.

- In post-lung transplant recipients, spirometry is usually normal and the presence of airway obstruction may indicate obliterative bronchiolitis.

Liver function

- Hepatic dysfunction may occur in all transplant patients, and is the most common cause of death in long-term kidney transplant survivors [26].
- Liver enzymes and coagulation profile should be checked. Measurement of plasma pre-albumin or galactose elimination capacity is also widely used [27,28].

Kidney function

- Because heart and lung transplant recipients require higher levels of immunosuppression, there seems to be a correlation with the greater occurrence of kidney dysfunction.
- It is estimated that at least 18% of liver recipients, 20% of lung recipients, and 32% of heart recipients will develop some degree of renal dysfunction at five years post-transplant [29].

Hematologic system

- Vascular thrombosis of the allograft can lead to serious consequences and eventual loss of the transplanted organ. Thrombophilic conditions can be found in various situations, including the hypercoagulable state of liver transplantation.
- On the other hand, a failing liver can lead to coagulopathy.
- After kidney transplantation, there may be a sudden increase in erythropoietin levels with the production of vast amounts of red blood cells that may cause peripheral vascular insufficiency or congestive heart failure [26].

Level of immunosuppression

- It is important to maintain immunosuppression at all times.
- In general, oral immunosuppression is preferred. Agents can be administered via a nasogastric tube, if suction is avoided.
- It may be difficult to achieve full immunosuppression when gastrointestinal absorption is impaired, such as with surgical ileus, small bowel obstruction, or diarrhea. Under these conditions, temporary conversion to intravenous formulation is acceptable with appropriate dose adjustments. However, the parenteral form may not always be available and some agents may need special concerns. Intravenous (IV) doses of azathioprine and corticosteroids need not change. On the other hand, corticosteroid doses can be increased as an emergency measure to treat acute rejection. When converting from the oral regimen, an IV dose of cyclosporine A should be reduced. IV preparations of cyclosporine can cause anaphylactic reactions, vasoconstriction, and hyperkalemia, and are not compatible with many plastic materials.
- In life-threatening situations such as severe infection not responding to aggressive treatment, it may be necessary to discontinue immunosuppression temporarily. The clinical course is followed closely with reinstitution of immunosuppression as soon as clinically possible.

Risk of postsurgical infection

- Antibiotic prophylaxis plays an important role in the perioperative management of post-transplant patients. Although these patients may be considered at higher risk of developing infectious complications, there is no evidence suggesting benefits of prolongation, or addition of routine antibiotic prophylaxis [24].
- Because of unusual clinical presentation, it is prudent to use culture reports for selecting proper antibiotics.
- It is recommended to avoid antibiotics that interact with immunosuppressive agents (Table 28.2) or have potential renal toxicity.

Adrenal insufficiency

- Patients who have received more than 20 mg/day of prednisolone or equivalent for more than three weeks in the preceding one year should be assumed to have hypothalamic–pituitary–adrenal axis suppression. However, patients are normally maintained on lower doses, usually 5–10 mg/day of prednisolone.
- Current recommendation is to let the patients who are on low-dose glucocorticoids receive their usual low dose in the perioperative period. Rarely, additional steroids to accommodate acute stress may be required [30].

Anesthetic considerations

Anesthetic technique

Various methods of anesthetic technique such as local, general, regional, and monitored anesthesia care have been used successfully in post-transplant patients.

- Main goal in the perioperative period is to prevent infection, avoid graft (and other organ) hypoperfusion and hypoxia, and prevent graft rejection.
- Patient's physical status, surgical procedure, specific risks related to intubation and mechanical ventilation, cardiovascular risks, and susceptibility of graft-to-fluid overload should be taken into consideration.
- If regional anesthesia is planned, bleeding risk should be ruled out by clotting studies and platelet count.
- Epidural anesthesia is preferred to spinal anesthesia for post-heart transplant patients, in whom profound hypotension and bradycardia should be avoided. Bleeding risk from possible collateral vessels in patients with portal hypertension, risks of catheter infection, and impaired intercostal muscle function should be kept in mind before the epidural.
- Because CNIs may cause neurotoxicity and decrease seizure threshold, it seems prudent to avoid hyperventilation.

Premedication

- Immunosuppressive agents should be administered and monitored daily.
- Standard premedication can be used in most cases.
- Anxiolytics are usually preferred (if at all) over opioids in post-lung transplant recipients to prevent respiratory depression.

Monitoring

Type of surgery, anesthetic plan, and availability of equipment determines the choice of perioperative monitoring techniques.

- In most cases, noninvasive standard monitoring (ECG, noninvasive blood pressure, pulse oximetry, end-tidal carbon dioxide, and temperature) is sufficient.
- Proper management of fluid status may require monitors that assess the volume status accurately. Dynamic parameters (e.g., pulse pressure variation or stroke volume variation) are theoretically better than static parameters (cardiovascular or pulmonary artery pressure).
- Invasive monitoring should be discussed according to risk and benefit and should be limited to the minimum with strict aseptic techniques.
- Use of antiseptic-impregnated catheters decreases catheter bacterial colonization and associated infections by over 60% in post-transplant patients [31].
- Superior vena cava stricture or thrombosis may interfere with the central venous pressure reading in post-heart transplant patients. The site of the internal jugular cannulation may be discussed with the transplant cardiologist if the right internal jugular vein is needed for biopsy of the transplanted heart.

Positioning

- Positioning of the patient requires extreme care, especially with the prone position. Patients are at risk for bone fractures.

Control of the airway

- Post-transplant patients have increased risk for aspiration.
- Delayed gastric emptying time and gastric atony respond to metoclopramide.
- Simple facemask or laryngeal mask ventilation should be avoided, except for short and non-complicated procedures.
- Oral intubation is preferred over nasal intubation because of the risks of infection and bleeding.
- Early extubation is highly recommended, as prolonged mechanical ventilation increases the risk of bacterial pneumonia.

Anesthetic agents

Intravenous agents

- Benzodiazepines should be used with caution where early extubation is required.
- Propofol is a safe induction agent, as long as one is aware of its potent vasodilatory effects and concomitant hypotension.
- Etomidate may be a better choice for unstable cardiovascular patients.
- Ketamine should be avoided in patients with renal impairment [32].

Inhalation agents

Isoflurane appears to be the preferred inhalation agent [33]. Sevoflurane and desflurane also appear safe, but there is a paucity of data.

Neuromuscular blocking agents

- Cyclosporine increases the block produced by non-depolarizing muscle relaxants.
- Succinylcholine (if not contraindicated) and atracurium after renal transplant, and atracurium or cisatracurium after liver transplantation are considered good choices [33].
- Rocuronium has been used safely in post-transplant patients and is also preferred for rapid sequence intubation where succinylcholine cannot be used.
- Pancuronium is excreted predominantly in urine and should not be used in kidney dysfunction patients, whereas vecuronium has also been used successfully.

Local anesthetic agents

- Bupivacaine is a widely used local anesthetic. Although renal impairment may result in increased risk of toxicity, it can be used safely in clinical doses [23].

Specific considerations

Post-heart transplantation

- If required, premedication can be prescribed as usual.
- One should be aware of pharmacological and pharmacodynamic changes associated with the denervated heart.
- Both general and regional anesthesia have been used safely.
- If neuraxial block is considered, preload must be carefully maintained.
- Intravenous anesthetic agents should be used with caution due to their vasodilatory effects. Propofol has been used safely in many euvolemic post-heart transplant patients [4].
- Although volatile anesthetics have some degree of myocardial depressant effects, they can be used safely.
- If intraoperative hemodynamic instability is expected, invasive monitoring including central venous or pulmonary artery catheterization is indicated. Noninvasive cardiac output monitoring is useful and transesophageal echocardiography provides assessment of the volume status and myocardial function. Again, monitors employing dynamic parameters for fluid responsiveness may be helpful.
- Amiodarone or verapamil are indicated for tachyarrythmias, whereas isoproterenol and epinephrine are the agents of choice for bradycardia.
- Transplanted hearts still respond to glucagon and phosphodiesterase inhibitors (milrinone, amrinone). Levosimendan, a calcium sensitizer, may improve cardiac function in post-heart transplant patients [34][35].

Post-lung transplantation

- Premedication with sedatives should be used with extreme caution in patients with marginal gas exchange or CO_2 retention. Anti-sialogogues are indicated if inspection of the airways is being performed.
- Post-lung transplant patients are vulnerable to fluid overload. Invasive monitoring may be necessary in cases of anticipated significant blood loss or large fluid shifts.

- Regional anesthesia provides some advantages over general anesthesia. It reduces the risk of airway trauma and aspiration while allowing earlier patient cooperation for postoperative pulmonary hygiene [4].
- If thoracic epidural blockade is used for postoperative pain relief, one should avoid dense intercostal muscle block. Peripheral nerve blocks are feasible and well tolerated. Patients whose respiratory reserve relies on the integrity of both hemi-diaphragms, inter-scalene brachial plexus block or deep cervical plexus block should be avoided due to the high incidence of phrenic nerve palsy with these blocks [16].
- Airway management in post-lung transplant patients is challenging. Mask ventilation or laryngeal mask airway can be used for short and simple procedures, but risks for silent aspiration should be kept in mind.
- Strict aseptic technique, use of air filters, sterile laryngoscopes, and breathing circuits are recommended. Oral intubation is preferred to nasal intubation. Moderate to deep anesthesia with gentle intubation is extremely helpful.
- Bilateral lung transplantation:
  - Cuff of the endotracheal tube should be placed just beyond the vocal cords to avoid trauma at the anastomotic site. Compliance of both lungs is normal; they are easy to ventilate.
  - One-lung ventilation can generally be performed with a double-lumen tube, a Univent tube, or bronchial blockers under fiberoptic bronchoscopic guidance to avoid trauma at the tracheobronchial anastomosis.
  - "Lung protective strategy" employing small tidal volume, higher respiratory rate, limiting the peak inspiratory pressure to 30–35 cmH_2O and PEEP of 5–8 cm of H_2O is recommended. It provides adequate gas exchange, lowers the stress to the surgical anastomosis with a decreased incidence of postoperative lung dysfunction [36].
- Mechanical ventilation of the single-lung transplant recipient is more complicated.
  - If the primary pathology was emphysema, the native lung is hyperinflated. It can be overinflated further if there is increased airway resistance or decreased compliance of the transplanted lung. This situation can result from sputum retention, intra-abdominal hypertension, prolonged use of the Trendelenberg position, and fluid overload.
  - If the native lung has restrictive pathology, lung expansion requires high airway pressure and may cause baro or volume trauma to the allograft. Differential lung ventilation with placement of a double-lumen tube and two ventilators may be considered. Special ventilation techniques, such as high-frequency jet ventilation, have been used in select cases, but not routinely [37].
  - Single-lung allograft receives the major part of ventilation and perfusion [4], and this should be kept in mind if the lateral decubitus position is mandated. In one-lung ventilation, if allograft deflation is required, hypoxemia is likely to occur.
- Extubation under deep anesthesia should be avoided due to risks of aspiration and retained secretions.

Post-liver transplantation

Because of denervation, the normal mechanism to maintain hepatic blood flow is impaired, making the liver allograft prone to ischemic injury. Therefore, intravascular

volume and systemic blood pressure should be kept normal [38]. One should avoid agents decreasing hepatic blood flow, such as propranolol and cimetidine.
- Newer inhalational agents appear safe; however, there is paucity of data. Isoflurane should be considered the volatile anesthetic of choice due to its decreased portal resistance effect and potentially improved portal blood flow [39].
- Increased splanchnic vascular resistance also impairs hepatic perfusion; therefore, light anesthesia, hypoxia, hypercapnia, high airway pressure, and excessive PEEP should be avoided [4].
- Epidural analgesia can be performed, provided coagulation parameters are normal.
- Immediately after liver transfusion, over-transfusion of blood products lead to hemoconcentration and may be associated with hepatic artery thrombosis. These patients should have minimal blood viscosity (hematocrit approximately 28%) [40].

Post-kidney transplantation

- Kidney transplant recipients may have normal serum creatinine, but the glomerular filtration rate is reduced. Therefore, they are still at risk for fluid and electrolyte imbalance, and reduced ability to metabolize or excrete drugs, leading to potential toxic accumulation.
- Agents not relying on renal function such as propofol, atracurium, and cis-atracurium are preferred. Meperidine and morphine should be used with caution.
- Isoflurane and desflurane are appropriate inhalation agents. Clinically used doses of sevoflurane also appear safe.
- Nephrotoxic and non-steroidal anti-inflammatory drugs should be avoided.
- Diuretics or liberal intravenous fluids must be administered after careful evaluation of the patient's volume status.
- Both regional and general anesthesia may be used. In patients with severe hypovolemia or uremic platelet dysfunction, central neuroaxial blockade should be used with caution.

Post-intestinal transplantation

- Common indications for intestinal transplantation include loss of intestinal function associated with a surgically shortened bowel, or nonsurgical factors such as motility disorders, absorptive insufficiencies, polyposis syndrome, or other tumors.
- Bowel motility usually returns to normal within 1–2 weeks, but gastric emptying time may be delayed for a longer period.
- Renal dysfunction may occur due to repeated insults from hypovolemia, immunosuppression, and antibiotics.
- Liver dysfunction is not uncommon is isolated small bowel transplantation.
- Patients are susceptible to infection due to impaired intestinal permeability and absorption because of denervation and lymphatic dysfunction [41].
- Ischemia, rejection, and enteritis may damage the intestinal mucosal barrier, resulting in bacterial translocation and subsequent sepsis.
- Graft rejection should be sought carefully. Presence of blood in the stools indicates rejection until proven otherwise. Graft surveillance relies on inspection of the stoma and distal ileum from routine endoscopy.

Total parenteral nutrition (TPN) is an issue that affects the patient's intravascular volume status and electrolyte level. With long-term TPN, infection and venous thrombosis may cause difficulties in gaining venous access.

Rapid-sequence induction is preferred if general anesthesia is chosen.

For abdominal surgery, difficult surgical dissection from adhesions is anticipated, resulting in prolonged operative time, major bleeding, and large fluid shifts. Appropriate venous access, invasive monitoring, blood product availability, and maintenance of body temperature should be planned.

Postoperative ventilation may be essential because these patients are often weak and debilitated. Epidural catheter insertion, if not contraindicated, is a good choice for postoperative pain control.

:onclusions

Vith advances in the perioperative care and transplant immunology, transplant recipients re living longer and leading almost normal lives. However, solid organ transplantation is a rade off. Transplant recipients suffer from chronic illness with multi-organ involvement nd poly-pharmacy is the rule. Stress of the transplant drains the patients emotionally. As nore and more transplant patients will require non-transplant surgical procedures, nesthesiologists need to understand the physiology of the transplant recipients and harmacology of the immunosuppressive agents. It is important to assess the function of he graft and other organs, and rule out rejection as well as infection before planning an nesthetic. Transplant specialists should be involved in managing immunosuppression, vhich should be maintained throughout the perioperative period. Emphasis should be iven to asepsis, early detection and prevention of infection, allograft rejection, and naintenance of allograft perfusion and oxygenation in the perioperative period.

₹eferences

Organ Procurement and Transplantation Network. Available from: www.optn.org (Accessed April 2013.)

Toivoven HJ. Anaesthesia for patient with a transplanted organ. *Acta Anaesthesiol Scand* 2000; **44**: 812–33.

Bristow MR. The surgically denervated, transplanted human heart. *Circulation* 1990; **82**: 658–60.

Keegan MT, Plevak DJ. The transplant recipient for nontransplant surgery. *Anesthesiol Clin North Am* 2004; **22**: 827–61.

Backman SB, Fox GS, Ralley FE. Pharmacological properties of the denervated heart. *Can J Anaesth* 1997; **44**: 900–1.

Beebe DS, Shumway SJ, Maddock R. Sinus arrest after intravenous neostigmine in two heart transplant recipients. *Anesth Analg* 1994; **78**: 779–82.

7. Sugita M, Ferraro P, Dagenais A, et al. Alveolar liquid clearance and sodium channel expression are decreased in transplanted canine lung. *Am J Respir Crit Care Med* 2003; **167**: 1440–50.

8. Haddow GR, Brock-Utne JG. A non-thoracic operation for patient with single lung transplantation. *Acta Anaesthesiol Scand* 1999; **43**: 960–3.

9. Cota AM, Midwinter MJ. Immunology of transplantation. *Anesth Intensive Care Med* 2009; **10**: 221–2.

10. Steiner RW, Awdishu L. Steroids in kidney transplant patients. *Semin Immunopathol* 2011; **33**: 157–67.

11. Floreth T, Bhorade SM, Ahya VN. Conventional and novel approaches to immunosuppression. *Clin Chest Med* 2011; **32**: 265–77.

12. Scherer MN, Banas B, Mantouvalou K, et al. Current concepts and perspectives of immunosuppression in organ transplantation. *Langenbecks Arch Surg* 2007; **392**: 511–23.

13. Fishman JA. Infection in solid-organ transplant recipients. *N Eng J Med* 2007; **357**: 2601–14.

14. Black AE. Anesthesia for pediatric patients who have had a transplant. *Int Anesthesiol Clin* 1995; **33**: 107–23.

15. Behrendt D, Ganz P, Fang JC. Cardiac allograft vasculopathy. *Curr Opin Cardiol* 2000; **15**: 422–9.

16. Feltracco P, Falasco G, Barbieri S, et al. Anesthetic considerations for nontransplant procedures in lung transplant patients. *J Clin Anesth* 2011; **23**: 508–16.

17. Buell JF, Gross TG, Woodle ES. Malignancy after transplantation. *Transplantation* 2005; **80**: S254–64.

18. Penn I. Cancers in renal transplant recipients. *Adv Ren Replace Ther* 2000; **7**: 147–56.

19. Hartevelt MM, Bavinck JN, Kootte AM, et al. Incidence of skin cancer after renal transplantation in the Netherlands. *Transplantation* 1990; **49**: 506–9.

20. Stewart JH, Buccianti G, Agodoa L, et al. Cancers of the kidney and urinary tract in patients on dialysis for end-stage renal disease: analysis of data from the United States, Europe, and Australia and New Zealand. *J Am Soc Nephrol* 2003; **14**: 197–207.

21. Denton MD, Magee CC, Ovuworie C, et al. Prevalence of renal cell carcinoma in patients with ESRD pre-transplantation: a pathologic analysis. *Kidney Int* 2002; **61**: 2201–9.

22. Goffin E, Devogelaer J-P. Bone disorders after organ transplantation. *Transplant Proc* 2005; **37**: 2832–3.

23. Black AE. Anesthesia for pediatric patients who have had a transplant. *Int Anesthesiol Clin* 1995; **33**: 107–23.

24. Gohh RY, Warren G. The preoperative evaluation of the transplanted patient for nontransplant surgery. *Surg Clin North Am* 2006; **86**: 1147–66.

25. Blasco LM, Parameshwa J, Vuylsteke A. Anaesthesia for noncardiac surgery in the heart transplant recipient. *Curr Opin Anaesthesiol* 2009; **22**: 109–13.

26. Rao VK. Posttransplant medical complications. *Surg Clin North Am* 1998; **78**: 113–32.

27. Rondana M, Milani L, Merkel C, et al. Value of prealbumin plasma levels as liver test. *Digestion* 1987: **37**: 72–8.

28. Salerno F, Borroni G, Moser P, et al. Prognostic value of the galactose test in predicting survival of patients with cirrhosis evaluated for liver transplantation. A prospective multicenter Italian study. *J Hepatol* 1996: **25**: 474–80.

29. Ojo AO, Held PJ, Port FK, et al. Chronic renal failure after transplantation of a nonrenal organ. *N Engl J Med* 2003; **349**: 931–40.

30. Bromberg JS, Baliga P, Cofer JB, et al. Stress steroids are not required for patient receiving a renal allograft and undergoing operation. *J Am Coll Surg* 1995; **180**: 532–

31. George SJ, Vuddamalay P, Boscoe MJ. Antiseptic-impregnated central venous catheters reduce the incidence of bacterial colonization and associated infection in immunocompromized transplant patients. *Eur J Anaesthesiol* 1997: **14**: 428–31.

32. Sear JW. Kidney transplants: induction an analgesic agents. *Int Anesthesiol Clin* 1995 **33**: 45–68.

33. Smith CE, Hunter JM. Anesthesia for rena transplantation: relaxants and volatiles. *In Anesthesiol Clin* 1995; **33**: 69–92.

34. Beiras-Fernandez A, Weis FC, Fuchs H, et al. Levosimendan treatment after primary organ failure in heart transplantation: a direct way to recovery? *Transplantation* 2006; **82**: 1101–3.

35. Beiras-Fernandez A, Weis FC, Kur F, et a Primary graft failure and Ca++ sensitizers after heart transplantation. *Transplant Pro* 2008; **40**: 951–2.

36. Samarutel J. Evidence-based medicine for lung-protective ventilation: the emperors

new clothes for doubtful recommendations? *Acta Anaesthesiol Scand* 2010; **54**: 42–5.

7. Panos L, Patterson GA, Demajo WA. The use of high-frequency jet ventilation during post-lung transplantation surgery. *J Cardiothorac Vasc Surg* 1993; **7**: 202–3.

8. Csete M, Sipher MJ. Management of the transplant patient for nontransplant procedures. *Adv Anesth* 1994; **11**: 407–31.

39. Keegan MT, Plevak DJ. Preoperative assessment of the patient with liver disease. *Am J Gastroenterol* 2005; **100**: 2116–27.

40. Tisone G, Gunson BK, Buckels JA, et al. Raised hematocrit: a contributing factor to hepatic artery thrombosis following liver transplantation. *Transplantation* 1988; **46**: 162–3.

41. Furukawa H, Reyes J, Abu-Elmagd K, et al. Intestinal transplantation at the University of Pittsburgh: six-year experience. *Transplant Proc* 1997; **29**: 688–9.

Index

Note: page numbers in *italics* refer to figures and tables